Clinical Management of Acute Lymphoblastic Leukemia

Mark R. Litzow • Elizabeth A. Raetz
Editors

Clinical Management of Acute Lymphoblastic Leukemia

From Bench to Bedside

Springer

Editors
Mark R. Litzow
Division of Hematology
Mayo Clinic
Rochester, MN, USA

Elizabeth A. Raetz
Department of Pediatrics
NYU Langone Health
New York, NY, USA

ISBN 978-3-030-85146-0 ISBN 978-3-030-85147-7 (eBook)
https://doi.org/10.1007/978-3-030-85147-7

This Springer imprint is published by the registered company Springer Nature Switzerland AG
The registered company address is: Gewerbestrasse 11, 6330 Cham, Switzerland

Preface

The genomic revolution has led to significant advances in understanding the genetic mechanisms underlying the pathophysiology of acute lymphoblastic leukemia (ALL). These studies in turn have identified new targets and treatment modalities for this challenging form of acute leukemia. They have also resulted in advances in our ability to detect minimal or measurable residual disease (MRD), which has enhanced our ability to prognosticate and tailor therapy.

In this textbook, entitled *Clinical Management of Acute Lymphoblastic Leukemia: From Bench to Bedside*, we have brought together noted experts in ALL to provide the reader with comprehensive information on the basic and translational science that underpins our new knowledge of the pathogenesis of ALL. Separate chapters on the genetics of B-cell and T-cell ALL highlight these new developments. A chapter on MRD assessment in ALL spotlights the translation of basic science discoveries to refinements in this essential prognostic tool.

We follow these exciting developments with multiple chapters highlighting advances in the treatment of B- and T-cell ALL across the age spectrum from infants to elderly adults. We also highlight the significant progress that has been seen in the treatment of children and adults with Philadelphia chromosome-positive ALL and highlight the management of the new entity of Philadelphia-like ALL. This part concludes with important chapters on the diagnosis and management of central nervous system ALL and the progress and challenges in the management of late sequelae of ALL therapy.

We conclude the book with an important part on new treatment modalities and highlight the tremendous advances that have been seen with development of monoclonal antibody-based and chimeric antigen receptor T-cell therapies. While advances in the treatment of T-cell ALL have lagged behind those in B-cell ALL, there are new agents on the horizon for this challenging subtype of ALL and we highlight these in a separate chapter. Finally, given all these new developments we conclude with updated information which refines the role of hematopoietic cell transplantation in both children and adults.

We hope readers will find this comprehensive textbook helpful as they confront the new opportunities and challenges of treating children and adults with ALL.

Rochester, MN, USA Mark R. Litzow
New York, NY, USA Elizabeth A. Raetz

Contents

Contributors

Anjali S. Advani Department of Leukemia, Taussig Cancer Institute, Cleveland Clinic, Cleveland, OH, USA

Liv Andrés-Jensen Department of Pediatrics and Adolescent Medicine, University Hospital Rigshospitalet, Copenhagen, Denmark

Institute of Clinical Medicine, Faculty of Health and Medical Sciences, University of Copenhagen, Copenhagen, Denmark

Colleen Annesley Department of Pediatrics, University of Washington, Seattle, WA, USA

Cancer and Blood Disorders Center, Seattle Children's Hospital, Seattle, WA, USA

Keith J. August Division of Pediatric Hematology/Oncology, Children's Mercy Hospital, Kansas City, MO, USA

Shimoli V. Barot Department of Internal Medicine, Cleveland Clinic, Cleveland, OH, USA

Erin H. Breese Department of Pediatrics, University of Cincinnati College of Medicine, Division of Oncology, Cancer and Blood Diseases Institute, Cincinnati Children's Hospital Medical Center, Cincinnati, OH, USA

Melissa A. Burns Department of Pediatric Oncology, Dana-Farber Cancer Institute, Harvard Medical School, Boston, MA, USA

Ryan D. Cassaday Department of Medicine, University of Washington School of Medicine, Seattle, WA, USA

Clinical Research Division, Fred Hutchinson Cancer Research Center, Seattle, WA, USA

Xueyan Chen Department of Laboratory Medicine and Pathology, University of Washington, Seattle, WA, USA

Adolfo Ferrando Institute for Cancer Genetics, Columbia University, New York, NY, USA

Rebecca Gardner Department of Pediatrics, University of Washington, Seattle, WA, USA

Cancer and Blood Disorders Center, Seattle Children's Hospital, Seattle, WA, USA

Francesca Gianni Institute for Cancer Genetics, Columbia University, New York, NY, USA

Nathan P. Gossai Department of Cancer and Blood Disorders, Children's Minnesota, Minneapolis, MN, USA

Erin M. Guest University of Missouri-Kansas City, Division of Pediatric Hematology/Oncology/Blood and Marrow Transplantation, Children's Mercy Kansas City, Kansas City, MO, USA

Laura E. Hogan Stony Brook Children's, Stony Brook, NY, USA

Christoffer Johansen Institute of Clinical Medicine, Faculty of Health and Medical Sciences, University of Copenhagen, Copenhagen, Denmark

Department of Oncology, University Hospital Rigshospitalet, Copenhagen, Denmark

Erik L. Kimble Department of Medicine, University of Washington School of Medicine, Seattle, WA, USA

Clinical Research Division, Fred Hutchinson Cancer Research Center, Seattle, WA, USA

Rishi S. Kotecha Department of Clinical Haematology, Oncology, Blood and Marrow Transplantation, Perth Children's Hospital, Perth, WA, Australia

Leukaemia Translational Research Laboratory, Telethon Kids Cancer Centre, Telethon Kids Institute, University of Western Australia, Perth, WA, Australia

Curtin Medical School, Curtin University, Perth, WA, Australia

Luke D. Maese Department of Pediatrics and Huntsman Cancer Institute, University of Utah, Salt Lake City, UT, USA

Jennifer L. McNeer Section of Pediatric Hematology/Oncology, The University of Chicago Comer Children's Hospital, Chicago, IL, USA

John C. Molina Pediatric Oncology Branch, Center for Cancer Research (CCR), National Cancer Institute (NCI), National Institutes of Health (NIH), Bethesda, MD, USA

Department of Pediatric Oncology, Johns Hopkins Hospital, Baltimore, MD, USA

Charles G. Mullighan Department of Pathology, Hematological Malignancies Program, St. Jude Children's Research Hospital, Memphis, TN, USA

Oliver G. Ottmann Division of Cancer and Genetics, School of Medicine, Cardiff University, Cardiff, UK

Sunil S. Raikar Department of Pediatrics, Aflac Cancer and Blood Disorders Center, Emory University and Children's Healthcare of Atlanta, Atlanta, GA, USA

Kathryn G. Roberts Department of Pathology, Hematological Malignancies Program, St. Jude Children's Research Hospital, Memphis, TN, USA

Eric S. Schafer Baylor College of Medicine, Texas Children's Cancer and Hematology Centers, Houston, TX, USA

Lauren D. Scherer Baylor College of Medicine, Texas Children's Cancer and Hematology Centers, Houston, TX, USA

Kjeld Schmiegelow Department of Pediatrics and Adolescent Medicine, University Hospital Rigshospitalet, Copenhagen, Denmark

Institute of Clinical Medicine, Faculty of Health and Medical Sciences, University of Copenhagen, Copenhagen, Denmark

Kirk R. Schultz Michael Cuccione Childhood Cancer Research Program, BC Children's Hospital and Research Institute, Vancouver, BC, Canada

Marc Schwartz Division of Hematology, University of Colorado, Aurora, CO, USA

Nirali N. Shah Pediatric Oncology Branch, Center for Cancer Research (CCR), National Cancer Institute (NCI), National Institutes of Health (NIH), Bethesda, MD, USA

Lewis B. Silverman Department of Pediatric Oncology, Dana-Farber Cancer Institute, Harvard Medical School, Boston, MA, USA

Divya Subburaj Pediatric Hematology/Oncology/BMT, BC Children's Hospital, Vancouver, BC, Canada

Sarah K Tasian Division of Oncology and Center for Childhood Cancer Research, Children's Hospital of Philadelphia, Philadelphia, PA, USA

Department of Pediatrics, Perelman School of Medicine at the University of Pennsylvania and Abramson Cancer Center, Philadelphia, PA, USA

David T. Teachey Division of Oncology, Department of Pediatrics, Center for Childhood Cancer Research, Children's Hospital of Philadelphia and Perelman School of Medicine, University of Pennsylvania, Philadelphia, PA, USA

Thai Hoa Tran Division of Pediatric Hematology-Oncology, Charles-Bruneau Cancer Center, CHU Sainte-Justine, Montreal, QC, Canada

Department of Pediatrics, University of Montreal, Montreal, QC, Canada

Matthew Wieduwilt University of Oklahoma, Stephenson Cancer Center, Oklahoma City, OK, USA

Brent L. Wood Department of Laboratory Medicine and Pathology, University of Washington, Seattle, WA, USA

Seattle Cancer Care Alliance, Seattle, WA, USA

Children's Hospital Los Angeles, Los Angeles, CA, USA

Part I
Translational Science

Chapter 1
Molecular Pathways and Targets in B-Cell Progenitor Acute Lymphoblastic Leukemia

Kathryn G. Roberts and Charles G. Mulligham

Introduction

Acute lymphoblastic leukemia (ALL) is a neoplasm of B- or T-lineage lymphoid progenitors, with B-cell precursor ALL (BCP-ALL) representing the more common lineage of disease in both children and adults. BCP-ALL comprises over 20 subtypes characterized by constellations of genetic alterations, including aneuploidy, chromosomal rearrangements, DNA copy number alterations, and sequence mutations and, typically, distinct gene expression profiles [1–3]. As described in this review, the subtypes of B-ALL show variability in the nature of the initiating lesion (e.g., single or multiple chromosomal rearrangements, sequence mutations, or aneuploidy), secondary genetic alterations, and outcome. The prevalence and prognosis of each subtype is age dependent. Moreover, there is growing appreciation of the role of germline coding and non-coding variants in predisposing to ALL, both in familial and sporadic cases, and, in some instances, predisposing to specific subtypes of ALL, a striking example being germline *TP53* alterations and low hypodiploid ALL [4]. In the majority of subtypes of B-ALL, secondary genomic alterations are important events required for leukemogenesis, and also influence the risk of relapse [5, 6] (Fig. 1.1). Indeed, it is now recognized that in the majority of cases of B-ALL, the disease is usually polyclonal at the time of diagnosis, and when relapse occurs, there is substantial genomic evolution with clonal rise and fall and mutational extinction, convergence, and emergence [7–9]. Herein, we review the genomic landscape of BCP-ALL, including discussion of the role of germline predisposition and the genetics of clonal evolution and relapse. This review will emphasize illustrative examples of recently defined subtypes of ALL and highlight

K. G. Roberts · C. G. Mullighan (✉)
Department of Pathology, Hematological Malignancies Program, St. Jude Children's Research Hospital, Memphis, TN, USA
e-mail: Kathryn.Roberts@STJUDE.ORG; Charles.Mullighan@STJUDE.ORG

M. R. Litzow, E. A. Raetz (eds.), *Clinical Management of Acute Lymphoblastic Leukemia*, https://doi.org/10.1007/978-3-030-85147-7_1

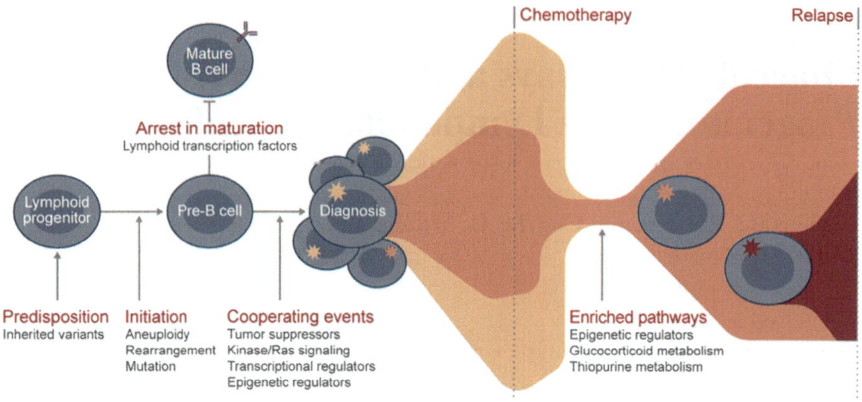

Fig. 1.1 Schema of the temporal pathogenesis of BCP-ALL

potential avenues for diagnostic implementation and therapeutic targeting of relapsed ALL with an emphasis on newly described entities and targets during the past decade.

Historic Aspects of Genetic and Genomic Classification of B-ALL

For many years, genetic classification of B-ALL was performed by cytogenetic karyotyping and complementary targeted fluorescence in situ hybridization (FISH) and molecular assays for specific chromosomal rearrangements and fusions [10]. These identified aneuploid B-ALL with high hyperdiploidy and hypodiploidy; chimeric fusions including *ETV6-RUNX1*, *BCR-ABL1*, and *TCF3-PBX1*; and rearrangement of *KMT2A* (*MLL*) in approximately two thirds of childhood ALL. Due to the low prevalence of high hyperdiploidy and *ETV6-RUNX1* in older individuals, over 50% of adult cases were unclassified [11]. This, coupled with the observation that many of these alterations were insufficient for leukemogenesis in experimental models, and the ability to detect several alterations at birth in cord blood or blood spots [12] years prior to the onset of leukemia, indicated that many cases of ALL had unidentified drivers and that collaborating genetic alterations are required for leukemogenesis in many cases.

The advent of microarray profiling of gene expression and DNA content (array-based comparative genomic hybridization, array-CGH, and single-nucleotide polymorphism (SNP) arrays) demonstrated that known subtypes of B-ALL exhibited relatively distinct gene expression profiles and could identify cases and subgroups that lacked a known driver [13–15]. SNP arrays identified multiple recurring DNA copy number alterations (CNA), particularly alterations in transcriptional regulators of lymphoid development (*PAX5, IKZF1*, *EBF1*), providing valuable insights into the nature of co-alterations in B-ALL [16, 17]. These approaches were largely incapable of robustly identifying subtype-defining new alterations, in part due to the limited ability to identify chromosomal rearrangements and chimeric fusion oncoproteins.

Transcriptome sequencing (RNA-seq) has been the most powerful single experimental approach in enabling a near-complete understanding of the molecular classification of B-ALL and the genomic drivers responsible. Although not able to fully identify all sequence and structural alterations, RNA-seq provides a wealth of data regarding gene expression, gene rearrangement, chromosomal aneuploidy, and mutations. The combination of all four data types has proven necessary in classifying B-ALL. The first advance in subtyping of B-ALL using RNA-seq was the identification of Ph-like (BCR-ABL1-like) ALL, a subtype first recognized using microarray gene expression profiling [18, 19], but requiring RNA-seq to resolve the remarkable diversity in genetic alterations, particularly chromosomal rearrangements resulting in enhancer hijacking and chimeric fusion oncoprotein formation, characteristic of this subtype of ALL [20, 21].

In the last 5 years, multiple groups from the USA, Europe, Japan, and China have generated or used B-ALL RNA-seq data to identify new targets of recurring rearrangement (e.g., *DUX4*, *MEF2D*, and *ZNF384*) associated with distinct gene expression profiles [22–29] and the presence of cases with alterations that phenocopy additional canonical B-ALL drivers, e.g., *ETV6-RUNX1*-like ALL [27]. Several of these subtypes have diverse rearrangements involving a single gene, some of which are cryptic and eluding classification by conventional cytogenetic analysis. Several large-scale B-ALL RNA-seq generation/aggregation studies encompassing up to almost 2000 samples enabled additional observations: additional, less prevalent subtypes driven by chromosomal rearrangements (e.g., rearrangement of *NUTM1* and *BCL2MYC/BCL6*), identification of subtypes driven by initiating sequence mutations rather than chromosomal rearrangements (e.g., PAX5 P80R and IKZF1 N159Y), and subtypes with relatively distinct gene expression but diverse alterations targeting a single gene (PAX5alt, with fusions, sequence mutations, and intragenic amplification of this DNA-binding transcription factor) [5, 6, 26, 29] (Fig. 1.2).

By extending these studies across the age spectrum, these data have been particularly valuable in defining the genetic basis of B-ALL in older individuals, which is more parsimonious in the repertoire of subtypes, and commonly driven by alterations that are now recognized as inherently high risk: *BCR-ABL1*, Ph-like, low hypodiploid, and *KMT2A*- rearranged ALL, providing a partial explanation for the historically poor outcomes of B-ALL in adults [30] (Fig. 1.3).

Collectively, these studies have enabled classification of over 90% of childhood and adult ALL cases (Table 1.1). A minority of cases remain unclassified, but their driver alterations will likely be identified by the application of WGS that can identify non-coding mutations and rearrangements that deregulate genes without generating a chimeric RNA molecule and thus are not detected by RNA-seq alone.

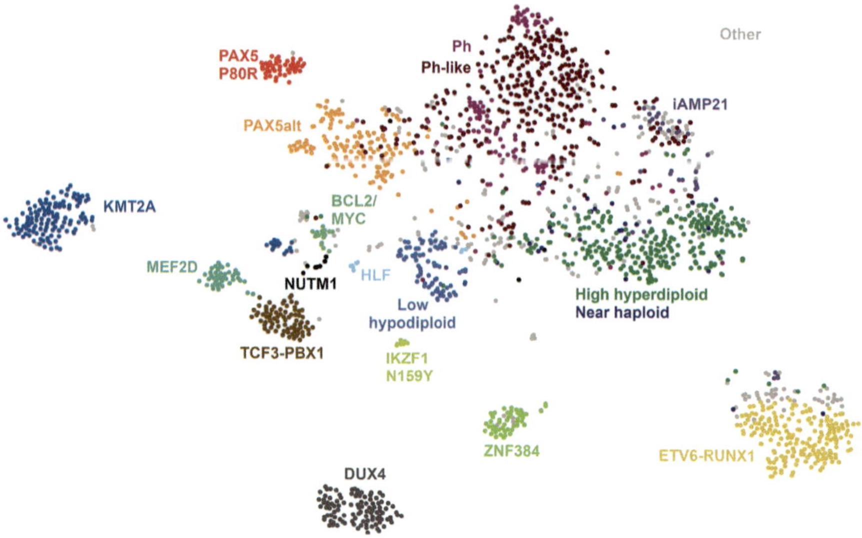

Fig. 1.2 t-SNE plot of gene expression data showing major B-cell precursor acute lymphoblastic leukemia (BCP-ALL) subtypes based on gene expression profiling of 1988 cases [5]. Each dot represents an individual case

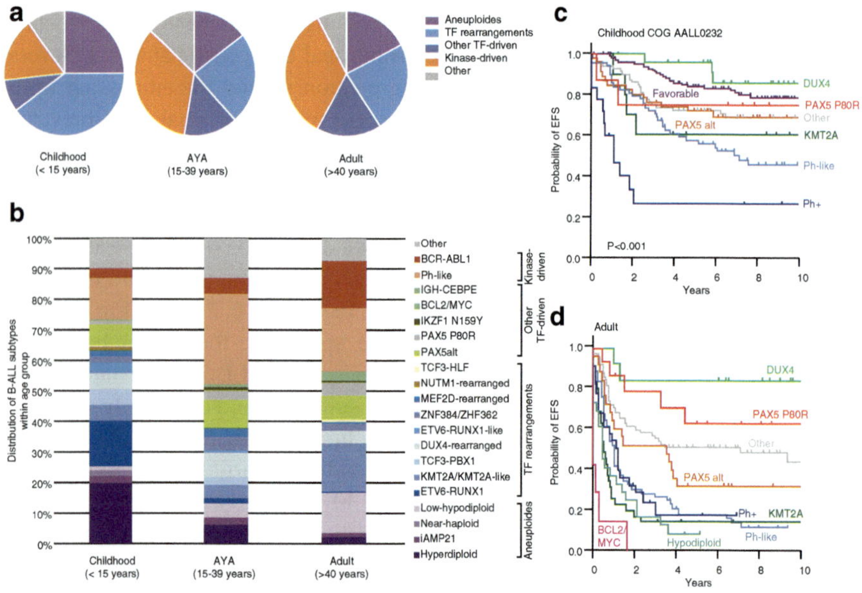

Fig. 1.3 Prevalence of each major subtype in B-cell precursor acute lymphoblastic leukemia (BCP-ALL) across age or risk. AYA, adolescent and young adult; SR, standard risk; HR, high risk. (**a**) Distribution of key groups of ALL according to age. (**b**) Cumulative prevalence of ALL subtypes by age. Outcome of selected subtypes for (**c**) high-risk childhood B-ALL and (**d**) adult ALL. (Data taken from Gu et al. [5])

Table 1.1 Genetic and clinical characteristics of B-ALL subtypes

Molecular subtype	Median age (years)	Peak prevalence	Genomic alterations	Characteristics	Therapeutic approach	Ref
High hyperdiploid (51–67 chromosomes)	4	Children (25%)	Ras pathway, FLT3, epigenetic modifiers	Excellent prognosis; association of *CREBBP* mutations with relapse; FLT3, Ras alterations	FLT3 inhibition?	[57, 59]
Low hypodiploid (32–39 chromosomes)	47	Adults (10–15%)	*IKZF2* deletion, biallelic *TP53* alterations	Poor prognosis; *TP53* alterations are commonly inherited in children, but not in adult	BCL2/BCL-XL inhibitors	[4, 67]
Near haploid (24–31 chromosomes)	5.4	< 3% in all ages	Ras pathway (*NF1*), *IKZF3* deletions	Intermediate prognosis; No loss of chromosome 21 is observed	BCL2/BCL-XL inhibitors	[4, 67]
iAMP21	10	< 3% in children and AYA	Gain of three or more extra copies of a region of chromosome 21 including *RUNX1*	Good prognosis with intensive therapy; low WBC at diagnosis; the germline Robertsonian translocation rob(15;21) or a germline ring chromosome 21 is associated with increased risk of iAMP21		[69, 70, 74]
ETV6-RUNX1	4	Children (25%)	Deletion of the non-rearranged *ETV6* allele, *PAX5* deletions, *WHSC1* mutations	Excellent prognosis; expression of CD27 and low/negative expression of CD44; acquired in utero		[16, 77]
ETV6-RUNX1-like ALL	3	Children (3%)	Alterations (fusions/deletions) in *ETV6*, *IKZF1*, *TCF3*	Intermediate to favorable prognosis; similar gene expression profile to *ETV6-RUNX1* ALL; expression of CD27 and low/negative expression of CD44		[5, 27, 76]
TCF3-PBX1	3	Children (8%)		Good prognosis; pre-B immunophenotype	ROR1, BCL2 inhibitors	[80, 183]
TCF3-HLF	15	< 1% in all ages	*PAX5* deletions, Ras pathway	Very poor prognosis, sensitivity to BCL2 inhibitors	BCL2 inhibitors	[88, 89]
KMT2A rearranged	40	Infants (80%) and adults (15%)	Ras pathway (subclonal), PI3K pathway	Poor prognosis; relation to therapy-related leukemia (topoisomerase II inhibitors); acquired in utero (infant ALL)	DOT1L, MENIN inhibitors	[92, 98, 99]
BCR-ABL1 (Ph+)	40–45	Adults (40–50%)	*IKZF1* alterations, *CDKN2A/B* deletions	Prognosis improved with TKI	Second-/third-generation TKI, rexinoids, FAK inhibitors	[43, 102, 108, 184, 185]

(continued)

Table 1.1

Molecular subtype	Median age (years)	Peak prevalence	Genomic alterations	Characteristics	Therapeutic approach	Ref
Ph-like	21	AYA (25–30%)	Multiple kinase alterations, *IKZF1* alterations, *CDKN2A/B* deletions	Poor prognosis, amenable to TKI therapy; similar gene expression profile to *BCR-ABL1* ALL	JAK, ABL1, TRK inhibitors; combination with PI3K, BCL2, BCL-XL inhibitors; CRLF2 CAR-T	[20, 116, 131, 133, 135, 139]
DUX4 rearranged	14.3	AYA (8%)	*ERG* deletions (polyclonal), *IKZF1* deletions, Ras pathway	Excellent prognosis; distinct immunophenotype (CD2 and CD371 positive)	Potentially deintensify therapy	[22–24, 140, 145]
MEF2D rearranged	14	AYA (7%)	Ras pathway	Intermediate to unfavorable prognosis; low or absent expression of CD10 and high expression of CD38	Bortezomib, panobinostat	[24, 145]
ZNF384 rearranged	15	AYA (5%)	Ras pathway, epigenetic modifiers	Peak age of onset and prognosis varies by fusion partners; low CD10 expression and aberrant CD13 and/or CD33 expression; frequent in childhood B/M MPAL	FLT3 inhibition	[22, 147, 148]
PAX5alt	10	Children (10%)	*PAX5* rearrangements	Intermediate prognosis; loss of heterozygosity or acquisition of compound heterozygosity of *PAX5*		
PAX5 P80R	22	Adults (4%)	Ras pathway, JAK-STAT pathway	Intermediate to favorable prognosis; association with dic(9:20)		[5, 159, 160, 186]
NUTM1 rearranged	3	Children (1%)		Excellent prognosis		[7]
IKZF1 N159Y		< 1% in all ages	Gain of whole chromosome 21	Retain non-mutated wild-type allele of *IKZF1*		[7]
BCL2/MYC rearranged	48	AYA and adults (3%)		Poor prognosis		[5]

Heritable Susceptibility to Leukemia

Several lines of evidence support genetic predisposition for many subtypes of BCP-ALL, including (a) Down syndrome and other rare constitutional syndromes with increased risks for leukemia; (b) kindreds with familial BCP-ALL; (c) genome-wide association studies (GWAS) that have identified non-coding DNA polymorphisms which influence risk of BCP-ALL; and (d) a growing number of genes harboring germline non-silent variants presumed to confer risk of sporadic HM.

Children with constitutional syndromes such as Down syndrome, Noonan syndrome, neurofibromatosis type 1, ataxia-telangiectasia, Fanconi anemia, and other bone marrow failure syndromes (severe congenital neutropenia, dyskeratosis congenita, Shwachman-Diamond syndrome, and Diamond-Blackfan anemia) have an increased risk of leukemia. The spectrum of risk is syndrome specific. For example, Down syndrome is associated with a markedly increased risk of AML and B-ALL; Noonan syndrome and neurofibromatosis type 1 have increased risk of JMML (discussed later in this chapter), ataxia-telangiectasia increases T-ALL risk, and bone marrow failure syndromes primarily increase risk of AML [31–34].

Familial cancer syndromes such as Li-Fraumeni syndrome, constitutional mismatch repair deficiency syndrome, or DNA repair syndromes (Bloom, Werner, Nijmegen breakage) have increased incidence of malignancy, including ALL in a proportion of cases [35, 36]. Familial BCP-ALL is uncommon, but genomic analyses of such kindreds has been tremendously informative by identifying non-silent germline variants in transcription factor and tumor suppressor genes segregating with ALL that in many cases are also present as germline events in sporadic BCP-ALL. Key examples are *TP53* germline mutations and low hypodiploid B-ALL, *ETV6* variants and hyperdiploid and *ETV6-RUNX1*-like ALL [37], and *PAX5* mutations and B-ALL with dicentric/isochromosome 9 [4, 38–40]. These susceptibility genes are targets of somatic mutation in ALL: *ETV6* and *PAX5* are rearranged, amplified, deleted, and mutated in B-ALL [5, 16]. Germline variants of *IKZF1* predispose to a syndrome with immunodeficiency, autoimmunity, and sporadic/familial BCP-ALL [41, 42]; somatic *IKZF1* alterations are enriched in *BCR-ABL1*, Ph-like, and *DUX4*-rearranged B-ALL [19, 23, 43].

Genome-wide association studies (GWAS) have identified at least 13 loci with primarily non-coding variants associated with BCP-ALL. The relative risk associated with these variants is modest compared with constitutional syndromes or familial leukemia. Risk variants are frequently at or near hematopoietic transcription factor or tumor suppressor gene loci, including *ARID5B, BAK1, CDKN2A/CDKN2B, BMI1-PIP4K2A, CEBPE, ELK3, ERG, GATA3, IGF2BP1, IKZF1 IKZF3*, *USP7*, and *LHPP* [36, 44, 45]. Several variants display ancestry and ALL subtype-specific associations, such as *GATA3* with Hispanics and Ph-like B-ALL, *ERG* with African Americans and *TCF3-PBX1* B-ALL, and *USP7* with African Americans and T-ALL with *TAL1* deregulation [46–48].

Genomic analyses have identified additional susceptibility variants in sporadic hyperdiploid B-ALL (*NBN*, *ETV6*, *FLT3*, *SH2B3*, and *CREBBP*), Down syndrome-associated B-ALL (*IKZF1*, *NBN*, *RTEL1*), and T-ALL (Fanconi-BRCA pathway mutations) [49–51].

Prenatal Origin of Leukemia

Several observations indicate that a proportion of childhood leukemia cases are initiated before birth [52–54]. Chromosomal translocations such as *ETV6-RUNX1* may be detected at birth in blood spots and cord blood, years before the clinical onset of leukemia, providing support for a multistep process of leukemogenesis. This is supported by genomic analyses of monozygotic, monochorionic twins concordant for leukemia, showing genetic identity of initiating lesions and discordance for secondary genetic alterations, indicating inter-twin, intrauterine transmission of leukemia [53, 55]. Evidence for in utero origin is strongest for *KMT2A*-rearranged and *ETV6-RUNX1* ALL. Anecdotal evidence supports in utero origin for other subtypes of B-ALL, including hyperdiploid and *ZNF384*-rearranged leukemia [56].

Aneuploid BCP-ALL: Hyperdiploidy, Hypodiploidy, and Intrachromosomal Amplification of Chromosome 21

High hyperdiploidy (51–67 chromosomes) comprises approximately 30% of pediatric BCP-ALL and is associated with a favorable prognosis (Table 1.1) [57]. High hyperdiploidy is characterized by a nonrandom gain of chromosomes, typically +X, +4, +6, +10, +14, +17, +18, and +21 [57]. In particular, combined gain of chromosome 4, 10, and 17 is associated with favorable prognosis [58]. Alterations involving the Ras pathway (*KRAS*, *NRAS*, *FLT3*, *PTPN11*) and epigenetic modifiers (*CREBBP*, *WHSC1*) are frequent genetic events, with deletions leading to enhancer hijacking and deregulation of FLT3 particularly common in high hyperdiploid ALL [57, 59]. These secondary genomic alterations and the gene expression profiles of high hyperdiploid and the near-haploid subset of hypodiploid ALL are similar, suggesting a common origin [60]. Low hyperdiploid cases (47–50 chromosomes) harbor a diverse range of chromosomal changes and alterations rather than representing a genetically distinct subtype of ALL.

Hypodiploid ALL comprises three subtypes, two of which have an unfavorable prognosis: near-haploid ALL (24–31 chromosomes) and low hypodiploid ALL (32–39 chromosomes) [61–63]. Notably, chromosome 21 is never lost in hypodiploid ALL nor in other forms of ALL, suggesting an essential role in tumor cell fitness [4]. High hypodiploid ALL (40–44 chromosomes) is genetically heterogeneous, is not a distinct subtype of B-ALL, and does not share the unfavorable outcome of the other two groups. Accurate identification of low/near-haploid ALL is important in view of the poor prognosis and inherited genetic basis of low hypodiploid ALL in children [4]. Duplication of the aneuploid genome, or masked hypodiploidy, is common and may be mistaken for high hyperdiploidy [64]. These entities can be distinguished by the patterns of chromosomal gain and loss of heterozygosity observed on cytogenetic or SNP array analysis: masked hypodiploidy typically has diploid and tetraploid chromosomes, whereas hyperdiploidy has a mixture of triploid and some tetraploid (e.g., 21, X); masked hypodiploid cases typically have LOH of the duplicated chromosomes. Flow cytometric analysis of DNA index frequently demonstrates peaks for both non-duplicated and masked clones in hypodiploid ALL, even if cytogenetic analysis demonstrates an apparently predominant masked clone.

Near-haploid ALL presents at a younger age and commonly exhibits alterations activating the Ras pathway (particularly *NF1*) and inactivating mutations/deletions of *IKZF3* (AIOLOS) [4]. Low hypodiploid ALL is rare but increases with age. Frequent secondary alterations include *IKZF2* (HELIOS), *RB1*, and *CDKN2A*/*CDKN2B*. The mechanistic differences between the IKAROS gene family members in leukemogenesis (*IKZF1* in kinase-driven and *DUX4*-rearranged leukemia and IKZF2/3 in hypodiploid ALL) remain to be determined. Importantly, almost all cases of low hypodiploid ALL in children and adults have biallelic alterations of *TP53* due to mutation (or less commonly focal deletion) and aneuploidy of the second chromosome [4]. In approximately half of pediatric cases (but not adult), the *TP53* mutations are germline, indicating that low hypodiploid ALL is a manifestation of Li-Fraumeni syndrome [4, 65]. Although still associated with an unfavorable prognosis, minimal residual disease (MRD) risk-stratified therapy has improved the outcome of hypodiploid ALL [66]. Hypodiploid ALL cells are sensitive to BCL2 inhibition, and BCL2 inhibitors are being evaluated in prospective clinical trials of newly diagnosed and relapsed/refractory ALL [67].

Intrachromosomal amplification of chromosome 21 (iAMP21) is more common in older children and is characterized by gain of three or more extra copies of a region of chromosome 21 including *RUNX1* generated by breakage-fusion-bridge cycles and chromothripsis [68–71]. The germline Robertsonian translocation rob(15;21) or a germline ring chromosome 21 is associated with a markedly elevated risk of iAMP21 [72]. Patients with iAMP21 usually lack other key cytogenetic alterations, although it is observed as a secondary event in *ETV6-RUNX1* and *BCR-ABL1* ALL in a minority of cases. Historically associated with an unfavorable outcome, intensive therapy improves prognosis [73, 74]. The key driver gene(s) located on chromosome 21 resulting in requirement for this chromosome in ALL, and mediating leukemogenesis in iAMP21 ALL, remains to be determined.

ETV6-RUNX1 and ETV6-RUNX1-Like ALL

The t(12:21)(p13:q22) translocation encodes *ETV6-RUNX1*, the most common fusion in BCP-ALL (20–25% in children) that is associated with a favorable prognosis [5, 75]. This translocation is frequently cryptic on cytogenetic analysis, and leukemic cells have a distinct immunophenotype (CD27 positive and CD44 low/negative) [76]. The *ETV6-RUNX1* fusion may be identified in umbilical cord blood and, thus, is considered to arise in utero as a leukemia-initiating alteration [75]. However, *ETV6-RUNX1* itself is insufficient to induce overt leukemia and requires the prolonged latency with additional genetic events including deletion of the non-rearranged *ETV6* allele, focal deletion of *PAX5*, and mutation of *WHSC1* [2, 16, 17, 75, 77]. This is supported by heterogeneity in the subclonal composition of *ETV6-RUNX1* ALL [75, 78, 79].

ETV6-RUNX1-like ALL exhibits a similar GEP and immunophenotype to *ETV6-RUNX1* ALL despite the lack of *ETV6-RUNX1* fusion [5, 6, 27, 76]. *ETV6-RUNX1*-like ALL is also most common in children and has relatively favorable outcome [27, 76]. This subtype includes several alternate rearrangements in *ETV6* (e.g., *ETV6-ELMO1*), *IKZF1* (e.g., *IKZF1-ETV6*), *TCF3* (e.g., *TCF3-FLI1*), and *FUS-ERG* as well as copy number alterations in *ETV6*, *IKZF1*, and *ARPP21*, suggesting that alteration of multiple ETS and other transcription factors are converging on the same mechanism of transformation (although not *ERG*, which is distinct in the *DUX4*-rearranged ALL) [5, 27, 76].

TCF3-PBX1 and TCF3-HLF BCP-ALL

The t(1;19)(q23;p13) translocation encoding *TCF3-PBX1* fusion is present in 5–6% of pediatric BCP-ALL and is associated with a pre-B in transition (cytoplasmic immunoglobulin heavy chain positive) immunophenotype [80]. Previously considered high risk due to higher central nervous system involvement and relapse [15, 81, 82], *TCF3-PBX1* ALL is classified as favorable or intermediate risk with current treatment regimens [83]. Conditional activation of *TCF3-PBX1* in B-cell progenitors results in enhanced self-renewal and eventual development of leukemia with *PAX5* deletion and activation of JAK-STAT or Ras signaling pathways [84]. Importantly, *TCF3-PBX1* ALL exhibits sensitivity to dasatinib and ponatinib, but not imatinib, which occurs as a result of inhibition of pre-BCR signaling by SRC kinases. Due to compensatory upregulation of *ROR1* expression, combination with ROR1 inhibition may enhance the sensitivity of dasatinib [85].

A variant of the t(1;19) translocation, t(17;19)(q22;p13), encodes the *TCF3-HLF* fusion, a rare subtype of ALL associated with an extremely poor prognosis [86, 87]. *TCF3-PBX1* and *TCF3-HLF* ALL have distinct gene expression profiles and mutational landscapes [88]. *TCF3-HLF* ALL exhibited stem cell and myeloid features with enrichment of *PAX5* deletions and alterations of Ras pathway genes [88]. The TCF-HLF fusion may act as a pioneer transcription factor, recruiting EP300 to activate MYC, with vulnerability to EP300 inhibition [89]. *TCF3-HLF* leukemic cells are sensitive to the BCL2 inhibitor venetoclax (ABT-199), representing a potential targeted therapeutic approach [88].

KMT2A-Rearranged ALL

KMT2A (*MLL*) on chromosome 11q23 is rearranged to more than 80 different partner genes, and these rearrangements describe a distinct subtype of leukemia with variable immunophenotype spanning ALL, AML, and mixed phenotype leukemia with both lymphoid and myeloid features and poor outcome [90]. *KMT2A*-rearranged BCP-ALL is typically of the pro-B phenotype, lacking CD10 expression, with co-expression of myeloid markers. Approximately 80% of *KMT2A*-rearranged ALL is observed in infants, in whom *KMT2A* rearrangement is acquired in utero. There is also a second peak in prevalence in adults, and more than 75% of cases are fused to *AFF1*. *KMT2A*-rearranged leukemia may also follow exposure to topoisomerase II inhibitors, with similar breakpoints to infant leukemia suggesting a common mechanism of leukemogenesis [91]. In infant ALL, the most commonly perturbed pathways include PI3K and Ras pathways [92–94]. *KMT2A* rearrangement results in assembly of a large multi-protein complex that results in aberrant transcriptional and epigenetic dysregulation via H3K79 methylation and recruitment of the H3K79 methyltransferase DOT1L, which interacts with multiple *KMT2A* rearrangement partners [95–97]. Multiple therapeutic approaches are being pursued, including inhibition of DOT1L, bromodomain, Menin, and the polycomb repressive complex [90, 97–99].

Kinase-Driven BCP-ALL: *BCR-ABL1* ALL and Ph-like ALL

The derivative chromosome 22, Philadelphia chromosome (Ph), arises from the reciprocal t(9;22)(q34;q11) translocation and encodes *BCR-ABL1* [7, 41, 100]. Although *BCR-ABL1* ALL is associated with poor prognosis, the addition of tyrosine kinase inhibitors (TKIs) to the conventional chemotherapy has improved outcome in children and adults [101–104]. In contrast to *BCR-ABL1*-positive chronic myeloid leukemia at chronic phase, *BCR-ABL1* ALL is characterized by a high frequency of secondary genetic alterations, particularly of the lymphoid transcription factor gene *IKZF1* and *CDKN2A/B* encoding the INK4/ARF cell cycle regulators [43, 105], and *IKZF1* alterations are associated with unfavorable outcome irrespective of TKI exposure [102, 105]. Moreover, mutations in the kinase domain of *ABL1* (most frequently T315I) induce TKI resistance and are more commonly observed in patients treated with TKI monotherapy or in adults treated with less intensive chemotherapy and less common in children treated with intensive chemotherapy [106]. Current treatment approaches to mitigate the poor outcome of *BCR-ABL1* ALL include frontline treatment with the third-generation TKI ponatinib with chemotherapy [101]. The adverse effect of *IKZF1* mutations in the pathogenesis of BCR-ABL1 ALL is in part due to loss of IKZF1 repression of stemness and cell-cell adhesion [107, 108]. This may be reversed by rexinoids (via agonism of rexinoid X receptor alpha, which induces expression of wild-type IKZF1) and focal adhesion kinase inhibitors (which inhibit downstream integrin signaling pathways) [108, 109].

Before consensus guidelines for MRD assessment in *BCR-ABL1* ALL were provided [110], several approaches have been tested for MRD monitoring (genome or transcriptome *BCR-ABL1* and Ig/TCR rearrangements) [111]. Importantly, some patients showed discrepancy of MRD results as assessed by measurement of Ig/TCR and *BCR-ABL1* transcript levels, due to the presence of the *BCR-ABL1* fusion in progenitors in addition to the blast population [111]. This *BCR-ABL1*-positive clonal hematopoiesis is suggestive of a CML-like disease exhibiting lymphoid blast crisis.

Ph-like or *BCR-ABL1*-like ALL exhibits a gene expression profile similar to *BCR-ABL1* ALL despite the lack of the *BCR-ABL1* fusion [18, 19]. The prevalence and outcome of Ph-like ALL are similar to those of *BCR-ABL1* ALL, increasing in incidence with age and associated with elevated MRD levels and/or higher rates of treatment failure [20, 112–118], although the prevalence of Ph-like ALL is higher than *BCR-ABL1* ALL in the adolescent and young adult (AYA) population [20, 117, 119, 120]. Similar to *BCR-ABL1* ALL, *IKZF1* alterations are common, which result in acquisition of stem cell-like features and poor responsiveness to TKI. The heterogeneous genetic alterations driving Ph-like ALL may be classified into four main groups (Table 1.2., Fig. 1.4): (1) alterations driving JAK-STAT signaling, including rearrangements and mutations/deletions of *CRLF2*, *JAK2*, *EPOR*, *TYK2*, *IL7R*, *SH2B3*, *JAK1*, *JAK3*, *TYK2*, and *IL2RB*; (2) fusions involving ABL-class genes (*ABL1*, *ABL2*, *CSF1R*, *LYN*, *PDGFRA*, *PDGFRB*); (3) mutations activating Ras signaling (*NRAS*, *KRAS*, *PTPN11*); and (4) less common fusions (*FLT3*, *FGFR1*, *NTRK3*) [2, 121, 122]. Of these, *CRLF2* alterations are found in almost half of Ph-like ALL in adolescents, young adults, and older adults, as well as in half of ALL associated with Down syndrome ALL [123–125]. These alterations are rearrangements of *CRLF2* to IGH or P2RY8 resulting in enhancer hijacking or promoter swapping, respectively, and aberrant expression of CRLF2 as part of a heterodimer with IL-7 receptor alpha. *CRLF2*-rearranged ALL commonly has concomitant alterations that facilitate JAK-STAT signaling pathway activation, including sequence mutations of Janus kinases (most commonly at R683 of the pseudokinase domain of JAK2), IL-7RA, and deletions of negative regulators of JAK-STAT signaling (*SH2B3* and *USP9X*) [126, 127]. *CRLF2* rearrangement is associated with Hispanic ancestry and a germline *GATA3* non-coding variant [46, 128].

Importantly, most kinase-activating alterations in Ph-like ALL can, theoretically, be targeted by FDA-approved TKIs: JAK-STAT signaling (JAK inhibition), ABL-class fusions (ABL inhibitor), and *FLT3* and *NTRK3* fusions (FLT3 and NTRK3 inhibitor) with emerging evidence of efficacy in human leukemia, although evidence for efficacy of TKIs, at least as monotherapy, is strongest for ABL1-class and ETV6-NTRK3 Ph-like ALL [20, 129–133]. In contrast JAK inhibitor monotherapy in preclinical and clinical studies of CRLF2-rearranged Ph-like ALL is less effective [134]. Combination of kinase inhibitors against multiple signaling shows synergistic effects in PDX models of *CRLF2/JAK* mutant (JAK and PI3K/mTOR inhibitors) and *ABL/PDGFR* mutant (dasatinib and PI3K/mTOR inhibitor) [135]. Several of these (ruxolitinib, imatinib, dasatinib, ponatinib) are being tested in frontline studies [120, 133, 136]. As kinase-activating lesions also drive signaling through additional signaling pathways (e.g., PI3K, MEK, etc.), it is likely that additional therapeutic approaches will be required for optimal therapeutic response. Additional therapeutic approaches include BCL2 inhibitors, which exhibit synergy with TKIs in preclinical models [137, 138], and chimeric antigen receptor T cells directed against CRLF2 [139].

Table 1.2 Kinase-activating alterations in Ph-like ALL

Category	Kinase gene	Representative alterations	Targeted therapy
JAK-STAT	*CRLF2*	Mutations (F232C), fusions (*CSF2RA, IGH, P2RY8*)	JAK inhibitor
	EPOR	Truncating rearrangement to enhancers (*IGH, IGK, LAIR1, THADA*)	JAK inhibitor
	TYK2	Fusions (*MYB, SMARCA4, ZNF430*)	TYK2 inhibitor
	TSLP	Fusions (*IQGAP2*)	JAK inhibitor
	SH2B3	Deletion/mutations	JAK inhibitor
	IL7RA	Mutations, indels	JAK inhibitor
	JAK1	Mutations (e.g., V658F)	JAK inhibitor
	JAK2	Mutations (of R683; most commonly R683G, also kinase domain mutations), fusions (*ATF7IP, BCR, EBF1, ETV6, HMBOX1, PAX5, PCM1, PPFIBP1, RFX3, SMU1, SNX29, SSBP2, STRN3, TERF2, TPR, USP25, WDR37, ZNF274, GOLGA5, SMU1, HMBOX1, SNX29, ZNF430*)	JAK inhibitor
	JAK3	Mutations (usually kinase domain)	JAK inhibitor
	IL2RB	Fusions (*MYH9*)	JAK inhibitor
	USP9X	USP9X-DDX3X interstitial deletion and fusion	JAK inhibitor
ABL	*ABL1*	Fusions (*CENPC, ETV6, FOXP1, LSM14A, MYO18B, NUP214, NUP153, RCSD1, RANBP2, SFPQ, SNX2, SPTAN1, ZMIZ1*)	Imatinib/dasatinib
	ABL2	Fusions (*ATF7IP, EBF1, ETV6, PAG1, RCSD1, SSBP2, TNIP1, ZEB2, ZC3HAV1, ZMYND8*)	Imatinib/dasatinib
	CSF1R	Fusions (*MEF2D, SSBP2, TBL1XR1*)	Imatinib/dasatinib
	LYN	Fusions (*GATAD2A, NCOR1*)	Imatinib/dasatinib
	PDGFRA	Fusions (*FIP1L1*)	Imatinib/dasatinib
	PDGFRB	Fusions (*ATF7IP, EBF1, ETV6, SNX29, SSBP2, TNIP1, ZEB2, ZMYND8*)	Imatinib/dasatinib
Ras	*NRAS*	Mutations	MEK inhibitor
	KRAS	Mutations	MEK inhibitor
	PTPN11	Mutations	MEK inhibitor
	NF1	Mutations/deletions	MEK inhibitor
	BRAF	Mutations	MEK inhibitor
	CBL	Fusions (*KANK1*)	MEK inhibitor
Other	*FLT3*	*FLT3*-ITD, fusions (*AMYM2*)	FLT3 inhibitor
	NTRK3	Fusions (*ETV6*)	NTRK3 inhibitor
	FGFR1	Fusions (*BCR, MYO18A*)	Ponatinib
	PTK2B	Fusions (*KDM6A, STAG2, TMEM2*)	FAK inhibitor
	DGKH	Fusions (*ZFAND3*)	
	BLNK	Fusions (*DNTT*)	

Clinical trials of TKI in Ph-like ALL include dasatinib (newly diagnosed, NCT03117751 and NCT03020030; relapsed, NCT02420717) and ruxolitinib (newly diagnosed, NCT02723994, NCT03571321, NCT03117751; relapsed, NCT02420717). Data updated from Gu et al. [5]

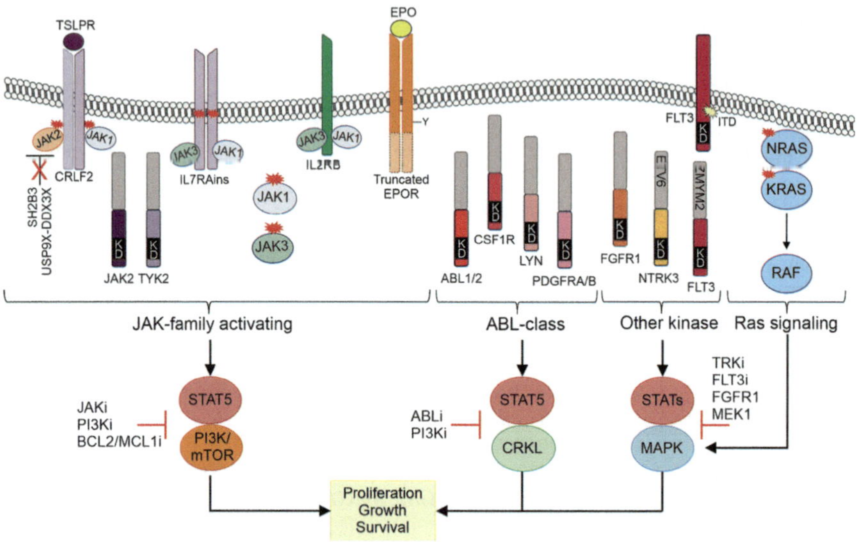

Fig. 1.4 Cartoon depicting targets of genetic alteration and type of mutation in Ph-like ALL

DUX4-Rearranged ALL

Rearrangement and overexpression of the homeobox transcription factor gene *DUX4* defines a distinct subgroup of BCP-ALL [5, 22, 23, 27]. This subtype also exhibits deregulation of the ETS family transcription factor *ERG* and comprises up to 5–10% of BCP-ALL with a slight peak in the AYA population. It has a distinct immunophenotype (CD2 and CD371 positive) and favorable outcome [140]. The pathogenesis of this form of leukemia is remarkable for the interrelated, sequential genetic events that deregulate two DNA-binding transcription factors characteristic of this disease (Fig. 1.5). Deregulation of *DUX4* is induced by rearrangement to strong enhancer elements, most commonly the immunoglobulin heavy chain (IGH) enhancer, which results in expression of a C-terminal truncated DUX4 protein that is not normally expressed in B cells [22, 23]. This truncated isoform of DUX4 then binds to an intragenic region of *ERG* resulting in transcriptional deregulation and expression of multiple aberrant coding and non-coding *ERG* isoforms and deletion of *ERG* in up to 70% of *DUX4*-rearranged cases [23]. One isoform is ERGalt, a C-terminal fragment which retains the DNA-binding and transactivating domain of ERG, that exerts a dominant negative effect and is transforming [23]. The deletions of *ERG* are commonly polyclonal [141], supporting a model in which an initiating rearrangement of *DUX4* results in gross transcriptional deregulation of ERG and primes the locus for RAG-mediated deletion. Loss of ERG activity, either through deletion and/or expression of ERGalt, cooperates with DUX4 deregulation in leukemogenesis [23, 141]. *DUX4* rearrangement is associated with a favorable outcome in children and adults, even with *IKZF1* deletion [142]. As clonal *ERG* deletions are

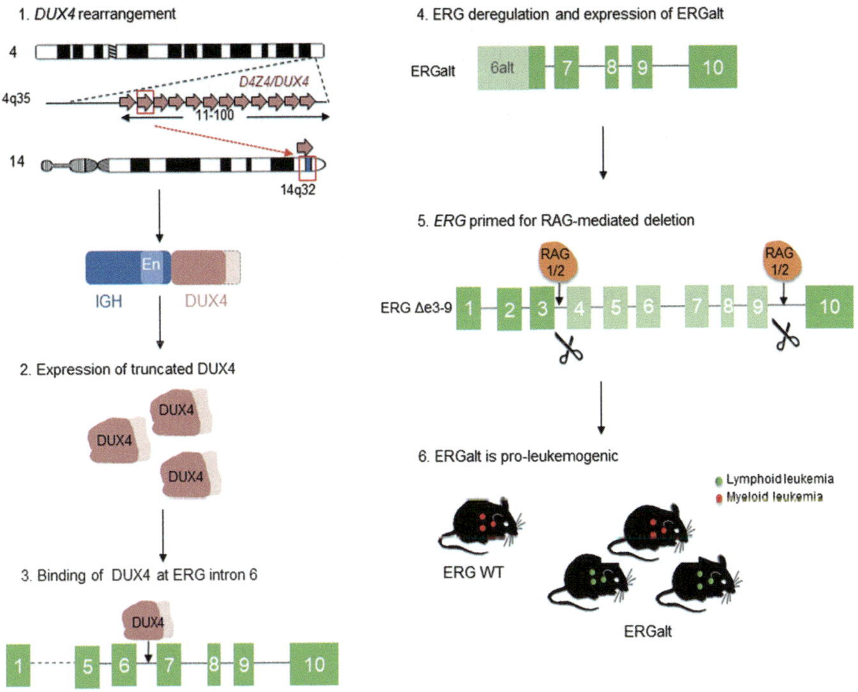

Fig. 1.5 Schema of the sequence of transcription factor alterations driving leukemogenesis in *DUX4*-rearranged ALL: rearrangement of DUX4 to strong enhancers results in deregulation of DUX4 expression with truncation of the C-terminus. This shortened form of DUX4 binds to intron 6 of *ERG*, resulting in gross transcriptional deregulation and expression of multiple coding, non-coding, and enhancer RNA species, including a C-terminal isoform initiated by a novel first exon, ERGalt. This aberrancy also permits deletion of *ERG* as a secondary event

not present in all *DUX4*-rearranged cases, the use of *ERG* deletion as a surrogate for this subtype, as is used in the definition of IKZF^{plus} [143], is suboptimal and should be avoided. Accurate identification of this favorable subtype of ALL requires identification of *DUX4* rearrangement (either directly or through identification of elevated *DUX4* expression) [23]. In this regard, detection of strong CD371 cell surface expression by flow cytometry might serve as a promising surrogate marker for this subtype [140].

MEF2D-Rearranged ALL

Rearrangement of *MEF2D* is associated with older age of onset and relatively inferior outcome due to early relapse [24, 26, 144, 145]. *MEF2D*-rearranged ALL is characterized by an aberrant immunophenotype (low or absent expression of CD10, high expression of CD38, and cytoplasmic μ-chain), mature B-ALL-like morphology, and distinct expression profiles. The N-terminal of *MEF2D* is fused to several partner genes, retaining its DNA-binding domain [24, 144, 145]. High expression of MEF2D fusion protein is induced by evasion from miRNA-mediated degradation [146] and results in transcriptional activation of MEF2D targets [24]. Dysregulated MEF2D targets include overexpression of HDAC9, which confers therapeutic sensitivity to HDAC inhibitors such as panobinostat [24].

ZNF384-Rearranged ALL

ZNF384 rearrangement defines a distinct subtype of leukemia that can be diagnosed as BCP-ALL or B/myeloid mixed phenotype acute leukemia (MPAL) [147]. ZNF384 is rearranged as the C-terminal partner to multiple genes, including the histone acetyltransferases and transcriptional regulators EP300 and CREBBP, SWI/SNF proteins SMARCA2 and ARID1B, and others (TAF15, EWSR1, TCF3, NIPBL, and CLTC) [5, 6, 22, 24–26, 29, 147–154]. The most common are EP300-ZNF384 (particularly in BCP-ALL) and TCF3-ZNF384 (in both BCP-ALL and B/myeloid MPAL). In BCP-ALL, peak age of onset and prognosis vary by fusion partners: *EP300-ZNF384* (median age 11, excellent outcome) and *TCF3-ZNF384* (median age 5, frequent late relapse) [5, 148, 155]. In contrast, *ZNF384*-rearranged ALL shows uniformly distinct immunophenotype (weak CD10 and aberrant CD13 and/or CD33 expression) and gene expression profiles [147, 148]. The secondary genomic alterations and gene expression profiles of *ZNF384*-rearranged BCP-ALL and MPAL cases are similar, and both have lineage plasticity at diagnosis and relapse (lymphoid disease to myeloid disease and vice versa) [147]. Transplantation of purified lymphoid or myeloid subpopulations of cells from *ZNF384*-rearranged leukemia showed that each subpopulation could reconstitute the immunophenotypic diversity of the primary leukemia, indicating that this plasticity is inherent to all leukemic cells [69]. These data support the notion that *ZNF384*-rearranged cases should be treated uniformly rather than tailoring therapy according to predominant lineage. In this regard, *FLT3* overexpression without mutation is characteristic of *ZNF384*-rearranged leukemia and in anecdotal reports can be targeted with the multi-kinase inhibitor sunitinib [156]. Due to the propensity of *ZNF384*-rearranged ALL to change lineage, CD19-directed CAR-T cell therapy may fail due to CD19-negative escape [147, 157, 158].

PAX5-Driven BCP-ALL: PAX5alt and PAX5 P80R

The paired box DNA-binding transcription factor PAX5 is required for B-cell lineage commitment and differentiation. *PAX5* alterations are important in the pathogenesis of BCP-ALL as initiating or cooperating lesions. These include (1) disease initiating alterations (PAX5 rearrangements in chimeric fusion oncoproteins and the P80R mutation [5, 16, 159–161], rearrangements/focal intragenic amplifications in *PAX5*-altered ALL [PAX5alt]) [5, 162], (2) secondary lesions (e.g., *PAX5* focal deletions in 30% of *ETV6-RUNX1* ALL [16, 77] and *PAX5* mutations in multiple subtypes), and (3) germline alterations that predispose to ALL [39]. In mouse models, *Pax5* heterozygosity cooperates with constitutive activation of the JAK-STAT pathway in the development of BCP-ALL, supporting its role as a haploinsufficient tumor suppressor [163].

PAX5alt is a subtype of BCP-ALL with similar leukemic cell gene expression profiles but diverse nature of underlying *PAX5* alterations. These include (1) cases with diverse (>20) *PAX5* rearrangements that typically preserve the N-terminal DNA-binding domain of PAX5, but with loss of the C-terminal transactivation domain, (2) cases with focal intragenic amplification of the *PAX5* DNA-binding paired domain (PAX5amp), and (3) cases with sequence mutations. Within this group, specific lesions are associated with variation in gene expression profile, for example, cases with *PAX5-ETV6* rearrangement, or compound heterozygosity for p.Arg38 and p.Arg140 mutations in the DNA-binding paired domain, have distinct gene expression profiles. PAX5alt is most common in children and the AYA population and is associated with intermediate outcome [5].

The PAX5 P80R subtype is characterized by the presence of the PAX5 P80R mutation with inactivation of the wild-type *PAX5* allele by deletion, loss-of-function mutation, or copy-neutral loss of heterozygosity [5, 159, 160]. Notably, heterozygous $Pax5^{P80R/+}$ knock-in mice develop transplantable BCP-ALL, with genetic inactivation of the wild-type *Pax5* allele [5]. Thus, biallelic *PAX5* alterations are a hallmark of this subtype, and sequence mutations of lymphoid transcription factors such as PAX5 P80R and IKZF1 N159Y (see below) may be initiating events in leukemogenesis. The prevalence of PAX5 P80R increases with age and is associated with intermediate to favorable prognosis [5, 159, 160]. Additional important cooperating lesions include structural rearrangements of chromosomal arms 9p and 20q, which associate with the presence of dic(9:20). Moreover, mutations in the Ras and JAK-STAT pathway members are particularly enriched, highlighting the potential for targeted therapies.

Other Subtypes of BCP-ALL

BCP-ALL with *NUTM1* rearrangements is a rare subtype observed exclusively in children [5, 6]. NUTM1 is a chromatin modifier, recruiting EP300 to increase local histone acetylation [164]. While the common partner, *BRD9-NUTM1*, is reported in BCP-ALL, *BRD4-NUTM1* is a hallmark of NUT midline carcinoma (NMC) and acts to repress differentiation in NMC by widespread repression of histone acetylation, indicating therapeutic approach with bromodomain and HDAC inhibitors. *NUTM1* is rearranged to multiple genes in BCP-ALL (and less commonly, T-ALL) [165] in addition to BRD9 [92, 166], including ACIN1 [24, 26, 92, 167, 168], AFF1 [6, 151], BPTF [165], CUX1 [24, 167], IKZF1 [6, 24, 27, 167],

SCL12A6 [6, 24, 167], and ZNF618 [6, 24, 29, 151], with emerging evidence that these fusions are enriched in non-*KMT2A*-rearranged BCR-ALL in infants [92, 168]. The potential for bromodomain inhibition as a therapeutic strategy has not yet been tested in *NUTM1*-rearranged BCP-ALL.

IKZF1 alterations, like *PAX5*, are also common across the spectrum of B-ALL (particularly in *BCR-ABL1*-positive, Ph-like, and *DUX4*-rearranged cases), but a specific mutation, IKZF1 p.Asn159Tyr, defines a subtype with gene expression profile [5, 6]. In this subtype, the non-mutated wild-type allele of *IKZF1* is retained, and most cases have concurrent gain of chromosome 21. Notably, this mutation is located at a residue that is critical for DNA binding of IKZF1 [169] and is also mutated in germline syndromes with immunodeficiency and autoimmunity [42, 170], although most commonly to serine but not tyrosine, suggesting genotype-phenotype variation of different IKZF1 mutations. The IKZF1 p.Asn159Tyr mutation induces misregulation of IKZF1 transcriptional activation, in part through distinctive nuclear mislocalization and enhanced intercellular adhesion [108].

Relapsed ALL

Genomic analyses of paired primary and relapsed ALL samples have revealed that these secondary mutations are acquired during disease progression with Darwinian patterns of selection, and highly branched clonal architectures, especially in early relapse (9–36 months) [8, 9, 78, 171–175]. Furthermore, chemotherapy of ALL has been postulated to induce bona fide drug resistance mutations including *NT5C2*, *PRPS1*, *NR3C1*, and *TP53* [9]. However, recent studies integrating genome sequencing of matched diagnosis and relapse samples, and xenografts propagated from these samples, coupled with drug sensitivity testing of the relapse fated clones have shown that relapse-fated subclones present at diagnosis commonly exhibit drug resistance prior to the administration of any therapy [174] (Fig. 1.6).

One of the representative relapse-specific somatic alterations is *CREBBP* alterations which occur in up to 20% of relapsed B-ALL and impair glucocorticoid sensitivity [60]. Early relapse is commonly associated with 6-MP resistance, as a result of *NT5C2* gain-of-function mutations [175–178], *PRPS1* mutations [179], and loss of *MSH6* [180]. *NT5C2* mutations confer resistance to purine analogs at the cost of impaired tumor cell growth and reduced leukemia-initiating cell activity [175]. While the development of NT5C2 inhibitors may be promising, several problems are anticipated such as the development of mutant specific inhibitors [176]. Importantly, *NT5C2* and *PRPS1* mutations are not detectable in primary samples even in a minor clone [7, 9, 175]. Other recurrent somatic alterations in relapsed ALL include mutations in [78] *SETD2*, *KDM6*, and *KMT2D* (*MLL2*) [9, 173, 181]. Tracking of these mutations as MRD may offer the opportunity to identify the relapse-fated clone early in disease evolution and modulate therapy accordingly to

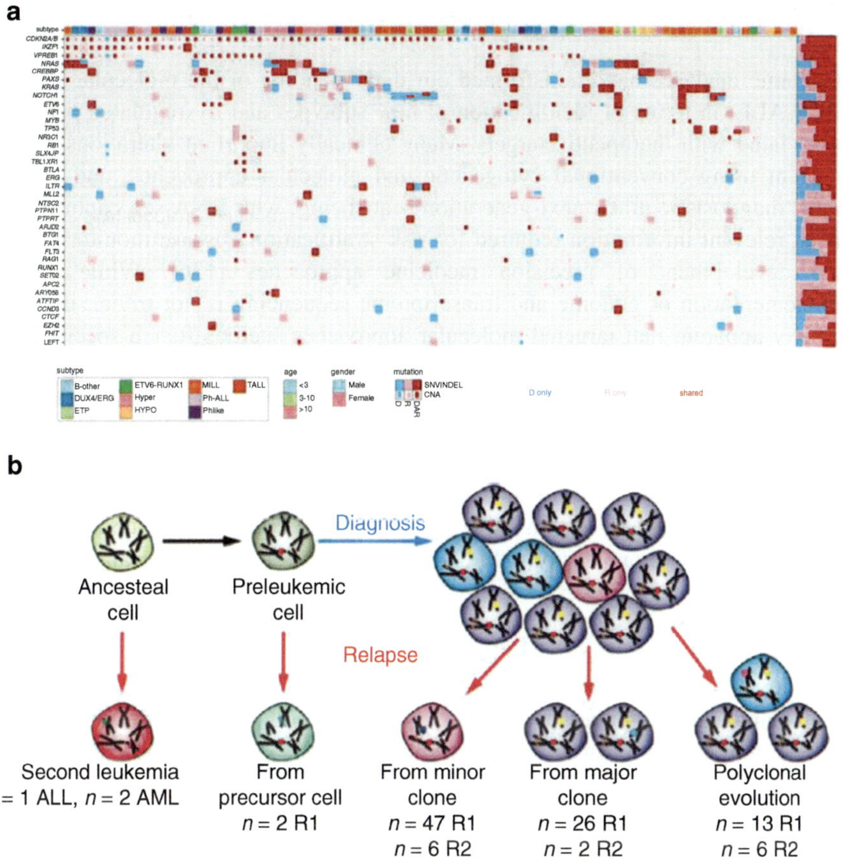

Fig. 1.6 (**a**) Oncoprint of the most common targets of mutation at relapse in childhood B- and T-ALL. (**b**) Patterns of clonal evolution in relapsed ALL. (Data taken from Waanders et al. [7])

circumvent relapse. Detailed, genome-wide analyses of large ALL cohorts have enabled several additional important observations: hypermutation becomes increasingly frequent during disease progression, is enriched in leukemic cells with mutations in mismatch repair genes and hypodiploidy, and results in a predicted increase in expressed neoantigen formation. Thus, strategies to promote autologous T cell reactivity may be efficacious in this setting. Secondly, careful analysis of the nature and structure of coding and non-coding sequence and structural variants has shown that most cases presumed to be second leukemias are indeed clonally related to the primary tumor, including cases with lineage shift/switch, indicating relapse from an ancestral, pre-diagnosis clone [7] (Fig. 1.6b). These observations confirm hypotheses from SNP array analyses of relapsed ALL [78] and are of therapeutic importance for disease monitoring and selection of therapy.

Summary

Genomic analyses have transformed our understanding of the molecular basis of BCP-ALL, in terms of identification of new subtypes and dysregulated pathways associated with therapeutic targets. Many clinically important alterations are not evident using conventional cytogenetic and molecular approaches, and optimal ALL diagnosis requires next-generation sequencing, with RNA-seq capturing the most relevant information required for risk stratification, disease monitoring, and the development of precision medicine approaches [136]. While clinical implementation of genome and transcriptome sequencing is not trivial, it is now clearly apparent that targeted molecular approaches such as fusion-specific PCR and exome/gene panel capture sequencing are not optimal as they do not capture the diversity of genomic alterations in ALL. Moreover, integrated genome, exome and transcriptome sequencing has been shown to have excellent sensitivity and specificity in detection of the various driver alterations in pediatric cancer [182]. Even if sequencing is not available, several key alterations can be detected by alternative approaches, such as flow cytometry for *CRLF2* (which correlates well with *CRLF2* overexpression) and FISH assays for gene rearrangements in Ph-like ALL.

These genomic discoveries are partly responsible for a wave of new therapeutic approaches entering the clinic in BCP-ALL including small molecules (TKI, BCL2 inhibitors, MEK inhibitors), antibody-based therapy (blinatumomab, inotuzumab), and cellular immunotherapy. Future challenges and opportunities include (1) determining the tumor intrinsic and extrinsic determinants of response in the era of targeted therapies and immunotherapy, (2) developing efficacious approaches to directly target transcription factor alterations that underlie over 50% of BCP-ALL, and (3) integrating genomic and functional genomic approaches to identify therapeutic vulnerabilities both in the research and clinical setting.

Acknowledgments The authors thank colleagues at St Jude Children's Research Hospital, the Children's Oncology Group, the NCI TARGET initiative, and colleagues for collaborative research described in this review. C.G.M. is supported by the St Jude Comprehensive Cancer Center Support Grant NCI P30 CA021765 and an NCI Outstanding Investigator Award R35 CA197695, the Henry Schueler 41&9 Foundation, a St. Baldrick's Foundation Robert J. Arceci Innovation Award (to C.G.M.), and the American Lebanese Syrian Associated Charities of St. Jude Children's Research Hospital.

Declaration of Competing Interest Charles Mullighan has received research funding from AbbVie, Pfizer, and Loxo Oncology and consulting fees from Illumina.

References

1. Iacobucci I, Mullighan CG. Genetic basis of acute lymphoblastic leukemia. J Clin Oncol. 2017;35(9):975–83.
2. Roberts KG, Mullighan CG. The biology of B-progenitor acute lymphoblastic leukemia. Cold Spring Harb Perspect Med. 2020;10(7):a03483.

3. Pui CH, Nichols KE, Yang JJ. Somatic and germline genomics in paediatric acute lymphoblastic leukaemia. Nat Rev Clin Oncol. 2019;16(4):227–40.
4. Holmfeldt L, Wei L, Diaz-Flores E, Walsh M, Zhang J, Ding L, et al. The genomic landscape of hypodiploid acute lymphoblastic leukemia. Nat Genet. 2013;45(3):242–52.
5. Gu Z, Churchman ML, Roberts KG, Moore I, Zhou X, Nakitandwe J, et al. PAX5-driven subtypes of B-progenitor acute lymphoblastic leukemia. Nat Genet. 2019;51(2):296–307.
6. Li JF, Dai YT, Lilljebjorn H, Shen SH, Cui BW, Bai L, et al. Transcriptional landscape of B cell precursor acute lymphoblastic leukemia based on an international study of 1,223 cases. Proc Natl Acad Sci U S A. 2018;115(50):E11711–e20.
7. Waanders E, Gu Z, Dobson SM, Antić Ž, Crawford JC, Ma X, et al. Mutational landscape and patterns of clonal evolution in relapsed pediatric acute lymphoblastic leukemia. Blood Cancer Discov. 2020;1(1):96–111.
8. Ma X, Edmonson M, Yergeau D, Muzny DM, Hampton OA, Rusch M, et al. Rise and fall of subclones from diagnosis to relapse in pediatric B-acute lymphoblastic leukaemia. Nat Commun. 2015;6:6604.
9. Li B, Brady SW, Ma X, Shen S, Zhang Y, Li Y, et al. Therapy-induced mutations drive the genomic landscape of relapsed acute lymphoblastic leukemia. Blood. 2020;135(1):41–55.
10. Harrison CJ, Foroni L. Cytogenetics and molecular genetics of acute lymphoblastic leukemia. Rev Clin Exp Hematol. 2002;6(2):91–113.
11. Stock W. Adolescents and young adults with acute lymphoblastic leukemia. Hematology Am Soc Hematol Educ Program. 2010;2010:21–9.
12. Gale KB, Ford AM, Repp R, Borkhardt A, Keller C, Eden OB, et al. Backtracking leukemia to birth: identification of clonotypic gene fusion sequences in neonatal blood spots. Proc Natl Acad Sci U S A. 1997;94(25):13950–4.
13. Yeoh EJ, Ross ME, Shurtleff SA, Williams WK, Patel D, Mahfouz R, et al. Classification, subtype discovery, and prediction of outcome in pediatric acute lymphoblastic leukemia by gene expression profiling. Cancer Cell. 2002;1(2):133–43.
14. Ross ME, Zhou X, Song G, Shurtleff SA, Girtman K, Williams WK, et al. Classification of pediatric acute lymphoblastic leukemia by gene expression profiling. Blood. 2003;102(8):2951–9.
15. Harvey RC, Mullighan CG, Wang X, Dobbin KK, Davidson GS, Bedrick EJ, et al. Identification of novel cluster groups in pediatric high-risk B-precursor acute lymphoblastic leukemia with gene expression profiling: correlation with genome-wide DNA copy number alterations, clinical characteristics, and outcome. Blood. 2010;116(23):4874–84.
16. Mullighan CG, Goorha S, Radtke I, Miller CB, Coustan-Smith E, Dalton JD, et al. Genome-wide analysis of genetic alterations in acute lymphoblastic leukaemia. Nature. 2007;446(7137):758–64.
17. Kuiper RP, Schoenmakers EF, van Reijmersdal SV, Hehir-Kwa JY, van Kessel AG, van Leeuwen FN, et al. High-resolution genomic profiling of childhood ALL reveals novel recurrent genetic lesions affecting pathways involved in lymphocyte differentiation and cell cycle progression. Leukemia. 2007;21(6):1258–66.
18. Den Boer ML, van Slegtenhorst M, De Menezes RX, Cheok MH, Buijs-Gladdines JG, Peters ST, et al. A subtype of childhood acute lymphoblastic leukaemia with poor treatment outcome: a genome-wide classification study. Lancet Oncol. 2009;10(2):125–34.
19. Mullighan CG, Su X, Zhang J, Radtke I, Phillips LA, Miller CB, et al. Deletion of IKZF1 and prognosis in acute lymphoblastic leukemia. N Engl J Med. 2009;360(5):470–80.
20. Roberts KG, Li Y, Payne-Turner D, Harvey RC, Yang YL, Pei D, et al. Targetable kinase-activating lesions in Ph-like acute lymphoblastic leukemia. N Engl J Med. 2014;371(11):1005–15.
21. Roberts KG, Morin RD, Zhang J, Hirst M, Zhao Y, Su X, et al. Genetic alterations activating kinase and cytokine receptor signaling in high-risk acute lymphoblastic leukemia. Cancer Cell. 2012;22(2):153–66.
22. Yasuda T, Tsuzuki S, Kawazu M, Hayakawa F, Kojima S, Ueno T, et al. Recurrent DUX4 fusions in B cell acute lymphoblastic leukemia of adolescents and young adults. Nat Genet. 2016;48(5):569–74.

23. Zhang J, McCastlain K, Yoshihara H, Xu B, Chang Y, Churchman ML, et al. Deregulation of DUX4 and ERG in acute lymphoblastic leukemia. Nat Genet. 2016;48(12):1481–9.
24. Gu Z, Churchman M, Roberts K, Li Y, Liu Y, Harvey RC, et al. Genomic analyses identify recurrent MEF2D fusions in acute lymphoblastic leukaemia. Nat Commun. 2016;7:13331.
25. Gocho Y, Kiyokawa N, Ichikawa H, Nakabayashi K, Osumi T, Ishibashi T, et al. A novel recurrent EP300-ZNF384 gene fusion in B-cell precursor acute lymphoblastic leukemia. Leukemia. 2015;29(12):2445–8.
26. Liu YF, Wang BY, Zhang WN, Huang JY, Li BS, Zhang M, et al. Genomic profiling of adult and pediatric B-cell acute lymphoblastic leukemia. EBioMedicine. 2016;8:173–83.
27. Lilljebjorn H, Henningsson R, Hyrenius-Wittsten A, Olsson L, Orsmark-Pietras C, von Palffy S, et al. Identification of ETV6-RUNX1-like and DUX4-rearranged subtypes in paediatric B-cell precursor acute lymphoblastic leukaemia. Nat Commun. 2016;7:11790.
28. Lilljebjorn H, Fioretos T. New oncogenic subtypes in pediatric B-cell precursor acute lymphoblastic leukemia. Blood. 2017;130(12):1395–401.
29. Zaliova M, Stuchly J, Winkowska L, Musilova A, Fiser K, Slamova M, et al. Genomic landscape of pediatric B-other acute lymphoblastic leukemia in a consecutive European cohort. Haematologica. 2019;104(7):1396–406.
30. Roberts KG. Genetics and prognosis of ALL in children vs adults. Hematology Am Soc Hematol Educ Program. 2018;2018(1):137–45.
31. Reiman A, Srinivasan V, Barone G, Last JI, Wootton LL, Davies EG, et al. Lymphoid tumours and breast cancer in ataxia telangiectasia; substantial protective effect of residual ATM kinase activity against childhood tumours. Br J Cancer. 2011;105(4):586–91.
32. Strullu M, Caye A, Lachenaud J, Cassinat B, Gazal S, Fenneteau O, et al. Juvenile myelomonocytic leukaemia and Noonan syndrome. J Med Genet. 2014;51(10):689–97.
33. Hasle H, Clemmensen IH, Mikkelsen M. Risks of leukaemia and solid tumours in individuals with Down's syndrome. Lancet. 2000;355(9199):165–9.
34. Rafei H, DiNardo CD. Hereditary myeloid malignancies. Best Pract Res Clin Haematol. 2019;32(2):163–76.
35. Plon SE, Lupo PJ. Genetic predisposition to childhood cancer in the genomic era. Annu Rev Genomics Hum Genet. 2019;20:241–63.
36. Gocho Y, Yang JJ. Genetic defects in hematopoietic transcription factors and predisposition to acute lymphoblastic leukemia. Blood. 2019;134(10):793–7.
37. Nishii R, Baskin-Doerfler R, Yang W, Oak N, Zhao X, Yang W, et al. Molecular basis of ETV6-mediated predisposition to childhood acute lymphoblastic leukemia. Blood. 2021;137(3):364–73.
38. Moriyama T, Metzger ML, Wu G, Nishii R, Qian M, Devidas M, et al. Germline genetic variation in ETV6 and risk of childhood acute lymphoblastic leukaemia: a systematic genetic study. Lancet Oncol. 2015;16(16):1659–66.
39. Shah S, Schrader KA, Waanders E, Timms AE, Vijai J, Miething C, et al. A recurrent germline PAX5 mutation confers susceptibility to pre-B cell acute lymphoblastic leukemia. Nat Genet. 2013;45(10):1226–31.
40. Noetzli L, Lo RW, Lee-Sherick AB, Callaghan M, Noris P, Savoia A, et al. Germline mutations in *ETV6* are associated with thrombocytopenia, red cell macrocytosis and predisposition to lymphoblastic leukemia. Nat Genet. 2015;47(5):535–8.
41. Churchman ML, Qian M, Te Kronnie G, Zhang R, Yang W, Zhang H, et al. Germline genetic IKZF1 variation and predisposition to childhood acute lymphoblastic leukemia. Cancer Cell. 2018;33(5):937–48.e8
42. Kuehn HS, Boisson B, Cunningham-Rundles C, Reichenbach J, Stray-Pedersen A, Gelfand EW, et al. Loss of B cells in patients with heterozygous mutations in IKAROS. N Engl J Med. 2016;374(11):1032–43.
43. Mullighan CG, Miller CB, Radtke I, Phillips LA, Dalton J, Ma J, et al. BCR-ABL1 lymphoblastic leukaemia is characterized by the deletion of Ikaros. Nature. 2008;453(7191):110–4.

44. Papaemmanuil E, Hosking FJ, Vijayakrishnan J, Price A, Olver B, Sheridan E, et al. Loci on 7p12.2, 10q21.2 and 14q11.2 are associated with risk of childhood acute lymphoblastic leukemia. Nat Genet. 2009;41(9):1006–10.
45. Trevino LR, Yang W, French D, Hunger SP, Carroll WL, Devidas M, et al. Germline genomic variants associated with childhood acute lymphoblastic leukemia. Nat Genet. 2009;41(9):1001–5.
46. Perez-Andreu V, Roberts KG, Harvey RC, Yang W, Cheng C, Pei D, et al. Inherited GATA3 variants are associated with Ph-like childhood acute lymphoblastic leukemia and risk of relapse. Nat Genet. 2013;45(12):1494–8.
47. Qian M, Xu H, Perez-Andreu V, Roberts KG, Zhang H, Yang W, et al. Novel susceptibility variants at the ERG locus for childhood acute lymphoblastic leukemia in Hispanics. Blood. 2019;133(7):724–9.
48. Qian M, Zhao X, Devidas M, Yang W, Gocho Y, Smith C, et al. Genome-wide association study of susceptibility loci for T-cell acute lymphoblastic leukemia in children. J Natl Cancer Inst. 2019;111(12):1350–7.
49. de Smith AJ, Lavoie G, Walsh KM, Aujla S, Evans E, Hansen HM, et al. Predisposing germline mutations in high hyperdiploid acute lymphoblastic leukemia in children. Genes Chromosomes Cancer. 2019;58(10):723–30.
50. Pouliot GP, Degar J, Hinze L, Kochupurakkal B, Vo CD, Burns MA, et al. Fanconi-BRCA pathway mutations in childhood T-cell acute lymphoblastic leukemia. PLoS One. 2019;14(11):e0221288.
51. Winer P, Muskens IS, Walsh KM, Vora A, Moorman AV, Wiemels JL, et al. Germline variants in predisposition genes in children with Down syndrome and acute lymphoblastic leukemia. Blood Adv. 2020;4(4):672–5.
52. Greaves M. Pre-natal origins of childhood leukemia. Rev Clin Exp Hematol. 2003;7(3):233–45.
53. Greaves MF, Maia AT, Wiemels JL, Ford AM. Leukemia in twins: lessons in natural history. Blood. 2003;102(7):2321–33.
54. Hein D, Borkhardt A, Fischer U. Insights into the prenatal origin of childhood acute lymphoblastic leukemia. Cancer Metastasis Rev. 2020;39(1):161–71.
55. Ma Y, Dobbins SE, Sherborne AL, Chubb D, Galbiati M, Cazzaniga G, et al. Developmental timing of mutations revealed by whole-genome sequencing of twins with acute lymphoblastic leukemia. Proc Natl Acad Sci U S A. 2013;110(18):7429–33.
56. Bueno C, Tejedor JR, Bashford-Rogers R, Gonzalez-Silva L, Valdes-Mas R, Agraz-Doblas A, et al. Natural history and cell of origin of TC F3-ZN F384 and PTPN11 mutations in monozygotic twins with concordant BCP-ALL. Blood. 2019;134(11):900–5.
57. Paulsson K, Lilljebjörn H, Biloglav A, Olsson L, Rissler M, Castor A, et al. The genomic landscape of high hyperdiploid childhood acute lymphoblastic leukemia. Nat Genet. 2015;47(6):672–6.
58. Sutcliffe MJ, Shuster JJ, Sather HN, Camitta BM, Pullen J, Schultz KR, et al. High concordance from independent studies by the Children's Cancer Group (CCG) and Pediatric Oncology Group (POG) associating favorable prognosis with combined trisomies 4, 10, and 17 in children with NCI Standard-Risk B-precursor Acute Lymphoblastic Leukemia: a Children's Oncology Group (COG) initiative. Leukemia. 2005;19(5):734–40.
59. Yang M, Safavi S, Woodward EL, Duployez N, Olsson-Arvidsson L, Ungerback J, et al. 13q12.2 deletions in acute lymphoblastic leukemia lead to upregulation of FLT3 through enhancer hijacking. Blood. 2020;136(8):946–56.
60. Mullighan CG, Zhang J, Kasper LH, Lerach S, Payne-Turner D, Phillips LA, et al. CREBBP mutations in relapsed acute lymphoblastic leukaemia. Nature. 2011;471(7337):235–9.
61. Pui CH, Williams DL, Raimondi SC, Rivera GK, Look AT, Dodge RK, et al. Hypodiploidy is associated with a poor prognosis in childhood acute lymphoblastic leukemia. Blood. 1987;70(1):247–53.

62. Harrison CJ, Moorman AV, Broadfield ZJ, Cheung KL, Harris RL, Reza Jalali G, et al. Three distinct subgroups of hypodiploidy in acute lymphoblastic leukaemia. Br J Haematol. 2004;125(5):552–9.
63. Nachman JB, Heerema NA, Sather H, Camitta B, Forestier E, Harrison CJ, et al. Outcome of treatment in children with hypodiploid acute lymphoblastic leukemia. Blood. 2007;110(4):1112–5.
64. Carroll AJ, Shago M, Mikhail FM, Raimondi SC, Hirsch BA, Loh ML, et al. Masked hypodiploidy: Hypodiploid acute lymphoblastic leukemia (ALL) mimicking hyperdiploid ALL in children: a report from the Children's Oncology Group. Cancer Genet. 2019;238:62–8.
65. Qian M, Cao X, Devidas M, Yang W, Cheng C, Dai Y, et al. TP53 germline variations influence the predisposition and prognosis of B-cell acute lymphoblastic leukemia in children. J Clin Oncol. 2018;36(6):591–9.
66. Mullighan CG, Jeha S, Pei D, Payne-Turner D, Coustan-Smith E, Roberts KG, et al. Outcome of children with hypodiploid ALL treated with risk-directed therapy based on MRD levels. Blood. 2015;126(26):2896–9.
67. Diaz-Flores E, Comeaux EQ, Kim KL, Melnik E, Beckman K, Davis KL, et al. Bcl-2 is a therapeutic target for hypodiploid B-lineage acute lymphoblastic leukemia. Cancer Res. 2019;79(9):2339–51.
68. Harrison CJ, Haas O, Harbott J, Biondi A, Stanulla M, Trka J, et al. Detection of prognostically relevant genetic abnormalities in childhood B-cell precursor acute lymphoblastic leukaemia: recommendations from the Biology and Diagnosis Committee of the International Berlin-Frankfurt-Munster study group. Br J Haematol. 2010;151(2):132–42.
69. Li Y, Schwab C, Ryan SL, Papaemmanuil E, Robinson HM, Jacobs P, et al. Constitutional and somatic rearrangement of chromosome 21 in acute lymphoblastic leukaemia. Nature. 2014;508(7494):98–102.
70. Harrison CJ, Moorman AV, Schwab C, Carroll AJ, Raetz EA, Devidas M, et al. An international study of intrachromosomal amplification of chromosome 21 (iAMP21): cytogenetic characterization and outcome. Leukemia. 2014;28(5):1015–21.
71. Moorman AV, Richards SM, Robinson HM, Strefford JC, Gibson BE, Kinsey SE, et al. Prognosis of children with acute lymphoblastic leukemia (ALL) and intrachromosomal amplification of chromosome 21 (iAMP21). Blood. 2007;109(6):2327–30.
72. Harrison CJ, Schwab C. Constitutional abnormalities of chromosome 21 predispose to iAMP21-acute lymphoblastic leukaemia. Eur J Med Genet. 2016;59(3):162–5.
73. Heerema NA, Carroll AJ, Devidas M, Loh ML, Borowitz MJ, Gastier-Foster JM, et al. Intrachromosomal amplification of chromosome 21 is associated with inferior outcomes in children with acute lymphoblastic leukemia treated in contemporary standard-risk Children's Oncology Group studies: a report from the Children's Oncology Group. J Clin Oncol. 2013;31(27):3397–402.
74. Moorman AV, Robinson H, Schwab C, Richards SM, Hancock J, Mitchell CD, et al. Risk-directed treatment intensification significantly reduces the risk of relapse among children and adolescents with acute lymphoblastic leukemia and intrachromosomal amplification of chromosome 21: a comparison of the MRC ALL97/99 and UKALL2003 trials. J Clin Oncol. 2013;31(27):3389–96.
75. Sundaresh A, Williams O. Mechanism of ETV6-RUNX1 leukemia. Adv Exp Med Biol. 2017;962:201–16.
76. Zaliova M, Kotrova M, Bresolin S, Stuchly J, Stary J, Hrusak O, et al. ETV6/RUNX1-like acute lymphoblastic leukemia: a novel B-cell precursor leukemia subtype associated with the CD27/CD44 immunophenotype. Genes Chromosomes Cancer. 2017;56(8):608–16.
77. Papaemmanuil E, Rapado I, Li Y, Potter NE, Wedge DC, Tubio J, et al. RAG-mediated recombination is the predominant driver of oncogenic rearrangement in ETV6-RUNX1 acute lymphoblastic leukemia. Nat Genet. 2014;46(2):116–25.
78. Mullighan CG, Phillips LA, Su X, Ma J, Miller CB, Shurtleff SA, et al. Genomic analysis of the clonal origins of relapsed acute lymphoblastic leukemia. Science. 2008;322(5906):1377–80.

79. Anderson K, Lutz C, van Delft FW, Bateman CM, Guo Y, Colman SM, et al. Genetic variegation of clonal architecture and propagating cells in leukaemia. Nature. 2011;469(7330):356–61.
80. Aspland SE, Bendall HH, Murre C. The role of E2A-PBX1 in leukemogenesis. Oncogene. 2001;20(40):5708–17.
81. Pui CH, Aur RJ, Bowman WP, Dahl GV, Dodge RK, George SL, et al. Failure of late intensification therapy to improve a poor result in childhood lymphoblastic leukemia. Cancer Res. 1984;44(8):3593–8.
82. Jeha S, Pei D, Raimondi SC, Onciu M, Campana D, Cheng C, et al. Increased risk for CNS relapse in pre-B cell leukemia with the t(1;19)/TCF3-PBX1. Leukemia. 2009;23(8):1406–9.
83. Jeha S, Pei D, Choi J, Cheng C, Sandlund JT, Coustan-Smith E, et al. Improved CNS control of childhood acute lymphoblastic leukemia without cranial irradiation: St Jude Total Therapy Study 16. J Clin Oncol. 2019;37(35):3377–91. JCO1901692
84. Duque-Afonso J, Feng J, Scherer F, Lin CH, Wong SH, Wang Z, et al. Comparative genomics reveals multistep pathogenesis of E2A-PBX1 acute lymphoblastic leukemia. J Clin Invest. 2015;125(9):3667–80.
85. Bicocca VT, Chang BH, Masouleh BK, Muschen M, Loriaux MM, Druker BJ, et al. Crosstalk between ROR1 and the Pre-B cell receptor promotes survival of t(1;19) acute lymphoblastic leukemia. Cancer Cell. 2012;22(5):656–67.
86. Panagopoulos I, Micci F, Thorsen J, Haugom L, Tierens A, Ulvmoen A, et al. A novel TCF3-HLF fusion transcript in acute lymphoblastic leukemia with a t(17;19)(q22;p13). Cancer Genet. 2012;205(12):669–72.
87. Hunger SP, Devaraj PE, Foroni L, Secker-Walker LM, Cleary ML. Two types of genomic rearrangements create alternative E2A-HLF fusion proteins in t(17;19)-ALL. Blood. 1994;83(10):2970–7.
88. Fischer U, Forster M, Rinaldi A, Risch T, Sungalee S, Warnatz HJ, et al. Genomics and drug profiling of fatal TCF3-HLF-positive acute lymphoblastic leukemia identifies recurrent mutation patterns and therapeutic options. Nat Genet. 2015;47(9):1020–9.
89. Huang Y, Mouttet B, Warnatz HJ, Risch T, Rietmann F, Frommelt F, et al. The leukemogenic TCF3-HLF complex rewires enhancers driving cellular identity and self-renewal conferring EP300 vulnerability. Cancer Cell. 2019;36(6):630–44.e9
90. Winters AC, Bernt KM. MLL-rearranged leukemias-an update on science and clinical approaches. Front Pediatr. 2017;5:4.
91. Pui CH, Relling MV. Topoisomerase II inhibitor-related acute myeloid leukaemia. Br J Haematol. 2000;109(1):13–23.
92. Andersson AK, Ma J, Wang J, Chen X, Gedman AL, Dang J, et al. The landscape of somatic mutations in infant MLL-rearranged acute lymphoblastic leukemias. Nat Genet. 2015;47(4):330–7.
93. Valentine MC, Linabery AM, Chasnoff S, Hughes AE, Mallaney C, Sanchez N, et al. Excess congenital non-synonymous variation in leukemia-associated genes in MLL- infant leukemia: a Children's Oncology Group report. Leukemia. 2014;28(6):1235–41.
94. Agraz-Doblas A, Bueno C, Bashford-Rogers R, Roy A, Schneider P, Bardini M, et al. Unraveling the cellular origin and clinical prognostic markers of infant B-cell acute lymphoblastic leukemia using genome-wide analysis. Haematologica. 2019;104(6):1176–88.
95. Bernt KM, Zhu N, Sinha AU, Vempati S, Faber J, Krivtsov AV, et al. MLL-rearranged leukemia is dependent on aberrant H3K79 methylation by DOT1L. Cancer Cell. 2011;20(1):66–78.
96. Krivtsov AV, Feng Z, Lemieux ME, Faber J, Vempati S, Sinha AU, et al. H3K79 methylation profiles define murine and human MLL-AF4 leukemias. Cancer Cell. 2008;14(5):355–68.
97. Chen CW, Koche RP, Sinha AU, Deshpande AJ, Zhu N, Eng R, et al. DOT1L inhibits SIRT1-mediated epigenetic silencing to maintain leukemic gene expression in MLL-rearranged leukemia. Nat Med. 2015;21(4):335–43.
98. Grembecka J, He S, Shi A, Purohit T, Muntean AG, Sorenson RJ, et al. Menin-MLL inhibitors reverse oncogenic activity of MLL fusion proteins in leukemia. Nat Chem Biol. 2012;8(3):277–84.

99. Krivtsov AV, Evans K, Gadrey JY, Eschle BK, Hatton C, Uckelmann HJ, et al. A Menin-MLL inhibitor induces specific chromatin changes and eradicates disease in models of MLL-rearranged leukemia. Cancer Cell. 2019;36(6):660–73.e11
100. Quintás-Cardama A, Cortes J. Molecular biology of bcr-abl1-positive chronic myeloid leukemia. Blood. 2009;113(8):1619–30.
101. Abou Dalle I, Jabbour E, Short NJ, Ravandi F. Treatment of Philadelphia chromosome-positive acute lymphoblastic leukemia. Curr Treat Options in Oncol. 2019;20(1):4.
102. Slayton WB, Schultz KR, Kairalla JA, Devidas M, Mi X, Pulsipher MA, et al. Dasatinib plus intensive chemotherapy in children, adolescents, and young adults with Philadelphia chromosome-positive acute lymphoblastic leukemia: results of Children's Oncology Group trial AALL0622. J Clin Oncol. 2018;36(22):2306–14. Jco2017767228
103. Schultz KR, Carroll A, Heerema NA, Bowman WP, Aledo A, Slayton WB, et al. Long-term follow-up of imatinib in pediatric Philadelphia chromosome-positive acute lymphoblastic leukemia: Children's Oncology Group study AALL0031. Leukemia. 2014;28(7):1467–71.
104. Shen S, Chen X, Cai J, Yu J, Gao J, Hu S, et al. Effect of dasatinib vs imatinib in the treatment of pediatric Philadelphia chromosome-positive acute lymphoblastic leukemia: a randomized clinical trial. JAMA Oncol. 2020;6(3):358–66.
105. Martinelli G, Iacobucci I, Storlazzi CT, Vignetti M, Paoloni F, Cilloni D, et al. IKZF1 (Ikaros) deletions in BCR-ABL1-positive acute lymphoblastic leukemia are associated with short disease-free survival and high rate of cumulative incidence of relapse: a GIMEMA AL WP report. J Clin Oncol. 2009;27(31):5202–7.
106. Chang BH, Willis SG, Stork L, Hunger SP, Carroll WL, Camitta BM, et al. Imatinib resistant BCR-ABL1 mutations at relapse in children with Ph+ ALL: a Children's Oncology Group (COG) study. Br J Haematol. 2012;157(4):507–10.
107. Joshi I, Yoshida T, Jena N, Qi X, Zhang J, Van Etten RA, et al. Loss of Ikaros DNA-binding function confers integrin-dependent survival on pre-B cells and progression to acute lymphoblastic leukemia. Nat Immunol. 2014;15(3):294–304.
108. Churchman ML, Low J, Qu C, Paietta EM, Kasper LH, Chang Y, et al. Efficacy of retinoids in IKZF1-mutated BCR-ABL1 acute lymphoblastic leukemia. Cancer Cell. 2015;28(3):343–56.
109. Churchman ML, Evans K, Richmond J, Robbins A, Jones L, Shapiro IM, et al. Synergism of FAK and tyrosine kinase inhibition in Ph+ B-ALL. JCI Insight. 2016;1(4):e86082.
110. Pfeifer H, Cazzaniga G, van der Velden VHJ, Cayuela JM, Schäfer B, Spinelli O, et al. Standardisation and consensus guidelines for minimal residual disease assessment in Philadelphia-positive acute lymphoblastic leukemia (Ph+ALL) by real-time quantitative reverse transcriptase PCR of e1a2 BCR-ABL1. Leukemia. 2019;33(8):1910–22.
111. Hovorkova L, Zaliova M, Venn NC, Bleckmann K, Trkova M, Potuckova E, et al. Monitoring of childhood ALL using BCR-ABL1 genomic breakpoints identifies a subgroup with CML-like biology. Blood. 2017;129(20):2771–81.
112. Herold T, Schneider S, Metzeler K, Neumann M, Hartmann L, Roberts KG, et al. Philadelphia chromosome-like acute lymphoblastic leukemia in adults have frequent IGH-CRLF2 and JAK2 mutations, persistence of minimal residual disease and poor prognosis. Haematologica. 2017;102(1):130–8.
113. Jain N, Roberts KG, Jabbour E, Patel K, Eterovic AK, Chen K, et al. Ph-like acute lymphoblastic leukemia: a high-risk subtype in adults. Blood. 2017;129(5):572–81.
114. Loh ML, Zhang J, Harvey RC, Roberts K, Payne-Turner D, Kang H, et al. Tyrosine kinome sequencing of pediatric acute lymphoblastic leukemia: a report from the Children's Oncology Group TARGET Project. Blood. 2013;121(3):485–8.
115. Reshmi SC, Harvey RC, Roberts KG, Stonerock E, Smith A, Jenkins H, et al. Targetable kinase gene fusions in high-risk B-ALL: a study from the Children's Oncology Group. Blood. 2017;129(25):3352–61.
116. Roberts KG, Gu Z, Payne-Turner D, McCastlain K, Harvey RC, Chen IM, et al. High frequency and poor outcome of Philadelphia chromosome-like acute lymphoblastic leukemia in adults. J Clin Oncol. 2017;35(4):394–401.

117. Roberts KG, Pei D, Campana D, Payne-Turner D, Li Y, Cheng C, et al. Outcomes of children with BCR-ABL1-like acute lymphoblastic leukemia treated with risk-directed therapy based on the levels of minimal residual disease. J Clin Oncol. 2014;32(27):3012–20.
118. Tasian SK, Hurtz C, Wertheim GB, Bailey NG, Lim MS, Harvey RC, et al. High incidence of Philadelphia chromosome-like acute lymphoblastic leukemia in older adults with B-ALL. Leukemia. 2017;31(4):981–4.
119. Roberts KG, Reshmi SC, Harvey RC, Chen IM, Patel K, Stonerock E, et al. Genomic and outcome analyses of Ph-like ALL in NCI standard-risk patients: a report from the Children's Oncology Group. Blood. 2018;132(8):815–24.
120. Tasian SK, Loh ML, Hunger SP. Philadelphia chromosome-like acute lymphoblastic leukemia. Blood. 2017;130(19):2064–72.
121. Roberts KG. Why and how to treat Ph-like ALL? Best Pract Res Clin Haematol. 2018;31(4):351–6.
122. Roberts KG. The biology of Philadelphia chromosome-like ALL. Best Pract Res Clin Haematol. 2017;30(3):212–21.
123. Russell LJ, Capasso M, Vater I, Moorman AV, Akasaka T, Harder L, et al. IGH translocations involving the pseudoautosomal region 1 (PAR1) of both sex chromosomes deregulate the cytokine receptor-like factor 2 (CRLF2) gene in B cell precursor acute lymphoblastic leukemia (BCP-ALL). Blood. 2008;112:787. (abstract)
124. Mullighan CG, Collins-Underwood JR, Phillips LA, Loudin MG, Liu W, Zhang J, et al. Rearrangement of CRLF2 in B-progenitor- and Down syndrome-associated acute lymphoblastic leukemia. Nat Genet. 2009;41(11):1243–6.
125. Hertzberg L, Vendramini E, Ganmore I, Cazzaniga G, Schmitz M, Chalker J, et al. Down syndrome acute lymphoblastic leukemia: a highly heterogeneous disease in which aberrant expression of CRLF2 is associated with mutated JAK2: a report from the iBFM Study Group. Blood. 2010;115(5):1006–17.
126. Russell LJ, Jones L, Enshaei A, Tonin S, Ryan SL, Eswaran J, et al. Characterisation of the genomic landscape of CRLF2-rearranged acute lymphoblastic leukemia. Genes Chromosomes Cancer. 2017;56(5):363–72.
127. Schwartzman O, Savino AM, Gombert M, Palmi C, Cario G, Schrappe M, et al. Suppressors and activators of JAK-STAT signaling at diagnosis and relapse of acute lymphoblastic leukemia in Down syndrome. Proc Natl Acad Sci U S A. 2017;114(20):E4030–E9.
128. Perez-Andreu V, Roberts KG, Xu H, Smith C, Zhang H, Yang W, et al. A genome-wide association study of susceptibility to acute lymphoblastic leukemia in adolescents and young adults. Blood. 2015;125(4):680–6.
129. Mullighan CG. How advanced are we in targeting novel subtypes of ALL? Best Pract Res Clin Haematol. 2019;32(4):101095.
130. Roberts KG, Janke LJ, Zhao Y, Seth A, Ma J, Finkelstein D, et al. ETV6-NTRK3 induces aggressive acute lymphoblastic leukemia highly sensitive to selective TRK inhibition. Blood. 2018;132(8):861–5.
131. Nardi V, Ku N, Frigault MJ, Dubuc AM, Tsai HK, Amrein PC, et al. Clinical response to larotrectinib in adult Philadelphia chromosome-like ALL with cryptic ETV6-NTRK3 rearrangement. Blood Adv. 2020;4(1):106–11.
132. Schewe DM, Lenk L, Vogiatzi F, Winterberg D, Rademacher AV, Buchmann S, et al. Larotrectinib in TRK fusion-positive pediatric B-cell acute lymphoblastic leukemia. Blood Adv. 2019;3(22):3499–502.
133. Tanasi I, Ba I, Sirvent N, Braun T, Cuccuini W, Ballerini P, et al. Efficacy of tyrosine kinase inhibitors in Ph-like acute lymphoblastic leukemia harboring ABL-class rearrangements. Blood. 2019;134(16):1351–5.
134. Maude SL, Tasian SK, Vincent T, Hall JW, Sheen C, Roberts KG, et al. Targeting JAK1/2 and mTOR in murine xenograft models of Ph-like acute lymphoblastic leukemia. Blood. 2012;120(17):3510–8.
135. Tasian SK, Teachey DT, Li Y, Shen F, Harvey RC, Chen IM, et al. Potent efficacy of combined PI3K/mTOR and JAK or ABL inhibition in murine xenograft models of Ph-like acute lymphoblastic leukemia. Blood. 2017;129(2):177–87.

136. Inaba H, Azzato EM, Mullighan CG. Integration of next-generation sequencing to treat acute lymphoblastic leukemia with targetable lesions: the St. Jude Children's Research Hospital approach. Front Pediatr. 2017;5:258.
137. Roberts KG, Yang YL, Payne-Turner D, Lin W, Files JK, Dickerson K, et al. Oncogenic role and therapeutic targeting of ABL-class and JAK-STAT activating kinase alterations in Ph-like ALL. Blood Adv. 2017;1(20):1657–71.
138. Moujalled DM, Hanna DT, Hediyeh-Zadeh S, Pomilio G, Brown L, Litalien V, et al. Cotargeting BCL-2 and MCL-1 in high-risk B-ALL. Blood Adv. 2020;4(12):2762–7.
139. Qin H, Cho M, Haso W, Zhang L, Tasian SK, Oo HZ, et al. Eradication of B-ALL using chimeric antigen receptor-expressing T cells targeting the TSLPR oncoprotein. Blood. 2015;126(5):629–39.
140. Schinnerl D, Mejstrikova E, Schumich A, Zaliova M, Fortschegger K, Nebral K, et al. CD371 cell surface expression: a unique feature of DUX4-rearranged acute lymphoblastic leukemia. Haematologica. 2019;104(8):e352–e5.
141. Zaliova M, Potuckova E, Hovorkova L, Musilova A, Winkowska L, Fiser K, et al. ERG deletions in childhood acute lymphoblastic leukemia with DUX4 rearrangements are mostly polyclonal, prognostically relevant and their detection rate strongly depends on screening method sensitivity. Haematologica. 2019;104(7):1407–16.
142. Zaliova M, Zimmermannova O, Dorge P, Eckert C, Moricke A, Zimmermann M, et al. ERG deletion is associated with CD2 and attenuates the negative impact of IKZF1 deletion in childhood acute lymphoblastic leukemia. Leukemia. 2014;28(1):182–5.
143. Stanulla M, Dagdan E, Zaliova M, Moricke A, Palmi C, Cazzaniga G, et al. IKZF1(plus) defines a new minimal residual disease-dependent very-poor prognostic profile in pediatric B-cell precursor acute lymphoblastic leukemia. J Clin Oncol. 2018;36(12):1240–9.
144. Ohki K, Kiyokawa N, Saito Y, Hirabayashi S, Nakabayashi K, Ichikawa H, et al. Clinical and molecular characteristics of MEF2D fusion-positive B-cell precursor acute lymphoblastic leukemia in childhood, including a novel translocation resulting in MEF2D-HNRNPH1 gene fusion. Haematologica. 2019;104(1):128–37.
145. Suzuki K, Okuno Y, Kawashima N, Muramatsu H, Okuno T, Wang X, et al. MEF2D-BCL9 fusion gene is associated with high-risk acute B-cell precursor lymphoblastic leukemia in adolescents. J Clin Oncol. 2016;34(28):3451–9.
146. Hirano D, Hayakawa F, Yasuda T, Tange N, Yamamoto H, Kojima Y, et al. Chromosomal translocation-mediated evasion from miRNA induces strong MEF2D fusion protein expression, causing inhibition of PAX5 transcriptional activity. Oncogene. 2019;38(13):2263–74.
147. Alexander TB, Gu Z, Iacobucci I, Dickerson K, Choi JK, Xu B, et al. The genetic basis and cell of origin of mixed phenotype acute leukaemia. Nature. 2018;562(7727):373–9.
148. Hirabayashi S, Ohki K, Nakabayashi K, Ichikawa H, Momozawa Y, Okamura K, et al. ZNF384-related fusion genes define a subgroup of childhood B-cell precursor acute lymphoblastic leukemia with a characteristic immunotype. Haematologica. 2017;102(1):118–29.
149. Kim J, Kim HS, Shin S, Lee ST, Choi JR. t(12;17)(p13;q12)/TAF15-ZNF384 rearrangement in acute lymphoblastic leukemia. Ann Lab Med. 2016;36(4):396–8.
150. Nyquist KB, Thorsen J, Zeller B, Haaland A, Troen G, Heim S, et al. Identification of the TAF15-ZNF384 fusion gene in two new cases of acute lymphoblastic leukemia with a t(12;17)(p13;q12). Cancer Genet. 2011;204(3):147–52.
151. Qian M, Zhang H, Kham SK, Liu S, Jiang C, Zhao X, et al. Whole-transcriptome sequencing identifies a distinct subtype of acute lymphoblastic leukemia with predominant genomic abnormalities of EP300 and CREBBP. Genome Res. 2017;27(2):185–95.
152. Shago M, Abla O, Hitzler J, Weitzman S, Abdelhaleem M. Frequency and outcome of pediatric acute lymphoblastic leukemia with ZNF384 gene rearrangements including a novel translocation resulting in an ARID1B/ZNF384 gene fusion. Pediatr Blood Cancer. 2016;63(11):1915–21.
153. Yamamoto K, Kawamoto S, Mizutani Y, Yakushijin K, Yamashita T, Nakamachi Y, et al. Mixed phenotype acute leukemia with t(12;17)(p13;q21)/TAF15-ZNF384 and other chromosome abnormalities. Cytogenet Genome Res. 2016;149(3):165–70.

154. Zhong CH, Prima V, Liang X, Frye C, McGavran L, Meltesen L, et al. E2A-ZNF384 and NOL1-E2A fusion created by a cryptic t(12;19)(p13.3; p13.3) in acute leukemia. Leukemia. 2008;22(4):723–9.
155. Hirabayashi S, Butler E, Ohki K, Kiyokawa N, Bergmann AK, Boer JM, et al. Acute lymphoblastic leukemia with zinc-finger protein 384 (ZNF384)-related rearrangements: a retrospective analysis from the Ponte Di Legno Childhood ALL Working Group. Blood. 2019;134(Supplement_1):652.
156. Griffith M, Griffith OL, Krysiak K, Skidmore ZL, Christopher MJ, Klco JM, et al. Comprehensive genomic analysis reveals FLT3 activation and a therapeutic strategy for a patient with relapsed adult B-lymphoblastic leukemia. Exp Hematol. 2016;44(7):603–13.
157. Oberley MJ, Gaynon PS, Bhojwani D, Pulsipher MA, Gardner RA, Hiemenz MC, et al. Myeloid lineage switch following chimeric antigen receptor T-cell therapy in a patient with TCF3-ZNF384 fusion-positive B-lymphoblastic leukemia. Pediatr Blood Cancer. 2018;65(9):e27265.
158. Novakova M, Zaliova M, Fiser K, Vakrmanova B, Slamova L, Musilova A, et al. DUX4r, ZNF384r and PAX5-P80R mutated B-cell precursor acute lymphoblastic leukemia frequently undergo monocytic switch. Haematologica. 2021;106(8):2066–75.
159. Passet M, Boissel N, Sigaux F, Saillard C, Bargetzi M, Ba I, et al. PAX5 P80R mutation identifies a novel subtype of B-cell precursor acute lymphoblastic leukemia with favorable outcome. Blood. 2019;133(3):280–4.
160. Bastian L, Schroeder MP, Eckert C, Schlee C, Tanchez JO, Kampf S, et al. PAX5 biallelic genomic alterations define a novel subgroup of B-cell precursor acute lymphoblastic leukemia. Leukemia. 2019;33(8):1895–909.
161. Nebral K, Denk D, Attarbaschi A, Konig M, Mann G, Haas OA, et al. Incidence and diversity of PAX5 fusion genes in childhood acute lymphoblastic leukemia. Leukemia. 2009;23(1):134–43.
162. Schwab C, Nebral K, Chilton L, Leschi C, Waanders E, Boer JM, et al. Intragenic amplification of PAX5: a novel subgroup in B-cell precursor acute lymphoblastic leukemia? Blood Adv. 2017;1(19):1473–7.
163. Dang J, Wei L, de Ridder J, Su X, Rust AG, Roberts KG, et al. Pax5 is a tumor suppressor in mouse mutagenesis models of acute lymphoblastic leukemia. Blood. 2015;125(23):3609–17.
164. French CA. NUT carcinoma: clinicopathologic features, pathogenesis, and treatment. Pathol Int. 2018;68(11):583–95.
165. Liu Y, Easton J, Shao Y, Maciaszek J, Wang Z, Wilkinson MR, et al. The genomic landscape of pediatric and young adult T-lineage acute lymphoblastic leukemia. Nat Genet. 2017;49(8):1211–8.
166. Nordlund J, Backlin CL, Zachariadis V, Cavelier L, Dahlberg J, Ofverholm I, et al. DNA methylation-based subtype prediction for pediatric acute lymphoblastic leukemia. Clin Epigenetics. 2015;7(1):11.
167. Hormann FM, Hoogkamer AQ, Beverloo HB, Boeree A, Dingjan I, Wattel MM, et al. NUTM1 is a recurrent fusion gene partner in B-cell precursor acute lymphoblastic leukemia associated with increased expression of genes on chromosome band 10p12.31-12.2. Haematologica. 2019;104(10):e455–e9.
168. Pincez T, Landry JR, Roussy M, Jouan L, Bilodeau M, Laramée L, et al. Cryptic recurrent ACIN1-NUTM1 fusions in non-KMT2A-rearranged infant acute lymphoblastic leukemia. Genes Chromosomes Cancer. 2020;59(2):125–30.
169. Cobb BS, Morales-Alcelay S, Kleiger G, Brown KE, Fisher AG, Smale ST. Targeting of Ikaros to pericentromeric heterochromatin by direct DNA binding. Genes Dev. 2000;14(17):2146–60.
170. Boutboul D, Kuehn HS, Van de Wyngaert Z, Niemela JE, Callebaut I, Stoddard J, et al. Dominant-negative IKZF1 mutations cause a T, B, and myeloid cell combined immunodeficiency. J Clin Invest. 2018;128(7):3071–87.
171. Kimura S, Seki M, Yoshida K, Shiraishi Y, Akiyama M, Koh K, et al. NOTCH1 pathway activating mutations and clonal evolution in pediatric T-cell acute lymphoblastic leukemia. Cancer Sci. 2019;110(2):784–94.

172. Ferrando AA, Lopez-Otin C. Clonal evolution in leukemia. Nat Med. 2017;23(10):1135–45.
173. Oshima K, Khiabanian H, da Silva-Almeida AC, Tzoneva G, Abate F, Ambesi-Impiombato A, et al. Mutational landscape, clonal evolution patterns, and role of RAS mutations in relapsed acute lymphoblastic leukemia. Proc Natl Acad Sci U S A. 2016;113(40):11306–11.
174. Dobson SM, Garcia-Prat L, Vanner RJ, Wintersinger J, Waanders E, Gu Z, et al. Relapse-fated latent diagnosis subclones in acute B lineage leukemia are drug tolerant and possess distinct metabolic programs. Cancer Discov. 2020;10(4):568–87.
175. Tzoneva G, Dieck CL, Oshima K, Ambesi-Impiombato A, Sanchez-Martin M, Madubata CJ, et al. Clonal evolution mechanisms in NT5C2 mutant-relapsed acute lymphoblastic leukaemia. Nature. 2018;553(7689):511–4.
176. Dieck CL, Ferrando A. Genetics and mechanisms of NT5C2-driven chemotherapy resistance in relapsed ALL. Blood. 2019;133(21):2263–8.
177. Meyer JA, Wang J, Hogan LE, Yang JJ, Dandekar S, Patel JP, et al. Relapse-specific mutations in NT5C2 in childhood acute lymphoblastic leukemia. Nat Genet. 2013;45(3):290–4.
178. Tzoneva G, Perez-Garcia A, Carpenter Z, Khiabanian H, Tosello V, Allegretta M, et al. Activating mutations in the NT5C2 nucleotidase gene drive chemotherapy resistance in relapsed ALL. Nat Med. 2013;19(3):368–71.
179. Li B, Li H, Bai Y, Kirschner-Schwabe R, Yang JJ, Chen Y, et al. Negative feedback-defective PRPS1 mutants drive thiopurine resistance in relapsed childhood ALL. Nat Med. 2015;21(6):563–71.
180. Evensen NA, Madhusoodhan PP, Meyer J, Saliba J, Chowdhury A, Araten DJ, et al. MSH6 haploinsufficiency at relapse contributes to the development of thiopurine resistance in pediatric B-lymphoblastic leukemia. Haematologica. 2018;103(5):830–9.
181. Mar BG, Bullinger LB, McLean KM, Grauman PV, Harris MH, Stevenson K, et al. Mutations in epigenetic regulators including SETD2 are gained during relapse in paediatric acute lymphoblastic leukaemia. Nat Commun. 2014;5:3469.
182. Rusch M, Nakitandwe J, Shurtleff S, Newman S, Zhang Z, Edmonson MN, et al. Clinical cancer genomic profiling by three-platform sequencing of whole genome, whole exome and transcriptome. Nat Commun. 2018;9(1):3962.
183. Karvonen H, Perttilä R, Niininen W, Hautanen V, Barker H, Murumägi A, et al. Wnt5a and ROR1 activate non-canonical Wnt signaling via RhoA in TCF3-PBX1 acute lymphoblastic leukemia and highlight new treatment strategies via Bcl-2 co-targeting. Oncogene. 2019;38(17):3288–300.
184. Churchman ML, Jones L, Evans K, Richmond J, Shapiro IM, Pachter JA, et al. Efficacy of focal adhesion kinase inhibition in combination with dasatinib in BCR-ABL1 acute lymphoblastic leukemia. Blood. 2015;126(23):3766.
185. Kantarjian HM, DeAngelo DJ, Stelljes M, Martinelli G, Liedtke M, Stock W, et al. Inotuzumab ozogamicin versus standard therapy for acute lymphoblastic leukemia. N Engl J Med. 2016;375(8):740–53.
186. Jung M, Schieck M, Hofmann W, Tauscher M, Lentes J, Bergmann A, et al. Frequency and prognostic impact of PAX5 p.P80R in pediatric acute lymphoblastic leukemia patients treated on an AIEOP-BFM acute lymphoblastic leukemia protocol. Genes Chromosomes Cancer. 2020;59(11):667–71.

Chapter 2
Genetic Mechanisms in T-Cell Acute Lymphoblastic Leukemia

Francesca Gianni and Adolfo Ferrando

T-Cell Lymphoblastic Leukemia: Clinical and Biological Features

T-cell acute lymphoblastic leukemia (T-ALL) is an immature lymphoid malignancy derived from the oncogenic transformation of early lymphoid precursors of the T-cell lineage. This disease accounts for 10–15% of pediatric and 20–25% of adult acute lymphoblastic leukemia cases [1, 2]. In children, the age of onset (9 years) is characteristically older than that of precursor B-cell ALL, which most frequently occurs between the ages of 2 and 5. Accordingly, T-ALL is frequently diagnosed in adolescents. In adults, there is a steady increase of incidence with age. In addition, male to female distribution shows a markedly higher prevalence in males than in females in patients under the age of 40 (Fig. 2.1a). At diagnosis T-ALL patients typically show high white cell counts in peripheral blood and signs and symptoms derived from blast infiltration in bone marrow (cytopenias) and lymphoid organs (lymphadenopathy, splenomegaly, and mediastinal thymic masses). It can also not infrequently cause meningeal infiltration in the central nervous system [3, 4].

Clinically, T-ALL associates with poor glucocorticoid sensitivity and higher rates of early relapse [5]. In fact, in early combination chemotherapy trials, T-ALL was recognized as a high-risk pediatric leukemia with long-term remission rates of about 10% only, compared with 40% for precursor B-cell ALL patients [4]. Today, cure rates for T-ALL patients treated in multicenter trials are close to 90% in children [6, 7] and 60% in adults [8, 9]. However, the prognosis of patients with primary resistant disease and in cases with relapsed leukemia remains exceedingly poor [10, 11].

F. Gianni · A. Ferrando (✉)
Institute for Cancer Genetics, Columbia University, New York, NY, USA
e-mail: fg2442@cumc.columbia.edu; af2196@columbia.edu

M. R. Litzow, E. A. Raetz (eds.), *Clinical Management of Acute Lymphoblastic Leukemia*, https://doi.org/10.1007/978-3-030-85147-7_2

T-ALL tumors are transcriptionally, genetically, immunophenotypically, and clinically heterogeneous with distinct clinico-biological groups defined by gene expression signatures related to their developmental arrest at different stages of thymocyte development (Fig. 2.1b, c) [12]. Among these, early T-cell precursor (ETP) leukemias show an early block at the CD4 CD8 double-negative stage of thymocyte development and are characterized by expression of a transcriptional program

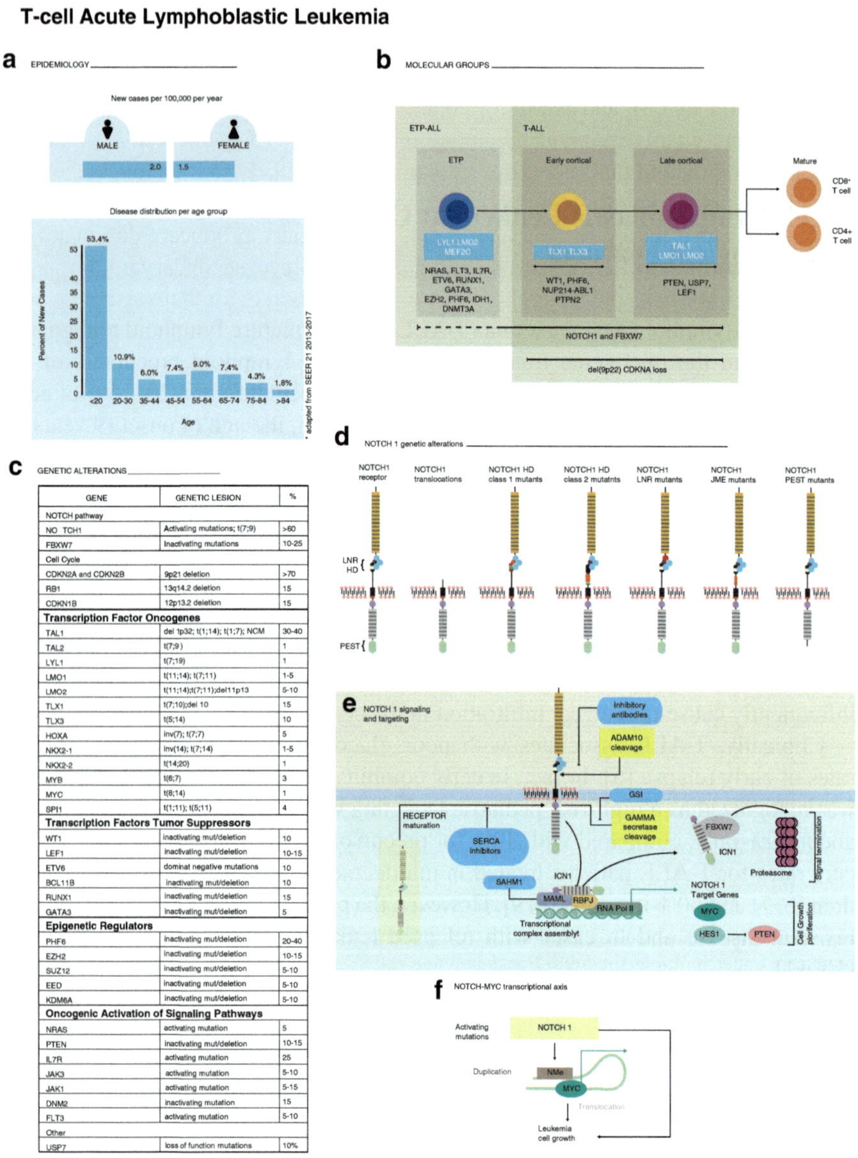

GENE	GENETIC LESION	%
NOTCH pathway		
NO TCH1	Activating mutations; t(7;9)	>60
FBXW7	Inactivating mutations	10-25
Cell Cycle		
CDKN2A and CDKN2B	9p21 deletion	>70
RB1	13q14.2 deletion	15
CDKN1B	12p13.2 deletion	15
Transcription Factor Oncogenes		
TAL1	del 1p32; t(1;14); t(1;7); NCM	30-40
TAL2	t(7;9)	1
LYL1	t(7;19)	1
LMO1	t(11;14); t(7;11)	1-5
LMO2	t(11;14);t(7;11);del11p13	5-10
TLX1	t(7;10);del 10	15
TLX3	t(5;14)	10
HOXA	inv(7); t(7;7)	5
NKX2-1	inv(14); t(7;14)	1-5
NKX2-2	t(14;20)	1
MYB	t(6;7)	3
MYC	t(8;14)	1
SPI1	t(1;11); t(5;11)	4
Transcription Factors Tumor Suppressors		
WT1	inactivating mut/deletion	10
LEF1	inactivating mut/deletion	10-15
ETV6	dominat negative mutations	10
BCL11B	inactivating mut/deletion	10
RUNX1	inactivating mut/deletion	15
GATA3	inactivating mut/deletion	5
Epigenetic Regulators		
PHF6	inactivating mut/deletion	20-40
EZH2	inactivating mut/deletion	10-15
SUZ12	inactivating mut/deletion	5-10
EED	inactivating mut/deletion	5-10
KDM6A	inactivating mut/deletion	5-10
Oncogenic Activation of Signaling Pathways		
NRAS	activating mutation	5
PTEN	inactivating mut/deletion	10-15
IL7R	activating mutation	25
JAK3	activating mutation	5-10
JAK1	activating mutation	5-15
DNM2	inactivating mutation	15
FLT3	activating mutation	5-10
Other		
USP7	loss of function mutations	10%

related to that of hematopoietic stem cells and myeloid progenitors [13, 14], while typical T-ALLs are transcriptionally related to more mature thymic populations (Fig. 2.1b) [12].

Oncogenic NOTCH1 in T-ALL

Early T-cell development represents the biological and conceptual framework of T-ALL transformation as the molecular mechanisms operating in T-ALL are closely related with signaling and developmental pathways governing cell proliferation, differentiation, survival, and metabolism during thymocyte development. In this context, thymic lymphoid precursors constitute the normal cell counterpart and probably the cell of origin of T-ALL. Among the different developmental pathways deregulated in T-ALL, NOTCH1 signaling plays a particularly prominent role. Activation of the NOTCH1 receptor by interaction with the thymic stroma instructs uncommitted early lymphoid progenitors in the thymus to differentiate into the T-cell lineage and supports thymocyte differentiation, growth, metabolism, and survival [15, 16]. In over 60% of T-ALL cases, NOTCH1 is aberrantly activated by oncogenic gain-of-function mutations resulting in ligand independent and prolonged NOTCH1

Fig. 2.1 T-ALL defining characteristics. (**a**) T-ALL accounts for 10–15% of pediatric and 20–25% of adult ALLs. Age of onset in children is around 9 years and adults show increased incidence with age. Prevalence of T-ALL is characteristically higher in males compared to females in patients under 40. (**b**) Molecular groups in T-ALL are defined by expression of transcription factor oncogenes and associated genetic lesions in close relationship with developmental arrest at different stages of thymocyte differentiation. (**c**) Genetic alterations responsible for thymocyte transformation prominently involve activation of NOTCH1 signaling, deregulation of cell cycle control, aberrant expression of transcription factor oncogenes, mutations in transcriptional regulators of early T-cell development, and mutations leading to disruption of epigenetic regulators and activation of the MAPK, JAK-STAT, and PI3K signaling pathways. (**d**) Genetic lesions in *NOTCH1* in T-ALL include mutations disrupting the HD-LNRR domains responsible to maintain the receptor inactive in absence of ligand engagement. Class 1 are proximal HD mutations and Class 2 are distal HD mutations. In addition, juxtamembrane expansion mutations (JME) displace the HD-LNRR complex away from the transmembrane region, and NOTCH1 translocations typically associate with deletion of the extracellular domains of NOTCH1. Deletions of the PEST domain in the C-terminus induce prolonged signaling as a result of impaired proteasomal degradation of activated NOTCH1 (ICN1). (**e**) Multiple components of NOTCH1 signaling can be inhibited by targeted therapies. NOTCH1 inhibitory antibodies block activation of the receptor by the ADAM10 protease. Gamma-secretase inhibitors (GSI) inhibit transmembrane cleavage by the gamma-secretase complex required for translocation of ICN1 to the nucleus. Inhibition of the ICN1-MAML1-RBPJ nuclear complex assembly by the SAHM1 peptide suppresses activation of NOTCH target genes, and inhibition of NOTCH1 precursor protein maturation in the trans-Golgi network can be achieved with inhibitors of the SERCA calcium channels. (**f**) The NOTCH-MYC transcriptional axis forms a feed-forward transcriptional circuitry that centrally supports leukemia cell growth. N-ME, a long-range distal *MYC* enhancer controlled by NOTCH1, links NOTCH1 activation and *MYC* expression in thymocyte development and leukemia

signaling (Fig. 2.1d) [17]. In addition about 1% of T-ALLs show aberrant *NOTCH1* expression and activity as a result of the t(7;9)(q34;q34.3) chromosomal translocation, which leads to the expression of a truncated and constitutively active form of the receptor (Fig. 2.1e) [18, 19]. NOTCH1 functions as a ligand-activated transcription factor and upon ligand engagement undergoes proteolytic cleavage by the ADAM10 metalloprotease and then by the γ-secretase aspartyl protease complex, which releases the intracellular portion of the receptor (ICN1) from the membrane and its translocation to the nucleus where it activates gene expression in association with the RBPJ DNA binding protein (Fig. 2.1e) [20–26]. *NOTCH1* mutations in T-ALL disrupt the negative regulatory region (NRR), which normally prevents cleavage by ADAM10 in the absence of ligand or truncates the C-terminal PEST domain responsible for the termination of ICN1 by proteasomal degradation (Fig. 2.1e) [17, 27]. In addition, mutations in F-box and WD repeat domain containing 7 (*FBXW7)* present in 10–25% of T-ALLs also result in prolonged NOTCH1 signaling by interfering with degradation of ICN1 [28–31]. Notably, leukemic transformation by NOTCH1 is dose dependent [32], and T-ALLs frequently show co-occurrence of both NRR and PEST *NOTCH1* mutations in cis, or a *NOTCH1* NRR-disrupting mutation in association with an *FBXW7* mutation (Fig. 2.1e) [17, 28–31].

Constitutively active NOTCH1 signaling promotes leukemia cell growth via direct upregulation of ribosome biosynthesis, protein translation, and nucleotide and amino acid metabolism [33], by promoting a protective heat shock protein-mediated stress response [34] and by upregulating the expression of the *MYC* oncogene, also a direct target of NOTCH1 (Figs. 2.1e, f) [33, 35]. In addition, *HES1*, an evolutionary conserved NOTCH1 target gene, supports NOTCH1-induced leukemia via upregulation of PI3K and NFKB pathways [36–38] and as negative regulator of apoptosis via transcriptional downregulation of the *BBC3* (PUMA) proapoptotic factor [39] and the glucocorticoid receptor [40]. Additional prominent NOTCH1 target genes involved in supporting leukemia cell growth and proliferation include the interleukin 7 receptor alpha chain (*IL7R*) [41] and *IGF1R* [42] receptors and cell cycle regulators such as *CCND3*, *CDK4*, and *CDK6* [43]. Finally, a role for NOTCH1 in T-ALL cell homing and migration has been linked with expression of the CCR5 and CCR9 [44] chemokine receptors, and NOTCH1-induced upregulation of *CCR7* in leukemia lymphoblasts may also favor meningeal infiltration [45].

Genetic Disruption of Cell Cycle Control

Genetic loss of the *CDKN2A P16/INK4A* and *P14/ARF* tumor suppressors in the short arm of chromosome 9 is found in over 70% of T-ALL cases [12, 46] leading to uncontrolled G1-S cell cycle progression and increased MDM2 activity resulting in impaired TP53 tumor suppressor function. In addition, deletions encompassing the *RB1* and *CDKN1B* cell cycle inhibitors can be found in approximately 15% of T-ALL cases [47, 48]. Moreover, about 6% of T-ALLs show activating mutations in *CCND3* [49], and 3% of cases harbor t(12;14)(p13;q11) and t(7;12)(q34;p13) translocations driving aberrantly high levels of *CCND2* expression [50], highlighting a major role for deregulated D type cyclin activity promoting G1-S cell cycle progression in T-cell transformation.

T-ALL Transcription Factor Oncogenes

Aberrant expression of *TAL1*, a developmentally important class II basic helix-loop-helix (bHLH) transcription factor, is found in 30–40% of T-ALL as result of local and intrachromosomal rearrangements and cis-acting intergenic mutations that create a de novo activating enhancer [51–53]. In addition, *LYL1*, *TAL2*, and *BHLHB1*, three TAL1-related class II bHLH factors, are also aberrantly expressed in rare cases as a result of chromosomal translocations [54–56]. Mechanistically, *TAL1* interferes with the function of the class I bHLH E-proteins (E2A/TCF3, HEB/TCF12, and E2-2/TCF4) disrupting the transcriptional programs that control T-cell differentiation [57–61]. In addition, *TAL1* together with *RUNX1* and *GATA3* forms self-reinforcing transcriptional positive autoregulatory loop, which in association with *MYB* drives T-ALL tumor initiation and maintenance [62]. Similarly, *LMO1* and *LMO2,* which encode bHLH-interacting LIM-only domain proteins, are aberrantly expressed in about 10% of T-ALL cases as a result of chromosomal translocations, cis-acting upstream deletions, and promoter and enhancer activating mutations [63–66]. LMO proteins form transcriptional complexes with *TAL1* and other bHLH factors in support of a common and cooperative role in T-ALL [67, 68]. Importantly, forced expression of these LMO factors induces stem cell-like self-renewal capacity in thymocytes [69, 70], which may underlie the development of LMO2-induced T-ALL in X-linked severe combined immunodeficiency patients undergoing retroviral-based gene therapy [71].

A separate group of T-ALLs show aberrant expression of oncogenic homeobox transcription factors. These include most prominently the *HOXA9* and *HOXA10* HOXA paralog genes and the *TLX1* and *TLX3* NK-L subclass of HOX transcription factors. *HOXA9* and *HOXA10* are activated in about 3% of T-ALL cases as a result of chromosomal rearrangements moving this paralog cluster into the vicinity of the *TCR* loci [72]. In addition, the *PICALM-MLLT10* oncogene generated as a result of the recurring t(10;11)(p13;q14-21) chromosomal translocation in 10% of T-ALLs [73], *KMT2-MLLT1* generated by the t(11;19)(q23;p13.3) rearrangement in 5% of T-ALL cases [74], and the *SET-NUP214* oncogene originating from a rare cryptic chromosome 9q deletion [75] all share in common a transcriptional program characterized by high levels of HOXA gene expression.

TLX1 is aberrantly expressed in T-ALLs with the t(10;14)(q24;q11) *TLX1-TCR* translocation [76, 77] present in about 5–10% of children and 30% of adult T-ALLs [12, 78]. In addition *TLX3* is most commonly activated as a result of the t(5;14)(q35;q32) *TLX3-BCL11B* translocation, which can be found in 20–25% of pediatric and 5% of adult T-ALL cases [12, 79]. Mechanistically, *TLX1* and *TLX3* regulate common direct target genes, and TLX1 and TLX3 leukemias share a common gene expression signature, which includes downregulation of numerous tumor suppressor genes also mutated in T-ALL such as *BCL11B*, *PHF6*, *RUNX1*, and *WT1* [80]. Similarly, *NKX2-1* and *NKX2-2*, two highly related homeobox genes, are rearranged and aberrantly expressed in about 5% of pediatric T-ALLs [81], and *NKX2-5* translocations to either *TCR* or *BCL11B* sites have been reported in occasional cases [82, 83].

The MYC transcription regulator functions as a central regulator of cell growth and proliferation downstream of NOTCH1 in thymocyte development and in T-ALL [33, 84]. In addition, about 1% of T-ALLs activate *MYC* as result of the t(8;14)(q24;q11) *MYC-TCR* translocation [85, 86]. Similarly, the t(6;7)(q23;q32) chromosomal translocation induces aberrant expression of the *MYB* leucine zipper transcription factor oncogene in about 2% of T-ALL cases, most commonly in young children under the age of 2 [87]. Moreover, activating mutations and focal duplications of the *MYB* locus are common in pediatric and adult T-ALLs [49, 88, 89]. Finally, different chromosomal rearrangements commonly inducing overexpression of the *SPI1* transcriptional regulator are present in 4% of pediatric T-ALLs, which seems to be associated with a poor prognosis [90].

Transcription Factor and Epigenetic Tumor Suppressors

Loss-of-function mutations and chromosomal deletions in T-ALL frequently involve epigenetic regulators and transcription factor genes with prominent roles in early T-cell development. Epigenetic regulators recurrently mutated in T-ALL include PRC2 complex genes (*EZH2*, *SUZ12*, and *EED*) [91, 92], the plant homeodomain-like factor *PHF6* [93], and *KDM6A*, a histone H3K27 demethylase [94, 95]. In addition epigenetic-disrupting mutations in *IDH1*, *IDH2*, and *DNMT3A* are frequently found in the ETP ALL group [14, 92]. Among these, loss of *PHF6* is the most common and can be found in about 20% of T-ALL cases [93] and in 20–25% of ETP leukemias [92]. PHF6 seems to actively participate in epigenetic regulation and interaction with the NuRD nucleosome repositioning and histone deacetylation complex [96, 97], but it is worth noting that it primarily localizes to the nucleolus where it participates in the control of ribosomal gene expression [98]. In T-ALL, *PHF6* mutations are an early tumor-initiating lesion, and knockout of *Phf6* in mice has been shown to induce increased self-renewal in hematopoietic stem cells and in NOTCH1-induced T-ALL models [99]. In addition, genetic lesions in the *EZH2, EED*, and *SUZ12* polycomb repressive complex 2 (PRC2) genes, responsible for epigenetic gene silencing via writing of the H3K27me3 epigenetic mark, are present in up to 25% of T-ALLs [91] and up to 42% of ETP leukemias. Conversely, mutations in the KDM6A, a H3K27me3 histone demethylase, are mutated in 5–15% of T-ALLs [94, 95].

Finally, mutations inactivating *RUNX1*, *ETV6*, and *GATA3*, transcription factors promoting thymocyte development, are associated with ETP leukemias [14, 92], and genetic alterations in *LEF1*, *WT1*, and *BCL11B* are predominantly found in early cortical T-ALLs with *TLX1* and *TLX3* translocations [80, 100, 101].

Mutational Activation of Oncogenic Signaling Pathways

About 5% of T-ALLs show chromosomal rearrangements resulting in *ABL1* fusion tyrosine kinase oncogenes including most frequently *NUP214-ABL1* [102] but also *EML1-ABL1* [103] and *ETV6-ABL1* [104]. In addition, activating mutations driving increased MAK, PI3K, and JAK-STAT signaling are recurrently found in T-ALL. Thus, canonical hotspot activating mutations in the *HRAS* and *KRAS* oncogenes are found in 10–15% of T-ALLs, particularly in ETP ALLs [49, 92], and genetic loss of the neurofibromatosis type 1 (*NF1*), a negative regulator of RAS signaling, occurs in 3% of cases [105]. Moreover, mutations driving constitutive PI3K activation can be found in about 30% of T-ALL samples [49]. Among these, loss of the *PTEN* tumor suppressor gene as a result of mutations and deletions is present in 10–15% of T-ALL cases [106]. In addition, the t(X;7)(q22;q34) and t(X;14)(q22;q11.2) translocations have been shown to induce overexpression of *IRS4* [107, 108], a signaling factor driving AKT activation [109]. Finally, activating mutations in *IL7R*, *JAK1*, *JAK3*, and *STAT5* resulting in constitutively active JAK-STAT signaling are present in about 25% of T-ALL cases [49, 110, 111] particularly in ETP leukemias [92]. Moreover, translocations targeting the zinc finger E-box-binding transcription factor *ZEB2* [112]; loss-of-function mutations in *DNM2*, which controls IL7 receptor trafficking; deletion of the *PTPN2* phosphatase; and mutations in *SH2B3*, a negative regulator of cytokine signaling, also result in increased JAK-STAT signaling [113–115]. Finally, about 8% of T-ALL cases show a recurrent R98S mutation in the ribosomal protein gene *RPL10*, with consequent changes in protein translation conductive of JAK-STAT signaling upregulation [116].

Association of Genetic Mutations and Chromosomal Rearrangements with Transcriptional and Biological Groups of T-ALL

T-ALL transformation is an orchestrated process in which cooperating mutations with convergent and complementary mechanisms of action associate defining distinct oncogenic pathways and molecular groups. ETP T-ALLs show a lower frequency of *NOTCH1* mutations and *CDKN2A* deletions and, in turn, show higher frequencies of mutations in signaling factors (e.g., *NRAS*, *FLT3*) and epigenetic regulators (e.g., *EZH2*, *IDH1*, *IDH2*, *DNMT3A*) commonly present in myeloid leukemias, as well as mutations in transcription factors governing hematopoietic and

T-cell development (e.g., *RUNX1*, *GATA3*, *ETV6*) [48, 92, 117]. In contrast, typical T-ALLs with an early cortical immunophenotype (CD1a, CD4, CD8 positive) are associated with activation of the *TLX1, TLX3, NKX2.1*, and *NKX2.2* transcription factor oncogenes and show a very high prevalence of *NOTCH1* mutations and *CDKN2A* deletions as well as an association with *PHF6* mutations, *BCL11B* and *WT1* mutations, and *NUP214-ABL1* rearrangements [12, 17, 81, 101, 102, 118]. Finally, T-ALLs with a more CD4-, CD8-, and CD3-positive late cortical thymocyte immunophenotype are characteristically associated with alterations resulting in aberrant expression of *TAL1* and *LMO* factors as well as with deletions and mutations in the *PTEN* tumor suppressor gene [12].

References

1. Pui CH, Mullighan CG, Evans WE, Relling MV. Pediatric acute lymphoblastic leukemia: where are we going and how do we get there? Blood. 2012;120(6):1165–74.
2. Dores GM, Devesa SS, Curtis RE, Linet MS, Morton LM. Acute leukemia incidence and patient survival among children and adults in the United States, 2001–2007. Blood. 2012;119(1):34–43.
3. Karrman K, Forestier E, Heyman M, Andersen MK, Autio K, Blennow E, et al. Clinical and cytogenetic features of a population-based consecutive series of 285 pediatric T-cell acute lymphoblastic leukemias: rare T-cell receptor gene rearrangements are associated with poor outcome. Genes Chromosomes Cancer. 2009;48(9):795–805.
4. Greaves MF, Janossy G, Peto J, Kay H. Immunologically defined subclasses of acute lymphoblastic leukaemia in children: their relationship to presentation features and prognosis. Br J Haematol. 1981;48(2):179–97.
5. Vrooman LM, Silverman LB. Childhood acute lymphoblastic leukemia: update on prognostic factors. Curr Opin Pediatr. 2009;21(1):1–8.
6. Hunger SP, Lu X, Devidas M, Camitta BM, Gaynon PS, Winick NJ, et al. Improved survival for children and adolescents with acute lymphoblastic leukemia between 1990 and 2005: a report from the Children's Oncology Group. J Clin Oncol. 2012;30(14):1663–9.
7. Conter V, Valsecchi MG, Parasole R, Putti MC, Locatelli F, Barisone E, et al. Childhood high-risk acute lymphoblastic leukemia in first remission: results after chemotherapy or transplant from the AIEOP ALL 2000 study. Blood. 2014;123(10):1470–8.
8. Stock W, Johnson JL, Stone RM, Kolitz JE, Powell BL, Wetzler M, et al. Dose intensification of daunorubicin and cytarabine during treatment of adult acute lymphoblastic leukemia: results of Cancer and Leukemia Group B Study 19802. Cancer. 2013;119(1):90–8.
9. Marks DI, Paietta EM, Moorman AV, Richards SM, Buck G, DeWald G, et al. T-cell acute lymphoblastic leukemia in adults: clinical features, immunophenotype, cytogenetics, and outcome from the large randomized prospective trial (UKALL XII/ECOG 2993). Blood. 2009;114(25):5136–45.
10. Einsiedel HG, von Stackelberg A, Hartmann R, Fengler R, Schrappe M, Janka-Schaub G, et al. Long-term outcome in children with relapsed ALL by risk-stratified salvage therapy: results of trial acute lymphoblastic leukemia-relapse study of the Berlin-Frankfurt-Munster Group 87. J Clin Oncol. 2005;23(31):7942–50.
11. Tallen G, Ratei R, Mann G, Kaspers G, Niggli F, Karachunsky A, et al. Long-term outcome in children with relapsed acute lymphoblastic leukemia after time-point and site-of-relapse stratification and intensified short-course multidrug chemotherapy: results of trial ALL-REZ BFM 90. J Clin Oncol. 2010;28(14):2339–47.

12. Ferrando AA, Neuberg DS, Staunton J, Loh ML, Huard C, Raimondi SC, et al. Gene expression signatures define novel oncogenic pathways in T cell acute lymphoblastic leukemia. Cancer Cell. 2002;1(1):75–87.
13. Coustan-Smith E, Mullighan CG, Onciu M, Behm FG, Raimondi SC, Pei D, et al. Early T-cell precursor leukaemia: a subtype of very high-risk acute lymphoblastic leukaemia. Lancet Oncol. 2009;10(2):147–56.
14. Van Vlierberghe P, Ambesi-Impiombato A, Perez-Garcia A, Haydu JE, Rigo I, Hadler M, et al. ETV6 mutations in early immature human T cell leukemias. J Exp Med. 2011;208(13):2571–9.
15. Radtke F, MacDonald HR, Tacchini-Cottier F. Regulation of innate and adaptive immunity by Notch. Nat Rev Immunol. 2013;13(6):427–37.
16. Radtke F, Wilson A, Stark G, Bauer M, van Meerwijk J, MacDonald HR, et al. Deficient T cell fate specification in mice with an induced inactivation of Notch1. Immunity. 1999;10(5):547–58.
17. Weng AP, Ferrando AA, Lee W, Morris JP, Silverman LB, Sanchez-Irizarry C, et al. Activating mutations of NOTCH1 in human T cell acute lymphoblastic leukemia. Science. 2004;306(5694):269–71.
18. Ellisen LW, Bird J, West DC, Soreng AL, Reynolds TC, Smith SD, et al. TAN-1, the human homolog of the Drosophila notch gene, is broken by chromosomal translocations in T lymphoblastic neoplasms. Cell. 1991;66(4):649–61.
19. Palomero T, Barnes KC, Real PJ, Glade Bender JL, Sulis ML, Murty VV, et al. CUTLL1, a novel human T-cell lymphoma cell line with t(7;9) rearrangement, aberrant NOTCH1 activation and high sensitivity to gamma-secretase inhibitors. Leukemia. 2006;20(7):1279–87.
20. De Strooper B, Annaert W, Cupers P, Saftig P, Craessaerts K, Mumm JS, et al. A presenilin-1-dependent gamma-secretase-like protease mediates release of Notch intracellular domain. Nature. 1999;398(6727):518–22.
21. Schroeter EH, Kisslinger JA, Kopan R. Notch-1 signalling requires ligand-induced proteolytic release of intracellular domain. Nature. 1998;393(6683):382–6.
22. Struhl G, Fitzgerald K, Greenwald I. Intrinsic activity of the Lin-12 and Notch intracellular domains in vivo. Cell. 1993;74(2):331–45.
23. Hsieh JJ, Henkel T, Salmon P, Robey E, Peterson MG, Hayward SD. Truncated mammalian Notch1 activates CBF1/RBPJk-repressed genes by a mechanism resembling that of Epstein-Barr virus EBNA2. Mol Cell Biol. 1996;16(3):952–9.
24. van Tetering G, van Diest P, Verlaan I, van der Wall E, Kopan R, Vooijs M. Metalloprotease ADAM10 is required for Notch1 site 2 cleavage. J Biol Chem. 2009;284(45):31018–27.
25. Dumortier A, Wilson A, MacDonald HR, Radtke F. Paradigms of notch signaling in mammals. Int J Hematol. 2005;82(4):277–84.
26. Wu L, Aster JC, Blacklow SC, Lake R, Artavanis-Tsakonas S, Griffin JD. MAML1, a human homologue of Drosophila mastermind, is a transcriptional co-activator for NOTCH receptors. Nat Genet. 2000;26(4):484–9.
27. Sulis ML, Williams O, Palomero T, Tosello V, Pallikuppam S, Real PJ, et al. NOTCH1 extracellular juxtamembrane expansion mutations in T-ALL. Blood. 2008;112(3):733–40.
28. O'Neil J, Grim J, Strack P, Rao S, Tibbitts D, Winter C, et al. FBW7 mutations in leukemic cells mediate NOTCH pathway activation and resistance to γ-secretase inhibitors. J Exp Med. 2007;204(8):1813–24.
29. Thompson BJ, Buonamici S, Sulis ML, Palomero T, Vilimas T, Basso G, et al. The SCFFBW7 ubiquitin ligase complex as a tumor suppressor in T cell leukemia. J Exp Med. 2007;204(8):1825–35.
30. Moberg KH, Bell DW, Wahrer DC, Haber DA, Hariharan IK. Archipelago regulates Cyclin E levels in Drosophila and is mutated in human cancer cell lines. Nature. 2001;413(6853):311–6.
31. Malyukova A, Dohda T, von der Lehr N, Akhoondi S, Corcoran M, Heyman M, et al. The tumor suppressor gene hCDC4 is frequently mutated in human T-cell acute lymphoblastic leukemia with functional consequences for Notch signaling. Cancer Res. 2007;67(12):5611–6.

32. Chiang MY, Xu L, Shestova O, Histen G, L'Heureux S, Romany C, et al. Leukemia-associated NOTCH1 alleles are weak tumor initiators but accelerate K-ras-initiated leukemia. J Clin Invest. 2008;118(9):3181–94.
33. Palomero T, Lim WK, Odom DT, Sulis ML, Real PJ, Margolin A, et al. NOTCH1 directly regulates c-MYC and activates a feed-forward-loop transcriptional network promoting leukemic cell growth. Proc Natl Acad Sci U S A. 2006;103(48):18261–6.
34. Kourtis N, Lazaris C, Hockemeyer K, Balandran JC, Jimenez AR, Mullenders J, et al. Oncogenic hijacking of the stress response machinery in T cell acute lymphoblastic leukemia. Nat Med. 2018;24(8):1157–66.
35. Herranz D, Ambesi-Impiombato A, Palomero T, Schnell SA, Belver L, Wendorff AA, et al. A NOTCH1-driven MYC enhancer promotes T cell development, transformation and acute lymphoblastic leukemia. Nat Med. 2014;20(10):1130–7.
36. Palomero T, Dominguez M, Ferrando AA. The role of the PTEN/AKT pathway in NOTCH1-induced leukemia. Cell Cycle. 2008;7(8):965–70.
37. Espinosa L, Cathelin S, D'Altri T, Trimarchi T, Statnikov A, Guiu J, et al. The Notch/Hes1 pathway sustains NF-kappaB activation through CYLD repression in T cell leukemia. Cancer Cell. 2010;18(3):268–81.
38. Wong GW, Knowles GC, Mak TW, Ferrando AA, Zuniga-Pflucker JC. HES1 opposes a PTEN-dependent check on survival, differentiation, and proliferation of TCRbeta-selected mouse thymocytes. Blood. 2012;120(7):1439–48.
39. Schnell SA, Ambesi-Impiombato A, Sanchez-Martin M, Belver L, Xu L, Qin Y, et al. Therapeutic targeting of HES1 transcriptional programs in T-ALL. Blood. 2015;125(18):2806–14.
40. Real PJ, Tosello V, Palomero T, Castillo M, Hernando E, de Stanchina E, et al. Gamma-secretase inhibitors reverse glucocorticoid resistance in T cell acute lymphoblastic leukemia. Nat Med. 2009;15(1):50–8.
41. Gonzalez-Garcia S, Garcia-Peydro M, Martin-Gayo E, Ballestar E, Esteller M, Bornstein R, et al. CSL-MAML-dependent Notch1 signaling controls T lineage-specific IL-7R{alpha} gene expression in early human thymopoiesis and leukemia. J Exp Med. 2009;206(4):779–91.
42. Medyouf H, Gusscott S, Wang H, Tseng JC, Wai C, Nemirovsky O, et al. High-level IGF1R expression is required for leukemia-initiating cell activity in T-ALL and is supported by Notch signaling. J Exp Med. 2011;208(9):1809–22.
43. Joshi I, Minter LM, Telfer J, Demarest RM, Capobianco AJ, Aster JC, et al. Notch signaling mediates G1/S cell-cycle progression in T cells via cyclin D3 and its dependent kinases. Blood. 2009;113(8):1689–98.
44. Mirandola L, Chiriva-Internati M, Montagna D, Locatelli F, Zecca M, Ranzani M, et al. Notch1 regulates chemotaxis and proliferation by controlling the CC-chemokine receptors 5 and 9 in T cell acute lymphoblastic leukaemia. J Pathol. 2012;226(5):713–22.
45. Buonamici S, Trimarchi T, Ruocco MG, Reavie L, Cathelin S, Mar BG, et al. CCR7 signalling as an essential regulator of CNS infiltration in T-cell leukaemia. Nature. 2009;459(7249):1000–4.
46. Hebert J, Cayuela JM, Berkeley J, Sigaux F. Candidate tumor-suppressor genes MTS1 (p16INK4A) and MTS2 (p15INK4B) display frequent homozygous deletions in primary cells from T- but not from B-cell lineage acute lymphoblastic leukemias. Blood. 1994;84(12):4038–44.
47. Mullighan CG, Goorha S, Radtke I, Miller CB, Coustan-Smith E, Dalton JD, et al. Genome-wide analysis of genetic alterations in acute lymphoblastic leukaemia. Nature. 2007;446(7137):758–64.
48. Van Vlierberghe P, Ambesi-Impiombato A, De Keersmaecker K, Hadler M, Paietta E, Tallman MS, et al. Prognostic relevance of integrated genetic profiling in adult T-cell acute lymphoblastic leukemia. Blood. 2013;122(1):74–82.
49. Liu Y, Easton J, Shao Y, Maciaszek J, Wang Z, Wilkinson MR, et al. The genomic landscape of pediatric and young adult T-lineage acute lymphoblastic leukemia. Nat Genet. 2017;49(8):1211–8.

50. Clappier E, Cuccuini W, Cayuela JM, Vecchione D, Baruchel A, Dombret H, et al. Cyclin D2 dysregulation by chromosomal translocations to TCR loci in T-cell acute lymphoblastic leukemias. Leukemia. 2006;20(1):82–6.
51. Bash RO, Hall S, Timmons CF, Crist WM, Amylon M, Smith RG, et al. Does activation of the TAL1 gene occur in a majority of patients with T-cell acute lymphoblastic leukemia? A Pediatric Oncology Group study. Blood. 1995;86(2):666–76.
52. Aplan PD, Lombardi DP, Ginsberg AM, Cossman J, Bertness VL, Kirsch IR. Disruption of the human SCL locus by "illegitimate" V-(D)-J recombinase activity. Science. 1990;250(4986):1426–9.
53. Mansour MR, Abraham BJ, Anders L, Berezovskaya A, Gutierrez A, Durbin AD, et al. Oncogene regulation. An oncogenic super-enhancer formed through somatic mutation of a noncoding intergenic element. Science. 2014;346(6215):1373–7.
54. Mellentin JD, Smith SD, Cleary ML. lyl-1, a novel gene altered by chromosomal translocation in T cell leukemia, codes for a protein with a helix-loop-helix DNA binding motif. Cell. 1989;58(1):77–83.
55. Xia Y, Brown L, Yang CY, Tsan JT, Siciliano MJ, Espinosa R 3rd, et al. TAL2, a helix-loop-helix gene activated by the (7;9)(q34;q32) translocation in human T-cell leukemia. Proc Natl Acad Sci U S A. 1991;88(24):11416–20.
56. Wang J, Jani-Sait SN, Escalon EA, Carroll AJ, de Jong PJ, Kirsch IR, et al. The t(14;21)(q11.2;q22) chromosomal translocation associated with T-cell acute lymphoblastic leukemia activates the BHLHB1 gene. Proc Natl Acad Sci U S A. 2000;97(7):3497–502.
57. Palomero T, Odom DT, O'Neil J, Ferrando AA, Margolin A, Neuberg DS, et al. Transcriptional regulatory networks downstream of TAL1/SCL in T-cell acute lymphoblastic leukemia. Blood. 2006;108(3):986–92.
58. Voronova AF, Lee F. The E2A and tal-1 helix-loop-helix proteins associate in vivo and are modulated by Id proteins during interleukin 6-induced myeloid differentiation. Proc Natl Acad Sci U S A. 1994;91(13):5952–6.
59. O'Neil J, Shank J, Cusson N, Murre C, Kelliher M. TAL1/SCL induces leukemia by inhibiting the transcriptional activity of E47/HEB. Cancer Cell. 2004;5(6):587–96.
60. Hsu HL, Wadman I, Baer R. Formation of in vivo complexes between the TAL1 and E2A polypeptides of leukemic T cells. Proc Natl Acad Sci U S A. 1994;91(8):3181–5.
61. Hsu HL, Cheng JT, Chen Q, Baer R. Enhancer-binding activity of the tal-1 oncoprotein in association with the E47/E12 helix-loop-helix proteins. Mol Cell Biol. 1991;11(6):3037–42.
62. Sanda T, Lawton LN, Barrasa MI, Fan ZP, Kohlhammer H, Gutierrez A, et al. Core transcriptional regulatory circuit controlled by the TAL1 complex in human T cell acute lymphoblastic leukemia. Cancer Cell. 2012;22(2):209–21.
63. Van Vlierberghe P, van Grotel M, Beverloo HB, Lee C, Helgason T, Buijs-Gladdines J, et al. The cryptic chromosomal deletion del(11)(p12p13) as a new activation mechanism of LMO2 in pediatric T cell acute lymphoblastic leukemia. Blood. 2006;108(10):3520–9.
64. Royer-Pokora B, Loos U, Ludwig WD. TTG-2, a new gene encoding a cysteine-rich protein with the LIM motif, is overexpressed in acute T-cell leukaemia with the t(11;14)(p13;q11). Oncogene. 1991;6(10):1887–93.
65. McGuire EA, Hockett RD, Pollock KM, Bartholdi MF, O'Brien SJ, Korsmeyer SJ. The t(11;14)(p15;q11) in a T-cell acute lymphoblastic leukemia cell line activates multiple transcripts, including Ttg-1, a gene encoding a potential zinc finger protein. Mol Cell Biol. 1989;9(5):2124–32.
66. Rahman S, Magnussen M, Leon TE, Farah N, Li Z, Abraham BJ, et al. Activation of the LMO2 oncogene through a somatically acquired neomorphic promoter in T-cell acute lymphoblastic leukemia. Blood. 2017;129(24):3221–6.
67. Larson RC, Lavenir I, Larson TA, Baer R, Warren AJ, Wadman I, et al. Protein dimerization between Lmo2 (Rbtn2) and Tal1 alters thymocyte development and potentiates T cell tumorigenesis in transgenic mice. EMBO J. 1996;15(5):1021–7.
68. Valge-Archer VE, Osada H, Warren AJ, Forster A, Li J, Baer R, et al. The LIM protein RBTN2 and the basic helix-loop-helix protein TAL1 are present in a complex in erythroid cells. Proc Natl Acad Sci U S A. 1994;91(18):8617–21.

69. Gerby B, Tremblay CS, Tremblay M, Rojas-Sutterlin S, Herblot S, Hebert J, et al. SCL, LMO1 and Notch1 reprogram thymocytes into self-renewing cells. PLoS Genet. 2014;10(12):e1004768.
70. McCormack MP, Young LF, Vasudevan S, de Graaf CA, Codrington R, Rabbitts TH, et al. The Lmo2 oncogene initiates leukemia in mice by inducing thymocyte self-renewal. Science. 2010;327(5967):879–83.
71. Hacein-Bey-Abina S, Von Kalle C, Schmidt M, McCormack MP, Wulffraat N, Leboulch P, et al. LMO2-associated clonal T cell proliferation in two patients after gene therapy for SCID-X1. Science. 2003;302(5644):415–9.
72. Soulier J, Clappier E, Cayuela JM, Regnault A, Garcia-Peydro M, Dombret H, et al. HOXA genes are included in genetic and biologic networks defining human acute T-cell leukemia (T-ALL). Blood. 2005;106(1):274–86.
73. Carlson KM, Vignon C, Bohlander S, Martinez-Climent JA, Le Beau MM, Rowley JD. Identification and molecular characterization of CALM/AF10fusion products in T cell acute lymphoblastic leukemia and acute myeloid leukemia. Leukemia. 2000;14(1):100–4.
74. Tkachuk DC, Kohler S, Cleary ML. Involvement of a homolog of Drosophila trithorax by 11q23 chromosomal translocations in acute leukemias. Cell. 1992;71(4):691–700.
75. Van Vlierberghe P, van Grotel M, Tchinda J, Lee C, Beverloo HB, van der Spek PJ, et al. The recurrent SET-NUP214 fusion as a new HOXA activation mechanism in pediatric T-cell acute lymphoblastic leukemia. Blood. 2008;111(9):4668–80.
76. Hatano M, Roberts CW, Minden M, Crist WM, Korsmeyer SJ. Deregulation of a homeobox gene, HOX11, by the t(10;14) in T cell leukemia. Science. 1991;253(5015):79–82.
77. Kennedy MA, Gonzalez-Sarmiento R, Kees UR, Lampert F, Dear N, Boehm T, et al. HOX11, a homeobox-containing T-cell oncogene on human chromosome 10q24. Proc Natl Acad Sci U S A. 1991;88(20):8900–4.
78. Ferrando AA, Neuberg DS, Dodge RK, Paietta E, Larson RA, Wiernik PH, et al. Prognostic importance of TLX1 (HOX11) oncogene expression in adults with T-cell acute lymphoblastic leukaemia. Lancet (London, England). 2004;363(9408):535–6.
79. Bernard OA, Busson-LeConiat M, Ballerini P, Mauchauffe M, Della Valle V, Monni R, et al. A new recurrent and specific cryptic translocation, t(5;14)(q35;q32), is associated with expression of the Hox11L2 gene in T acute lymphoblastic leukemia. Leukemia. 2001;15(10):1495–504.
80. Della Gatta G, Palomero T, Perez-Garcia A, Ambesi-Impiombato A, Bansal M, Carpenter ZW, et al. Reverse engineering of TLX oncogenic transcriptional networks identifies RUNX1 as tumor suppressor in T-ALL. Nat Med. 2012;18(3):436–40.
81. Homminga I, Pieters R, Langerak Anton W, de Rooi JJ, Stubbs A, Verstegen M, et al. Integrated transcript and genome analyses reveal NKX2-1 and MEF2C as potential oncogenes in T cell acute lymphoblastic leukemia. Cancer Cell. 2011;19(4):484–97.
82. Nagel S, Kaufmann M, Drexler HG, MacLeod RA. The cardiac homeobox gene NKX2-5 is deregulated by juxtaposition with BCL11B in pediatric T-ALL cell lines via a novel t(5;14)(q35.1;q32.2). Cancer Res. 2003;63(17):5329–34.
83. Przybylski GK, Dik WA, Grabarczyk P, Wanzeck J, Chudobska P, Jankowski K, et al. The effect of a novel recombination between the homeobox gene NKX2-5 and the TRD locus in T-cell acute lymphoblastic leukemia on activation of the NKX2-5 gene. Haematologica. 2006;91(3):317–21.
84. Herranz D, Ambesi-Impiombato A, Sudderth J, Sanchez-Martin M, Belver L, Tosello V, et al. Metabolic reprogramming induces resistance to anti-NOTCH1 therapies in T cell acute lymphoblastic leukemia. Nat Med. 2015;21(10):1182–9.
85. Erikson J, Finger L, Sun L, ar-Rushdi A, Nishikura K, Minowada J, et al. Deregulation of c-myc by translocation of the alpha-locus of the T-cell receptor in T-cell leukemias. Science. 1986;232(4752):884–6.
86. Finger LR, Harvey RC, Moore RC, Showe LC, Croce CM. A common mechanism of chromosomal translocation in T- and B-cell neoplasia. Science. 1986;234(4779):982–5.

87. Clappier E, Cuccuini W, Kalota A, Crinquette A, Cayuela JM, Dik WA, et al. The C-MYB locus is involved in chromosomal translocation and genomic duplications in human T-cell acute leukemia (T-ALL), the translocation defining a new T-ALL subtype in very young children. Blood. 2007;110(4):1251–61.
88. Lahortiga I, De Keersmaecker K, Van Vlierberghe P, Graux C, Cauwelier B, Lambert F, et al. Duplication of the MYB oncogene in T cell acute lymphoblastic leukemia. Nat Genet. 2007;39(5):593–5.
89. O'Neil J, Tchinda J, Gutierrez A, Moreau L, Maser RS, Wong KK, et al. Alu elements mediate MYB gene tandem duplication in human T-ALL. J Exp Med. 2007;204(13):3059–66.
90. Seki M, Kimura S, Isobe T, Yoshida K, Ueno H, Nakajima-Takagi Y, et al. Recurrent SPI1 (PU.1) fusions in high-risk pediatric T cell acute lymphoblastic leukemia. Nat Genet. 2017;49(8):1274–81.
91. Ntziachristos P, Tsirigos A, Van Vlierberghe P, Nedjic J, Trimarchi T, Flaherty MS, et al. Genetic inactivation of the polycomb repressive complex 2 in T cell acute lymphoblastic leukemia. Nat Med. 2012;18(2):298–301.
92. Zhang J, Ding L, Holmfeldt L, Wu G, Heatley SL, Payne-Turner D, et al. The genetic basis of early T-cell precursor acute lymphoblastic leukaemia. Nature. 2012;481(7380):157–63.
93. Van Vlierberghe P, Palomero T, Khiabanian H, Van der Meulen J, Castillo M, Van Roy N, et al. PHF6 mutations in T-cell acute lymphoblastic leukemia. Nat Genet. 2010;42(4):338–42.
94. Ntziachristos P, Tsirigos A, Welstead GG, Trimarchi T, Bakogianni S, Xu L, et al. Contrasting roles of histone 3 lysine 27 demethylases in acute lymphoblastic leukaemia. Nature. 2014;514(7523):513–7.
95. Van der Meulen J, Sanghvi V, Mavrakis K, Durinck K, Fang F, Matthijssens F, et al. The H3K27me3 demethylase UTX is a gender-specific tumor suppressor in T-cell acute lymphoblastic leukemia. Blood. 2015;125(1):13–21.
96. Liu Z, Li F, Zhang B, Li S, Wu J, Shi Y. Structural basis of plant homeodomain finger 6 (PHF6) recognition by the retinoblastoma binding protein 4 (RBBP4) component of the nucleosome remodeling and deacetylase (NuRD) complex. J Biol Chem. 2015;290(10):6630–8.
97. Todd MA, Picketts DJ. PHF6 interacts with the nucleosome remodeling and deacetylation (NuRD) complex. J Proteome Res. 2012;11(8):4326–37.
98. Wang J, Leung JW, Gong Z, Feng L, Shi X, Chen J. PHF6 regulates cell cycle progression by suppressing ribosomal RNA synthesis. J Biol Chem. 2013;288(5):3174–83.
99. Wendorff AA, Quinn SA, Rashkovan M, Madubata CJ, Ambesi-Impiombato A, Litzow MR, et al. Phf6 loss enhances HSC self-renewal driving tumor initiation and leukemia stem cell activity in T-ALL. Cancer Discov. 2019;9(3):436–51.
100. Gutierrez A, Sanda T, Ma W, Zhang J, Grebliunaite R, Dahlberg S, et al. Inactivation of LEF1 in T-cell acute lymphoblastic leukemia. Blood. 2010;115(14):2845–51.
101. De Keersmaecker K, Real PJ, Gatta GD, Palomero T, Sulis ML, Tosello V, et al. The TLX1 oncogene drives aneuploidy in T cell transformation. Nat Med. 2010;16(11):1321–7.
102. Graux C, Cools J, Melotte C, Quentmeier H, Ferrando A, Levine R, et al. Fusion of NUP214 to ABL1 on amplified episomes in T-cell acute lymphoblastic leukemia. Nat Genet. 2004;36(10):1084–9.
103. De Keersmaecker K, Graux C, Odero MD, Mentens N, Somers R, Maertens J, et al. Fusion of EML1 to ABL1 in T-cell acute lymphoblastic leukemia with cryptic t(9;14)(q34;q32). Blood. 2005;105(12):4849–52.
104. Van Limbergen H, Beverloo HB, van Drunen E, Janssens A, Hahlen K, Poppe B, et al. Molecular cytogenetic and clinical findings in ETV6/ABL1-positive leukemia. Genes Chromosomes Cancer. 2001;30(3):274–82.
105. Balgobind BV, Van Vlierberghe P, van den Ouweland AM, Beverloo HB, Terlouw-Kromosoeto JN, van Wering ER, et al. Leukemia-associated NF1 inactivation in patients with pediatric T-ALL and AML lacking evidence for neurofibromatosis. Blood. 2008;111(8):4322–8.
106. Palomero T, Sulis ML, Cortina M, Real PJ, Barnes K, Ciofani M, et al. Mutational loss of PTEN induces resistance to NOTCH1 inhibition in T-cell leukemia. Nat Med. 2007;13(10):1203–10.

107. Karrman K, Kjeldsen E, Lassen C, Isaksson M, Davidsson J, Andersson A, et al. The t(X;7)(q22;q34) in paediatric T-cell acute lymphoblastic leukaemia results in overexpression of the insulin receptor substrate 4 gene through illegitimate recombination with the T-cell receptor beta locus. Br J Haematol. 2009;144(4):546–51.
108. Kang DH, Kim SH, Jun JW, Lee YW, Shin HB, Ahn JY, et al. Simultaneous translocation of both TCR loci (14q11) with rare partner loci (Xq22 and 12p13) in a case of T-lymphoblastic leukemia. Ann Lab Med. 2012;32(3):220–4.
109. Uchida T, Myers MG Jr, White MF. IRS-4 mediates protein kinase B signaling during insulin stimulation without promoting antiapoptosis. Mol Cell Biol. 2000;20(1):126–38.
110. Shochat C, Tal N, Bandapalli OR, Palmi C, Ganmore I, te Kronnie G, et al. Gain-of-function mutations in interleukin-7 receptor-alpha (IL7R) in childhood acute lymphoblastic leukemias. J Exp Med. 2011;208(5):901–8.
111. Zenatti PP, Ribeiro D, Li W, Zuurbier L, Silva MC, Paganin M, et al. Oncogenic IL7R gain-of-function mutations in childhood T-cell acute lymphoblastic leukemia. Nat Genet. 2011;43(10):932–9.
112. Goossens S, Radaelli E, Blanchet O, Durinck K, Van der Meulen J, Peirs S, et al. ZEB2 drives immature T-cell lymphoblastic leukaemia development via enhanced tumour-initiating potential and IL-7 receptor signalling. Nat Commun. 2015;6:5794.
113. Tremblay CS, Brown FC, Collett M, Saw J, Chiu SK, Sonderegger SE, et al. Loss-of-function mutations of Dynamin 2 promote T-ALL by enhancing IL-7 signalling. Leukemia. 2016;30(10):1993–2001.
114. Kleppe M, Soulier J, Asnafi V, Mentens N, Hornakova T, Knoops L, et al. PTPN2 negatively regulates oncogenic JAK1 in T-cell acute lymphoblastic leukemia. Blood. 2011;117(26):7090–8.
115. Perez-Garcia A, Ambesi-Impiombato A, Hadler M, Rigo I, LeDuc CA, Kelly K, et al. Genetic loss of SH2B3 in acute lymphoblastic leukemia. Blood. 2013;122(14):2425–32.
116. Girardi T, Vereecke S, Sulima SO, Khan Y, Fancello L, Briggs JW, et al. The T-cell leukemia-associated ribosomal RPL10 R98S mutation enhances JAK-STAT signaling. Leukemia. 2018;32(3):809–19.
117. Neumann M, Heesch S, Schlee C, Schwartz S, Gokbuget N, Hoelzer D, et al. Whole-exome sequencing in adult ETP-ALL reveals a high rate of DNMT3A mutations. Blood. 2013;121(23):4749–52.
118. Tosello V, Mansour MR, Barnes K, Paganin M, Sulis ML, Jenkinson S, et al. WT1 mutations in T-ALL. Blood. 2009;114(5):1038–45.

Chapter 3
Minimal Residual Disease in Acute Lymphoblastic Leukemia: Techniques and Application

Xueyan Chen and Brent L. Wood

Introduction

Acute lymphoblastic leukemia (ALL) is a heterogeneous group of diseases with different clinical, phenotypic, and genetic features and variable response to therapy. ALL predominantly occurs in children but affects adults as well. The estimated annual incidence of ALL is 1–4.75 cases per 100,000 people [1, 2]. In newly diagnosed pediatric ALL, 80–85% of cases have a precursor B-cell phenotype (B-ALL), and 12–15% have a precursor T-cell phenotype (T-ALL) [1, 3].

With contemporary chemotherapy protocols, the survival rates among children and adolescence with ALL have improved substantially over the past several decades. Pediatric ALL has been considered a highly curable disease, with 5-year event-free survival (EFS) above 85% [4, 5]. Outcomes for T-ALL, historically inferior to B-ALL, have also significantly improved with recent advances in therapy, with 5-year EFS over 85% [6–8].

A significant reason for the improvement in outcome for ALL is the implementation of risk-stratified therapy based on patient characteristics and types of leukemia as well as response to therapy [4, 9, 10]. Minimal or measurable residual disease (MRD), measured by sensitive methods at various time points post-induction

X. Chen
Department of Laboratory Medicine and Pathology, University of Washington, Seattle, WA, USA
e-mail: xchen1@uw.edu

B. L. Wood (✉)
Department of Laboratory Medicine and Pathology, University of Washington, Seattle, WA, USA

Seattle Cancer Care Alliance, Seattle, WA, USA

Children's Hospital Los Angeles, Los Angeles, CA, USA
e-mail: Bwood@chla.usc.edu

M. R. Litzow, E. A. Raetz (eds.), *Clinical Management of Acute Lymphoblastic Leukemia*, https://doi.org/10.1007/978-3-030-85147-7_3

therapy, represents the integration of biological features of leukemia, patient characteristics, and chemotherapy regimens, which together determine treatment efficacy. In both pediatric and adult ALL, MRD status is the most powerful prognostic factor and highly predictive of relapse, superseding other historically relevant factors including age, white blood cell count, and cytogenetics [11–25]. MRD has proven utility in risk group assignment and informing tailored management of patients, including intensification or reduction of chemotherapy, hematopoietic stem cell transplantation (HSCT), and novel therapies.

Given the unequivocal prognostic impact of MRD by numerous studies, it is essential to develop sensitive, accurate, and standardized methods for MRD detection and monitoring. The assessment of MRD has evolved substantially over the past decade with improvements in technology. Currently, MRD in ALL is most commonly evaluated by multiparametric flow cytometry and real-time quantitative polymerase chain reaction (RQ-PCR)-based methods. Most recently, new molecular methods, such as high-throughput sequencing (HTS), have evolved into routine laboratory tools to improve the sensitivity and specificity of MRD detection and to enhance prognostication.

Concept of MRD

Current multiagent regimens allow the majority of patients with ALL to achieve durable remission. Traditionally, treatment response is determined by morphology-based methods and clinical criteria [26]. However, many patients achieving morphologic remission ultimately relapse, indicating that morphology-based methods are neither sensitive nor specific enough to detect low levels of leukemic blasts. Highly sensitive methods are required to better assess the reduction in disease burden and to recognize impending relapse.

The first report of detection of morphologically non-evident residual disease in leukemia was published nearly four decades ago, which identified residual leukemic cells in the bone marrow of patients with T-ALL using fluorochrome-conjugated antisera by fluorescence microscopy [27]. That led to the introduction of the fundamental concept of MRD which is used to describe the presence of leukemic blasts after therapy at a level below the limit of conventional cytomorphologic detection (<5% of blasts). It is estimated that MRD is present in 33–47% of adult patients with B-ALL following induction therapy [28]. On the basis of the independent and high prognostic value of MRD for outcome seen in numerous studies, there is a strong rationale to incorporate MRD status into the criteria to define treatment response. The Consensus Development Workshop on MRD from major European study groups established a standardized description of MRD-based response, including "complete MRD response," "MRD persistence," and "MRD reappearance," which allows a standardized assessment of response to treatment and for comparison of MRD results between different treatment protocols [29]. The definition of remission has gradually evolved; recent studies have proposed to use both morphology and MRD when assessing remission [30, 31]. The current risk stratification strategy in ALL combines conventional risk factors and MRD into a decision algorithm.

Techniques for MRD Detection

To be clinically informative, optimal MRD assays should reliably discriminate leukemic blasts from normal lymphoid cells with high sensitivity consistently during the course of therapy, facilitate a timely report of results, and allow wide implementation with interlaboratory standardization. Multiparametric flow cytometry to identify leukemic blasts by immunophenotypic aberrancy and RQ-PCR-based methods to detect leukemia-specific rearranged immunoglobulin (IG) and T-cell receptor genes (TCR) are the most commonly used MRD assays in clinical practice [32]. Reverse transcriptase quantitative PCR (RT-qPCR) amplification of oncogenic fusion transcripts from balanced chromosome translocation is less commonly used because the identifiable fusion transcripts are only present in a subset of ALL. With recent advances in HTS, much effort has been devoted to the development of HTS-based MRD assays and their implementation in clinical practice. Currently, multiparametric flow cytometry and RQ-PCR analysis of IG/TCR gene rearrangements are informative in >95% of patients with Ph-negative B-ALL and T-ALL. While RT-qPCR-based testing of BCR/ABL1 fusion is a commonly used method for MRD monitoring in Ph-positive B-ALL [33, 34], a persistent signal may not correlate with outcome due to the presence of the translocation in preleukemic stem cells or mature forms derived from those stem cells, so supplementation by another method is now increasingly common.

Multiparametric Flow Cytometry

Methodological Principles of MRD Detection by Flow Cytometry

Discriminating leukemic blasts from normal lymphoid progenitors relies on the immunophenotypic principle that the antigen expression patterns on the normal lymphoid progenitors through all stages of differentiation are highly reproducible and differ from those seen on leukemic blasts, which have altered patterns of antigen expression resulting from underlying genetic mutations [35]. At present, this fundamental principle is applied in two related methodological approaches for MRD detection by flow cytometry.

The first approach is based on identification of a combination of antigens with aberrant expression patterns on the leukemic blasts, designated "leukemia-associated immunophenotypes" (LAIPs) that are not observed in normal lymphoid progenitors [36]. The main types of LAIPs include asynchronous antigen expression, cross-lineage antigen expression, antigen overexpression/underexpression, and ectopic phenotypes [19, 37]. LAIPs are first identified at diagnosis, using an antibody panel to define regions in multiparametric space that are occupied by leukemic blasts but not normal lymphoid cells. Following treatment, the informative antibody panel identified at diagnosis is used on post-therapy samples, and any leukemic blasts present in the predefined LAIP regions are considered as MRD. Leukemic blasts may have multiple LAIPs recognized in the diagnostic sample, all of which should be carefully followed in the subsequent samples to improve sensitivity and specificity of MRD detection. The increased number of fluorochromes and the ability to analyze more antigens simultaneously would in principle improve the confidence of identification of a leukemic blast population with specific LAIPs.

Although it has been successfully applied in some studies, this strategy has some limitations. First, LAIPs of leukemic clones are not always stable throughout the therapy [38–41], likely due to leukemic blast heterogeneity and subclone selection. One study observed a change of expression of at least one antigen in 69% of the cases with B-ALL between diagnostic and relapsed samples [38]. Such immunophenotypic shifts may lead to false-negative results, if rigid gating strategy with defined regions is used to identify MRD. Second, the immunophenotype of the background normal lymphoid progenitors and leukemic blasts may be altered under the influence of therapeutic drugs [38, 42–44]. It has been shown that steroid treatment in patients with B-ALL can induce immunophenotypic modulation of leukemic blasts including downregulation of immature antigens CD10 and CD34 and upregulation of mature antigens CD20 and CD45. In T-ALL, immaturity-associated antigens, such as TdT, CD99, and CD34, were dramatically reduced during therapy, while lineage-associated markers remained relatively stable [45]. Similarly, the immunophenotype of normal lymphoid progenitors may also change, causing it to appear in the regions predefined for abnormal blasts which results in a false-positive result. In addition, noise from nonspecific binding of reagents can be present in some samples and be counted as part of the LAIP, resulting in a false-positive result. Lastly, this method is entirely dependent on the LAIPs identified at diagnosis. Without the prerequisite knowledge of diagnostic LAIPs, an individualized antibody panel cannot be constructed to define regions for precise MRD detection. This requirement will have significant impact on its application in reference laboratories and tertiary care centers, where only post-therapy samples are available.

An alternative approach, known as "difference from normal," relies on the theory that the immunophenotype of the leukemic blasts differs from the spectrum of antigenic expression patterns on normal lymphoid cells of similar lineage and maturational stage [46, 47]. At initial diagnosis, this method establishes the specific immunophenotype of leukemic blasts, similar to the identification of LAIPs. As such, this method is a superset of the LAIP approach. In the post-therapy samples, all progenitor populations at varying maturation stages are evaluated to look for discrete populations having immunophenotypic aberrancies that deviate from the antigenic patterns of normal progenitors (Fig. 3.1). The immunophenotype identified in the diagnostic sample can be used as a starting point for post-therapy assessment, but diagnostic LAIPs to define regions for MRD are not required by the "difference from normal" approach. A standard antibody panel emphasizing normal

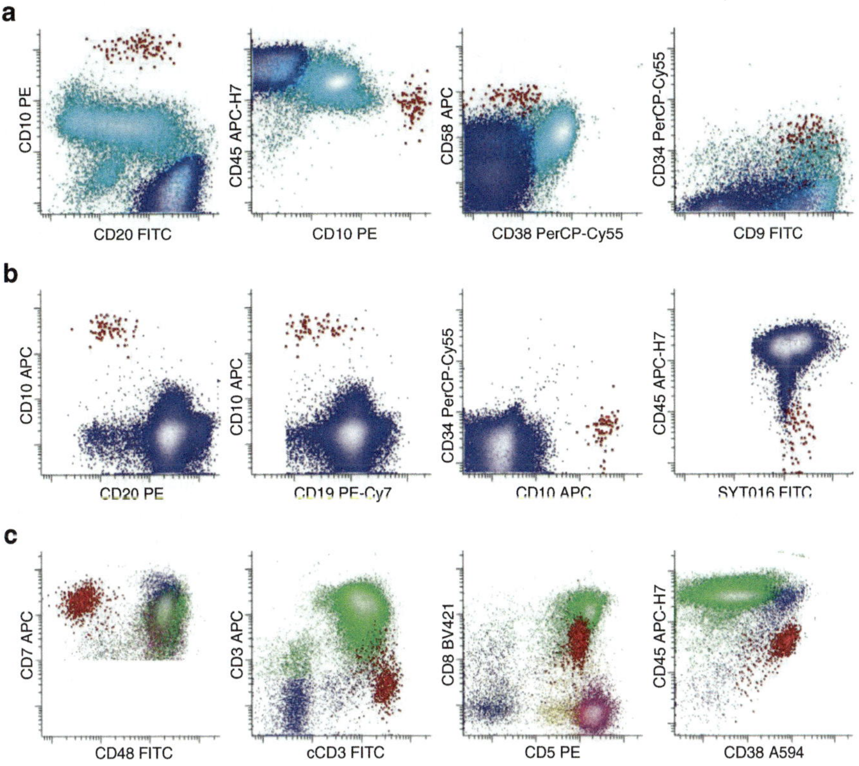

Fig. 3.1 The detection of MRD for acute lymphoblastic leukemia (ALL) following induction therapy by flow cytometry. Bone marrow (**a**, **c**) or peripheral blood (**b**) post-induction therapy was analyzed with an informative antibody panel. The antibody combination allows the identification of residual leukemic blasts by deviation from normal lymphoid progenitors based on lineage and maturational stage

(**a**) B-ALL MRD. The leukemic blasts (red) that represent MRD are characterized by abnormal expression of CD9 (uniform), CD10 (increased), CD34 (slightly increased), CD38 (decreased), CD45 (slightly decreased), and CD58 (increased) relative to immature normal B-cell precursors (cyan) of similar maturational stage. The mature B cells are colored in blue. The population is enumerated at 0.011% of total nucleated cells and 0.023% of nucleated mononuclear cells

(**b**) B-ALL MRD (day 8 post-induction therapy). The leukemic blasts (red) that represent MRD are characterized by abnormal expression of CD10 (increased), CD19 (decreased), CD34 (slightly increased), and CD45 (decreased) comparing to normal immature B-cell precursors, which should not be present in the peripheral blood at this time point. The mature B cells are colored in blue. The population is enumerated at 0.02% of total nucleated cells

(**c**) T-ALL MRD. The leukemic blasts (red) that represent MRD are characterized by abnormal expression of CD3 (absent on the surface, present in the cytoplasm), CD5 (slightly decreased), CD7 (slightly increased), CD8, CD38 (increased), and CD48 (absent) relative to mature T cells (green and pink). The population is enumerated at 0.33% of white cells and 1.1% of nucleated mononuclear cells

patterns of lymphoid maturation and including aberrant antigens commonly identified in LAIPs, rather than individualized antibody panels for LAIPs, can be implemented, which are important factors to consider especially for reference laboratory testing. Immunophenotypic shifts on leukemic blasts during therapy, which may have an impact on MRD detection by LAIP evaluation, do not affect MRD recognition by the "difference from normal" approach in a majority of cases. Despite all these advantages over the LAIP method, "difference from normal" does require extensive expert knowledge of antigenic expression patterns on lymphoid progenitors during normal differentiation and regeneration, making interlaboratory standardization and implementation of data interpretation challenging.

In clinical practice, an integrated strategy using components of both methods simultaneously is commonly applied to improve diagnostic accuracy. Flow cytometry assay sensitivity is largely dependent on the number of events acquired, the antibody panels used, and the degree of immunophenotypic deviation of the leukemic blasts from normal progenitors. Despite the fact that the recommended number of events for acquisition and the number of events to define a clonal leukemic blast population vary significantly among laboratories, a sensitivity of 0.01% can be achieved in a large majority of B-ALL and T-ALL. Assay sensitivity can also vary at different time points post-therapy as some abnormal immunophenotypes may be challenging to differentiate from immunophenotypic aberrancies associated with active marrow regeneration. In a sample with a large number of normal lymphoid progenitors, assay sensitivity may be significantly reduced unless the leukemic population shows prominent abnormalities.

Flow Cytometry Antibody Panels

Desirable MRD assays should have minimal antibody interaction and provide high fluorescence intensities on leukemic blasts with low background. Although there is no consensus on antibody panel selection, different combinations have been tested in B-ALL MRD detection [17, 48–52]. The optimal antibody panels for B-ALL MRD would facilitate identification of leukemic blasts with aberrant, immature immunophenotypes that deviate from normal lymphoid cells. The selection of antibodies for T-ALL MRD emphasizes the ability to identify immunophenotypic features of immature T cells distinct from mature T and NK cells, as the presence of immature T cells in peripheral blood or bone marrow strongly suggests MRD (Table 3.1) [45, 47]. The reagent panels for T-ALL MRD are less well defined and validated because of the low frequency of the disease.

The Children's Oncology Group (COG) assay uses two 6-color reagent combinations for identification of leukemic blasts, and a third reagent combination containing a DNA/RNA binding dye (Syto16) provides a nucleated cell denominator for enumeration (Table 3.1) [12]. Residual leukemic blasts are enumerated as the percentage of total nucleated mononuclear cells, excluding maturing granulocytic cells and including nucleated erythroid cells. MRD measured by the COG assay is highly prognostic in pediatric B-ALL and useful in risk stratification and

Table 3.1 Antibody panels for the detection of MRD in acute lymphoblastic leukemia (ALL)

A. Antibody panels recommended by Euro-Flow Consortium for B-ALL MRD									
	PB	PO	FITC	PE	PerCP5.5	PE-Cy7	APC	APC C750	
1	CD20	CD45	CD81	CD66c/ CD123	CD34	CD19	CD10	CD38	
2	CD20	CD45	CD81	CD73/ CD304	CD34	CD19	CD10	CD38	
B. COG antibody panels for B-ALL MRD									
	FITC	PE	PerCP5.5	PE-Cy7	APC	APC-H7			
1	CD20	CD10	CD38	CD19	CD58	CD45			
2	CD9	CD13 + 33	CD34	CD19	CD10	CD45			
3	Syto16		CD3	CD19	CD71	CD45			
C. COG antibody panels for B-ALL MRD at day 8 post induction (peripheral blood only)									
	FITC	PE	PerCP5.5	PE-Cy7	APC	APC-H7			
	Syto16	CD20	CD34	CD19	CD10	CD45			
D. Antibody panels for B-ALL MRD in patients post anti-CD19 therapy									
	BV421	BV510	FITC	PE	PerCP5.5	PE-Cy7	APC	APC-H7	
	CD10	CD38	CD66b	CD22	CD34	CD20	CD24	CD45	
E. COG antibody panels for T-ALL MRD									
	V450/ BV421	FITC	PE	PE-CF594	PE-Cy5	PE-Cy7	A594	APC	APC-H7
1	CD16	cCD3	CD7		CD56	CD5	CD38	sCD3	CD45
2	CD8	CD48	CD5	CD34	CD56 + 16	CD3	CD4	CD7	CD45
3	Syto16		CD7		CD56	CD3		CD71	CD45

A594 Alexa Fluor 594, *APC* allophycocyanin, *FITC* fluorescein isothiocyanate, *PE* phycoerytherin, *PE-Cy5* PE-cyanine-5, *PE-Cy7* PE-cyanine-7, *PerCP5.5* PerCP-Cy5.5, *PO* pacific orange

risk-directed therapy [12] and has been implemented in a standardized manner in a network of more than 20 laboratories internationally.

Recently, the EuroFlow Consortium described a fully standardized 2 tube, 8-color antibody panel for B-ALL MRD testing (Table 3.1) after multiple rounds of multicenter optimization, which allowed separation between leukemic blasts and normal lymphoid progenitors in >99% of the patients [53]. In samples with sufficient cells (>4 million) analyzed, flow cytometric MRD assay reached a sensitivity of ≤0.001% (10^{-5}), similar to RQ-PCR-based method. The concordance between flow cytometric and RQ-PCR-based MRD data was 98% (97% for samples with MRD < 0.01%).

Over the past several years, immunotherapy has been introduced to patients with relapsed/refractory B-ALL and demonstrated encouraging results. Both chimeric antigen receptor-expressing T cells (CAR-T cells) and bi-specific T-cell engager (BiTE) directed against B-cell marker CD19 deplete both normal B cells and leukemic blasts expressing CD19 [54–58]. As a principal reagent to identify B cells,

CD19 alone is insufficient to enrich for B cells after anti-CD19-targeted therapy. In this context, other B-cell markers must be incorporated to allow for B-cell identification and MRD detection. A novel flow cytometric assay using both CD22 and CD24 as alternative gating reagents for B cells has been described and validated in the setting of immunotherapy targeting CD19 or CD22 (Table 3.1) [59]. The proposed combination showed a good correlation with the standard flow cytometric assay for B-ALL MRD detection and successfully identifies both CD19-positive and CD19-negative leukemic blasts.

Real-Time Quantitative PCR

IG and TCR genes undergo rearrangements during early stages of B and T lymphocyte maturation. Leukemic blasts in ALL originate from one single lymphoid progenitor and therefore carry the same clonally rearranged IG and TCR genes. RQ-PCR-based MRD testing relies on identification of clonally rearranged IG and TCR genes which represent unique sequences in individual leukemic blasts among normal lymphoid cells expressing rearranged genes with different sequences [60]. While IG rearrangements are more frequently detected in B-ALL and TCR rearrangements more commonly found in T-ALL, both B-ALL and T-ALL leukemic blasts can display cross-lineage rearrangement [61, 62]. Clonal IG heavy chain (IGH) and TCR gamma (TCRG) gene rearrangements can be detected in >90% of B-ALL and T-ALL [63, 64]. Approximately 70% of clonal IGH rearrangements are preserved in relapsed B-ALL [65, 66], whereas ~90% of rearrangements are preserved in relapsed T-ALL [67]. Therefore, it is recommended that at least two independent clonal IG/TCR markers are used for MRD detection to reduce false-negative results [68]. With additional PCR targets [such as IG kappa, incomplete IGH, TCR beta (TCRB), TCR delta (TCRD), etc.], 90–95% of ALL patients can be monitored by at least two sensitive MRD targets [60, 64]. This assay generally reaches a sensitivity of 0.01–0.001% (10^{-4}–10^{-5}).

RQ-PCR-based MRD testing is a complex, multistep process. The specific IG or TCR gene rearrangements are sequenced at diagnosis for target identification, allele-specific oligonucleotide (ASO) primers designed complimentary to the unique patient or leukemic-specific junctional region sequences are synthesized, and RQ-PCR conditions are optimized for each target. The ASO primers are then applied to post-therapy samples to identify patient-specific IG/TCR gene rearrangements, and quantification of MRD is achieved by comparing the amplified product to a standard curve established from amplification of serial dilution of a control gene [69]. As a result, the RQ-PCR-based method is time-consuming and laborious and requires extensive knowledge and expertise; therefore, standardization and quality control of the assay are critical for correct interpretation of data and to allow interlaboratory comparison of MRD results. This method has been thoroughly standardized via international collaboration through the efforts of the Euro-MRD groups, with established guidelines for determination of quantitative range, sensitivity, specificity, and reproducibility for each assay [29, 60, 70].

In addition to IG and TCR gene rearrangements, leukemic-specific gene fusion transcripts, such as *BCR/ABL1* and *MLL* rearrangements, are found in one third of ALL and can also be used as targets for quantitative measurement of residual leukemic cells at mRNA level by RT-qPCR [29]. This assay uses the same primer/probe combination for all patients and is more sensitive (up to 10^{-6}) than DNA-based assay as many copies of mRNA can be present in a leukemic blast.

High-Throughput Next-Generation Sequencing (HTS)

With recent advances in sequencing technology, HTS has become an emerging tool for MRD detection with improved sensitivity compared to flow cytometry and RQ-PCR and has demonstrated a potential as a diagnostic platform. This technique has high-level multiplexing capacity that allows for simultaneous amplification of all possible combinations of the rearranged IG or TCR loci using consensus primers. At diagnosis, HTS detects patient-specific index clonal IG/TCR gene rearrangements using universal primers. The same procedure is applied to the posttreatment samples to identify the index sequences and quantify MRD, eliminating the requirement for patient-specific ASO primers [14]. In addition, HTS can detect small neoplastic subclones present after therapy not identified by flow cytometry or RQ-PCR and monitor clonal evolution that is the source of false-negative results seen with RQ-PCR-based methods. Leukemic clones detected by HTS at relapse can be genetically identical to, evolved from, or completely distinct from diagnostic clones [71]. In theory, HTS-based techniques can reach a sensitivity below 10^{-5} for MRD detection. Some studies using commercial assays have claimed an even lower limit of MRD detection of 10^{-6}–10^{-7} in B-ALL [72, 73].

HTS offers higher sensitivity and precision than other MRD techniques and has been applied to MRD monitoring in ALL. In one cohort of T-ALL, HTS identified at least one clonal TCRB or TCRG rearrangements in 81% of pretreatment samples. At day 29, HTS showed greater sensitivity and specificity than flow cytometry in MRD assessment by detecting the original clonal TCRB sequences [74]. The absence of clonal TCRB rearrangements was associated with early thymic precursor (ETP) or near-ETP subtypes, where rearrangement of TCR had not yet occurred. Similarly in B-ALL, HTS of IGH genes detected clonal IGH rearrangements in 95% of diagnostic samples and successfully identified MRD in day 29 posttreatment samples with a tenfold increase in the lower limit of detection as compared to flow cytometry [75]. These findings suggest the potential clinical utility of HTS in MRD monitoring and risk stratification. Prospective studies will be needed to compare the predictive values of MRD by HTS and standard methods. As HTS becomes more applicable and affordable, consensus guidelines for data interpretation and its clinical use are expected before implementation in ALL MRD surveillance.

Comparison of Methods for MRD Detection

The advantages and logistical challenges associated with different MRD techniques are outlined in Table 3.2. The choice of MRD techniques is mainly dependent on the clinical trial design and available resources. The major advantages of flow cytometry are general applicability to all ALL, wide availability of the assay, rapid reporting of the results allowing for prompt decision making, and simultaneous assessment

Table 3.2 Advantages and limitations of MRD techniques in acute lymphoblastic leukemia (ALL)

	Multiparametric flow cytometry	Real-time quantitative PCR	Reverse transcriptase quantitative PCR	High-throughput sequencing
Target	Leukemia-associated immunophenotypes or "difference from normal" approach	IG/TCR gene rearrangements	Leukemic fusion transcripts	IG/TCR gene rearrangements
Applicability	Essentially all ALL	>95% of ALL	25–40% of B-ALL, 10–15% of T-ALL	>95% of ALL
Sensitivity	3–4 colors: 0.1–0.01%	0.01–0.001%	0.01–0.001%	0.0001%
	6–10 colors: 0.01–0.001%			
Specimen	Viable cells	DNA	RNA	DNA
Turn-around time	1–2 days	~ 4 weeks	1–3 days	1–2 weeks
Availability	Widely available	Widely available in Europe	Widely available	Largely experimental, limited availability
Cost	Moderate expense	More expensive	Moderate expense	Most expensive
Advantages	Rapid resulting	High sensitivity	Rapid resulting	High sensitivity
	Direct quantification	Thorough standardization	High sensitivity	Readily standardized
	Identifies and monitors therapeutic targets	Clinically validated role in risk stratification and treatment decisions by various clinical trials	Does not require patient-specific assays	Detects subclones and clonal evolution
	Provides information on cellular composition		Targets stable during treatment	Provides information on physiological B/T-cell repertoire
				Does not require patient-specific assays

Table 3.2 (continued)

	Multiparametric flow cytometry	Real-time quantitative PCR	Reverse transcriptase quantitative PCR	High-throughput sequencing
Disadvantages	Inadequate interlaboratory standardization	High cost	Only applicable to ALL harboring detectable fusion transcripts	High cost
	Requires expert knowledge for data interpretation	Requires diagnostic sample to identify patient-specific IG/TCR gene rearrangements	Limited standardization	Requires diagnostic sample to identify patient-specific index IG/TCR gene rearrangements
	False negativity resulting from immunophenotypic shifts or confounding regenerating progenitors	Requires construction of patient-specific primers	Instability of RNA	Requires complex bioinformatics
		Time consuming and labor intensive	Uncertain quantification of leukemic blasts	Limited clinical validation
		False negativity resulting from clonal evolution		

of cellular characteristics required for targeted therapies. Unlike RQ-PCR that requires patient-specific primers, flow cytometry uses standardized antibody panels for essentially all patients. The main challenge in performing MRD detection by flow cytometry is the lack of reproducibility across laboratories due to considerable variability in instrumentation, reagents and procedures, data analysis software, and reporting [76, 77]. Because the data interpretation is inherently subjective, expert knowledge of normal and regenerative antigenic expression pattern of lymphoid progenitors and experience with immunophenotypic shifts post-therapy are required for accurate data interpretation. Therefore, interlaboratory standardization of methodologies is necessary to ensure comparability of MRD results between different laboratories and treatment protocols. As shown for the COG assay, training the laboratories to use a standardized assay, along with systemic education and feedback on MRD data interpretation, can reduce discordance among interpreters [78]. The recent technical innovations including flow cytometers that allow for more colors and automated data analysis [79] could improve sensitivity, specificity, and time effectiveness of MRD detection.

RQ-PCR-based MRD assay is the gold standard method in ALL and has been extensively optimized and standardized in Europe. Although it is labor-intensive, time-consuming, and expensive, RQ-PCR analysis of IG/TCR rearrangement for MRD is 1-log more sensitive (10^{-4}–10^{-5}) than that achieved by standard flow cytometry [52, 80, 81]. This assay requires a laborious initial characterization of IG/TCR gene rearrangements in leukemic blasts and construction of patient-specific ASO primers for posttreatment testing, making it challenging and expensive in a routine clinical setting. Other limitations include false-negative results due to clonal evolution or emergence of a new clone and false-positive results caused by nonspecific amplification of IG/TCR genes in background lymphoid progenitors [82]. Currently, MRD assessment by flow cytometry is the standard of care in ALL in the United States, whereas RQ-PCR-based testing is commonly used in European clinical trials.

Most studies have shown that flow cytometry and RQ-PCR analysis of IG or TCR rearrangements generate concordant MRD measurements, for MRD levels >0.01% [48, 52, 80, 83–85]. The discordant cases were frequently seen with low levels of MRD (<0.01%), mostly flow-negative/RQ-PCR-positive. The discordance can be explained by the higher sensitivity of the RQ-PCR assay, presence of nonviable blasts detected by RQ-PCR but not by flow cytometry, nonspecific amplification of normal DNA resulting in false-positive RQ-PCR results, immunophenotypic changes post-therapy, and the presence of confounding regenerating blasts which may reduce the sensitivity of flow cytometry. In B-ALL, the concordance between flow cytometry and RQ-PCR was time point-dependent; most discordance was found at day 33 post-therapy (70% concordant), as compared with day 15 (86% concordant) and day 78 (87% concordant) [52]. Patients with discordant MRD results at day 33 had an intermediate clinical outcome much closer to concordantly negative cases than to the concordantly positive cases, suggesting that the presence of very low level of discordant MRD at day 33 is not strongly predictive of outcome.

HTS platforms may mitigate some of the limitations of flow cytometry and RQ-PCR. Similar to RQ-PCR, a sample containing a relatively large number (>5%) of leukemic blasts is required for identification of clonally rearranged IG/TCR gene index sequences. Importantly, HTS uses a standardized assay with multiplexed primers for both diagnostic and subsequent samples and is therefore less laborious and time-consuming than standard RQ-PCR assays. HTS has the ability to detect minor subclones and monitor clonal evolution, reducing false-negative results seen by RQ-PCR assays. In addition, HTS also allows the evaluation of the heterogeneity of the normal lymphoid repertoire. Comparing to flow cytometry, HTS is less likely to be affected by immunophenotypic shifts and the presence of regenerating blasts, and data interpretation is less subjective. Nevertheless, flow cytometry provides more rapid reporting than either RQ-PCR or HTS, which is important when rapid clinical decision-making is needed, e.g., at End of Induction (EOI).

Early studies have suggested a higher analytic sensitivity of MRD detection at 10^{-6}–10^{-7} in B-ALL by HTS than that can be achieved by flow cytometry and RQ-PCR [73]. Subsequent studies further demonstrated HTS could detect MRD in posttreatment samples that was not identified by flow cytometry in both B-ALL [75] and T-ALL [74]. In both studies, the MRD results were highly concordant between HTS and flow cytometry at the limit of detection of 0.01%. HTS additionally detected very low levels of MRD not identified by flow cytometry in a significant subset of patients. Comparing with RQ-PCR, MRD results in B-ALL by both methods were concordant in 85–96% of patients [73, 86]. Using an MRD threshold of 0.01%, HTS was comparable to flow cytometry in predicting outcome and risk stratification [87]. Despite these promising results, clinical relevance of MRD measured by HTS needs to be further defined in randomized trials before implementation of HTS into routine MRD monitoring and risk stratification.

Clinical Application of MRD

Multiple published trials have demonstrated the indispensible prognostic value of MRD in both pediatric and adult ALL regardless of disease subtype, therapeutic regimen, method and timing of MRD assessment, and threshold of MRD cutoff [88]. As a result, MRD status has been incorporated into clinical trials to assess response to initial treatment, for subsequent MRD-based risk stratification, and to direct future therapy. It is important to recognize that the clinical impact of MRD is strictly dependent on the timing of MRD assessment and MRD threshold for decision-making determined by therapeutic protocols. Therefore, MRD data cannot be directly extrapolated from one treatment regimen to another but rather must be evaluated under the same therapeutic conditions.

Prognostic Implication of MRD

MRD in Frontline Chemotherapy

Many studies unanimously support the significant prognostic impact of MRD in ALL, and therefore MRD serves as a critical component for risk stratification. The first large-scale prospective study AIEOP-BFM-ALL2000 in childhood and adolescent B-ALL introduced standardized assessment of MRD by RQ-PCR (sensitive of at least 10^{-4}) at two time points for risk stratification [9]. MRD negativity at day 33 post-induction is the strongest predictor for excellent 5-year EFS, and high levels of MRD ($\geq 10^{-3}$) at day 78 are highly predictive of relapse. Similar conclusions were drawn in pediatric patients with T-ALL enrolled in the same protocol [89]. Other study groups confirmed the independent prognostic impact of MRD, however, using different timing and methods of MRD testing and different cutoff values of MRD [11, 12, 18, 90, 91]. In a Swedish multicenter study, a MRD level ≥0.1% at day 29 quantified by both flow cytometry and RQ-PCR predicted high risk of relapse in children with B-ALL [81]. In T-ALL, MRD detected by RQ-PCR was superior to flow cytometry in predicting relapse.

The independent prognostic effect of MRD is also recognized in adult ALL using RQ-PCR [16, 25, 92] or flow cytometry [15]. Conventional prognostic factors lose their prognostic value when MRD status was included in the analysis [16, 25]. A retrospective study of adults with MRD-positive ALL ($\geq 10^{-4}$) by flow cytometry or RQ-PCR who received standard treatment of care between 2000 and 2014 was recently performed using the European ALL study group database [93]. The data showed relatively short relapse free survival (RFS) and overall survival (OS) in patients with MRD-positive ALL, particularly at higher MRD levels, while lower baseline MRD level was a strong predictor for better RFS. Early complete molecular response during induction therapy was associated with an excellent outcome [94].

Several studies have assessed the prognostic utility of HTS-based monitoring for MRD and have reported that MRD measured by HTS predicts risk of relapse in both pediatric [73, 86, 95] and adult ALL [96]. In the recent COG studies AALL0331 and AALL0232, using a MRD threshold of 0.01%, HTS was equivalent to flow cytometry in its ability for risk stratification in childhood B-ALL at EOI [87]. Reducing the threshold of HTS below 0.01% at EOI did not improve risk stratification in general but allowed identification of a small subset (19.9%) of standard-risk MRD-negative patients who had an outstanding outcome and required no further therapy. Although low-positive MRD ($<10^{-4}$) and high-positive MRD ($\geq 10^{-4}$) were similarly associated with decreased leukemia-free survival [95], HTS provided opportunity to identify additional patients with MRD who would benefit with intensified therapy. Despite enhanced sensitivity of HTS to $<10^{-6}$, the clinically actionable MRD threshold for most patients appears to be unchanged. Comparison of the clinical utility of these methods should be addressed in prospective studies before definite adoption of HTS to replace other methods in MRD quantification for optimal risk stratification.

MRD in Pre- and Post-hematopoietic Cell Transplant

The prognostic impact of MRD status prior to hematopoietic cell transplant (HCT) is well established in children and adults [72, 97–101]. Many studies have also explored the importance of post-HCT MRD status, and all demonstrated that any evidence of MRD is significantly associated with increased risk of relapse [99, 100, 102–105]. Studies have also been performed to evaluate whether more sensitive HTS better predicts relapse than standard methods in the setting of pre- and post-HCT. In a small cohort of adult B-ALL patients, MRD detected by HTS within 30 days prior to HCT predicts post-HCT relapse [100]. After HCT, MRD $\geq 10^{-6}$ detected in blood samples had shown a 100% positive predictive value for relapse. Comparing to flow cytometry, pre- and post-HCT MRD detected by HTS predicts relapse and survival more accurately than 6-color flow cytometry in pediatric patients with B-ALL [72]. Therefore, post-HCT MRD monitoring by HTS is useful in detecting impending relapse for early intervention before overt relapse.

MRD In Ph-Positive ALL

Ph-positive B-ALL accounts for about 25% of adult ALL [1]. While MRD is the most significant prognostic factor in Ph-negative ALL, the utility of MRD assessment in Ph-positive is not well defined. In patients treated with frontline chemotherapy combined with tyrosine kinase inhibitors (TKI), complete molecular response measured by RT-qPCR at 3 months was associated with superior RFS and OS even without HCT compared with those with lesser molecular response [106, 107]. The French GRAAPH-2003 study, however, showed that early MRD evaluation did not significantly influence OS and disease-free survival [108]. The French GRAAPH-2005 study further confirmed that early MRD response was less discriminant than WBC [109]. HCT improved outcome in patients with persistent MRD, but patients who achieved major molecular response did not benefit from HCT. To explore the predictive value of MRD in the setting of HCT, recent studies on Ph-positive ALL patients treated with chemotherapy and TKI support the prognostic relevance of MRD before HCT [110, 111]. Achieving a complete molecular response prior to HCT significantly reduced the risk of relapse after HCT. Future prospective studies using MRD-based stratification may be necessary to clarify remaining issues and shed light on optimal management in Ph-positive ALL.

MRD in Targeted Therapy

In the era of immunotherapy, MRD assessment can recognize patients that may benefit from novel therapeutic agents, in particular, in patients who are not candidates for HCT. Inotuzumab ozogamicin directed against CD22 [112], BiTE blinatumomab [58, 113], and CAR-T cells directed against CD19 [55, 56] have been used in relapsed/refractory ALL and have shown to improve survival, in part mediated through inducing complete MRD response. The FDA has approved the use of blinatumomab in childhood and adult ALL patients with MRD $\geq$ 0.1% in first or second CR based on a phase 2 trial [114]. Of 116 patients evaluated, patients who achieved MRD negativity (78%) had significantly longer RFS and OS than patients with persistent MRD. In a subsequent large phase 3 study randomizing Ph-negative relapsed/refractory ALL patients between blinatumomab and standard of care salvage chemotherapy, patients receiving blinatumomab had significantly higher rates of complete remission (CR) and negative MRD status and longer EFS and OS than with chemotherapy [115]. This is the first time the FDA used MRD endpoint as the basis for approval of a therapeutic agent. Regarding anti-CD19 CAR-T cells, several groups have shown that most of the responding patients became negative and maintain this status for several months or years [56, 116–118]. However, relapse rates are high even in patients achieving MRD negativity, different from frontline chemotherapy. After CAR-T therapy, MRD appears to be insufficient to predict long-term remissions. High-sensitivity MRD assays and early time point testing may be necessary to identify a subset of patients with rapid and deep response and good prognosis. The prognostic relevance of MRD in the setting of novel therapies needs to be further elucidated in clinical trials.

Therapeutic Implication of MRD

Although there are profound differences in trial design, methods and timing of MRD testing, and threshold for MRD-directed therapy, the major prospective studies have provided strong evidence that risk-directed therapy based on the presence of MRD improves survival and reduces the relapse rate in intermediate- and high-risk pediatric ALL [7, 12, 119–122]. MRD levels at various time points post-therapy have been validated to predict relapse and incorporated into post-remission therapy regimen, including therapy intensification and HCT [123]. Similarly in adult ALL, high-risk patients with unfavorable MRD status can benefit from more intensive therapy, such as HCT, with significantly improved EFS and OS [15, 25, 92, 124].

On the other hand, MRD may be used to identify good responders that may benefit from treatment de-escalation to reduce toxicity [125, 126]. In MRC UKALL 2003 study of pediatric and young adult ALL, there was no significant difference in EFS in low-risk patients defined by MRD status at EOI (undetectable or $<10^{-4}$) who received one or two delayed intensification courses [125], implying that treatment reduction is feasible for low-risk patients. HCT does not appear to be beneficial in patients with low levels of or no detectable MRD and therefore should be avoided [15, 25].

It is very likely that MRD has different clinical and therapeutic meanings dependent on the underlying biology and genotype. Genome sequencing of pre- and post-treatment childhood B-ALL identifies two distinct evolutionary patterns, a highly dynamic pattern and a quasi-inert evolutionary pattern, governing early and late relapse, respectively [127]. If confirmed in other cohorts, these findings have clinical implications and emphasize the need for adapted treatment strategies to prevent therapeutic escape.

Practical Issues

Specimen Types for MRD Testing

MRD is tested and quantified in either peripheral blood or bone marrow, although the sample type has an apparent impact on assay sensitivity. MRD levels show a strong correlation in paired peripheral blood and bone marrow in T-ALL, but poor correlation in B-ALL with lower levels of MRD detected in peripheral blood [128, 129]. Therefore, bone marrow is the preferred sample to achieve optimal sensitivity for MRD detection in B-ALL. Recent studies demonstrate that although paired peripheral blood and bone marrow samples showed comparable clonal distribution in most of patients with B-ALL, the peripheral blood does not consistently represent the clonal composition in the bone marrow, further implicating the importance of sample selection in MRD detection [130, 131].

Timing and Methods for MRD Assessment

MRD is a time point- and context-dependent variable that has different prognostic implications at different time points following treatment. Although there is a lack of full agreement on optimal timing and methods of MRD assessment, in B-ALL a threshold of 0.01% at EOI is commonly used to identify patients with a greater risk of relapse and is largely technology independent. In T-ALL the data are less robust, but a threshold of 0.01–0.1% at the End of Consolidation therapy appears to identify poor-risk patients, in part a reflection of slower leukemic blast clearance in T-ALL compared with B-ALL. In addition, the MRD threshold to identify poor-risk patients appears dependent on the underlying biology, for example, an MRD threshold of 0.1% at EOI is optimal to identify poor-risk patients within the pediatric standard-risk B-ALL cohort having double trisomies, while an MRD threshold of 0.01% provides similar risk stratification for the remaining pediatric standard-risk patients [132, 133]. Based on the intent of MRD assessment, a general strategy for MRD testing will likely require more than one technology. At early time points (EOI), flow cytometry or RQ-PCR-based methods, if applicable, can provide adequate sensitivity and rapid resulting for prompt decision-making. Further from therapy, especially post-remission surveillance, a high-sensitivity assay, such as HTS, is desirable as it is more likely that any level of MRD will be associated with a higher risk of overt hematologic relapse.

MRD Monitoring Post-remission

There is no consensus regarding the clinically appropriate interval for MRD monitoring in patients who are in remission and no longer receiving therapy. Given the different rates of response to therapy and different relapse kinetics of various leukemia subtypes, the schedule of MRD monitoring may vary significantly. In the German Multicenter ALL (GMALL) trial, the utility of MRD as an indicator of impending relapse was prospectively evaluated in 105 MRD-negative patients by RQ-PCR with a 3-month interval after consolidation [22]. Thirteen of 15 patients (89%) with MRD detected within the quantitative range of RQ-PCR subsequently relapsed after a median interval of 4.1 months, indicating that MRD positivity during early phase of post-consolidation is predictive of subsequent hematologic relapse. Base on these data, molecular relapse defined as conversion to quantifiable

MRD by RQ-PCR led to salvage therapy prior to hematologic relapse in GMALL trial. As to the length of MRD monitoring, a follow-up of 12 months after the end of the first year of therapy with 3-month interval seems adequate to detect most of the patients who later relapsed. A recent study confirmed the previous findings by demonstrating MRD positivity detected by flow cytometry at any time points after achieving CR was associated with a high risk of relapse in a series of 546 MRD-negative ALL patients [134]. This study monitored MRD at the time of CR and at ~3-month interval thereafter. MRD was detected in 55 patients with a median of 14 months, and 44 of 55 patients (80%) subsequently developed hematologic relapse after a median of 3 months. These findings support the concept that MRD detected in CR can predict hematologic relapse, making post-remission MRD monitoring necessary if pre-emptive intervention is planned.

MRD as a Surrogate Endpoint for Outcomes

There is a clinical need to identify novel endpoints that facilitate the assessment of drug efficacy at early stages than those allowed by conventional endpoints. To be considered, alteration in surrogate endpoints must reflect changes in outcomes. Although MRD is strongly correlated with outcomes in ALL for drugs in current use [88] and available at an early time point, it cannot reflect the long-term therapeutic or toxic effects of drugs. Several studies have indicated MRD response does not reflect the effect of drugs on outcomes [135, 136]. For the first time, a meta-analysis of individual data from two large phase 3 trials for childhood ALL [8, 135] was performed to formally evaluate whether MRD status at EOI frontline treatment is an accurate surrogate endpoint for EFS [137]. While the analysis confirmed the strong prognostic effect of early MRD response on EFS regardless of treatment, MRD at EOI was found to be a poor surrogate for treatment effect on EFS at the trial level. As MRD is commonly used for risk stratification in ALL, subsequent treatment is modulated based on MRD itself and may attenuate potential surrogacy. The data suggests the limitation of a powerful prognostic factor in being a surrogate endpoint in the setting of frontline ALL treatment. Using MRD as a primary endpoint for accelerated approval of a novel drug would require demonstration of a direct linkage between a change in therapy based on MRD and traditional clinical endpoints, such as EFS and OS.

Summary

MRD has emerged as a strong independent predictor of outcomes in pediatric and adult ALL. MRD monitoring provides an assessment of response to therapy that is more informative than that provided by morphologic evaluation. Novel techniques, such as HTS, have the potential to overcome the limitations of standard flow cytometry and RQ-PCR-based methods, although reporting is not yet rapid enough for early clinical decision-making. MRD status post-therapy is crucial for risk assessment and for determining those patients that may benefit from therapeutic reduction or intensification to improve clinical outcome. However, the prognostic significance of MRD is dependent on the clinical scenario, leukemic biology, and timing of MRD testing. Disease and treatment-specific protocols should dictate the schedule of MRD monitoring, the optimal methods for MRD detection, and the cutoff value for MRD status, to ensure optimal risk stratification and personalized therapy. Integration of complex genetic information and MRD is likely to increasingly drive personalized clinical protocols. Future prospective studies are ultimately needed to prove the efficacy of MRD-adapted treatment in randomized trials.

Acknowledgments Funding source: none

Conflict of Interest Statement All authors declare that they have no conflict of interest.

References

1. Swerdlow SH, Campo E, Harris NL, et al. WHO classification of tumours of haematopoietic and lymphoid tissues. Revised 4th ed. Lyon: International Agency for Research on Cancer; 2017.
2. Redaelli A, Laskin BL, Stephens JM, et al. A systematic literature review of the clinical and epidemiological burden of acute lymphoblastic leukaemia (ALL). Eur J Cancer Care. 2005;14:53–62.
3. Raetz EA, Teachey DT. T-cell acute lymphoblastic leukemia. Hematology Am Soc Hematol Educ Program. 2016;2016:580–8.
4. Hunger SP, Lu X, Devidas M, et al. Improved survival for children and adolescents with acute lymphoblastic leukemia between 1990 and 2005: a report from the Children's Oncology Group. J Clin Oncol. 2012;30:1663–9.
5. Pui CH, Campana D, Pei D, et al. Treating childhood acute lymphoblastic leukemia without cranial irradiation. N Engl J Med. 2009;360:2730–41.
6. Patrick K, Wade R, Goulden N, et al. Outcome for children and young people with early T-cell precursor acute lymphoblastic leukaemia treated on a contemporary protocol, UKALL 2003. Br J Haematol. 2014;166:421–4.
7. Vora A, Goulden N, Mitchell C, et al. Augmented post-remission therapy for a minimal residual disease-defined high-risk subgroup of children and young people with clinical standard-risk and intermediate-risk acute lymphoblastic leukaemia (UKALL 2003): a randomised controlled trial. Lancet Oncol. 2014;15:809–18.
8. Moricke A, Zimmermann M, Valsecchi MG, et al. Dexamethasone vs prednisone in induction treatment of pediatric ALL: results of the randomized trial AIEOP-BFM ALL 2000. Blood. 2016;127:2101–12.
9. Conter V, Bartram CR, Valsecchi MG, et al. Molecular response to treatment redefines all prognostic factors in children and adolescents with B-cell precursor acute lymphoblastic leukemia: results in 3184 patients of the AIEOP-BFM ALL 2000 study. Blood. 2010;115:3206–14.
10. Moricke A, Reiter A, Zimmermann M, et al. Risk-adjusted therapy of acute lymphoblastic leukemia can decrease treatment burden and improve survival: treatment results of 2169 unselected pediatric and adolescent patients enrolled in the trial ALL-BFM 95. Blood. 2008;111:4477–89.

11. Borowitz MJ, Devidas M, Hunger SP, et al. Clinical significance of minimal residual disease in childhood acute lymphoblastic leukemia and its relationship to other prognostic factors: a Children's Oncology Group study. Blood. 2008;111:5477–85.
12. Borowitz MJ, Wood BL, Devidas M, et al. Prognostic significance of minimal residual disease in high risk B-ALL: a report from Children's Oncology Group study AALL0232. Blood. 2015;126:964–71.
13. Bruggemann M, Raff T, Flohr T, et al. Clinical significance of minimal residual disease quantification in adult patients with standard-risk acute lymphoblastic leukemia. Blood. 2006;107:1116–23.
14. van Dongen JJ, van der Velden VH, Bruggemann M, et al. Minimal residual disease diagnostics in acute lymphoblastic leukemia: need for sensitive, fast, and standardized technologies. Blood. 2015;125:3996–4009.
15. Ribera JM, Oriol A, Morgades M, et al. Treatment of high-risk Philadelphia chromosome-negative acute lymphoblastic leukemia in adolescents and adults according to early cytologic response and minimal residual disease after consolidation assessed by flow cytometry: final results of the PETHEMA ALL-AR-03 trial. J Clin Oncol. 2014;32:1595–604.
16. Beldjord K, Chevret S, Asnafi V, et al. Oncogenetics and minimal residual disease are independent outcome predictors in adult patients with acute lymphoblastic leukemia. Blood. 2014;123:3739–49.
17. Bjorklund E, Mazur J, Soderhall S, et al. Flow cytometric follow-up of minimal residual disease in bone marrow gives prognostic information in children with acute lymphoblastic leukemia. Leukemia. 2003;17:138–48.
18. Coustan-Smith E, Sancho J, Hancock ML, et al. Clinical importance of minimal residual disease in childhood acute lymphoblastic leukemia. Blood. 2000;96:2691–6.
19. Dworzak MN, Froschl G, Printz D, et al. Prognostic significance and modalities of flow cytometric minimal residual disease detection in childhood acute lymphoblastic leukemia. Blood. 2002;99:1952–8.
20. Ciudad J, San Miguel JF, Lopez-Berges MC, et al. Prognostic value of immunophenotypic detection of minimal residual disease in acute lymphoblastic leukemia. J Clin Oncol. 1998;16:3774–81.
21. Mortuza FY, Papaioannou M, Moreira IM, et al. Minimal residual disease tests provide an independent predictor of clinical outcome in adult acute lymphoblastic leukemia. J Clin Oncol. 2002;20:1094–104.
22. Raff T, Gokbuget N, Luschen S, et al. Molecular relapse in adult standard-risk ALL patients detected by prospective MRD monitoring during and after maintenance treatment: data from the GMALL 06/99 and 07/03 trials. Blood. 2007;109:910–5.
23. Krampera M, Vitale A, Vincenzi C, et al. Outcome prediction by immunophenotypic minimal residual disease detection in adult T-cell acute lymphoblastic leukaemia. Br J Haematol. 2003;120:74–9.
24. Panzer-Grumayer ER, Schneider M, Panzer S, et al. Rapid molecular response during early induction chemotherapy predicts a good outcome in childhood acute lymphoblastic leukemia. Blood. 2000;95:790–4.
25. Dhedin N, Huynh A, Maury S, et al. Role of allogeneic stem cell transplantation in adult patients with Ph-negative acute lymphoblastic leukemia. Blood. 2015;125:2486–96.
26. Pui CH, Robison LL, Look AT. Acute lymphoblastic leukaemia. Lancet. 2008;371:1030–43.
27. Bradstock KF, Janossy G, Tidman N, et al. Immunological monitoring of residual disease in treated thymic acute lymphoblastic leukaemia. Leuk Res. 1981;5:301–9.
28. Pigneux A, Montesinos P, Cong Z, et al. Testing for minimal residual disease in adults with acute lymphoblastic leukemia in Europe: a clinician survey. BMC Cancer. 2018;18:1100.
29. Bruggemann M, Schrauder A, Raff T, et al. Standardized MRD quantification in European ALL trials: proceedings of the second international symposium on MRD assessment in Kiel, Germany, 18–20 September 2008. Leukemia. 2010;24:521–35.

30. Gupta S, Devidas M, Loh ML, et al. Flow-cytometric vs. -morphologic assessment of remission in childhood acute lymphoblastic leukemia: a report from the Children's Oncology roup (COG). Leukemia. 2018;32:1370–9.
31. O'Connor D, Moorman AV, Wade R, et al. Use of minimal residual disease assessment to redefine induction failure in pediatric acute lymphoblastic leukemia. J Clin Oncol. 2017;35:660–7.
32. Kroger N, Bacher U, Bader P, et al. NCI first international workshop on the biology, prevention, and treatment of relapse after allogeneic hematopoietic stem cell transplantation: report from the committee on disease-specific methods and strategies for monitoring relapse following allogeneic stem cell transplantation. Part I: methods, acute leukemias, and myelodysplastic syndromes. Biol Blood Marrow Transplant. 2010;16:1187–211.
33. Hovorkova L, Zaliova M, Venn NC, et al. Monitoring of childhood ALL using BCR-ABL1 genomic breakpoints identifies a subgroup with CML-like biology. Blood. 2017;129:2771–81.
34. Zaliova M, Fronkova E, Krejcikova K, et al. Quantification of fusion transcript reveals a subgroup with distinct biological properties and predicts relapse in BCR/ABL-positive ALL: implications for residual disease monitoring. Leukemia. 2009;23:944–51.
35. Wood BL. Principles of minimal residual disease detection for hematopoietic neoplasms by flow cytometry. Cytometry B Clin Cytom. 2016;90:47–53.
36. Coustan-Smith E, Behm FG, Sanchez J, et al. Immunological detection of minimal residual disease in children with acute lymphoblastic leukaemia. Lancet. 1998;351:550–4.
37. Vidriales MB, Perez JJ, Lopez-Berges MC, et al. Minimal residual disease in adolescent (older than 14 years) and adult acute lymphoblastic leukemias: early immunophenotypic evaluation has high clinical value. Blood. 2003;101:4695–700.
38. Borowitz MJ, Pullen DJ, Winick N, et al. Comparison of diagnostic and relapse flow cytometry phenotypes in childhood acute lymphoblastic leukemia: implications for residual disease detection: a report from the Children's Oncology Group. Cytometry B Clin Cytom. 2005;68:18–24.
39. Guglielmi C, Cordone I, Boecklin F, et al. Immunophenotype of adult and childhood acute lymphoblastic leukemia: changes at first relapse and clinico-prognostic implications. Leukemia. 1997;11:1501–7.
40. Lucio P, Gaipa G, van Lochem EG, et al. BIOMED-I concerted action report: flow cytometric immunophenotyping of precursor B-ALL with standardized triple-stainings. BIOMED-1 concerted action investigation of minimal residual disease in acute leukemia: international standardization and clinical evaluation. Leukemia. 2001;15:1185–92.
41. Hur M, Chang YH, Lee DS, et al. Immunophenotypic and cytogenetic changes in acute leukaemia at relapse. Clin Lab Haematol. 2001;23:173–9.
42. Gaipa G, Basso G, Aliprandi S, et al. Prednisone induces immunophenotypic modulation of CD10 and CD34 in nonapoptotic B-cell precursor acute lymphoblastic leukemia cells. Cytometry B Clin Cytom. 2008;74:150–5.
43. Gaipa G, Basso G, Maglia O, et al. Drug-induced immunophenotypic modulation in childhood ALL: implications for minimal residual disease detection. Leukemia. 2005;19:49–56.
44. Dworzak MN, Gaipa G, Schumich A, et al. Modulation of antigen expression in B-cell precursor acute lymphoblastic leukemia during induction therapy is partly transient: evidence for a drug-induced regulatory phenomenon. Results of the AIEOP-BFM-ALL-FLOW-MRD-Study Group. Cytometry B Clin Cytom. 2010;78:147–53.
45. Roshal M, Fromm JR, Winter S, et al. Immaturity associated antigens are lost during induction for T cell lymphoblastic leukemia: implications for minimal residual disease detection. Cytometry B Clin Cytom. 2010;78:139–46.
46. Wood B. Multicolor immunophenotyping: human immune system hematopoiesis. Methods Cell Biol. 2004;75:559–76.
47. Wood BL. Flow cytometric monitoring of residual disease in acute leukemia. Methods Mol Biol. 2013;999:123–36.

48. Karawajew L, Dworzak M, Ratei R, et al. Minimal residual disease analysis by eight-color flow cytometry in relapsed childhood acute lymphoblastic leukemia. Haematologica. 2015;100:935–44.
49. Shaver AC, Greig BW, Mosse CA, et al. B-ALL minimal residual disease flow cytometry: an application of a novel method for optimization of a single-tube model. Am J Clin Pathol. 2015;143:716–24.
50. Dworzak MN, Gaipa G, Ratei R, et al. Standardization of flow cytometric minimal residual disease evaluation in acute lymphoblastic leukemia: multicentric assessment is feasible. Cytometry B Clin Cytom. 2008;74:331–40.
51. Coustan-Smith E, Song G, Clark C, et al. New markers for minimal residual disease detection in acute lymphoblastic leukemia. Blood. 2011;117:6267–76.
52. Gaipa G, Cazzaniga G, Valsecchi MG, et al. Time point-dependent concordance of flow cytometry and real-time quantitative polymerase chain reaction for minimal residual disease detection in childhood acute lymphoblastic leukemia. Haematologica. 2012;97:1582–93.
53. Theunissen P, Mejstrikova E, Sedek L, et al. Standardized flow cytometry for highly sensitive MRD measurements in B-cell acute lymphoblastic leukemia. Blood. 2017;129:347–57.
54. Topp MS, Gockbuget N, Stein AS. Correction to Lancet Oncol 2015; 16: 60, 61. Safety and activity of blinatumomab for adult patients with relapsed or refractory B-precursor acute lymphoblastic leukaemia: a multi-centre, single-arm, phase 2 study. Lancet Oncol. 2015;16:e158.
55. Maude SL, Teachey DT, Porter DL, et al. CD19-targeted chimeric antigen receptor T-cell therapy for acute lymphoblastic leukemia. Blood. 2015;125:4017–23.
56. Maude SL, Frey N, Shaw PA, et al. Chimeric antigen receptor T cells for sustained remissions in leukemia. N Engl J Med. 2014;371:1507–17.
57. Zhu M, Wu B, Brandl C, et al. Blinatumomab, a bispecific T-cell engager (BiTE((R))) for CD-19 targeted cancer immunotherapy: clinical pharmacology and its implications. Clin Pharmacokinet. 2016;55:1271–88.
58. Zugmaier G, Gokbuget N, Klinger M, et al. Long-term survival and T-cell kinetics in relapsed/refractory ALL patients who achieved MRD response after blinatumomab treatment. Blood. 2015;126:2578–84.
59. Cherian S, Miller V, McCullouch V, et al. A novel flow cytometric assay for detection of residual disease in patients with B-lymphoblastic leukemia/lymphoma post anti-CD19 therapy. Cytometry B Clin Cytom. 2018;94:112–20.
60. van der Velden VH, Cazzaniga G, Schrauder A, et al. Analysis of minimal residual disease by Ig/TCR gene rearrangements: guidelines for interpretation of real-time quantitative PCR data. Leukemia. 2007;21:604–11.
61. Szczepanski T, Beishuizen A, Pongers-Willemse MJ, et al. Cross-lineage T cell receptor gene rearrangements occur in more than ninety percent of childhood precursor-B acute lymphoblastic leukemias: alternative PCR targets for detection of minimal residual disease. Leukemia. 1999;13:196–205.
62. van Dongen JJ, Langerak AW, Bruggemann M, et al. Design and standardization of PCR primers and protocols for detection of clonal immunoglobulin and T-cell receptor gene recombinations in suspect lymphoproliferations: report of the BIOMED-2 concerted action BMH4-CT98-3936. Leukemia. 2003;17:2257–317.
63. Bruggemann M, van der Velden VH, Raff T, et al. Rearranged T-cell receptor beta genes represent powerful targets for quantification of minimal residual disease in childhood and adult T-cell acute lymphoblastic leukemia. Leukemia. 2004;18:709–19.
64. van der Velden VH, Szczepanski T, Wijkhuijs JM, et al. Age-related patterns of immunoglobulin and T-cell receptor gene rearrangements in precursor-B-ALL: implications for detection of minimal residual disease. Leukemia. 2003;17:1834–44.
65. Szczepanski T, Willemse MJ, Brinkhof B, et al. Comparative analysis of Ig and TCR gene rearrangements at diagnosis and at relapse of childhood precursor-B-ALL provides improved strategies for selection of stable PCR targets for monitoring of minimal residual disease. Blood. 2002;99:2315–23.

66. Germano G, del Giudice L, Palatron S, et al. Clonality profile in relapsed precursor-B-ALL children by GeneScan and sequencing analyses. Consequences on minimal residual disease monitoring. Leukemia. 2003;17:1573–82.
67. Szczepanski T, van der Velden VH, Raff T, et al. Comparative analysis of T-cell receptor gene rearrangements at diagnosis and relapse of T-cell acute lymphoblastic leukemia (T-ALL) shows high stability of clonal markers for monitoring of minimal residual disease and reveals the occurrence of second T-ALL. Leukemia. 2003;17:2149–56.
68. Szczepanski T. Why and how to quantify minimal residual disease in acute lymphoblastic leukemia? Leukemia. 2007;21:622–6.
69. Pongers-Willemse MJ, Verhagen OJ, Tibbe GJ, et al. Real-time quantitative PCR for the detection of minimal residual disease in acute lymphoblastic leukemia using junctional region specific TaqMan probes. Leukemia. 1998;12:2006–14.
70. van der Velden VH, Panzer-Grumayer ER, Cazzaniga G, et al. Optimization of PCR-based minimal residual disease diagnostics for childhood acute lymphoblastic leukemia in a multicenter setting. Leukemia. 2007;21:706–13.
71. Bashford-Rogers RJ, Nicolaou KA, Bartram J, et al. Eye on the B-ALL: B-cell receptor repertoires reveal persistence of numerous B-lymphoblastic leukemia subclones from diagnosis to relapse. Leukemia. 2016;30:2312–21.
72. Pulsipher MA, Carlson C, Langholz B, et al. IgH-V(D)J NGS-MRD measurement pre- and early post-allotransplant defines very low- and very high-risk ALL patients. Blood. 2015;125:3501–8.
73. Faham M, Zheng J, Moorhead M, et al. Deep-sequencing approach for minimal residual disease detection in acute lymphoblastic leukemia. Blood. 2012;120:5173–80.
74. Wu D, Sherwood A, Fromm JR, et al. High-throughput sequencing detects minimal residual disease in acute T lymphoblastic leukemia. Sci Transl Med. 2012;4:134ra63.
75. Wu D, Emerson RO, Sherwood A, et al. Detection of minimal residual disease in B lymphoblastic leukemia by high-throughput sequencing of IGH. Clin Cancer Res. 2014;20:4540–8.
76. van Dongen JJ, Orfao A, EuroFlow C. EuroFlow: resetting leukemia and lymphoma immunophenotyping. Basis for companion diagnostics and personalized medicine. Leukemia. 2012;26:1899–907.
77. Wood BL, Arroz M, Barnett D, et al. 2006 Bethesda international consensus recommendations on the immunophenotypic analysis of hematolymphoid neoplasia by flow cytometry: optimal reagents and reporting for the flow cytometric diagnosis of hematopoietic neoplasia. Cytometry B Clin Cytom. 2007;72(Suppl 1):S14–22.
78. Keeney M, Wood BL, Hedley BD, et al. A QA program for MRD testing demonstrates that systematic education can reduce discordance among experienced interpreters. Cytometry B Clin Cytom. 2018;94:239–49.
79. DiGiuseppe JA, Tadmor MD, Pe'er D. Detection of minimal residual disease in B lymphoblastic leukemia using viSNE. Cytometry B Clin Cytom. 2015;88:294–304.
80. Ryan J, Quinn F, Meunier A, et al. Minimal residual disease detection in childhood acute lymphoblastic leukaemia patients at multiple time-points reveals high levels of concordance between molecular and immunophenotypic approaches. Br J Haematol. 2009;144:107–15.
81. Thorn I, Forestier E, Botling J, et al. Minimal residual disease assessment in childhood acute lymphoblastic leukaemia: a Swedish multi-centre study comparing real-time polymerase chain reaction and multicolour flow cytometry. Br J Haematol. 2011;152:743–53.
82. van der Velden VH, Wijkhuijs JM, van Dongen JJ. Non-specific amplification of patient-specific Ig/TCR gene rearrangements depends on the time point during therapy: implications for minimal residual disease monitoring. Leukemia. 2008;22:641–4.
83. Kerst G, Kreyenberg H, Roth C, et al. Concurrent detection of minimal residual disease (MRD) in childhood acute lymphoblastic leukaemia by flow cytometry and real-time PCR. Br J Haematol. 2005;128:774–82.
84. Neale GA, Coustan-Smith E, Stow P, et al. Comparative analysis of flow cytometry and polymerase chain reaction for the detection of minimal residual disease in childhood acute lymphoblastic leukemia. Leukemia. 2004;18:934–8.

85. Denys B, van der Sluijs-Gelling AJ, Homburg C, et al. Improved flow cytometric detection of minimal residual disease in childhood acute lymphoblastic leukemia. Leukemia. 2013;27:635–41.
86. Kotrova M, Muzikova K, Mejstrikova E, et al. The predictive strength of next-generation sequencing MRD detection for relapse compared with current methods in childhood ALL. Blood. 2015;126:1045–7.
87. Wood B, Wu D, Crossley B, et al. Measurable residual disease detection by high-throughput sequencing improves risk stratification for pediatric B-ALL. Blood. 2018;131:1350–9.
88. Berry DA, Zhou S, Higley H, et al. Association of minimal residual disease with clinical outcome in pediatric and adult acute lymphoblastic leukemia: a meta-analysis. JAMA Oncol. 2017;3(7):e170580.
89. Schrappe M, Valsecchi MG, Bartram CR, et al. Late MRD response determines relapse risk overall and in subsets of childhood T-cell ALL: results of the AIEOP-BFM-ALL 2000 study. Blood. 2011;118:2077–84.
90. van Dongen JJ, Seriu T, Panzer-Grumayer ER, et al. Prognostic value of minimal residual disease in acute lymphoblastic leukaemia in childhood. Lancet. 1998;352:1731–8.
91. Eckert C, Hagedorn N, Sramkova L, et al. Monitoring minimal residual disease in children with high-risk relapses of acute lymphoblastic leukemia: prognostic relevance of early and late assessment. Leukemia. 2015;29:1648–55.
92. Gokbuget N, Kneba M, Raff T, et al. Adult patients with acute lymphoblastic leukemia and molecular failure display a poor prognosis and are candidates for stem cell transplantation and targeted therapies. Blood. 2012;120:1868–76.
93. Gokbuget N, Dombret H, Giebel S, et al. Minimal residual disease level predicts outcome in adults with Ph-negative B-precursor acute lymphoblastic leukemia. Hematology. 2019;24:337–48.
94. Salek C, Folber F, Fronkova E, et al. Early MRD response as a prognostic factor in adult patients with acute lymphoblastic leukemia. Eur J Haematol. 2016;96:276–84.
95. Sekiya Y, Xu Y, Muramatsu H, et al. Clinical utility of next-generation sequencing-based minimal residual disease in paediatric B-cell acute lymphoblastic leukaemia. Br J Haematol. 2017;176:248–57.
96. Torra OS, Othus M, Williamson DW, et al. Minimal residual disease detection by next generation sequencing in adult B-cell acute lymphoblastic leukemia (ALL) patients treated on SWOG trial S0333. Blood. 2014;124:2399.
97. Campana D, Leung W. Clinical significance of minimal residual disease in patients with acute leukaemia undergoing haematopoietic stem cell transplantation. Br J Haematol. 2013;162:147–61.
98. Bader P, Kreyenberg H, Henze GH, et al. Prognostic value of minimal residual disease quantification before allogeneic stem-cell transplantation in relapsed childhood acute lymphoblastic leukemia: the ALL-REZ BFM Study Group. J Clin Oncol. 2009;27:377–84.
99. Bar M, Wood BL, Radich JP, et al. Impact of minimal residual disease, detected by flow cytometry, on outcome of myeloablative hematopoietic cell transplantation for acute lymphoblastic leukemia. Leuk Res Treatment. 2014;2014:421723.
100. Logan AC, Vashi N, Faham M, et al. Immunoglobulin and T cell receptor gene high-throughput sequencing quantifies minimal residual disease in acute lymphoblastic leukemia and predicts post-transplantation relapse and survival. Biol Blood Marrow Transplant. 2014;20:1307–13.
101. Terwey TH, Hemmati PG, Nagy M, et al. Comparison of chimerism and minimal residual disease monitoring for relapse prediction after allogeneic stem cell transplantation for adult acute lymphoblastic leukemia. Biol Blood Marrow Transplant. 2014;20:1522–9.
102. Miglino M, Berisso G, Grasso R, et al. Allogeneic bone marrow transplantation (BMT) for adults with acute lymphoblastic leukemia (ALL): predictive role of minimal residual disease monitoring on relapse. Bone Marrow Transplant. 2002;30:579–85.
103. Uzunel M, Jaksch M, Mattsson J, et al. Minimal residual disease detection after allogeneic stem cell transplantation is correlated to relapse in patients with acute lymphoblastic leukaemia. Br J Haematol. 2003;122:788–94.

104. Spinelli O, Peruta B, Tosi M, et al. Clearance of minimal residual disease after allogeneic stem cell transplantation and the prediction of the clinical outcome of adult patients with high-risk acute lymphoblastic leukemia. Haematologica. 2007;92:612–8.
105. Bader P, Kreyenberg H, von Stackelberg A, et al. Monitoring of minimal residual disease after allogeneic stem-cell transplantation in relapsed childhood acute lymphoblastic leukemia allows for the identification of impending relapse: results of the ALL-BFM-SCT 2003 trial. J Clin Oncol. 2015;33:1275–84.
106. Ravandi F, Jorgensen JL, Thomas DA, et al. Detection of MRD may predict the outcome of patients with Philadelphia chromosome-positive ALL treated with tyrosine kinase inhibitors plus chemotherapy. Blood. 2013;122:1214–21.
107. Short NJ, Jabbour E, Sasaki K, et al. Impact of complete molecular response on survival in patients with Philadelphia chromosome-positive acute lymphoblastic leukemia. Blood. 2016;128:504–7.
108. Tanguy-Schmidt A, Rousselot P, Chalandon Y, et al. Long-term follow-up of the imatinib GRAAPH-2003 study in newly diagnosed patients with de novo Philadelphia chromosome-positive acute lymphoblastic leukemia: a GRAALL study. Biol Blood Marrow Transplant. 2013;19:150–5.
109. Chalandon Y, Thomas X, Hayette S, et al. Randomized study of reduced-intensity chemotherapy combined with imatinib in adults with Ph-positive acute lymphoblastic leukemia. Blood. 2015;125:3711–9.
110. Lussana F, Intermesoli T, Gianni F, et al. Achieving molecular remission before allogeneic stem cell transplantation in adult patients with Philadelphia chromosome-positive acute lymphoblastic leukemia: impact on relapse and long-term outcome. Biol Blood Marrow Transplant. 2016;22:1983–7.
111. Nishiwaki S, Imai K, Mizuta S, et al. Impact of MRD and TKI on allogeneic hematopoietic cell transplantation for Ph+ALL: a study from the adult ALL WG of the JSHCT. Bone Marrow Transplant. 2016;51:43–50.
112. Kantarjian HM, DeAngelo DJ, Stelljes M, et al. Inotuzumab ozogamicin versus standard therapy for acute lymphoblastic leukemia. N Engl J Med. 2016;375:740–53.
113. Topp MS, Gokbuget N, Stein AS, et al. Safety and activity of blinatumomab for adult patients with relapsed or refractory B-precursor acute lymphoblastic leukaemia: a multicentre, single-arm, phase 2 study. Lancet Oncol. 2015;16:57–66.
114. Gokbuget N, Dombret H, Bonifacio M, et al. Blinatumomab for minimal residual disease in adults with B-cell precursor acute lymphoblastic leukemia. Blood. 2018;131:1522–31.
115. Kantarjian H, Stein A, Gokbuget N, et al. Blinatumomab versus chemotherapy for advanced acute lymphoblastic leukemia. N Engl J Med. 2017;376:836–47.
116. Davila ML, Riviere I, Wang X, et al. Efficacy and toxicity management of 19-28z CAR T cell therapy in B cell acute lymphoblastic leukemia. Sci Transl Med. 2014;6:224ra25.
117. Lee DW, Kochenderfer JN, Stetler-Stevenson M, et al. T cells expressing CD19 chimeric antigen receptors for acute lymphoblastic leukaemia in children and young adults: a phase 1 dose-escalation trial. Lancet. 2015;385:517–28.
118. Gardner RA, Finney O, Annesley C, et al. Intent-to-treat leukemia remission by CD19 CAR T cells of defined formulation and dose in children and young adults. Blood. 2017;129:3322–31.
119. Mullighan CG, Jeha S, Pei D, et al. Outcome of children with hypodiploid ALL treated with risk-directed therapy based on MRD levels. Blood. 2015;126:2896–9.
120. Roberts KG, Pei D, Campana D, et al. Outcomes of children with BCR-ABL1-like acute lymphoblastic leukemia treated with risk-directed therapy based on the levels of minimal residual disease. J Clin Oncol. 2014;32:3012–20.
121. Eckert C, Henze G, Seeger K, et al. Use of allogeneic hematopoietic stem-cell transplantation based on minimal residual disease response improves outcomes for children with relapsed acute lymphoblastic leukemia in the intermediate-risk group. J Clin Oncol. 2013;31:2736–42.
122. Pui CH, Pei D, Coustan-Smith E, et al. Clinical utility of sequential minimal residual disease measurements in the context of risk-based therapy in childhood acute lymphoblastic leukaemia: a prospective study. Lancet Oncol. 2015;16:465–74.

123. Campana D. Minimal residual disease monitoring in childhood acute lymphoblastic leukemia. Curr Opin Hematol. 2012;19:313–8.
124. Bassan R, Spinelli O, Oldani E, et al. Improved risk classification for risk-specific therapy based on the molecular study of minimal residual disease (MRD) in adult acute lymphoblastic leukemia (ALL). Blood. 2009;113:4153–62.
125. Vora A, Goulden N, Wade R, et al. Treatment reduction for children and young adults with low-risk acute lymphoblastic leukaemia defined by minimal residual disease (UKALL 2003): a randomised controlled trial. Lancet Oncol. 2013;14:199–209.
126. Pieters R, de Groot-Kruseman H, Van der Velden V, et al. Successful therapy reduction and intensification for childhood acute lymphoblastic leukemia based on minimal residual disease monitoring: study ALL10 from the Dutch Childhood Oncology Group. J Clin Oncol. 2016;34:2591–601.
127. Spinella JF, Richer C, Cassart P, et al. Mutational dynamics of early and late relapsed childhood ALL: rapid clonal expansion and long-term dormancy. Blood Adv. 2018;2:177–88.
128. van der Velden VH, Jacobs DC, Wijkhuijs AJ, et al. Minimal residual disease levels in bone marrow and peripheral blood are comparable in children with T cell acute lymphoblastic leukemia (ALL), but not in precursor-B-ALL. Leukemia. 2002;16:1432–6.
129. Volejnikova J, Mejstrikova E, Valova T, et al. Minimal residual disease in peripheral blood at day 15 identifies a subgroup of childhood B-cell precursor acute lymphoblastic leukemia with superior prognosis. Haematologica. 2011;96:1815–21.
130. Theunissen PMJ, van Zessen D, Stubbs AP, et al. Antigen receptor sequencing of paired bone marrow samples shows homogeneous distribution of acute lymphoblastic leukemia subclones. Haematologica. 2017;102:1869–77.
131. Fries C, Adlowitz DG, Spence JM, et al. Acute lymphoblastic leukemia clonal distribution between bone marrow and peripheral blood. Pediatr Blood Cancer. 2020;67:e28280.
132. Borowitz MJ, Pullen DJ, Shuster JJ, et al. Minimal residual disease detection in childhood precursor-B-cell acute lymphoblastic leukemia: relation to other risk factors. A Children's Oncology Group study. Leukemia. 2003;17:1566–72.
133. O'Connor D, Enshaei A, Bartram J, et al. Genotype-Specific Minimal Residual Disease Interpretation Improves Stratification in Pediatric Acute Lymphoblastic Leukemia. J Clin Oncol. 2018;36:34–43.
134. Pemmaraju N, Kantarjian H, Jorgensen JL, et al. Significance of recurrence of minimal residual disease detected by multi-parameter flow cytometry in patients with acute lymphoblastic leukemia in morphological remission. Am J Hematol. 2017;92:279–85.
135. Larsen EC, Devidas M, Chen S, et al. Dexamethasone and high-dose methotrexate improve outcome for children and young adults with high-risk B-acute lymphoblastic leukemia: a report from Children's Oncology Group Study AALL0232. J Clin Oncol. 2016;34:2380–8.
136. Parker C, Waters R, Leighton C, et al. Effect of mitoxantrone on outcome of children with first relapse of acute lymphoblastic leukaemia (ALL R3): an open-label randomised trial. Lancet. 2010;376:2009–17.
137. Galimberti S, Devidas M, Lucenti A, et al. Validation of minimal residual disease as surrogate endpoint for event-free survival in childhood acute lymphoblastic leukemia. JNCI Cancer Spectr. 2018;2:pky069.

Part II
Therapeutics

Chapter 4
Treatment of Pediatric B- and T-Cell Acute Lymphoblastic Leukemia

Laura E. Hogan, Luke D. Maese, Keith J. August, and Jennifer L. McNeer

Introduction/Epidemiology

Acute lymphoblastic leukemia (ALL) is the fourth most common leukemia after acute myeloid leukemia (AML), chronic lymphocytic leukemia (CLL), and chronic myeloid leukemia (CML), with an estimated 64,200 new cases worldwide in 2017 and 5930 new cases in the USA in 2019 [1, 2]. Half of the cases occur in children, making it the most common childhood cancer. There are 30 cases per million in those under the age of 20 in the USA, and approximately 3000 children are diagnosed annually [1, 3]. B-cell ALL (B-ALL) and T-cell ALL (T-ALL) are the primary immunophenotypes diagnosed in children, accounting for 85% and 15% of childhood ALL, respectively. B-ALL is more prevalent in Caucasian (35.6 cases per million) and Hispanic (40.9 per million) populations compared to black (14.8 per million) populations, and the peak age range at diagnosis is 2–5 years [4]. T-ALL on the other hand has a 1.7-fold higher incidence in black children compared to

L. E. Hogan
Stony Brook Children's, Stony Brook, NY, USA
e-mail: Laura.Hogan@stonybrookmedicine.edu

L. D. Maese
Department of Pediatrics and Huntsman Cancer Institute, University of Utah, Salt Lake City, UT, USA
e-mail: luke.maese@hsc.utah.edu

K. J. August
Division of Pediatric Hematology/Oncology, Children's Mercy Hospital, Kansas City, MO, USA
e-mail: kjaugust@cmh.edu

J. L. McNeer (✉)
Section of Pediatric Hematology/Oncology, The University of Chicago Comer Children's Hospital, Chicago, IL, USA
e-mail: jmcneer@peds.bsd.uchicago.edu

M. R. Litzow, E. A. Raetz (eds.), *Clinical Management of Acute Lymphoblastic Leukemia*, https://doi.org/10.1007/978-3-030-85147-7_4

Caucasian children on a series of Children's Cancer Group (CCG) clinical trials [5–7]. The incidence of T-ALL also increases with age, with T-ALL comprising 25% of ALL diagnoses in those ≥20 years of age [6–8]. Through careful disease characterization and risk stratification of patients, cure rates for both B-ALL and T-ALL have increased tremendously over the past several decades.

Currently over 90% of children diagnosed with ALL in the USA are ultimately cured of their disease [3, 9, 10]. Despite high cure rates, disease that is refractory to upfront therapy or that relapses after initial remission continues to be a significant challenge, as salvage rates for these children remain suboptimal. Often these children require hematopoietic stem cell transplant (HSCT) for cure, which carries a high rate of treatment-related morbidity and mortality and a significant burden of late effects. In recent years there has been remarkable development of effective immunotherapies and other targeted treatments. These therapies carry the promise of continued improvement in outcomes, ideally with less toxicity, and are being incorporated into treatment regimens for newly diagnosed patients.

Biology

B-ALL

The field of cancer cytogenetics began with the identification of the Philadelphia chromosome in patients with CML and the subsequent discovery of the hallmark pathogenic translocation between chromosomes 9 and 22 encountered in this disease [11]. Since then, a number of such translocations have been described, with breakpoints characterized in increasingly fine detail. These translocations are now recognized as drivers of ALL development and, for B-ALL, are a component of the risk stratification used to guide treatment. The backbone of leukemia cytogenetic analysis remains G-banding to produce a cytogenetic karyotype, which identifies many of the relevant chromosome abnormalities in B-ALL [12]. Fluorescence in situ hybridization (FISH) and reverse transcription polymerase chain reaction (RT-PCR) complement karyotypic analysis as means to identify more cryptic aberrations [12].

Certain somatic chromosomal aberrations within leukemic blasts are considered favorable and are associated with improved outcomes (Table 4.1). Such changes include a translocation between chromosomes 12 and 21 [t(12;21)(p13;q22)]/*ETV6-RUNX1*, or high hyperdiploidy defined as a modal chromosome number of 51–65 chromosomes, particularly if there are trisomies of chromosomes 4 and 10 [13, 14]. Other abnormalities such as t(9;22)(q34;q11.2)/*BCR-ABL1*/Philadelphia chromosome-positive (Ph+), hypodiploidy (modal chromosome number <44), intrachromosomal amplification of chromosome 21 (iAMP21), 11q23/*KMT2A* rearrangements, t(17;19)(q21-q22;p13), or the *IGH* translocations and *CRLF2* rearrangements found in Philadelphia chromosome-like (Ph-like, see below) B-ALL

Table 4.1 Cytogenetic abnormalities in B-ALL

Favorable	Unfavorable	Intermediate but recurrent
t(12;21)(p13;q22); *ETV6-RUNX1*	11q23 Rearrangements; *KMT2A*-R t(4;11)(q21;q23)	t(1;19)(q23;p13.3); *TCF3-PBX1*
High hyperdiploidy (51–65 chromosomes) Double trisomy of chromosomes 4 and 10	Hypodiploidy (modal number <44 or DNA Index <0.81)	Other trisomies
	iAMP21	
	t(9;22)(q34;q11.1); *BCR-ABL*	
	t(17;19)(q21-q22;p13.3)	
	IGH@ translocations and *CRLF2* rearrangements associated with Ph-like B-ALL	

indicate higher risk disease and worse outcomes [12–20]. Also frequently present are changes that are considered of intermediate risk, such as t(1;19)(q23;p13.3)/*TCF3-PBX1* and trisomies of various other chromosomes [12, 21].

The prevalence of genomic lesions in B-ALL varies by age. For example, *KMT2A* rearrangements, in particular t(4;11)(q21;q23), are frequently observed in infant ALL and harbor a poor prognosis [22, 23]. On the other hand, more than half of children between the ages of 1 and 10 years are found to have favorable cytogenetics, namely, t(12;21) or high hyperdiploidy [12, 14]. As the age at diagnosis increases, unfavorable cytogenetic findings become more prevalent. The incidence of Ph+ B-ALL increases in adolescents, as do aberrations such as *IGH* translocations and *CRLF2* rearrangements that can be associated with Ph-like B-ALL [12, 21]. Cytogenetic findings are incorporated into risk stratification strategies, along with features such as age and white blood cell count (WBC) at presentation, and disease response [24–27].

In addition to analysis of chromosomal changes in leukemic blasts, molecular findings are becoming increasingly important in disease categorization and treatment allocation. The most clinically relevant discovery to date has been that of Ph-like B-ALL, first described in 2009. This subset of B-ALL has a gene expression profile similar to that of Ph+ B-ALL, but without the presence of a BCR-ABL fusion protein [28, 29]. In addition to *IKZF1* deletions, which are also found in Ph+ B-ALL, Ph-like disease is characterized by various aberrations in cytokine receptor and tyrosine kinase pathways potentially targetable by tyrosine kinase inhibitors (TKIs) [30]. Patients with Ph-like B-ALL tend to fare worse than those without this gene signature, similar to the outcomes of Ph+ disease prior to the incorporation of TKIs into treatment regimens. Studies incorporating these targeted agents into treatment regimens for Ph-like B-ALL are ongoing [30, 31].

Other works have led to the discovery of germline predictors of familial leukemia risk as well as predisposition to unique drug metabolism or toxicity profiles. It is now well-established that low-hypodiploid B-ALL is nearly universally associated with mutations in the *TP53* gene, half of which are germline [32, 33]. Hypodiploid B-ALL is a known manifestation of Li-Fraumeni syndrome (LFS), and all such patients should be referred for genetic counseling and germline *TP53* testing [34]. This knowledge also carries implications for treatment regimens, as the historical trend to recommend hematopoietic stem cell transplant (HSCT) in first remission (CR1) for these patients may unnecessarily put them at risk for second malignant neoplasms (SMN) if high doses of alkylators, topoisomerase inhibitors or radiation are included in conditioning regimens. Recent analyses indicate, however, that HSCT is not beneficial to these patients and innovative treatment approaches are required [35, 36].

The interrogation of genomic variants in ALL has expanded not only our understanding of disease biology but also that of host variants impacting susceptibility to ALL, disease response/outcomes, drug metabolism, and toxicity. Historically, apart from LFS, predisposition to ALL was associated with rare genetic syndromes including Bloom, Nijmegen breakage, Wiskott-Aldrich, and ataxia-telangiectasia. However, with the advent of improved germline genomic characterization, several new syndromes predisposing to ALL resulting from pathogenic mutations in *ETV6* and *PAX5* have been identified with more surely to come [34]. In addition to these known pathogenic mutations, genomic studies now reveal additional risk loci that predispose to the development of ALL and may predict response to therapy [37]. Germline single-nucleotide polymorphisms (SNPs) have been identified that are predictive of the presence of minimal residual disease (MRD) during early therapy as well as relapse risk independent of MRD [38, 39]. SNPs have also been found to be predictive of antileukemic drug pharmacokinetics, which likely play a role in disease response and drug toxicity [37, 38, 40]. Only a small number of these SNPs are currently utilized to guide antileukemic drug dosing, namely, variants of *TPMT* and *NUDT15*, which encode thiopurine S-methyltransferase and nucleotide triphosphate diphosphatase, respectively. Patients with variants in these genes are more susceptible to the myelosuppressive effects of mercaptopurine, especially if those variants are homozygous, and dose modifications for mercaptopurine are built into current leukemia protocols [41–45].

T-ALL

Similar to B-ALL, cytogenetic analysis has provided insight into the pathogenicity of chromosomal translocations and rearrangements in T-ALL [46], but a significantly better understanding of T-ALL biology has evolved with the advent of molecular diagnostics. Gene expression profiling has led to the identification of aberrantly expressed transcription factor oncogenes, and more recently, genome- and transcriptome-wide sequencing have provided a more comprehensive understanding of T-ALL pathogenesis [47, 48].

As our understanding of the biology of T-ALL has expanded, several themes have emerged. First, the array of genetic alterations is widely diverse with over 100 driver gene mutations, and individual cases of T-ALL frequently contain greater than ten biologically relevant genomic lesions [47, 49, 50]. Second, although alterations are diverse, they can be grouped into several common categories. Chromosomal translocations, most commonly involving the T-cell receptor (TCR) on chromosomes 7 and 14 and several proto-oncogenes, define a large subgroup. This group is further classified according to partner proto-oncogenes and dysregulated gene expression patterns that further delineate T-ALL subtypes. The most common subtypes according to these characterizations are *TAL1* (30–35%), *TLX3* (20–25%), *HOXA* (5–15%), *TLX1* (5–10%), *LMO2/LYL1* (5–10%), *NKX2-1* (14%), *LMO1/2* (3–10%), *TAL2* (1–3%) [47, 51].

T-ALL can also be sub-classified according to the affected biologic mechanism. Transcriptional regulation with mutations identified in over 20 genes, primarily in the genes listed above, is impacted in over 90% of cases [47, 49]. Cell cycle progression and tumor suppressor pathways are altered in over 80% of cases with *CDKN2A/B* (70–80%) being most commonly mutated [47, 51]. Within the context of T-ALL, the NOTCH signaling pathway plays an important role in promoting T-cell lineage commitment, cell growth, and proliferation. This pathway is altered in nearly 80% of cases, with *NOTCH1* (60–70%) and *FBXW7* (10–30%) being the most commonly mutated genes [47, 52]. Epigenetic lesions are also prevalent, occurring in nearly 70% of cases [47, 49]. Genes involved in DNA methylation (*DNMT3A*), histone methylation (*EED, EZH2, KMD6A, SUZ12*), histone acetylation (*PHF6*), and ubiquitination (*USP7*) have all been found mutated in cases of T-ALL [53, 54]. Other oncogenic signaling pathways such as PI3K-AKT, JAK-STAT, and Ras-MAPK are also implicated in T-ALL pathogenesis with at least one of these affected in up to 70% of patients [47]. Although these pathways are unique, aberrant interleukin-7 (IL-7) signaling is a driver of all three [49]. Gene mutations involving these pathways lead to dysregulated kinase signaling and proliferation of T-ALL.

While the biologic understanding of T-ALL has expanded exponentially in the past decade, this has not translated into significant modifications of risk classification. Unlike in B-ALL, in which biologic characterizations have been converted into clearly defined risk categories, T-ALL subtypes as defined above are not independently associated with outcome [55]. Identified aberrant signaling pathways provide insight into potential future treatment with targeted agents; however evidence that these mutations significantly impact survival is limited. The presence of *NOTCH1* and/or *FBXW7* mutations has been correlated with nominal improvements in outcomes [56]. Biallelic TCRγ deletions were initially found to be associated with a poor response to induction chemotherapy and inferior outcomes in a small group of patients; however a recent investigation of this aberration in a larger cohort confirmed the slow response to chemotherapy, but this did not translate into significant survival differences [57, 58].

Prognostic Factors

At the time of diagnosis and over the course of early phases of treatment, patient and disease characteristics are utilized to risk-stratify patients and tailor therapy accordingly. Patient age and WBC at diagnosis have been long-standing features incorporated into risk stratification algorithms for patients with B-ALL. Infants with ALL have very aggressive disease, are treated according to protocols specific for this age group, and are reviewed in a separate chapter in this book. For non-infant children, age ≥10 years and/or WBC ≥50,000/μL indicate higher-risk disease according to National Cancer Institute (NCI) risk classification guidelines [24]. These features maintain significance on multivariate analyses that incorporate biology and disease response into models predictive of outcomes [24, 26, 27]. In T-ALL, age and WBC at diagnosis are not so clearly prognostic in children, as many pediatric cooperative groups have demonstrated a lack of strong association of outcomes with these features [59–61]. In contrast, a large adult cooperative group study showed an association between traditional prognostic factors including elevated WBC count (>100,000/μL) and age (>35 years old) and inferior outcomes [62]. Historically, T-ALL was considered a more aggressive disease, with inferior outcomes compared to B-ALL. However, with intense Berlin-Frankfurt-Münster (BFM)-based therapy for all T-ALL patients, regardless of presenting features, current outcomes have become quite similar to those of patients with B-ALL [63, 64].

As described above, chromosomal aberrations within B-ALL blasts can be categorized as favorable, unfavorable, or intermediate, with therapy adjusted accordingly. Patients with favorable genetics and good disease response have excellent outcomes with current BFM-based therapy, even for those patients considered NCI high risk at diagnosis [65–67]. Unfavorable genetic findings, however, are an indication to intensify therapy, and historically certain genetic subgroups have undergone HSCT in CR1, even if they had a good response to initial therapy. Over time the use of HSCT in CR1 has decreased, with current practice utilizing disease response as a better indicator of those patients who require this level of intensification [68]. Therapy is not currently risk-adjusted based on cytogenetic or genomic findings in T-ALL.

Finally, regardless of immunophenotype, minimal residual disease (MRD) assessment at early time points is the most significant predictor of outcome [25–27]. This is particularly true in T-ALL due to the lack of other informative prognostic factors [69]. Patients with B-ALL and MRD that persists at a level of ≥0.01% after consolidation therapy (~12 weeks of treatment) fare poorly (5-year disease-free survival (DFS) 39 ± 7%), and this is generally an indication to intensify therapy, often with HSCT in CR1 [26], though clinical trials are currently underway to determine whether chimeric antigen receptor T-cell receptor therapy (CAR-T therapy) may afford at least similar outcomes (NCT03876769). While flow cytometry and polymerase chain reaction (PCR) are the most common methods to assess MRD, more sensitive methodologies, such as high-throughput sequencing, are now being explored as a means to detect lower levels of MRD in patients who have no disease detectable by current standard approaches [70]. The role of this more sensitive assay in risk stratification algorithms is currently being investigated.

The kinetics of disease response to therapy in T-ALL differ from that of B-ALL, as slower blast clearance is much more common in the former. In the AIEOP-BFM ALL 2000 trial, bone marrow MRD measured by PCR at day 78 was highly prognostic, with T-ALL patients who did not achieve an MRD level of <0.1% having a 7-year event free survival (EFS) of 49.8% (SE 5.1%) compared to 80.6% (SE 2.3%) for those patients who were positive at the end of induction (day 33) but <0.1% by day 78 [61]. This slow clearance is principally evident in early T-cell precursor (ETP) ALL where end-induction MRD by flow cytometry is >0.01% in over 80% of patients [71, 72]. Until recently, ETP-ALL was thought to portend a worse outcome compared to other T-ALL; however it has now been shown that contemporary treatment regimens abrogate this risk [72]. For those patients with ETP-ALL, the same time point of day 78 is useful for prognosis, as those with MRD ≥0.1% at day 78 had a 5-year EFS of 46.9% (SE 8.8%), while those that had detectable MRD at either day 33 or 78, but at a level <0.1% by day 78, had a 5 year EFS of 65.6% (SE 5.9%) on the AIEOP-BFM-ALL 2000 study [61].

In the future, T-ALL will likely be risk stratified by combining response to therapy (MRD assessment) with mutational analysis. In the FRALLE2000T study, patients were identified as genetically low risk if they had mutations in *NOTCH1* or *FBXW7* with wild-type *RAS* and *PTEN* and genetically high risk if mutations were found in *RAS* or *PTEN* [73]. Genetically low-risk patients had a cumulative incidence of relapse (CIR) of 11% compared to 36% in the high-risk group. Importantly, this result was independent of MRD measured at day 35. A risk stratification strategy using this genetic algorithm combined with MRD results and initial WBC was extremely successful at identifying a low-risk population of children with T-ALL who had a 5-year CIR of only 1.7%.

Disease Management and Treatment Strategy

This section will be limited to a general description of therapeutic approaches and rationale for patients with B-ALL and T-ALL. Please see the relevant chapters for discussion of particular groups such as Ph+ and Ph-like B-ALL, as well as prophylaxis and control of central nervous system (CNS) disease and the treatment of ALL in infants.

The treatment of ALL occurs in sequential blocks, or phases of therapy (Fig. 4.1). Most cooperative groups utilize an approach pioneered by the BFM study group [74], beginning with a remission induction phase (referred to as "protocol IA" in Europe), followed by consolidation therapy/protocol IB. Induction therapy varies slightly across cooperative group and consortium protocols but generally includes vincristine, a corticosteroid, asparaginase, and, depending on the treating group and risk designation, an anthracycline. BFM-based consolidation therapy consists of cyclophosphamide, cytarabine, and 6-mercaptopurine, with the Children's Oncology

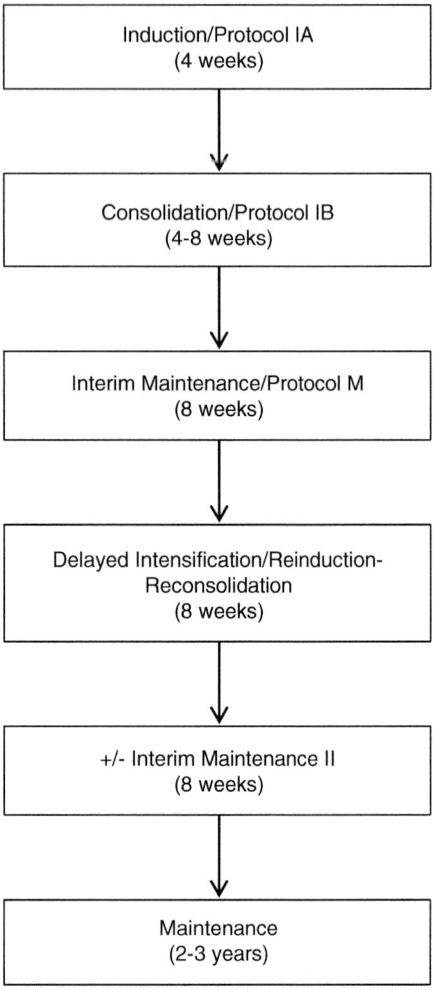

Fig. 4.1 Treatment phases for acute lymphoblastic leukemia

Group (COG) also including vincristine and asparaginase during periods of myelosuppression ("augmented" BFM, aBFM). The COG uses a less intense consolidation for patients with standard-risk B-ALL, which consists largely of oral mercaptopurine and intrathecal chemotherapy.

The use of glucocorticoids varies across treatment protocols, with both dexamethasone and prednisone used to treat ALL (Table 4.2). Dexamethasone has higher potency and increased CNS penetration but is also associated with increases in toxicity, specifically a higher infection rate, and an increased incidence of osteonecrosis. Therefore the increased efficacy must be balanced with the potential for more side and late effects. In the AIEOP-BFM-ALL 2000 trial, children with ALL were randomized to receive either prednisone or dexamethasone as the induction steroid following a 7-day prednisone pre-phase. Pediatric patients randomized to the

Table 4.2 Studies for newly diagnosed patients

Study question	Study	Patient population[a]	Significant findings	
Dexamethasone versus prednisone	AIEOP-BFM ALL 2000 [75]	B- and T-ALL (1–18 years)	*Relapse risk* DEX 13.7% PRED 21.3%	*T-ALL overall survival* DEX 80.8% PRED 76.2%
	UKALL97/99 [76]	B- and T-ALL (1–18 years)	*5-year CNS relapse rate* DEX-based induction 2.5% PRED-based induction 5%	
	AALL0232 [78]	B-ALL (1–9 years)	*5-year EFS* DH 91.2% PH 80.8%	DC 83.2% PC 82.1%
Capizzi-MTX versus HD-MTX	AALL0232 [78]	B-ALL (>1 and <31 years)	*5-year EFS* HD-MTX 79.6% C-MTX 75.2%	*5-year OS* HD-MTX 88.9% C-MTX 86.1%
	AALL0434 [64]	T-ALL (>1 and <31 years)	*5-year DFS* HD-MTX 85.3% C-MTX 91.5%	*5-year OS* HD-MTX 89.4% C-MTX 93.7%
Omission of CNS radiation	EORTC-CLG 58951 [80]	B- and T-ALL (<18 years)	Isolated T-ALL CNS relapse rate 5.3% Total T-ALL relapse rate involving CNS 8.5%	
	SJCRH Total Therapy XV [81]	B- and T-ALL (≥1 and ≤18 years)	Isolated CNS relapse rate 8.1%	
	UKALL 2003 [82]	B- and T-ALL (1–24 years)	CNS relapse rate 3.5%	
Addition of nelarabine to chemotherapy	AALL0434 [63]	T-ALL (>1 and <31 years)	*4-year DFS* Nelarabine 88.9% No nelarabine 83.3%	
Pediatric-inspired therapy for AYAs with ALL	C10403 [90]	B- and T-ALL (16–39 years)	3-year EFS 59% 3-year OS 73%	
	DFCI 01-175 [91]	B- and T-ALL (18–50 years)	4-year DFS 69% (of those reaching CR) 4-year OS 67% (all patients)	

DEX dexamethasone, *PRED* prednisone, *C-MTX* Capizzi-methotrexate, *HD-MTX* high-dose methotrexate, *DH* DEX with HD-MTX, *DC* DEX with C-MTX, *PH* PRED with HD-MTX, *PC* PRED with C-MTX, *CNS* central nervous system, *EFS* event-free survival, *DFS* disease-free survival, *OS* overall survival, *AYA* adolescent and young adult, *CR* complete remission

[a]Population relative to this chapter and table, which may be a subset of all eligible patients

dexamethasone arm had a decreased risk of relapse compared to prednisone (13.7% vs. 21.3%, p = 0.024) that did not translate into an overall survival benefit due to increases in toxicity [75]. Notably, patients with T-ALL who demonstrated a good prednisone response defined as peripheral blood absolute blast count <1000 after 7 days had the largest survival benefit with an overall survival of 91.4% for dexamethasone compared to 82.6% with prednisone. The benefit of dexamethasone in preventing CNS relapses was demonstrated in the UKALL97/99 trials. The administration of dexamethasone rather than prednisone during induction therapy reduced the rate of CNS relapse in children with both B- and T-ALL from 5% at 5 years to 2.5% [76]. These studies support the notion that for T-ALL, dexamethasone is the superior steroid. For patients with B-ALL on the other hand, the superiority of dexamethasone is not so clear [77], and the choice of corticosteroid in various phases of therapy is, to some extent, guided by patient age. The COG study AALL0232 was designed to compare dexamethasone versus prednisone in induction therapy for patients with high-risk (HR) B-ALL, but the randomization was halted in patients ≥10 years of age due to excessive rates of osteonecrosis. While dexamethasone was superior in young patients, it did not confer greater efficacy in adolescents [78]. Taken together, these data highlight the complexity of steroid choices which are guided by age, leukemia immunophenotype, and cooperative group preference.

The initial intense phases of therapy are followed by interim maintenance (IM)/protocol M, which consists largely of intravenous methotrexate (MTX) given in escalating low doses without leucovorin rescue (Esc-MTX) with or without two doses of pegylated-asparaginase (PEG) known as Capizzi-style methotrexate (C-MTX) or in intermediate/high doses with leucovorin rescue (HD-MTX). Vincristine is administered as well during this phase, as is mercaptopurine in high-risk protocols that utilize HD-MTX. In the USA, patients with NCI standard-risk (SR) B-ALL without adverse features treated according to COG protocols do not receive HD-MTX during interim maintenance, as clear survival benefits have not been demonstrated in this group [66]. On the other hand, patients with NCI HR B-ALL do benefit from treatment with HD-MTX in IM, including patients with NCI SR B-ALL with adverse biologic features or slow disease response (Table 4.2). On COG study AALL0232, which randomized NCI HR patients to HD-MTX versus C-MTX, 5-year EFS was 79.6 ± 1.6% vs 75.2 ± 1.7% (p = 0.008), and 5-year OS was 88.9 ± 1.2% vs. 86.1 ± 1.4% (p = 0.025) [78].

In a similar comparison for patients with T-ALL, COG study AALL0434 evaluated the optimal delivery of MTX during IM (Table 4.2). Notably this trial enrolled a total of 1562 patients, making it the largest study ever conducted in pediatric T-ALL to date [64]. Enrolled patients were allocated to receive either five doses of C-MTX with vincristine or four doses of HD-MTX (5 g/m^2/dose) along with vincristine and mercaptopurine during the IM phase. The 5-year DFS and OS for the patients randomized to the C-MTX arm were 91.5 ± 3.3% and 93.7 ± 2.9%, which were superior to outcomes on the HD-MTX arm: 85.3 ± 4.2% and 89.4 ± 3.8%, respectively (P = 0.005 for DFS and P = 0.04 for OS). Notably, CNS relapses were more frequent in the patients on the HD-MTX arm with 23 total relapses compared to only 6 on the C-MTX arm. It is important to note that patients on the HD-MTX arm received cranial radiation at a later time point in therapy compared to those on the C-MTX arm and it is unclear whether this difference in timing impacted CNS relapse rates.

Subsequently, there is another phase of intense therapy (delayed intensification), composed of reinduction and reconsolidation phases, with substitutions of chemotherapeutics within drug classes to address drug resistance that may be arising, such as 6-thioguanine for 6-mercaptopurine and doxorubicin for daunorubicin. Some protocols include a second IM phase using Esc-MTX or C-MTX. Debate continues regarding the benefits of this second IM phase. All protocols call for a prolonged maintenance phase consisting largely of oral antimetabolite therapy.

CNS Therapy

Dedicated treatment of the CNS with intensive intrathecal chemotherapy begins during induction and continues throughout therapy. Patients with overt CNS disease at diagnosis are often treated with cranial irradiation, although the current trend has been to decrease significantly, or even omit, radiation therapy for as many patients as possible. CNS therapy is especially important for patients with T-ALL who experience a higher rate of CNS relapse compared to their counterparts with B-ALL. To compensate for this increased risk, many treatment protocols attempt to intensify CNS-directed therapy in T-ALL, with strategies that are heterogenous and widely varied across protocols. A meta-analysis of 78 studies found no difference in event-free survival using four CNS radiation strategies in children with T-ALL: CNS radiation for everyone, risk-directed CNS radiation, CNS radiation only for patients with evidence of CNS involvement of their leukemia (CNS positive patients), and no CNS radiation for all patients [79]. In the EORTC-CLG 58951 study, CNS radiation was omitted for 296 children with T-ALL, with an isolated CNS relapse rate of 5.3% and a total rate of 8.5% for all relapses involving the CNS [80]. The St. Jude Children's Research Hospital Total Therapy XV study also treated 76 children with T-ALL without any CNS radiation with an isolated CNS relapse rate of 8.1% [81]. The UKALL 2003 study treated 388 children with T-ALL without cranial radiation, and the CNS relapse rate was only 3.5% [82]. Knowing that younger patients are at high risk for long-term complications associated with CNS radiation such as neurocognitive impairment, secondary malignancies, and endocrinopathies, limiting cranial radiation to as few children as possible is critical. Methods of intensifying CNS treatment without cranial radiation in children with T-ALL include optimizing intrathecal therapy with the use of additional intrathecal treatments or triple intrathecal chemotherapy, using dexamethasone as the preferred corticosteroid, and intensifying asparaginase therapy. More recently, the benefit of nelarabine has been demonstrated for patients with T-ALL, especially for control of CNS disease (Table 4.2) [63]. Nelarabine is a purine nucleoside analog prodrug of ara-G that selectively incorporates into the DNA of T cells leading to the inhibition of DNA synthesis and can be considered targeted therapy for T-cell disease. In addition to the methotrexate randomization described above, COG AALL0434 randomized patients to receive or not receive six 5-day courses of nelarabine incorporated into a BFM-based chemotherapy backbone. The 4-year DFS for patients randomized to nelarabine was 88.9% ± 2.2% compared to 83.3% ± 2.5% for those who did not receive nelarabine ($p = 0.0332$). In particular, nelarabine significantly decreased the rate of CNS relapses, without significant increases in neurotoxicity compared to standard chemotherapy.

Adolescents and Young Adults

While treatment of certain patient groups is discussed in different chapters of this book, treatment of adolescents and young adults (AYAs) with ALL will be commented on briefly here. A number of retrospective studies have demonstrated improved outcomes for AYAs when treated using pediatric-inspired protocols, rather than adult protocols [83–89]. This finding led to several prospective studies applying pediatric-inspired therapy to young adults (Table 4.2). The Cancer and Acute Leukemia Group B 10403 study (C10403), conducted from 2007 to 2012, treated patients between the ages of 16–39 years with the superior arm of the most recent COG study for B-ALL (COG AALL0232). The 3-year EFS was 59% (95% CI 54–65%) and overall survival (OS) 73% (95% CI 68–78%), significantly better than historical controls (3-year OS 55%) [90]. Similarly, Dana-Farber Cancer Institute (DFCI) used a pediatric regimen for the treatment of patients 18–50 years of age, with a 4-year disease-free survival (DFS) of 69% (95% CI 56–78%) for those patients achieving complete remission (CR, 78 of 92 patients). Of all eligible patients, the 4-year OS was 67% (95% CI 56–76%), significantly better than the historical survival rates of <50% [91]. Studies such as these have confirmed the improved outcomes for AYAs with ALL when treated using a pediatric approach, but outcomes for AYAs are still worse than those of their pediatric counterparts. The cause of this difference in outcome is likely multifactorial, with treatment setting, disease biology, compliance with chemotherapy regimens, and increased toxicity rates all notable contributing factors. T-ALL is more common in the AYA population and has until recently portended a worse prognosis. Cytogenetic abnormalities in B-ALL shift toward more unfavorable profiles at older ages, with a lower incidence of t(12;21)/ETV6-RUNX1 fusion or hyperdiploidy, but more frequent iAMP21 or t(9;22)/BCR-ABL fusion [14, 92]. Finally, Ph-like disease reaches a peak in the AYA age group, conferring worse outcomes [28–30, 93].

Treatment setting likely plays a role in outcomes, as AYAs seek care both in pediatric and adult settings. Importantly, pediatric settings tend to have a broader array of psychosocial services for patients, and these services are particularly important for AYAs [94]. This type of support likely contributes to improved adherence with chemotherapy regimens, which is greatly important given that adherence to the oral chemotherapy that comprises the bulk of the prolonged maintenance phase of therapy has been demonstrated to contribute significantly to patient outcomes. Non-adherence (taking <90% of prescribed maintenance antimetabolite therapy) is associated with a significantly increased relapse risk (HR = 3.9, p = 0.01) [95, 96]. Factors that adversely impact adherence include level of education and presence of a parent or other caregiver to supervise medication administration, both of which can be surmised to affect the AYA population. While no adherence studies specific to the AYA ALL population have been conducted to date, the Alliance for Clinical Trials A041501 study (NCT03150693) has an embedded adherence objective, evaluating adherence to oral maintenance chemotherapy in an AYA ALL population. Overall, familiarity with the intricacies of the disease and psychosocial needs of AYAs with ALL is important, as outcomes are worse for patients treated at non-specialized cancer centers when compared to patients treated at NCI-designated Comprehensive Cancer Centers or COG sites (15–21 years, HR = 1.9, p = 0.005; 22–29 years, HR = 2.6, p < 0.001; 30–39 years, HR = 3.0, p < 0.001) [97].

Recurrent Disease

Despite remarkable survival improvements in newly diagnosed children with B-ALL, treatment of the 10–15% of patients who experience relapse after initial therapy remains a challenge [3, 98, 99]. While SR B-ALL patients have excellent 5-year EFS rates, approximately twice as many children are diagnosed with SR B-ALL as compared to HR B-ALL. Thus, children with SR B-ALL still account for approximately half of B-ALL relapses [100]. Most children with relapsed B-ALL will not be cured, and this remains a leading cause of death in young people, with a 5-year OS of approximately 35–50% following relapse [99–105].

The most important predictors of outcome after B-ALL relapse are length of initial remission, site of relapse, and disease clearance upon reinduction therapy [101–103, 106–110]. These factors are used to stratify patients into high-risk (HR), intermediate-risk (IR), and low-risk (LR) relapses. Patients who relapse early (<36 months from diagnosis) in the bone marrow have dismal outcomes that approach 15% long-term survival, while those who relapse late (>36 months from diagnosis) have approximately a 40–70% rate of salvage [104, 111–114]. The best outcomes occur in patients with late (>18 months from diagnosis) extramedullary relapses, in whom survival rates approach 80% [100, 115, 116]. The importance of end of reinduction MRD has also been demonstrated in the relapse population, with those patients positive for MRD at this time point having inferior outcomes compared to patients with no residual disease [108, 109, 114, 117, 118]. This is especially true for those patients with late bone marrow (>36 months from diagnosis) or extramedullary (>18 months from diagnosis) relapses [114, 117].

Current approaches to relapsed ALL share many similarities to frontline therapy. All patients, regardless of relapse site, require systemic chemotherapy for reinduction using many of the same drugs as for newly diagnosed patients, although generally at increased intensity. For those patients considered to have HR or IR relapses, post-reinduction chemotherapy or immunotherapy followed by HSCT is considered the best chance for cure [100, 119]. Even with this approach, outcomes in patients that have an early marrow relapse and remain MRD positive at the end of reinduction are dismal, with EFS rates of 3–10%, though subsequent clearance of MRD is significantly better when immunotherapy is utilized following reinduction chemotherapy [119, 120]. The longer-term impact of this on EFS remains to be seen. Better outcomes are observed with later relapses, especially if MRD is negative at the end of reinduction. Long-term survival rates for patients with late marrow relapses who are MRD negative at the end of reinduction approach 90% [114]. Patients with late isolated extramedullary relapses who are MRD negative at the end of reinduction also have good outcomes [116, 121]. The majority of these patients with so-called LR relapses can be cured with chemotherapy alone and therefore are not allocated to HSCT in second remission. Outcomes after second or greater relapse, however, are even worse, with 2-year EFS ranging from 10% to 40% for second to eighth salvage therapy [122, 123].

Children with T-ALL that is refractory to treatment or who experience a relapse after achieving remission have exceptionally poor outcomes, and despite aggressive regimens, post-reinduction CR rates have been exceedingly low for children with T-ALL. For example, only two out of seven patients with T-ALL achieved a CR after induction on the COG study AALL01P2 in which the reinduction regimen included an intensification of PEG and a substitution of idarubicin as the anthracycline until excess toxicity rates led to a return to doxorubicin [117]. The addition of bortezomib to an intensive reinduction platform on COG study AALL07P1 improved the CR rate to 68% ± 10% in 22 patients with T-ALL (Table 4.3) [120]. Prior to the successful integration of nelarabine into upfront T-ALL therapy, nelarabine was evaluated in a number of clinical trials for patients with relapsed T-ALL. A COG phase II study of nelarabine in children with first or greater T-cell relapse demonstrated an overall response rate (ORR) of 55% (95% CI 38–72%) for those patients with first relapse and 27% (95% CI 11–43%) for those with second relapse (Table 4.3) [124]. A phase IV observational study reported a similar ORR of 39.3% using nelarabine as a single agent [125]. As nelarabine was well tolerated by the majority of children with relapsed T-ALL and induced remission as a single agent, it has also been studied in combination with other conventional chemotherapy agents. A Therapeutic Advances in Childhood Leukemia (TACL) treatment regimen using nelarabine combined with cyclophosphamide and etoposide reported a CR in four of nine patients with relapsed/refractory T-ALL treated (44%) at varying dose levels (Table 4.3) [126].

For children with T-ALL that achieve a second CR with reinduction therapy, HSCT is considered to be the only curative treatment, though long-term survival rates remain poor. A review of the Center for International Blood and Marrow Transplant Research database identified 229 children with T-ALL who underwent HSCT in second remission. Allogeneic HSCT following a myeloablative conditioning regimen led to a 3-year OS rate of 48% (95% CI 41–55%) [127]. Treatment failures were primarily due to relapse in 30% (95% CI 24–37%) of the patients, with an additional 24% (95% CI 18–30%) experiencing treatment-related mortality by 3 years.

Table 4.3 Studies for patients with relapsed disease

	Study	Patient population[a]	Significant findings	
T-ALL studies	AALL07P1 [120] (bortezomib + chemotherapy)	Relapsed T-ALL (≥1 and ≤31 years)	T-ALL CR rate 68%	
	P9673 [124] (Nelarabine)	Relapsed T-ALL (<21 years)	*Overall response rate* First relapse 55% ≥Second relapse 27%	
	T2008-002 [126] (nelarabine/cyclophosphamide/etoposide)	Relapsed/refractory T-ALL (1–21 years)	T-ALL CR rate 44%	
Blinatumomab studies	AALL1121 [128] (blinatumomab)	Relapsed/refractory B-ALL (<18 years)	CR rate 39%	
	AALL1331 [119] (blinatumomab ± chemotherapy)	Relapsed B-ALL (≥1 and <31 years)	*2 year DFS* *(HR/IR patients)* Blinatumomab 59.3% No blinatumomab 41%	*2-year OS* *(HR/IR patients)* Blinatumomab 79.4% No blinatumomab 59.2%
Inotuzumab studies	INO-VATE [129] (inotuzumab vs. chemotherapy)	Relapsed/refractory B-ALL (≥18 years)	*CR rates* Inotuzumab 80.7% Chemotherapy 33.3%	*MRD-negative rates* Inotuzumab 78.4% Chemotherapy 28.1%
	AALL1621 [131] (inotuzumab)	Relapsed/refractory B-ALL (≥1 and <22 years)	CR rate 58.3% MRD negative (of those in CR) 65.5%	
CAR-T studies	Pedi CART19 [132] (tisagenlecleucel)	Relapsed/refractory B-ALL (1–24 years)	CR rate 90%	
	ELIANA [133] (tisagenlecleucel)	Relapsed/refractory B-ALL (<25 years)	CR rate 81%, all MRD negative 12-month EFS 50%	

CR complete remission, *DFS* disease-free survival, *OS* overall survival, *HR* high risk, *IR* intermediate risk, *MRD* minimal residual disease
[a]Population relative to this chapter and table, which may be a subset of all eligible patients

Novel Therapies

B-ALL

Several novel therapies have shown great promise in R/R B-ALL. Blinatumomab is a bispecific T-cell engager targeting CD19 that has shown to be highly effective in the treatment of R/R B-cell malignancies. In 2016, the US Food and Drug Administration (FDA) approved blinatumomab for children with R/R B-ALL. In 2018, the FDA expanded the approval to treat persistent MRD as well. In a phase 2 study of pediatric patients, 39% of R/R patients achieved CR with single-agent blinatumomab within the first two cycles (Table 4.3) [128]. Of those in remission, 52% were also MRD negative. The COG recently completed a randomized phase 3 study of blinatumomab plus chemotherapy in first relapse of B-ALL (Table 4.3) [119]. The HR/IR randomization was closed early by the Data and Safety Monitoring Committee after finding that the experimental arm (arm B) receiving two blocks of post-induction blinatumomab in place of chemotherapy blocks had improved DFS, superior OS, lower toxicity, and superior MRD clearance compared to patients treated with chemotherapy alone (arm A). The 2-year DFS and OS were 41.0% ± 6% and 59.2% ± 6% for arm A compared to 59.3% ± 5.4% and 79.4% ± 4.5% for arm B ($p = 0.05$ for DFS, $p = 0.005$ for OS). Among patients with detectable MRD (≥0.01%) at the completion of block 1 chemotherapy, the proportion that achieved undetectable MRD (<0.01%) after chemotherapy block 2 (arm A) compared to blinatumomab cycle 1 (arm B) was 29% vs. 76%.

Inotuzumab ozogamicin (InO) is an antibody-drug conjugate (ADC) composed of a humanized IgG monoclonal CD22-targeted antibody linked to calicheamicin, an antitumor antibiotic. In a randomized phase 3 trial of adults with relapsed CD22+ ALL, patients were randomized to receive single-agent InO or standard chemotherapy, and InO was found to be superior to chemotherapy, with a CR rate for InO of 80.7% (95% CI 72.1–87.7%) compared to 33.3% (95% CI 24.0–43.7%) for the chemotherapy group ($p < 0.001$, Table 4.3) [129]. Additionally, 78.4% (95% CI 68.4–86.5%) of patients were in an MRD-negative CR/complete response with incomplete hematologic recovery (CRi) with InO, compared with only 28.1% (95% CI 13.7–46.7%) in the chemotherapy group ($p < 0.001$). In 2017, the FDA approved InO for adults with R/R B-ALL. In a retrospective review of 51 heavily pretreated children with R/R ALL that received InO, 67% achieved CR/CRi and 71% of those in remission achieved an MRD negative status [130]. More recently the COG conducted a phase 2 trial of single-agent InO in 48 children and young adults with B-ALL in second relapse or first relapse refractory to initial reinduction therapy (Table 4.3) [131]. The CR/CRi rate after one cycle in this heavily pretreated population was 58.3% (95% CI 43.2–72.4%), with 65.5% of these patients MRD negative. In all of these studies, InO was safe and well tolerated. The most concerning toxicity is sinusoidal obstruction syndrome (SOS), which appears to be most associated with HSCT after InO therapy [130, 131].

Chimeric antigen receptors (CARs) are molecules that combine an antigen receptor with one or more intracellular T-cell signaling domains. Using gene transfer, CARs can be integrated into the genome of T cells, redirecting them to target specific tumor antigens. Briefly, a patient's T cells are collected via leukapheresis and transduced with a viral construct coding for a CAR. The transduced T cells are then infused into the patient. The most studied CARs in ALL target the CD19 antigen on B cells, resulting in remission rates of 67–93% in adult and pediatric patients with heavily pretreated R/R ALL [132–137]. Thirty patients were treated on a phase 1–2a study of CTL019 (now known as tisagenlecleucel) conducted at Children's Hospital of Philadelphia and achieved a CR rate of 90% in R/R B-ALL (Table 4.3). In a separate phase 2, multicenter study of tisagenlecleucel in 75 pediatric and young adults with R/R B-ALL, 81% (95% CI 71–89%) of patients achieved remission, with MRD negativity in all responding patients. At 12 months, the EFS was 50% (95% CI 35–64%, Table 4.3) [132, 133]. Tisagenlecleucel was approved by the FDA in August 2017 for pediatric and young adults with refractory B-ALL or B-ALL in second or greater relapse.

CAR-T cell therapy is associated with potentially life-threatening cytokine release syndrome (CRS) and neurologic toxicity. These complications are consistent across various CAR-T cell products and result from the activation and expansion of CAR-T cells in vivo [132–138]. Severe CRS may require treatment with tocilizumab, a monoclonal antibody against the interleukin-6 (IL-6) receptor, or the use of steroids [139, 140]. Neurologic events include encephalopathy, delirium, focal deficits, word finding difficulties, and seizures. The neurologic toxicities tend to be self-limited but are worse in patients with a high disease burden and more severe CRS [140, 141].

T-ALL

Bortezomib is a first-generation proteasome inhibitor that is biologically active in T-ALL and selectively inhibits the 26S proteasome [142]. Treatment with bortezomib results in the inhibition of the degradation of proteins involved in cell cycle regulation, transcription factor activation, and apoptosis [143]. Bortezomib sensitizes malignant cells to the effects of chemotherapy and may help to overcome resistance to chemotherapy, particularly to glucocorticoids [144]. As discussed earlier, in a phase 2 study conducted by COG for children with ALL in first relapse, the addition of bortezomib to standard reinduction chemotherapy led to an encouraging CR rate of 68% ± 10% in children with T-ALL [120]. Bortezomib combined with chemotherapy had been under investigation for children and adolescents with newly diagnosed T-ALL by COG (AALL1231, NCT02112916), but the study was closed prematurely after release of results from the prior COG study (AALL0434) that demonstrated the impact of nelarabine on outcomes for T-ALL [63].

Daratumumab is a monoclonal antibody targeting CD38 that is approved for adult patients with multiple myeloma and has led to promising preclinical responses in T-ALL xenografts [145]. In 21 children with T-ALL, CD38 was readily expressed with high levels of expression persisting during continued treatment with chemotherapy [145]. Daratumumab combined with chemotherapy is currently being evaluated in early phase trials in children and adolescents with recurrent T-ALL (NCT03384654).

Gamma secretase inhibitors (GSIs) are a promising potential new therapy for children with T-ALL as well. GSIs target *NOTCH1* activation in T-ALL by reducing levels of intracellular *NOTCH1* and downregulating target genes [146]. Activation of the *NOTCH1* pathway is the most commonly identified recurrent genetic aberration identified in pediatric T-ALL and is found in 56% of cases [147]. GSIs also can reverse corticosteroid resistance, which is commonly identified in relapsed T-ALL samples [148, 149]. GSIs remain in clinical trials due to unacceptable toxicity, primarily gastrointestinal [150]. Other potential targeted treatment options for children with relapsed T-ALL that are being investigated include mTOR inhibitors (NCT03328104), BCL-2 inhibitors (NCT03181126), JAK-STAT pathway inhibitors, and CDK4/6 inhibitors (NCT03792256, NCT03515200, NCT03740334).

Late Effects

Many late effect studies for ALL focus on survivors who were treated decades ago. These studies have shown a wide spectrum of late effects including second malignancies, cardiac dysfunction, short stature, cataracts, and neurocognitive impairments [151]. Adult survivors of childhood ALL treated in the 1970s and 1980s also appear to be at a higher risk of developing metabolic syndrome, which predisposes to coronary artery disease and stroke [152]. In the Childhood Cancer Survivor Study (CCSS), ALL patients treated between 1970 and 1986 reported higher rates of chronic medical conditions, mental health problems, functional impairment, and activity limitations compared to siblings [153]. Additionally, compared to age-, year-, and sex-matched rates in the US population, the CCSS found that ALL survivors were at increased risk of early mortality (15.2 times more likely to die of subsequent cancer, 7 times more likely to die from cardiac-related events, and 2.6 times more likely to die from other medical causes) [154]. In an effort to reduce toxicity, these findings have led to changes in treatment approaches in the modern era. The majority of newly diagnosed patients are treated without cranial radiation or high cumulative dose of anthracyclines, alkylating agents, or epipodophyllotoxins. Despite these modifications, patients treated on contemporary ALL protocols remain at risk for long-term sequelae, with neurocognitive deficits, cardiac dysfunction, and skeletal toxicities such as osteonecrosis and low bone mineral density.

The high doses (24–28 Gy) of cranial radiation therapy (CRT) used in treatment regimens in the 1970s led to low intelligence quotients and high rates of learning disabilities in ALL survivors of that era. Long-term survivors who received 24 Gy of CRT developed impairments in immediate and delayed memory, suggestive of early cognitive aging [155–157]. Thus, a major goal of eliminating CRT in childhood ALL was to avoid neurocognitive late effects. Unfortunately, other

CNS-directed therapies used in place of CRT, such as intensive intrathecal chemotherapy and high-dose MTX, can also lead to cognitive impairments. Therefore, even without CRT there are impairments in intelligence and difficulties with attention, memory, processing speed, and executive function in survivors of childhood ALL [158–160]. Children with T-ALL are at particular risk, since they have higher rates of CNS disease at diagnosis and higher rates of CNS relapse. Thus, a greater proportion of children with T-ALL receive CRT compared to those diagnosed with B-ALL.

Anthracyclines cause a dose-dependent irreversible loss of cardiomyocytes and reduce left ventricular wall thickness and mass. This can lead to decreased left ventricular fractional shortening and subsequent cardiomyopathy, intracardiac conduction deficits, heart failure, myocardial infarction, valvar/pericardial disease, and hypertension [161–166]. To address this, studies have been conducted evaluating dexrazoxane, a chemoprotectant which decreases tissue damage by chelating intracellular iron and decreasing oxygen free radicals. It has been demonstrated to provide long-term cardioprotection without sacrificing oncologic efficacy and is now being more readily incorporated into treatment regimens containing high cumulative doses of anthracyclines to mitigate these late effects [167, 168].

Osteonecrosis is bone damage resulting from a temporary or permanent loss of blood supply that can ultimately lead to collapse of the joint surface depending on its location. Osteonecrosis typically presents during treatment, but symptoms can persist for years after therapy completion and may result in the need for orthopedic surgical intervention. Risk factors for the development of osteonecrosis include high cumulative glucocorticoid dose and older age [169–171]. In particular, dexamethasone is associated with a higher risk than prednisone, particularly in adolescents, and this has led to therapy modifications in ALL protocols, namely, the use of alternating week dexamethasone during the delayed intensification phase of therapy, as well as a preference for prednisone rather than dexamethasone during certain treatment phases for adolescents [78, 170–172]. Regardless of such modifications, increased rates of osteoporosis and osteopenia are seen in ALL survivors [173–175], with a dose-dependent decrease in bone mineral density after exposure to methotrexate and corticosteroids [174].

Future Directions

While the majority of children with either B- or T-ALL are cured, there is a need to define better treatment for the 10–20% currently not cured, especially those with T-ALL in whom outcomes following relapse remain dismal. Future approaches must avoid additional toxicities for those who will be cured without further intensification of therapy. One approach toward achieving this goal is to improve our current risk stratification systems. Assessment of MRD by either flow cytometry or qPCR remains the most powerful predictor of outcome in ALL, but relapses still occur in patients considered MRD negative at early treatment time points. Enhancing the sensitivity to detect MRD may identify patient populations who would benefit from further intensification of upfront therapy. Using DNA-based high-throughput sequencing (HTS) of the immunoglobulin heavy chain (IgH), MRD at a threshold of 1.0×10^{-6} can be detected in B-ALL, which is significantly lower than the level of detection by flow cytometry and previously found to be more predictive of relapse than a qPCR-based MRD [70, 176, 177]. HTS to measure MRD is currently being investigated by the COG in the standard-risk B-ALL protocol AALL1731 (NCT03914625). As noted earlier, disease response is currently our best tool for risk stratification in T-cell disease, but efforts are ongoing to better understand the underlying molecular abnormalities, which may be incorporated in future risk stratification algorithms as well.

Another future approach will be optimal incorporation of targeted and immunotherapeutic treatment strategies. This is of paramount importance in T-ALL where the development of these approaches has lagged behind that of B-ALL. Contemporary approaches to improve outcomes for newly diagnosed patients involve bringing active immunotherapies in the R/R setting to upfront treatment regimens. For B-ALL this includes blinatumomab, inotuzumab, and tisagenlecleucel, both in pediatric and adult cooperative groups. Furthermore, TKIs are routinely incorporated into the treatment of patients with Ph+ ALL and are now being studied prospectively in patients with Ph-like ALL. Finally, strategies to improve current immunotherapeutic success in R/R B-ALL include the addition of checkpoint inhibitors to blinatumomab and CAR-T therapy, as well as expansion of CAR-T technology to include novel/multiple antigen targets, as well as ways to improve their persistence and overcome resistance by leukemic cells. In T-ALL, there are fewer new alternatives, but recent success with nelarabine has conferred optimism, and as noted above there are promising new therapies such as bortezomib and daratumumab under investigation.

References

1. Siegel RL, Miller KD, Jemal A. Cancer statistics, 2019. CA Cancer J Clin. 2019;69(1):7–34.
2. James SL, Abate D, Abate KH, Abay SM, Abbafati C, Abbasi N, et al. Global, regional, and national incidence, prevalence, and years lived with disability for 354 diseases and injuries for 195 countries and territories, 1990–2017: a systematic analysis for the Global Burden of Disease Study 2017. Lancet. 2018;392(10159):1789–858.
3. Hunger SP, Mullighan CG. Acute lymphoblastic leukemia in children. N Engl J Med. 2015;373(16):1541–52.
4. Lim JY, Bhatia S, Robison LL, Yang JJ. Genomics of racial and ethnic disparities in childhood acute lymphoblastic leukemia. Cancer. 2014;120(7):955–62.
5. Bhatia S, Sather HN, Heerema NA, Trigg ME, Gaynon PS, Robison LL. Racial and ethnic differences in survival of children with acute lymphoblastic leukemia. Blood. 2002;100(6):1957–64.
6. Murthy GSG, Narra R, Dhakal B, Hamadani M, Michaelis LC, Atallah E. Incidence and outcomes of T-cell acute lymphoblastic leukemia (T-ALL) in United States. Blood J Am Soc Hematol. 2017;130:2575.

7. Teachey DT, Pui C-H. Comparative features and outcomes between paediatric T-cell and B-cell acute lymphoblastic leukaemia. Lancet Oncol. 2019;20(3):e142–e54.
8. Pui C-H, Relling MV, Downing JR. Acute lymphoblastic leukemia. N Engl J Med. 2004;350(15):1535–48.
9. Hunger SP, Lu X, Devidas M, Camitta BM, Gaynon PS, Winick NJ, et al. Improved survival for children and adolescents with acute lymphoblastic leukemia between 1990 and 2005: a report from the Children's Oncology Group. J Clin Oncol. 2012;30(14):1663–9.
10. Pui CH, Yang JJ, Hunger SP, Pieters R, Schrappe M, Biondi A, et al. Childhood acute lymphoblastic leukemia: progress through collaboration. J Clin Oncol. 2015;33(27):2938–48.
11. Chandra HS, Heisterkamp NC, Hungerford A, Morrissette JJ, Nowell PC, Rowley JD, et al. Philadelphia chromosome symposium: commemoration of the 50th anniversary of the discovery of the Ph chromosome. Cancer Genet. 2011;204(4):171–9.
12. Moorman AV. The clinical relevance of chromosomal and genomic abnormalities in B-cell precursor acute lymphoblastic leukaemia. Blood Rev. 2012;26(3):123–35.
13. Moorman AV, Enshaei A, Schwab C, Wade R, Chilton L, Elliott A, et al. A novel integrated cytogenetic and genomic classification refines risk stratification in pediatric acute lymphoblastic leukemia. Blood. 2014;124(9):1434–44.
14. Harrison CJ. Cytogenetics of paediatric and adolescent acute lymphoblastic leukaemia. Br J Haematol. 2009;144(2):147–56.
15. Heerema NA, Nachman JB, Sather HN, Sensel MG, Lee MK, Hutchinson R, et al. Hypodiploidy with less than 45 chromosomes confers adverse risk in childhood acute lymphoblastic leukemia: a report from the Children's Cancer Group. Blood. 1999;94(12):4036–45.
16. Heerema NA, Carroll AJ, Devidas M, Loh ML, Borowitz MJ, Gastier-Foster JM, et al. Intrachromosomal amplification of chromosome 21 is associated with inferior outcomes in children with acute lymphoblastic leukemia treated in contemporary standard-risk Children's Oncology Group studies: a report from the Children's Oncology Group. J Clin Oncol. 2013;31(27):3397–402.
17. Harrison CJ, Moorman AV, Broadfield ZJ, Cheung KL, Harris RL, Reza Jalali G, et al. Three distinct subgroups of hypodiploidy in acute lymphoblastic leukaemia. Br J Haematol. 2004;125(5):552–9.
18. Harrison CJ, Moorman AV, Schwab C, Carroll AJ, Raetz EA, Devidas M, et al. An international study of intrachromosomal amplification of chromosome 21 (iAMP21): cytogenetic characterization and outcome. Leukemia. 2014;28(5):1015–21.
19. Moorman AV, Richards SM, Robinson HM, Strefford JC, Gibson BE, Kinsey SE, et al. Prognosis of children with acute lymphoblastic leukemia (ALL) and intrachromosomal amplification of chromosome 21 (iAMP21). Blood. 2007;109(6):2327–30.
20. Roberts KG, Pei D, Campana D, Payne-Turner D, Li Y, Cheng C, et al. Outcomes of children with BCR-ABL1–like acute lymphoblastic leukemia treated with risk-directed therapy based on the levels of minimal residual disease. J Clin Oncol. 2014;32(27):3012–20.
21. Moorman AV. New and emerging prognostic and predictive genetic biomarkers in B-cell precursor acute lymphoblastic leukemia. Haematologica. 2016;101(4):407–16.
22. Pieters R, De Lorenzo P, Ancliffe P, Aversa LA, Brethon B, Biondi A, et al. Outcome of infants younger than 1 year with acute lymphoblastic leukemia treated with the interfant-06 protocol: results from an international phase III randomized study. J Clin Oncol. 2019;37(25):2246–56.
23. Brown P, Pieters R, Biondi A. How I treat infant leukemia. Blood. 2019;133(3):205–14.
24. Smith M, Arthur D, Camitta B, Carroll AJ, Crist W, Gaynon P, et al. Uniform approach to risk classification and treatment assignment for children with acute lymphoblastic leukemia. J Clin Oncol. 1996;14(1):18–24.
25. Borowitz MJ, Devidas M, Hunger SP, Bowman WP, Carroll AJ, Carroll WL, et al. Clinical significance of minimal residual disease in childhood acute lymphoblastic leukemia and its relationship to other prognostic factors: a Children's Oncology Group study. Blood. 2008;111(12):5477–85.

26. Borowitz MJ, Wood BL, Devidas M, Loh ML, Raetz EA, Salzer WL, et al. Prognostic significance of minimal residual disease in high risk B-ALL: a report from Children's Oncology Group study AALL0232. Blood. 2015;126(8):964–71.
27. Conter V, Bartram CR, Valsecchi MG, Schrauder A, Panzer-Grümayer R, Möricke A, et al. Molecular response to treatment redefines all prognostic factors in children and adolescents with B-cell precursor acute lymphoblastic leukemia: results in 3184 patients of the AIEOP-BFM ALL 2000 study. Blood. 2010;115(16):3206–14.
28. Mullighan CG, Su X, Zhang J, Radtke I, Phillips LA, Miller CB, et al. Deletion of IKZF1 and prognosis in acute lymphoblastic leukemia. N Engl J Med. 2009;360(5):470–80.
29. Den Boer ML, van Slegtenhorst M, De Menezes RX, Cheok MH, Buijs-Gladdines JG, Peters ST, et al. A subtype of childhood acute lymphoblastic leukaemia with poor treatment outcome: a genome-wide classification study. Lancet Oncol. 2009;10(2):125–34.
30. Roberts KG, Li Y, Payne-Turner D, Harvey RC, Yang YL, Pei D, et al. Targetable kinase-activating lesions in Ph-like acute lymphoblastic leukemia. N Engl J Med. 2014;371(11):1005–15.
31. Tasian SK, Loh ML, Hunger SP. Philadelphia chromosome-like acute lymphoblastic leukemia. Blood. 2017;130(19):2064–72.
32. Holmfeldt L, Wei L, Diaz-Flores E, Walsh M, Zhang J, Ding L, et al. The genomic landscape of hypodiploid acute lymphoblastic leukemia. Nat Genet. 2013;45(3):242–52.
33. Mühlbacher V, Zenger M, Schnittger S, Weissmann S, Kunze F, Kohlmann A, et al. Acute lymphoblastic leukemia with low hypodiploid/near triploid karyotype is a specific clinical entity and exhibits a very high TP53 mutation frequency of 93%. Genes Chromosomes Cancer. 2014;53(6):524–36.
34. Porter CC, Druley TE, Erez A, Kuiper RP, Onel K, Schiffman JD, et al. Recommendations for surveillance for children with leukemia-predisposing conditions. Clin Cancer Res. 2017;23(11):e14–22.
35. McNeer JL, Devidas M, Dai Y, Carroll AJ, Heerema NA, Gastier-Foster JM, et al. Hematopoietic stem-cell transplantation does not improve the poor outcome of children with Hypodiploid acute lymphoblastic leukemia: a report from Children's Oncology Group. J Clin Oncol. 2019;37(10):780–9.
36. Pui CH, Rebora P, Schrappe M, Attarbaschi A, Baruchel A, Basso G, et al. Outcome of children with hypodiploid acute lymphoblastic leukemia: a retrospective multinational study. J Clin Oncol. 2019;37(10):770–9.
37. Pui CH, Nichols KE, Yang JJ. Somatic and germline genomics in paediatric acute lymphoblastic leukaemia. Nat Rev Clin Oncol. 2019;16(4):227–40.
38. Yang JJ, Cheng C, Yang W, Pei D, Cao X, Fan Y, et al. Genome-wide interrogation of germline genetic variation associated with treatment response in childhood acute lymphoblastic leukemia. JAMA. 2009;301(4):393–403.
39. Yang JJ, Cheng C, Devidas M, Cao X, Campana D, Yang W, et al. Genome-wide association study identifies germline polymorphisms associated with relapse of childhood acute lymphoblastic leukemia. Blood. 2012;120(20):4197–204.
40. Relling MV, Yang W, Das S, Cook EH, Rosner GL, Neel M, et al. Pharmacogenetic risk factors for osteonecrosis of the hip among children with leukemia. J Clin Oncol. 2004;22(19):3930–6.
41. Moriyama T, Nishii R, Perez-Andreu V, Yang W, Klussmann FA, Zhao X, et al. NUDT15 polymorphisms alter thiopurine metabolism and hematopoietic toxicity. Nat Genet. 2016;48(4):367–73.
42. Nishii R, Moriyama T, Janke LJ, Yang W, Suiter CC, Lin TN, et al. Preclinical evaluation of NUDT15-guided thiopurine therapy and its effects on toxicity and antileukemic efficacy. Blood. 2018;131(22):2466–74.
43. Relling MV, Schwab M, Whirl-Carrillo M, Suarez-Kurtz G, Pui CH, Stein CM, et al. Clinical pharmacogenetics implementation consortium guideline for thiopurine dosing based on TPMT and NUDT15 genotypes: 2018 update. Clin Pharmacol Ther. 2019;105(5):1095–105.

44. Yang JJ, Landier W, Yang W, Liu C, Hageman L, Cheng C, et al. Inherited NUDT15 variant is a genetic determinant of mercaptopurine intolerance in children with acute lymphoblastic leukemia. J Clin Oncol. 2015;33(11):1235–42.
45. McLeod HL, Krynetski EY, Relling MV, Evans WE. Genetic polymorphism of thiopurine methyltransferase and its clinical relevance for childhood acute lymphoblastic leukemia. Leukemia. 2000;14(4):567–72.
46. Raimondi SC, Behm FG, Roberson PK, Pui C-H, Rivera GK, Murphy S, et al. Cytogenetics of childhood T-cell leukemia. Blood. 1988;72(5):1560–6.
47. Liu Y, Easton J, Shao Y, Maciaszek J, Wang Z, Wilkinson MR, et al. The genomic landscape of pediatric and young adult T-lineage acute lymphoblastic leukemia. Nat Genet. 2017;49(8):1211.
48. Ferrando AA, Neuberg DS, Staunton J, Loh ML, Huard C, Raimondi SC, et al. Gene expression signatures define novel oncogenic pathways in T cell acute lymphoblastic leukemia. Cancer Cell. 2002;1(1):75–87.
49. Girardi T, Vicente C, Cools J, De Keersmaecker K. The genetics and molecular biology of T-ALL. Blood J Am Soc Hematol. 2017;129(9):1113–23.
50. Durinck K, Goossens S, Peirs S, Wallaert A, Van Loocke W, Matthijssens F, et al. Novel biological insights in T-cell acute lymphoblastic leukemia. Exp Hematol. 2015;43(8):625–39.
51. Belver L, Ferrando A. The genetics and mechanisms of T cell acute lymphoblastic leukaemia. Nat Rev Cancer. 2016;16(8):494.
52. Sanchez-Martin M, Ferrando A. The NOTCH1-MYC highway toward T-cell acute lymphoblastic leukemia. Blood J Am Soc Hematol. 2017;129(9):1124–33.
53. Huether R, Dong L, Chen X, Wu G, Parker M, Wei L, et al. The landscape of somatic mutations in epigenetic regulators across 1,000 paediatric cancer genomes. Nat Commun. 2014;5:3630.
54. Peirs S, Van der Meulen J, Van de Walle I, Taghon T, Speleman F, Poppe B, et al. Epigenetics in T-cell acute lymphoblastic leukemia. Immunol Rev. 2015;263(1):50–67.
55. van Grotel M, Meijerink JP, van Wering ER, Langerak AW, Beverloo HB, Buijs-Gladdines J, et al. Prognostic significance of molecular-cytogenetic abnormalities in pediatric T-ALL is not explained by immunophenotypic differences. Leukemia. 2008;22(1):124.
56. Jenkinson S, Koo K, Mansour M, Goulden N, Vora A, Mitchell C, et al. Impact of NOTCH1/FBXW7 mutations on outcome in pediatric T-cell acute lymphoblastic leukemia patients treated on the MRC UKALL 2003 trial. Leukemia. 2013;27(1):41.
57. Gutierrez A, Dahlberg SE, Neuberg DS, Zhang J, Grebliunaite R, Sanda T, et al. Absence of biallelic TCRγ deletion predicts early treatment failure in pediatric T-cell acute lymphoblastic leukemia. J Clin Oncol. 2010;28(24):3816.
58. Farah N, Kirkwood AA, Rahman S, Leon T, Jenkinson S, Gale RE, et al. Prognostic impact of the absence of biallelic deletion at the TRG locus for pediatric patients with T-cell acute lymphoblastic leukemia treated on the Medical Research Council UK Acute Lymphoblastic Leukemia 2003 trial. Haematologica. 2018;103(7):e288–e92.
59. Hastings C, Gaynon PS, Nachman JB, Sather HN, Lu X, Devidas M, et al. Increased post-induction intensification improves outcome in children and adolescents with a markedly elevated white blood cell count (≥200 × 10(9) /l) with T cell acute lymphoblastic leukaemia but not B cell disease: a report from the Children's Oncology Group. Br J Haematol. 2015;168(4):533–46.
60. Patrick K, Vora A. Update on biology and treatment of T-cell acute lymphoblastic leukaemia. Curr Opin Pediatr. 2015;27(1):44–9.
61. Schrappe M, Valsecchi MG, Bartram CR, Schrauder A, Panzer-Grümayer R, Möricke A, et al. Late MRD response determines relapse risk overall and in subsets of childhood T-cell ALL: results of the AIEOP-BFM-ALL 2000 study. Blood. 2011;118(8):2077–84.
62. Marks DI, Paietta EM, Moorman AV, Richards SM, Buck G, DeWald G, et al. T-cell acute lymphoblastic leukemia in adults: clinical features, immunophenotype, cytogenetics, and

outcome from the large randomized prospective trial (UKALL XII/ECOG 2993). Blood. 2009;114(25):5136–45.
63. Dunsmore K, Winter S, Devidas M, Wood B, Esiashvili N, Eisenberg N, et al. COG AALL0434: a randomized trial testing nelarabine in newly diagnosed T-cell malignancy. Pediatr Blood Cancer. 2018;65(S2):e27455.
64. Winter SS, Dunsmore KP, Devidas M, Wood BL, Esiashvili N, Chen Z, et al. Improved survival for children and young adults with T-lineage acute lymphoblastic leukemia: results from the Children's Oncology Group AALL0434 methotrexate randomization. J Clin Oncol. 2018;36(29):2926–34.
65. Raetz E, Loh ML, Devidas M, Maloney K, Larsen EC, Mattano LA, et al. Genetic and response-based risk classification identifies a subgroup of NCI high risk childhood B-lymphoblastic leukemia (HR B-ALL) with outstanding outcomes: a report from the Children's Oncology Group (COG). ASH Meeting Abstracts. 2015;126:807.
66. Maloney KW, Devidas M, Wang C, Mattano LA, Friedmann AM, Buckley P, et al. Outcome in children with standard-risk B-cell acute lymphoblastic leukemia: results of Children's Oncology Group trial AALL0331. J Clin Oncol. 2019;38(6):602–12. JCO1901086
67. Mattano LA, Devidas M, Friedmann AM, Raetz EA, Loh M, Buckley P, et al. Outstanding outcome for children with standard-risk low (SR-Low) acute lymphoblastic leukemia (ALL) and no benefit to intensified PEG-asparaginase (PEG-ASNase) therapy: results of Children's Oncology Group (COG) study AALL0331. Blood. 2014;124(21):793.
68. Merli P, Algeri M, Del Bufalo F, Locatelli F. Hematopoietic stem cell transplantation in pediatric acute lymphoblastic leukemia. Curr Hematol Malig Rep. 2019;14(2):94–105.
69. Pullen J, Shuster JJ, Link M, Borowitz M, Amylon M, Carroll AJ, et al. Significance of commonly used prognostic factors differs for children with T cell acute lymphocytic leukemia (ALL), as compared to those with B-precursor ALL. A Pediatric Oncology Group (POG) study. Leukemia. 1999;13(11):1696–707.
70. Wood B, Wu D, Crossley B, Dai Y, Williamson D, Gawad C, et al. Measurable residual disease detection by high-throughput sequencing improves risk stratification for pediatric B-ALL. Blood. 2018;131(12):1350–9.
71. Raetz EA, Teachey DT. T-cell acute lymphoblastic leukemia. Hematology Am Soc Hematol Educ Program. 2016;2016(1):580–8.
72. Wood BL, Winter SS, Dunsmore KP, Devidas M, Chen S, Asselin B, et al. T-lymphoblastic leukemia (T-ALL) shows excellent outcome, lack of significance of the early thymic precursor (ETP) immunophenotype, and validation of the prognostic value of end-induction minimal residual disease (MRD) in Children's Oncology Group (COG) study AALL0434. Blood. 2014;124(21):1.
73. Petit A, Trinquand A, Chevret S, Ballerini P, Cayuela J-M, Grardel N, et al. Oncogenetic mutations combined with MRD improve outcome prediction in pediatric T-cell acute lymphoblastic leukemia. Blood. 2018;131(3):289–300.
74. Henze G, Langermann HJ, Brämswig J, Breu H, Gadner H, Schellong G, et al. The BFM 76/79 acute lymphoblastic leukemia therapy study (author's transl). Klin Padiatr. 1981;193(3):145–54.
75. Möricke A, Zimmermann M, Valsecchi MG, Stanulla M, Biondi A, Mann G, et al. Dexamethasone vs prednisone in induction treatment of pediatric ALL: results of the randomized trial AIEOP-BFM ALL 2000. Blood. 2016;127(17):2101–12.
76. Mitchell CD, Richards SM, Kinsey SE, Lilleyman J, Vora A, Eden TOB, et al. Benefit of dexamethasone compared with prednisolone for childhood acute lymphoblastic leukaemia: results of the UK Medical Research Council ALL97 randomized trial. Br J Haematol. 2005;129(6):734–45.
77. McNeer JL, Nachman JB. The optimal use of steroids in paediatric acute lymphoblastic leukaemia: no easy answers. Br J Haematol. 2010;149(5):638–52.
78. Larsen EC, Devidas M, Chen S, Salzer WL, Raetz EA, Loh ML, et al. Dexamethasone and high-dose methotrexate improve outcome for children and young adults with high-risk B-acute

lymphoblastic leukemia: a report from Children's Oncology Group study AALL0232. J Clin Oncol. 2016;34(20):2380–8.
79. Kelly MJ, Trikalinos TA, Dahabreh IJ, Gianferante M, Parsons SK. Cranial radiation for pediatric T-lineage acute lymphoblastic leukemia: a systematic review and meta-analysis. Am J Hematol. 2014;89(10):992–7.
80. De Moerloose B, Suciu S, Ferster A, Mazingue FO, Sirvent N, Costa V, et al. Low CNS relapse incidence without radiotherapy and improvement of outcome: results of subsequent EORTC-CLG 58881 and 58951 trials in pediatric T-cell acute lymphoblastic leukemia (ALL). Blood. 2012;120(21):133.
81. Pui C-H, Campana D, Pei D, Bowman WP, Sandlund JT, Kaste SC, et al. Treating childhood acute lymphoblastic leukemia without cranial irradiation. N Engl J Med. 2009;360(26):2730–41.
82. Patrick K, Wade R, Goulden N, Mitchell C, Rowntree C, Hancock J, et al. Improved outcome for children and young people with T-acute lymphoblastic leukaemia: results of the UKALL 2003 trial. Blood. 2014;124(21):3702.
83. Stock W, La M, Sanford B, Bloomfield CD, Vardiman JW, Gaynon P, et al. What determines the outcomes for adolescents and young adults with acute lymphoblastic leukemia treated on cooperative group protocols? A comparison of Children's Cancer Group and Cancer and Leukemia Group B studies. Blood. 2008;112(5):1646–54.
84. Nachman JB, La MK, Hunger SP, Heerema NA, Gaynon PS, Hastings C, et al. Young adults with acute lymphoblastic leukemia have an excellent outcome with chemotherapy alone and benefit from intensive postinduction treatment: a report from the Children's Oncology Group. J Clin Oncol. 2009;27(31):5189–94.
85. Boissel N, Auclerc MF, Lhéritier V, Perel Y, Thomas X, Leblanc T, et al. Should adolescents with acute lymphoblastic leukemia be treated as old children or young adults? Comparison of the French FRALLE-93 and LALA-94 trials. J Clin Oncol. 2003;21(5):774–80.
86. de Bont JM, Holt B, Dekker AW, van der Does-van den Berg A, Sonneveld P, Pieters R. Significant difference in outcome for adolescents with acute lymphoblastic leukemia treated on pediatric vs adult protocols in the Netherlands. Leukemia. 2004;18(12):2032–5.
87. Hallböök H, Gustafsson G, Smedmyr B, Söderhäll S, Heyman M, Group SAALL, et al. Treatment outcome in young adults and children >10 years of age with acute lymphoblastic leukemia in Sweden: a comparison between a pediatric protocol and an adult protocol. Cancer. 2006;107(7):1551–61.
88. Ramanujachar R, Richards S, Hann I, Goldstone A, Mitchell C, Vora A, et al. Adolescents with acute lymphoblastic leukaemia: outcome on UK national paediatric (ALL97) and adult (UKALLXII/E2993) trials. Pediatr Blood Cancer. 2007;48(3):254–61.
89. Ribera JM, Oriol A, Sanz MA, Tormo M, Fernández-Abellán P, del Potro E, et al. Comparison of the results of the treatment of adolescents and young adults with standard-risk acute lymphoblastic leukemia with the Programa Español de Tratamiento en Hematología pediatric-based protocol ALL-96. J Clin Oncol. 2008;26(11):1843–9.
90. Stock W, Luger SM, Advani AS, Yin J, Harvey RC, Mullighan CG, et al. A pediatric regimen for older adolescents and young adults with acute lymphoblastic leukemia: results of CALGB 10403. Blood. 2019;133(14):1548–59.
91. DeAngelo DJ, Stevenson KE, Dahlberg SE, Silverman LB, Couban S, Supko JG, et al. Long-term outcome of a pediatric-inspired regimen used for adults aged 18-50 years with newly diagnosed acute lymphoblastic leukemia. Leukemia. 2015;29(3):526–34.
92. Möricke A, Zimmermann M, Reiter A, Gadner H, Odenwald E, Harbott J, et al. Prognostic impact of age in children and adolescents with acute lymphoblastic leukemia: data from the trials ALL-BFM 86, 90, and 95. Klin Padiatr. 2005;217(6):310–20.
93. Herold T, Baldus CD, Gökbuget N. Ph-like acute lymphoblastic leukemia in older adults. N Engl J Med. 2014;371(23):2235.
94. Smith AW, Seibel NL, Lewis DR, Albritton KH, Blair DF, Blanke CD, et al. Next steps for adolescent and young adult oncology workshop: an update on progress and recommendations for the future. Cancer. 2016;122(7):988–99.

95. Bhatia S, Landier W, Hageman L, Kim H, Chen Y, Crews KR, et al. 6MP adherence in a multiracial cohort of children with acute lymphoblastic leukemia: a Children's Oncology Group study. Blood. 2014;124(15):2345–53.
96. Landier W, Hageman L, Chen Y, Kornegay N, Evans WE, Bostrom BC, et al. Mercaptopurine ingestion habits, red cell thioguanine nucleotide levels, and relapse risk in children with acute lymphoblastic leukemia: a report from the Children's Oncology Group study AALL03N1. J Clin Oncol. 2017;35(15):1730–6.
97. Wolfson J, Sun CL, Wyatt L, Stock W, Bhatia S. Adolescents and young adults with acute lymphoblastic leukemia and acute myeloid leukemia: impact of care at specialized cancer centers on survival outcome. Cancer Epidemiol Biomark Prev. 2017;26(3):312–20.
98. Bhojwani D, Pui CH. Relapsed childhood acute lymphoblastic leukaemia. Lancet Oncol. 2013;14(6):e205–17.
99. Ko RH, Ji L, Barnette P, Bostrom B, Hutchinson R, Raetz E, et al. Outcome of patients treated for relapsed or refractory acute lymphoblastic leukemia: a Therapeutic Advances in Childhood Leukemia Consortium study. J Clin Oncol. 2010;28(4):648–54.
100. Nguyen K, Devidas M, Cheng SC, La M, Raetz EA, Carroll WL, et al. Factors influencing survival after relapse from acute lymphoblastic leukemia: a Children's Oncology Group study. Leukemia. 2008;22(12):2142–50.
101. Tallen G, Ratei R, Mann G, Kaspers G, Niggli F, Karachunsky A, et al. Long-term outcome in children with relapsed acute lymphoblastic leukemia after time-point and site-of-relapse stratification and intensified short-course multidrug chemotherapy: results of trial ALL-REZ BFM 90. J Clin Oncol. 2010;28(14):2339–47.
102. Parker C, Waters R, Leighton C, Hancock J, Sutton R, Moorman AV, et al. Effect of mitoxantrone on outcome of children with first relapse of acute lymphoblastic leukaemia (ALL R3): an open-label randomised trial. Lancet. 2010;376(9757):2009–17.
103. Raetz EA, Cairo MS, Borowitz MJ, Blaney SM, Krailo MD, Leil TA, et al. Chemoimmunotherapy reinduction with epratuzumab in children with acute lymphoblastic leukemia in marrow relapse: a Children's Oncology Group Pilot Study. J Clin Oncol. 2008;26(22):3756–62.
104. Freyer DR, Devidas M, La M, Carroll WL, Gaynon PS, Hunger SP, et al. Postrelapse survival in childhood acute lymphoblastic leukemia is independent of initial treatment intensity: a report from the Children's Oncology Group. Blood. 2011;117(11):3010–5.
105. Oskarsson T, Söderhäll S, Arvidson J, Forestier E, Montgomery S, Bottai M, et al. Relapsed childhood acute lymphoblastic leukemia in the Nordic countries: prognostic factors, treatment and outcome. Haematologica. 2016;101(1):68–76.
106. Locatelli F, Schrappe M, Bernardo ME, Rutella S. How I treat relapsed childhood acute lymphoblastic leukemia. Blood. 2012;120(14):2807–16.
107. Locatelli F, Moretta F, Rutella S. Management of relapsed acute lymphoblastic leukemia in childhood with conventional and innovative approaches. Curr Opin Oncol. 2013;25(6):707–15.
108. Paganin M, Zecca M, Fabbri G, Polato K, Biondi A, Rizzari C, et al. Minimal residual disease is an important predictive factor of outcome in children with relapsed 'high-risk' acute lymphoblastic leukemia. Leukemia. 2008;22(12):2193–200.
109. Eckert C, Biondi A, Seeger K, Cazzaniga G, Hartmann R, Beyermann B, et al. Prognostic value of minimal residual disease in relapsed childhood acute lymphoblastic leukaemia. Lancet. 2001;358(9289):1239–41.
110. Coustan-Smith E, Gajjar A, Hijiya N, Razzouk BI, Ribeiro RC, Rivera GK, et al. Clinical significance of minimal residual disease in childhood acute lymphoblastic leukemia after first relapse. Leukemia. 2004;18(3):499–504.
111. Eapen M, Zhang MJ, Devidas M, Raetz E, Barredo JC, Ritchey AK, et al. Outcomes after HLA-matched sibling transplantation or chemotherapy in children with acute lymphoblastic leukemia in a second remission after an isolated central nervous system relapse: a collaborative study of the Children's Oncology Group and the Center for International Blood and Marrow Transplant Research. Leukemia. 2008;22(2):281–6.

112. Pulsipher MA, Langholz B, Wall DA, Schultz KR, Bunin N, Carroll W, et al. Risk factors and timing of relapse after allogeneic transplantation in pediatric ALL: for whom and when should interventions be tested? Bone Marrow Transplant. 2015;50(9):1173–9.
113. Bhatla T, Jones CL, Meyer JA, Vitanza NA, Raetz EA, Carroll WL. The biology of relapsed acute lymphoblastic leukemia: opportunities for therapeutic interventions. J Pediatr Hematol Oncol. 2014;36(6):413–8.
114. Lew G, Lu X, Yanofsky R, Rheingold SR, Whitlock J, Gulig SD, et al. The significance of minimal residual disease (MRD) in relapsed childhood B-lymphoblastic leukemia (B-ALL): a report from Children's Oncology Group (COG) protocol AALL0433. J Clin Oncol. 2014;32:10014.
115. Raetz EA, Bhatla T. Where do we stand in the treatment of relapsed acute lymphoblastic leukemia? Hematology Am Soc Hematol Educ Program. 2012;2012:129–36.
116. Barredo JC, Devidas M, Lauer SJ, Billett A, Marymont M, Pullen J, et al. Isolated CNS relapse of acute lymphoblastic leukemia treated with intensive systemic chemotherapy and delayed CNS radiation: a Pediatric Oncology Group study. J Clin Oncol. 2006;24(19):3142–9.
117. Raetz EA, Borowitz MJ, Devidas M, Linda SB, Hunger SP, Winick NJ, et al. Reinduction platform for children with first marrow relapse of acute lymphoblastic leukemia: a Children's Oncology Group study. J Clin Oncol. 2008;26(24):3971–8.
118. Attarbaschi A, Mann G, Panzer-Grümayer R, Röttgers S, Steiner M, König M, et al. Minimal residual disease values discriminate between low and high relapse risk in children with B-cell precursor acute lymphoblastic leukemia and an intrachromosomal amplification of chromosome 21: the Austrian and German acute lymphoblastic leukemia Berlin-Frankfurt-Munster (ALL-BFM) trials. J Clin Oncol. 2008;26(18):3046–50.
119. Brown PA, Ji L, Xu X, Devidas M, Hogan L, Borowitz MJ, et al. A randomized phase 3 trial of blinatumomab vs. chemotherapy as post-reinduction therapy in high and intermediate risk (HR/IR) first relapse of B-acute lymphoblastic leukemia (B-ALL) in children and adolescents/young adults (AYAs) demonstrates superior efficacy and tolerability of blinatumomab: a report from Children's Oncology Group study AALL1331. Blood. 2019;134:LBA-1.
120. Horton TM, Whitlock JA, Lu X, O'Brien MM, Borowitz MJ, Devidas M, et al. Bortezomib reinduction chemotherapy in high-risk ALL in first relapse: a report from the Children's Oncology Group. Br J Haematol. 2019;186(2):274–85.
121. Ritchey AK, Pollock BH, Lauer SJ, Andejeski Y, Barredo J, Buchanan GR. Improved survival of children with isolated CNS relapse of acute lymphoblastic leukemia: a pediatric oncology group study. J Clin Oncol. 1999;17(12):3745–52.
122. Sun W, Triche T, Malvar J, Gaynon P, Sposto R, Yang X, et al. A phase 1 study of azacitidine combined with chemotherapy in childhood leukemia: a report from the TACL consortium. Blood. 2018;131(10):1145–8.
123. Reismüller B, Peters C, Dworzak MN, Pötschger U, Urban C, Meister B, et al. Outcome of children and adolescents with a second or third relapse of acute lymphoblastic leukemia (ALL): a population-based analysis of the Austrian ALL-BFM (Berlin-Frankfurt-Münster) study group. J Pediatr Hematol Oncol. 2013;35(5):e200–4.
124. Berg SL, Blaney SM, Devidas M, Lampkin TA, Murgo A, Bernstein M, et al. Phase II study of nelarabine (compound 506U78) in children and young adults with refractory T-cell malignancies: a report from the Children's Oncology Group. J Clin Oncol. 2005;23(15):3376–82.
125. Zwaan CM, Kowalczyk J, Schmitt C, Bielorai B, Russo MW, Woessner M, et al. Safety and efficacy of nelarabine in children and young adults with relapsed or refractory T-lineage acute lymphoblastic leukaemia or T-lineage lymphoblastic lymphoma: results of a phase 4 study. Br J Haematol. 2017;179(2):284–93.
126. Whitlock J, dalla Pozza L, Goldberg JM, Silverman LB, Ziegler DS, Attarbaschi A, et al. Nelarabine in combination with etoposide and cyclophosphamide is active in first relapse of childhood T-acute lymphocytic leukemia (T-ALL) and T-lymphoblastic lymphoma (T-LL). Blood. 2014;124(21):795.
127. Burke MJ, Verneris MR, Le Rademacher J, He W, Abdel-Azim H, Abraham AA, et al. Transplant outcomes for children with T cell acute lymphoblastic leukemia in second remis-

sion: a report from the Center for International Blood and Marrow Transplant Research. Biol Blood Marrow Transplant. 2015;21(12):2154–9.
128. von Stackelberg A, Locatelli F, Zugmaier G, Handgretinger R, Trippett TM, Rizzari C, et al. Phase I/phase II study of blinatumomab in pediatric patients with relapsed/refractory acute lymphoblastic leukemia. J Clin Oncol. 2016;34(36):4381–9.
129. Kantarjian HM, DeAngelo DJ, Stelljes M, Martinelli G, Liedtke M, Stock W, et al. Inotuzumab ozogamicin versus standard therapy for acute lymphoblastic leukemia. N Engl J Med. 2016;375(8):740–53.
130. Bhojwani D, Sposto R, Shah N, Rodriguez V, O'Brien MM, McNeer JL, et al. Inotuzumab ozogamicin in pediatric patients with relapsed/refractory acute lymphoblastic leukemia. J Clin Oncol (ASCO Annual Meeting Abstracts). 2017;35:10512.
131. O'Brien MM, Ji L, Shah NN, Rheingold SR, Bhojwani D, Yi JS, et al. A phase 2 trial of Inotuzumab Ozogamicin (InO) in children and young adults with relapsed or refractory (R/R) CD22+ B-acute lymphoblastic leukemia (B-ALL): results from Children's Oncology Group Protocol AALL1621. Blood. 2019;134:741.
132. Maude SL, Frey N, Shaw PA, Aplenc R, Barrett DM, Bunin NJ, et al. Chimeric antigen receptor T cells for sustained remissions in leukemia. N Engl J Med. 2014;371(16):1507–17.
133. Maude SL, Laetsch TW, Buechner J, Rives S, Boyer M, Bittencourt H, et al. Tisagenlecleucel in children and young adults with B-cell lymphoblastic leukemia. N Engl J Med. 2018;378(5):439–48.
134. Lee DW, Kochenderfer JN, Stetler-Stevenson M, Cui YK, Delbrook C, Feldman SA, et al. T cells expressing CD19 chimeric antigen receptors for acute lymphoblastic leukaemia in children and young adults: a phase 1 dose-escalation trial. Lancet. 2015;385(9967):517–28.
135. Gardner RA, Finney O, Annesley C, Brakke H, Summers C, Leger K, et al. Intent-to-treat leukemia remission by CD19 CAR T cells of defined formulation and dose in children and young adults. Blood. 2017;129(25):3322–31.
136. Park JH, Rivière I, Gonen M, Wang X, Sénéchal B, Curran KJ, et al. Long-term follow-up of CD19 CAR therapy in acute lymphoblastic leukemia. N Engl J Med. 2018;378(5):449–59.
137. Turtle CJ, Hanafi LA, Berger C, Gooley TA, Cherian S, Hudecek M, et al. CD19 CAR-T cells of defined CD4+:CD8+ composition in adult B cell ALL patients. J Clin Invest. 2016;126(6):2123–38.
138. Frey NV. Chimeric antigen receptor T cells for acute lymphoblastic leukemia. Am J Hematol. 2019;94(S1):S24–S7.
139. Kotch C, Barrett D, Teachey DT. Tocilizumab for the treatment of chimeric antigen receptor T cell-induced cytokine release syndrome. Expert Rev Clin Immunol. 2019;15(8):813–22.
140. Hirayama AV, Turtle CJ. Toxicities of CD19 CAR-T cell immunotherapy. Am J Hematol. 2019;94(S1):S42–S9.
141. Hay KA. Cytokine release syndrome and neurotoxicity after CD19 chimeric antigen receptor-modified (CAR-) T cell therapy. Br J Haematol. 2018;183(3):364–74.
142. Koyama D, Kikuchi J, Hiraoka N, Wada T, Kurosawa H, Chiba S, et al. Proteasome inhibitors exert cytotoxicity and increase chemosensitivity via transcriptional repression of Notch1 in T-cell acute lymphoblastic leukemia. Leukemia. 2014;28(6):1216–26.
143. Jackson G, Einsele H, Moreau P, Miguel JS. Bortezomib, a novel proteasome inhibitor, in the treatment of hematologic malignancies. Cancer Treat Rev. 2005;31(8):591–602.
144. Horton TM, Gannavarapu A, Blaney SM, D'Argenio DZ, Plon SE, Berg SL. Bortezomib interactions with chemotherapy agents in acute leukemia in vitro. Cancer Chemother Pharmacol. 2006;58(1):13–23.
145. Bride KL, Vincent TL, Im SY, Aplenc R, Barrett DM, Carroll WL, et al. Preclinical efficacy of daratumumab in T-cell acute lymphoblastic leukemia. Blood. 2018;131(9):995–9.
146. Palomero T, Lim WK, Odom DT, Sulis ML, Real PJ, Margolin A, et al. NOTCH1 directly regulates c-MYC and activates a feed-forward-loop transcriptional network promoting leukemic cell growth. Proc Natl Acad Sci. 2006;103(48):18261–6.

147. Weng AP, Ferrando AA, Lee W, Morris JP, Silverman LB, Sanchez-Irizarry C, et al. Activating mutations of NOTCH1 in human T cell acute lymphoblastic leukemia. Science. 2004;306(5694):269–71.
148. Li Y, Buijs-Gladdines JGCAM, Canté-Barrett K, Stubbs AP, Vroegindeweij EM, Smits WK, et al. IL-7 receptor mutations and steroid resistance in pediatric T cell acute lymphoblastic leukemia: a genome sequencing study. PLoS Med. 2016;13(12):e1002200.
149. Real PJ, Tosello V, Palomero T, Castillo M, Hernando E, de Stanchina E, et al. γ-Secretase inhibitors reverse glucocorticoid resistance in T cell acute lymphoblastic leukemia. Nat Med. 2009;15(1):50–8.
150. Habets RA, de Bock CE, Serneels L, Lodewijckx I, Verbeke D, Nittner D, et al. Safe targeting of T cell acute lymphoblastic leukemia by pathology-specific NOTCH inhibition. Sci Transl Med. 2019;11(494):eaau6246.
151. Silverman LB. Balancing cure and long-term risks in acute lymphoblastic leukemia. Hematology Am Soc Hematol Educ Program. 2014;2014(1):190–7.
152. Nottage KA, Ness KK, Li C, Srivastava D, Robison LL, Hudson MM. Metabolic syndrome and cardiovascular risk among long-term survivors of acute lymphoblastic leukaemia – from the St. Jude Lifetime Cohort. Br J Haematol. 2014;165(3):364–74.
153. Mody R, Li S, Dover DC, Sallan S, Leisenring W, Oeffinger KC, et al. Twenty-five-year follow-up among survivors of childhood acute lymphoblastic leukemia: a report from the Childhood Cancer Survivor Study. Blood. 2008;111(12):5515–23.
154. Armstrong GT, Liu Q, Yasui Y, Neglia JP, Leisenring W, Robison LL, et al. Late mortality among 5-year survivors of childhood cancer: a summary from the Childhood Cancer Survivor Study. J Clin Oncol. 2009;27(14):2328–38.
155. Waber DP, Gioia G, Paccia J, Sherman B, Dinklage D, Sollee N, et al. Sex differences in cognitive processing in children treated with CNS prophylaxis for acute lymphoblastic leukemia. J Pediatr Psychol. 1990;15(1):105–22.
156. Butler RW, Hill JM, Steinherz PG, Meyers PA, Finlay JL. Neuropsychologic effects of cranial irradiation, intrathecal methotrexate, and systemic methotrexate in childhood cancer. J Clin Oncol. 1994;12(12):2621–9.
157. Armstrong GT, Reddick WE, Petersen RC, Santucci A, Zhang N, Srivastava D, et al. Evaluation of memory impairment in aging adult survivors of childhood acute lymphoblastic leukemia treated with cranial radiotherapy. J Natl Cancer Inst. 2013;105(12):899–907.
158. Pui CH, Campana D, Pei D, Bowman WP, Sandlund JT, Kaste SC, et al. Treating childhood acute lymphoblastic leukemia without cranial irradiation. N Engl J Med. 2009;360(26):2730–41.
159. Krull KR, Zhang N, Santucci A, Srivastava DK, Krasin MJ, Kun LE, et al. Long-term decline in intelligence among adult survivors of childhood acute lymphoblastic leukemia treated with cranial radiation. Blood. 2013;122(4):550–3.
160. Cheung YT, Krull KR. Neurocognitive outcomes in long-term survivors of childhood acute lymphoblastic leukemia treated on contemporary treatment protocols: a systematic review. Neurosci Biobehav Rev. 2015;53:108–20.
161. Lipshultz SE, Colan SD, Gelber RD, Perez-Atayde AR, Sallan SE, Sanders SP. Late cardiac effects of doxorubicin therapy for acute lymphoblastic leukemia in childhood. N Engl J Med. 1991;324(12):808–15.
162. Lipshultz SE, Lipsitz SR, Sallan SE, Dalton VM, Mone SM, Gelber RD, et al. Chronic progressive cardiac dysfunction years after doxorubicin therapy for childhood acute lymphoblastic leukemia. J Clin Oncol. 2005;23(12):2629–36.
163. Lipshultz SE, Wong JC, Lipsitz SR, Simbre VC, Zareba KM, Galpechian V, et al. Frequency of clinically unsuspected myocardial injury at a children's hospital. Am Heart J. 2006;151(4):916–22.
164. Bansal N, Amdani S, Lipshultz ER, Lipshultz SE. Chemotherapy-induced cardiotoxicity in children. Expert Opin Drug Metab Toxicol. 2017;13(8):817–32.
165. Goorin AM, Chauvenet AR, Perez-Atayde AR, Cruz J, McKone R, Lipshultz SE. Initial congestive heart failure, six to ten years after doxorubicin chemotherapy for childhood cancer. J Pediatr. 1990;116(1):144–7.

166. Mulrooney DA, Yeazel MW, Kawashima T, Mertens AC, Mitby P, Stovall M, et al. Cardiac outcomes in a cohort of adult survivors of childhood and adolescent cancer: retrospective analysis of the Childhood Cancer Survivor Study cohort. BMJ. 2009;339:b4606.
167. Lipshultz SE, Franco VI, Miller TL, Colan SD, Sallan SE. Cardiovascular disease in adult survivors of childhood cancer. Annu Rev Med. 2015;66:161–76.
168. Lipshultz SE, Scully RE, Lipsitz SR, Sallan SE, Silverman LB, Miller TL, et al. Assessment of dexrazoxane as a cardioprotectant in doxorubicin-treated children with high-risk acute lymphoblastic leukaemia: long-term follow-up of a prospective, randomised, multicentre trial. Lancet Oncol. 2010;11(10):950–61.
169. te Winkel ML, Pieters R, Hop WC, de Groot-Kruseman HA, Lequin MH, van der Sluis IM, et al. Prospective study on incidence, risk factors, and long-term outcome of osteonecrosis in pediatric acute lymphoblastic leukemia. J Clin Oncol. 2011;29(31):4143–50.
170. Vrooman LM, Stevenson KE, Supko JG, O'Brien J, Dahlberg SE, Asselin BL, et al. Postinduction dexamethasone and individualized dosing of Escherichia Coli L-asparaginase each improve outcome of children and adolescents with newly diagnosed acute lymphoblastic leukemia: results from a randomized study--Dana-Farber Cancer Institute ALL Consortium Protocol 00-01. J Clin Oncol. 2013;31(9):1202–10.
171. Mattano LA, Devidas M, Nachman JB, Sather HN, Hunger SP, Steinherz PG, et al. Effect of alternate-week versus continuous dexamethasone scheduling on the risk of osteonecrosis in paediatric patients with acute lymphoblastic leukaemia: results from the CCG-1961 randomised cohort trial. Lancet Oncol. 2012;13(9):906–15.
172. Mattano LA, Sather HN, Trigg ME, Nachman JB. Osteonecrosis as a complication of treating acute lymphoblastic leukemia in children: a report from the Children's Cancer Group. J Clin Oncol. 2000;18(18):3262–72.
173. Essig S, Li Q, Chen Y, Hitzler J, Leisenring W, Greenberg M, et al. Risk of late effects of treatment in children newly diagnosed with standard-risk acute lymphoblastic leukaemia: a report from the Childhood Cancer Survivor Study cohort. Lancet Oncol. 2014;15(8):841–51.
174. Mandel K, Atkinson S, Barr RD, Pencharz P. Skeletal morbidity in childhood acute lymphoblastic leukemia. J Clin Oncol. 2004;22(7):1215–21.
175. Vitanza NA, Hogan LE, Zhang G, Parker RI. The progression of bone mineral density abnormalities after chemotherapy for childhood acute lymphoblastic leukemia. J Pediatr Hematol Oncol. 2015;37(5):356–61.
176. Wu D, Emerson RO, Sherwood A, Loh ML, Angiolillo A, Howie B, et al. Detection of minimal residual disease in B lymphoblastic leukemia by high-throughput sequencing of IGH. Clin Cancer Res. 2014;20(17):4540–8.
177. Kotrova M, Muzikova K, Mejstrikova E, Novakova M, Bakardjieva-Mihaylova V, Fiser K, et al. The predictive strength of next-generation sequencing MRD detection for relapse compared with current methods in childhood ALL. Blood. 2015;126(8):1045–7.

Chapter 5
Treatment of Adult B- and T-Cell Acute Lymphoblastic Leukemia: An Overview of Current Treatments and Novel Advances

Shimoli V. Barot and Anjali S. Advani

Clinical Case I

A 52 year-old woman presents with night sweats, fatigue, easy bruising, and dyspnea on exertion. Past medical history is notable for hypertension. Complete blood count (CBC) at presentation is as follows: white blood cell (WBC) count 11×10^9/L, hemoglobin 7.3 g/dL, and platelets 42×10^9/L. Bone marrow aspirate/biopsy demonstrates 90% blasts. Flow cytometry is positive for CD10, CD19, CD22, CD34, CD79a, HLA-DR, and TdT, diagnostic for pre-B-ALL. She is CD20- and has a normal karyotype. Tissue typing confirms a HLA-matched compatible sibling. Reverse transcriptase polymerase chain reaction (RT-PCR) for *BCR-ABL1* is negative. Testing for the Ph-like signature is negative for any ABL class fusions or JAK pathway alterations. Therefore, she does not have any high-risk features.

Risk Stratification

Accurate risk stratification is a key aspect in the management of ALL. It aids in determining optimal initial treatment and consideration of HSCT. Historically, the MRC UKALLXII/ECOG E2993 study [5] found that factors at diagnosis predictive of overall survival (OS) and disease-free survival (DFS) were age (P = 0.001), WBC count $<30 \times 10^9$/L for B-lineage or $< 100 \times 10^9$/L for T-lineage (P = 0.001), and immunophenotype, T-lineage vs. B-lineage (P = 0.001). With improved

S. V. Barot
Department of Internal Medicine, Cleveland Clinic, Cleveland, OH, USA
e-mail: barots@ccf.org

A. S. Advani (✉)
Department of Leukemia, Taussig Cancer Institute, Cleveland Clinic, Cleveland, OH, USA
e-mail: advania@ccf.org

M. R. Litzow, E. A. Raetz (eds.), *Clinical Management of Acute Lymphoblastic Leukemia*, https://doi.org/10.1007/978-3-030-85147-7_5

understanding of the genetic landscape of ALL, recurrent cytogenetic and molecular abnormalities have been identified. These have now become more crucial in the prognosis and management of ALL [6–10]. One of these cytogenetic aberrations is the presence of the Ph chromosome (t[9;22][q34;q11]). It accounts for about 25% of adult ALL and 50% of cases in older adults. It has an aggressive clinical course with high risk of relapse [11]. However, the development of tyrosine kinase inhibitors (TKIs) has revolutionized the management of these patients and is discussed in a separate chapter. Some other adverse genetic abnormalities in ALL include complex karyotype (≥5 chromosomal abnormalities), intrachromosomal amplification of chromosome 21 (iAMP21), t(v;14)(v;q32)-*IGH*-r, low hypodiploidy/near triploidy, t(4;11)(q21;q23)-*KMT2A-AFF1*, and other *MLL* translocations. Conversely, t(12;21)(p13;q22)(ETV6–RUNX1), which is observed almost exclusively in children, and hyperdiploidy have significantly better outcomes (Fig. 5.1 and Table 5.1).

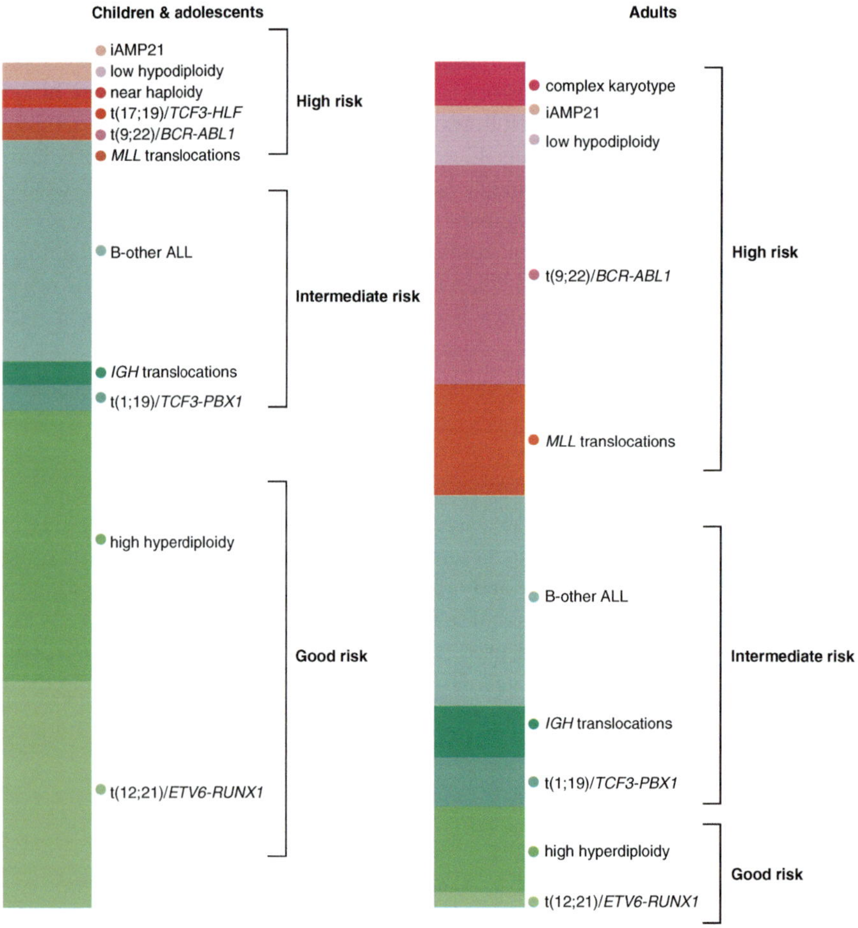

Fig. 5.1 Recurrent cytogenetic and molecular abnormalities in ALL. (Used with permission: Moorman [140])

Table 5.1 Common recurrent cytogenetic abnormalities in pediatric and adult B-ALL [130]

Risk groups	Cytogenetic abnormalities	Clinical significance	Frequency
Good risk	Hyperdiploidy (>50 chromosomes)	Favorable prognosis	25–30% in children; 7–8% in adults
	t(12;21)/*ETV-RUNX1*	Favorable prognosis in children, undetermined in adults	25% in children; 0–4% in adults
Intermediate risk	t(1;19)/*E2A-PBX1*	Intermediate to favorable prognosis	1–6% in children; 1–3% in adults
	t(5;14)/*IL3-IGH*	Intermediate	Rare
Poor risk	t(9;22)/*BCR-ABL1*	Poor prognosis	1–3% in children; 25–30% in adults
	t(v;11q23)/*KMT2A (MLL)* rearrangements	Poor prognosis	2/3 in infants; 1–2% in older children; 4–9% in adults
	Hypodiploidy (<44 chromosomes)	Poor prognosis	6% in children, 7–8% in adults

In 2009, a new subtype of ALL called Ph-like or *BCR/ABL1*-like ALL was identified which expresses a genomic signature reminiscent of *BCR/ABL1* in the absence of the *BCR/ABL1* fusion [12–14]. Ph-like ALL is detected in about 10% of children, 25% of AYAs, and 20–30% of adults. It is associated with poor chemotherapy response, high MRD, and significantly inferior outcomes [15–19]. Ninety-one percent of these patients harbor genetic alterations activating tyrosine kinase signaling. *CRLF2* rearrangements occur in up to 60% of adolescents and adults. ABL-class fusions are present in approximately 10–15% of children and adults. Other alterations include *JAK2* or *EPOR* rearrangements and mutations activating JAK-STAT or Ras signaling pathways [20]. Utilization of early HSCT, mAbs, and targeted therapies with kinase inhibitors is currently under investigation for Ph-like ALL and is discussed in a separate chapter.

Clinical Case I (Continued)

The patient is started on induction chemotherapy according to the CALGB 19802 protocol.

Treatment

The standard management approach in adult B-ALL consists of multi-agent chemotherapy administered over 2–3 years. Various protocols have been developed based on pediatric regimens. However, overall treatment consists of four integral components:

- Induction phase
- Consolidation phase

- Maintenance phase
- CNS prophylaxis and/or treatment

Induction Chemotherapy

The aim of the initial induction phase is to achieve CR which is defined as <5% blasts in the bone marrow and disease eradication at the molecular level (MRD negativity). Induction therapies are given over 4–6 weeks and typically involve either a four-drug regimen of vincristine, anthracycline, corticosteroid, and L-asparaginase or a five-drug regimen adding cyclophosphamide.

Anthracyclines Cancer and Leukemia Group B (CALGB) 7612 [21] evaluated the addition of daunorubicin to an induction regimen of vincristine, prednisone, and L-asparaginase. CR was observed in 83% vs. 47% (P = 0.003) of patients, and it established the role of an anthracycline in induction therapy.

Corticosteroids Historically, prednisone was utilized in induction regimens. However, trials comparing dexamethasone vs. prednisone showed that dexamethasone was associated with a significantly improved event-free survival (EFS) and a lower risk of CNS relapse in children [22, 23]. This is because dexamethasone penetrates the blood-brain barrier (BBB) more effectively [24]. However, dexamethasone has been associated with a higher rate of infection-related deaths and avascular necrosis especially in AYAs and adults [25, 26].

L-Asparaginase Asparaginase is an enzyme that breaks down extracellular asparagine into aspartic acid and ammonia. Depletion of extracellular asparagine inhibits the growth of ALL cells. Four-agent induction with intensive asparaginase therapy improved EFS in childhood ALL [27]. Similarly, in adults, the CALGB 9511 [28] used PEG-asparaginase and determined that patients who achieved effective plasma asparagine depletion have improved median OS (31% vs. 13%). However, adverse effects associated with asparaginase include thrombosis, pancreatitis, hyperglycemia, hepatotoxicity, immunogenicity, and infusion reactions.

Cyclophosphamide The Gruppo Italiano Malattie EMatologiche dell'Adulto (GIMEMA) 0288 [29] evaluated the addition of cyclophosphamide to a conventional four-drug induction of vincristine, prednisone, daunorubicin, and asparaginase. The addition of cyclophosphamide significantly influenced CR achievement in a multivariate analysis.

Some of the commonly used regimens combining these drugs are:

- *CALGB 8811 (Larson 1995) and 9111 (Larson 1998) regimen*

  Based on the success of pediatric regimens, the CALGB 8811 [30] utilized an intensive five-drug chemotherapy program of cyclophosphamide, daunorubicin, vincristine, prednisone, and L-asparaginase for induction in 197 adults. A CR was achieved in 85% of patients, the median survival was 36 months, and the median remission duration was 29 months. However, the CNS prophylaxis in this regimen incorporated cranial radiation which has largely fallen out of favor due to complications such as neurocognitive decline, endocrine abnormalities, and brain necrosis [31].

A major difficulty with these intensive chemotherapy regimens is prolonged myelosuppression. Hence, the CALGB 9111 [32] evaluated the benefit of recombinant human granulocyte colony-stimulating factor (G-CSF) support in shortening the neutrophil recovery time and allowing the use of dose-intensive regimens with acceptable toxicity. Patients in the G-CSF group had significantly shorter durations of neutropenia and thrombocytopenia and fewer days in the hospital. They also had a higher CR rate and fewer deaths during induction.

- *CALGB 19802 regimen*

  CALGB 19802 [33] tested dose intensification of daunorubicin and cytarabine (ara-c) as well as the use of high-dose intravenous, oral, and intrathecal MTX as a substitute to cranial radiation for CNS prophylaxis. The intensification of daunorubicin and ara-c failed to result in an overall improvement in DFS or OS compared with historical CALGB studies. However, intensive systemic, oral, and intrathecal MTX and ara-c dosing could effectively replace CNS radiation based on the results.

- *Hyper-CVAD (hyperfractionated cyclophosphamide, vincristine, doxorubicin [Adriamycin], and dexamethasone)*

  Hyper-CVAD (hyperfractionated cyclophosphamide, vincristine, doxorubicin [Adriamycin], and dexamethasone), a dose-intensive two-phase chemotherapy regimen, was developed at the MD Anderson Cancer Center. The dose-intensive phase consists of four cycles of hyper-CVAD alternating with four cycles of high-dose MTX and ara-c. It also includes a risk-stratified schedule of CNS prophylaxis with intrathecal MTX and intrathecal ara-c as well as supportive care with antibiotic prophylaxis and G-CSF therapy. Maintenance therapy consists of 6-mercaptopurine (6-MP, Purinethol), vincristine (Oncovin), MTX, and prednisone (POMP) for 2 years. The phase II trial of a hyper-CVAD-based regimen reported an excellent 91% CR rate and a 39% 5-year OS. A subsequent retrospective review from the same center with further follow-up reported an increased mortality during induction with advanced patient age (2% vs. 15% for <60 or ≥60 years, respectively) [34, 35]. The chief drawback of administering this regimen is the increased myelosuppression and the increased necessity for longer hospital admission.

- *MRC UKALL XII/ECOG 2993 regimen*

  In one of the largest multicenter prospective trials conducted to date, 1521 adolescent and adult patients received induction therapy consisting of vincristine, daunorubicin, prednisone, and L-asparaginase for 4 weeks (phase I) followed by cyclophosphamide, ara-c, oral 6-MP, and intrathecal MTX for 4 weeks (phase II). With a CR rate of 91% and OS of 45% for patients who achieved CR, this induction regimen is highly efficacious [5].

- Regimens commonly used in older adults include the GRAALL-SA1 regimen [36], GMALL regimen [37], PETHEMA-based regimen [38], Modified DFCI 91-01 protocol [39], and others (Table 5.2). The treatment of elderly patients with ALL is discussed in a separate chapter.

Central Nervous System Prophylaxis and/or Treatment

Prior to the use of CNS prophylaxis, about 75% of recurrences in children involved the CNS [40]. In adults, CNS involvement at the time of presentation is uncommon (5–7%) [41, 42]. However, CNS relapse occurs in about 30% of patients who have achieved a CR [43]. CNS prophylaxis is thus imperative, and the method used should be congruent with the studies investigating the particular regimen. The modalities include CNS radiation, intrathecal chemotherapy, and systemic high-dose therapy with MTX and/or ara-c [44].

Radiation is an effective form of CNS-directed therapy but is frequently associated with long-term adverse effects, such as secondary neoplasms, endocrinopathy, neurocognitive dysfunction, and neurotoxicity [31]. In a CNS prophylaxis study of adults who received intrathecal and systemic therapy, the frequency of CNS recurrence was similar to that observed in protocols that included cranial radiation [45]. Similarly, Pui et al. concluded that a combination of early intensive systemic and intrathecal chemotherapy allows omission of cranial radiation [24]. Systemic chemotherapy alone is limited for CNS prophylaxis given the poor penetration of drugs in the BBB. The ability of ara-c and MTX to penetrate the BBB makes them useful agents [46]. However, maintaining prolonged therapeutic concentrations in the CSF requires high doses which frequently lead to toxicity. Hence, intrathecal chemotherapy is now used widely, because it allows

Table 5.2 Commonly used regimens in adult ALL

Number	Trial	Number of patients	Rate of CR (%)	Reference
1	CALGB 8811	197	85	[30]
2	CALGB 9111	198	85	[32]
3	CALGB 19802	161	80	[33]
4	EORTC ALL-3	340	74	[131]
5	GIMEMA 0288	767	82	[29]
6	GIMEMA 0496	450	80	[9]
7	GMALL 05	1163	83	[132]
8	JALSG ALL 93	263	78	[133]
9	LALA 87	572	76	[134]
10	LALA 94	922	84	[62]
11	MDACC	288	92	[34]
12	MRC UKALL XII/ECOG E2993	1521	91	[5]
13	PETHEMA ALL 93	222	82	[103]
14	UCSF	109	88	[135]

direct intra-CSF treatment and a sustained therapeutic drug concentration in the CSF. The various regimens used are MTX in mono- or triple-therapy with ara-c and steroids, and their effectiveness has been established in various studies [47–49]. This is further elaborated in a separate chapter.

Addition of Monoclonal Antibodies for CD20+ ALL

The CD20 antigen is present on 30–50% of B-ALL blasts and was previously associated with an adverse prognosis [50]. Currently, the addition of rituximab, a mAb against CD20, to chemotherapy has improved OS in adult patients <60 years of age with CD20+ ALL [51, 52]. In contrast, older adults (≥60 years) did not appear to benefit from the addition of rituximab. In a recent study, 209 patients (18–59 years) with newly diagnosed CD20+ B-ALL were randomly assigned to receive chemotherapy ±16–18 infusions of rituximab spanning induction through maintenance. EFS was longer in the rituximab group than in the control ($P = 0.04$), and the 2-year EFS rates were 65% vs. 52%, respectively [50]. Given this data, incorporation of rituximab with chemotherapy has become standard of care for newly diagnosed CD20+ B-ALL in patients <60 years of age.

Ofatumumab, a type I human antibody that targets a different CD20 epitope compared to rituximab, induces more potent antibody-dependent and complement-mediated cell death and is being evaluated in clinical trials [53, 54]. Similarly, obinutuzumab, a novel type II glycoengineered humanized anti-CD20 mAb, working primarily by inducing direct cell death and antibody-dependent cell-mediated cytotoxicity is being investigated as well [55].

Clinical Case I (Continued)

The patient completes induction chemotherapy according to the CALGB 19802 protocol without significant complications. Bone marrow biopsy on day 28 demonstrates a CR with no detectable MRD by multicolor flow cytometry (MFC). At this stage, a decision is made not to proceed to HSCT given her MRD negative status and lack of high-risk features. She continues consolidation/maintenance chemotherapy per protocol.

Minimal Residual Disease

With any of the above induction regimens, about 85–90% of newly diagnosed adults will achieve CR. However, patients in initial clinical and morphologic CR can have persistent leukemia cells below the detection limits of conventional cytomorphologic testing. This is defined as minimal residual disease. A study on molecular MRD analysis carried out by the German Multicenter Study Group for Adult ALL (GMALL) on 580 patients demonstrated that the molecular response to standard induction and consolidation treatment was the only significant prognostic factor for remission duration and survival in both standard-risk and high-risk groups [56]. These data have been confirmed by other groups, regardless of the cutoff values, MRD technique, timing of MRD analysis, and target patient population [57, 58]. The three most widely used techniques are RT-PCR, MFC, and next-generation sequencing (NGS). EuroFlow-based next-generation flow cytometry and high-throughput sequencing of Ig/TCR are also used [59]. The clonoSEQ assay is an in vitro diagnostic that uses multiplex PCR and NGS to identify and quantify certain gene sequences in DNA extracted from the bone marrow of ALL patients. It is capable of detecting MRD at levels below 1 in one million cells and received FDA approval in September 2018 [60]. Although the timing of MRD assessment in adult ALL varies in different studies, it is commonly accepted that the initial measurement should be performed upon completion of induction therapy. Thereafter, ongoing MRD monitoring is extremely important since the presence of MRD $>10^{-4}$ is consistently predictive of subsequent hematologic relapse at every stage of the disease as seen in the GMALL studies [61]. MRD is now widely accepted and is regarded today as the most important prognostic factor in the management of childhood and adult ALL. It is further discussed in a separate chapter.

Consolidation/Intensification Chemotherapy

The primary aim of post-remission therapy is therefore to eradicate MRD. The three main approaches are chemotherapy, autologous HSCT, and allogeneic HSCT.

The French LALA-87 [62] investigated the use of allogeneic HSCT, autologous HSCT, or consolidation chemotherapy in 436 patients in first remission. Fifteen to forty-year-old patients with an HLA-identical sibling underwent a matched sibling HSCT. Those 40–50-year-old patients without an HLA-identical sibling were randomly assigned treatment with either autologous HSCT or chemotherapy. All patients >50 years were treated with chemotherapy alone. This trial demonstrated a significant superiority of allogeneic HSCT in high-risk ALL patients (defined as CNS-positive ALL; presence of Ph chromosome, t(4;11), t(1;19), or other abnormalities involving 11q23 rearrangements; a WBC count $>30 \times 10^9/L$; and patients who did not achieve CR after one course of chemotherapy). Similarly, there was a trend in favor of autologous HSCT over chemotherapy in high-risk patients. Conversely, allogeneic HSCT was not superior to autologous HSCT or chemotherapy in standard-risk ALL.

The International MRC UKALLXII/ECOG E2993 was the largest prospective study of 1484 patients to evaluate the role of allogeneic HSCT in first remission [63]. All patients aged 15–55 years with an HLA-matched sibling donor were assigned to receive an allogeneic HSCT in first CR, whereas those without a compatible sibling donor were randomized to receive either autologous HSCT or prolonged chemotherapy. Five-year OS for patients with and without a donor was

53% vs. 45% (P = 0.02) indicating the superiority of allogeneic HSCT overall. For the high-risk patients (defined as patients >35 years; those with a high WBC count at presentation of $\geq 30 \times 10^9$/L for B-lineage and $\geq 100 \times 10^9$/L for T-lineage; and Ph chromosome positive), relapse rate was significantly reduced (63% vs. 37%; $P \leq 0.001$). However, unexpectedly, the 5-year OS was not significantly superior (41% vs. 35%; P = 0.2) secondary to HSCT-associated toxicities. In contrast, for the standard-risk patients, having a donor was associated with significantly superior OS (62% vs. 52%; P = 0.02) and reduced relapse rate (49% vs. 24%; $P \leq 0.001$). Additionally, an autologous transplantation was found to be less effective than conventional consolidation/maintenance chemotherapy in all patients.

These data have been further validated in a meta-analysis of 13 trials with 2648 patients which concluded that allogeneic HSCT was superior to autologous HSCT or chemotherapy for patients with ALL in first remission and the survival advantage was of greater statistical significance for patients with standard-risk than with high-risk ALL [64]. Similarly, Gupta et al. analyzed data from 13 studies including 2962 patients and found no benefit of autologous HSCT in comparison to chemotherapy for adults in first remission but found that allogeneic HSCT improved survival for patients <35 years of age [65]. It is important to note that the younger patients in these original studies were not treated with pediatric regimens and currently AYA patients achieve better outcomes on pediatric regimens than conventional adult regimens.

In conclusion, for patients with high-risk features and persistent MRD and patients with relapsed/refractory disease, allogeneic HSCT offers the best chance for a durable response. However, it is important to take into account the risk/benefit ratio with higher morbidity and mortality associated with allogeneic HSCT. Patients at standard risk who achieve and maintain molecular remission can be treated with consolidation/maintenance chemotherapy including the AYA population given the improved outcomes with the current pediatric regimens.

Maintenance Chemotherapy

Maintenance therapy is a standard component of ALL management and is given for 2–3 years after consolidation beyond which it has not been shown to have benefit [66]. The most commonly used drugs are 6-MP, MTX, vincristine, and prednisone. CNS prophylaxis is continued during this time in some regimens, particularly pediatric protocols.

Clinical Case I (Continued)

She relapses 2.5 years from diagnosis and after receiving maintenance therapy. CBC is as follows: WBC 12×10^9/L, hemoglobin 6.6 g/dL, and platelets 15×10^9/L. Her bone marrow is completely replaced with lymphoblasts with the original immunophenotype. She is treated with blinatumomab and achieves a second remission. Thereafter, she undergoes HSCT from her sibling donor.

Relapsed/Refractory Disease

While 85–90% of patients achieve remission after induction therapy, there is a subset that is refractory to induction therapy. Additionally, despite a high frequency of CR, relapses are common and overall long-term survival is poor in adults [3]. Once patients relapse, the only hope of curative therapy is successful re-induction followed by allogeneic HSCT. Thus, attaining a CR to bridge patients to HSCT is currently the goal of salvage therapies. Re-induction regimens include standard or novel chemotherapeutic agents or immunotherapies (Fig. 5.2).

Liposomal Vincristine

Vincristine sulfate liposome injection (VSLI) encapsulates vincristine in a sphingomyelin/cholesterol envelope for targeted delivery, increased efficacy, and lower neurotoxicity. In August 2012, VSLI received FDA approval for relapsed/refractory

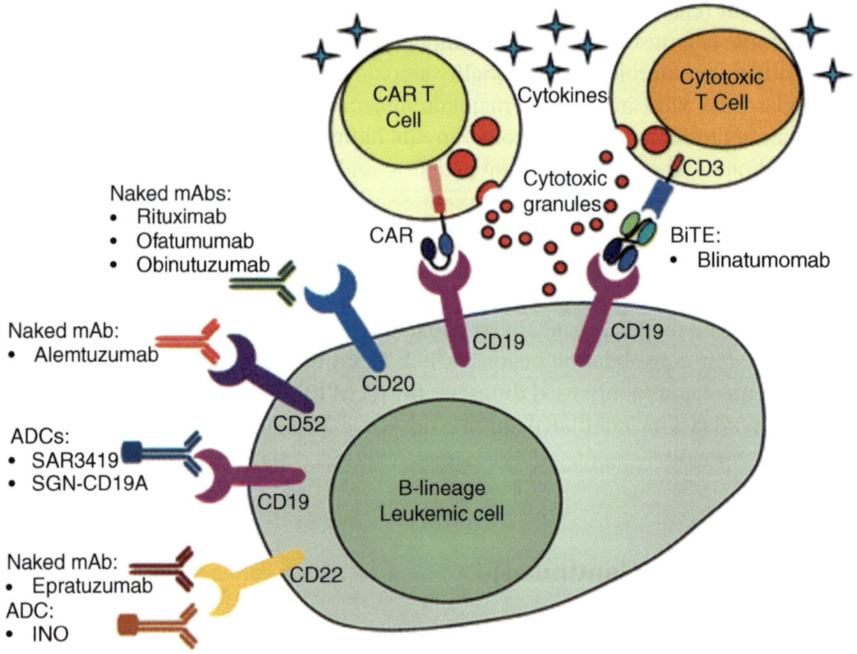

Fig. 5.2 Novel immunotherapies in ALL. mAb monoclonal antibody, ADC antibody-drug conjugate, INO inotuzumab ozogamicin, BiTE bispecific T-cell engager, CAR chimeric antigen receptor. (Used with permission: Wei et al. [141])

ALL based on a phase II trial in which overall response rate (ORR) with VSLI monotherapy was 35% and 20% of the patients achieved a CR/complete response with incomplete hematologic recovery (CRi). Nineteen percent of the complete responders were successfully bridged to HSCT [67].

Clofarabine

Clofarabine is a deoxyadenosine analog approved by the FDA for the treatment of younger patients (1–21 years) with relapsed/refractory ALL [68]. In adults, phase I/II trials demonstrated an ORR of 17% [69]. A similar 17% rate of CR/CRi was observed among patients treated with clofarabine combined with ara-c [70]. In a study from GRAALL, adult patients with relapsed/refractory ALL were treated with clofarabine in combination with conventional chemotherapy (ENDEVOL cohort) or a more intensive regimen (VANDEVOL cohort) yielding a CR rate of 50% vs. 41% and median OS of 6.5 months [71].

Blinatumomab

Blinatumomab is a bi-specific T-cell engager (BiTE) mAb construct that binds simultaneously to CD3+ cytotoxic T cells and to CD19+ ALL blasts. This facilitates the patient's T cells to recognize and eliminate CD19+ ALL blasts.

In a phase II clinical trial with blinatumomab for relapsed/refractory B-ALL, the CR/CRi rate was 69% after the first two cycles and 88% of responders achieved a molecular remission [72]. A separate multicenter phase II study demonstrated that 43% patients achieved a CR/CRi after only 2 cycles of treatment with blinatumomab with a median OS of 6.1 months [73]. Based on these results, blinatumomab was approved by the FDA in December 2014 for patients with relapsed/refractory pre-B-ALL. Thereafter, the phase III TOWER trial of 405 adults with heavily pretreated pre-B-ALL found that treatment with blinatumomab resulted in significantly improved CR rates and longer OS than standard chemotherapy. 6 month EFS rates were 31% vs. 12% and median remission duration was 7.3 vs. 4.6 months for blinatumomab vs. chemotherapy respectively [74].

Blinatumomab is also currently approved for pre-B-ALL in first or second remission with MRD ≥0.1% based on the multicenter BLAST trial [75] in which 78% of patients achieved a complete MRD response. The relapse-free survival was 54% at 18 months and the median OS was 36.5 months. Importantly, MRD responders had longer relapse-free survival (23.6 vs. 5.7 months; $P = 0.002$) and OS (38.9 vs. 12.5 months; $P = 0.002$) compared with MRD non-responders. At present, blinatumomab is also being investigated for use in frontline therapy of newly diagnosed B-ALL and in combination with other therapies [76–81].

Inotuzumab Ozogamicin

Inotuzumab ozogamicin (InO) is an antibody-drug conjugate composed of a humanized anti-CD22 mAb conjugated to the cytotoxic agent calicheamicin. It binds with high affinity to CD22, a cell-surface antigen expressed by >90% of B-cell blasts in nearly all patients with B-ALL. The antibody-drug conjugate is then rapidly internalized, and subsequent intracellular release of unconjugated calicheamicin leads to apoptosis via its binding to and cleavage of double-stranded DNA [82].

The phase III INO-VATE trial compared InO with one of three standard chemotherapy regimens, FLAG (fludarabine, ara-c, and G-CSF), ara-c+mitoxantrone, and single-agent ara-c, and found that the risk of progression or death was reduced by 55% with InO vs. standard chemotherapy. 80.7% vs. 29.4% of patients achieved CR/CRi, and 78.4% vs. 28.1% of responders attained MRD negativity with InO vs. chemotherapy. The CR/CRi rates for first and second salvage therapy were 87.7% and 66.7%, respectively (vs. 28.8% and 30.6% in the chemotherapy arm) [83, 84]. Based on these results, InO was FDA approved for relapsed/refractory pre-B-ALL in August 2017. At present, studies are underway using InO in frontline therapy, in MRD, and in combination with various agents [85–88].

Both blinatumomab and InO have comparable response rates. However, due to a short half-life, blinatumomab requires a continuous infusion. The major adverse effects include infusion reactions as well as the potentially fatal cytokine release syndrome (CRS) and neurological toxicities. Neurological events can include tremor, dizziness, confusion, and aphasia. Significant CRS was reported in 2% of patients and generally occurs with the first treatment [73]. It is treated by interrupting/permanently discontinuing the infusion and using corticosteroids.

Conversely, InO can be given weekly. The most frequent adverse effect is myelosuppression. InO is associated with hepatotoxicity and most commonly grade 1 or 2 liver-related laboratory abnormalities. Importantly, the INO-VATE trial reported a higher rate of veno-occlusive disease (VOD)/sinusoidal obstruction syndrome (SOS) in the InO arm (11% vs. 1%). Patients at increased risk of SOS include age ≥65 years, history of HSCT before InO treatment, history of liver disease, longer duration of InO exposure, and conditioning regimens containing two alkylating agents, especially those containing thiotepa. Studies have emphasized the importance of medical history and implementing risk reduction strategies in patients undergoing HSCT after InO [89].

CAR-T (Tisagenlecleucel)

CAR T-cell therapy is a revolutionary treatment in which T cells are genetically engineered to express chimeric antigen receptors specifically directed toward antigens on a patient's tumor cells and then infused back into the patient where they attack and kill the cancer cells.

In August 2017, the FDA approved the anti-CD19 CAR T-cell agent tisagenlecleucel for the treatment of patients up to 25 years of age with relapsed/refractory B-ALL based on the results of the ELIANA global multicenter trial of 75 patients (3–21 years). Eighty-one percent of patients had an ORR within the first 3 months and 100% achieved MRD-negative status. Persistence of tisagenlecleucel in the blood was observed for as long as 20 months leading to a durable relapse-free survival rate of 80% at 6 months and 59% at 12 months, and only 9% of patients proceeded to allogeneic HSCT [90]. However, growing experience has revealed that remissions may be short in a substantial number of patients owing to poor persistence and/or resistance from antigen loss or modulation. Improved strategies and newer CAR-Ts are being developed to overcome this hurdle [91].

In a phase I trial, 53 adults with relapsed/refractory B-ALL received one infusion of 19-28z CAR-T cells, which expressed a second-generation CD19-specific CAR, and 83% of patients achieved CR. Median EFS was 6.1 months and median OS was 12.9 months. Other studies have also reported similar results, but it has not yet been approved in the adult population [92, 93].

Toxicities, which can be fatal, include CRS, B-cell aplasia, and cerebral edema. Tocilizumab, a recombinant humanized mAb against the interleukin-6 receptor (IL-6R), has been FDA approved for the treatment of severe/life-threatening CRS resulting from CAR T-cell therapy in patients ≥2 years of age. In clinical trials, 69% of patients with CAR T-cell therapy-related CRS had complete resolution within 2 weeks after receiving one to two doses of tocilizumab [94].

Venetoclax/Navitoclax

Venetoclax is a highly selective BCL-2 inhibitor. Navitoclax is a BCL-2/BCL-X_L/BCL-$_W$ inhibitor, but prolonged thrombocytopenia limits its continuous use at higher doses. The combination aims for synergistic activity against BCL-2 with reduction in the limiting adverse effect from navitoclax. A phase I, multicenter study (NCT03181126) is currently evaluating venetoclax+navitoclax and chemotherapy (PEG-asparaginase, vincristine, dexamethasone) in relapsed/refractory ALL. Based on preliminary data, the ORR was 56% (20/36) in the total population with best responses of CR/CRi/CR with incomplete platelet recovery (CRp) in 18 patients. Of the 18 patients with CR/CRi/CRp, 10 (56%) had undetectable MRD. The preliminary efficacy data is promising in this heavily pretreated population [95].

Clinical Case II

A 22-year-old man presents with fever, weight loss, fatigue, and abdominal pain. He has no past medical history. CBC at presentation is as follows: WBC 21 × 10^9/L, hemoglobin 7.1 g/dL, and platelets 33 × 10^9/L. Hepatosplenomegaly is present.

Bone marrow biopsy is consistent with the diagnosis of precursor B-ALL. He is CD20- and cytogenetics show a normal male karyotype. RT-PCR for *BCR-ABL1* and Ph-like signature testing is negative. FISH is negative for recurrent genetic abnormalities.

Approach to a Young Adult

At the intersection between children and older adults is the population of AYAs. Their disease biology, management, and psychosocial factors are unique and require a distinct approach.

Risk Stratification

In an analysis of 21,626 ALL cases diagnosed between 1990 and 2005 and treated with Children's Oncology Group (COG) regimen, survival rates decreased significantly with increasing age at diagnosis regardless of treatment era (94.1% for ages 1–10, 84.7% for ages 10–15, and 75.9% for ages 15–22 years in the 2000–2005 cohort) [1]. An explanation for this is the primary differences in the frequency of the recurrent genetic alterations between children and adults with ALL [96, 97]. The most significant of these is the poor-risk Ph chromosome which is observed in 2–5% of children vs. 30% of adults. iAMP21 is present in 2% of childhood ALL, is more frequent in older children and adolescents, and is associated with a higher risk of relapse. *IgH* rearrangements are more frequent in the AYA population and are also associated with unfavorable outcomes. Additionally, the t(12;21)(p13;q22)(ETV6–RUNX1), associated with good prognosis, is observed in 25% of children vs. 3% of adults. Similarly, a hyperdiploid karyotype (>50 chromosomes) is found in 30–40% of children vs. 2–10% of adults. Hence, as age increases, there is a progressive rise in the prevalence of ALL genetic subtypes with poor prognosis, whereas subtypes with favorable outcomes become less common [98]. Therefore, relative to children, AYAs tend to present with higher rates of unfavorable genetic abnormalities and thus have inferior outcomes.

Clinical Case II (Continued)

The patient is started on induction chemotherapy according to the pediatric-based C10403 protocol.

Treatment

Adult treatment regimens typically include intensive use of myelosuppressive agents and allogeneic HSCT in first remission. Conversely, pediatric regimens focus on the Berlin-Frankfurt-Munster (BFM) backbone of vincristine, daunorubicin, prednisone, asparaginase, early and frequent CNS prophylaxis with intrathecal ara-c/MTX, and prolonged maintenance therapy. Because an AYA patient may be viewed as either an older child or a younger adult, AYAs were historically treated with either pediatric or adult ALL protocols based on the population most often seen by the treating oncologist. These inconsistencies led to the first comparisons of pediatric and adult regimens in the AYA population (Tables 5.3a and 5.3b).

- *Berlin-Frankfurt-Munster (BFM) Regimen*

  Stock et al. [99] performed a retrospective comparison of 321 adolescents aged 16–20 years who were treated on consecutive trials in either the Children's Cancer Group (CCG) using the BFM pediatric-style regimen or the CALGB adult-style regimen from 1988 to 2001. CR rates were 90% and identical in both arms. However, CCG adolescents had a 63% EFS and 67% OS at 7 years vs. 34% and 46% ($P < 0.001$), respectively, in the CALGB. Comparison of the regimens demonstrated that CCG adolescents received earlier and more intensive CNS prophylaxis and higher cumulative doses of non-myelosuppressive agents. Subsequently, similar results were also reported by several other groups [100–102].
- *PETHEMA (Programa Español de Tratamiento en Hematología) Pediatric-Based Protocol ALL-96*

  Retrospective studies consistently demonstrated that AYAs have better outcomes when treated with pediatric protocols, but prospective studies were scarce,

Table 5.3a Adult versus pediatric regimens for adolescent and young adults

Country	Adult regimen	EFS	Pediatric regimen	EFS	Reference
USA	CALGB	34	CCG	63	[99]
France	LALA94	41	FRALLE93	67	[100]
UK	UK ALL XII	49	ALL97	65	[136]
Finland	FLGN	60	NOPHO	67	[137]
Netherland	HOVON	34	DCOG	69	[138]
Italy	GIMEMA	71	AEIOP	80	[139]

Table 5.3b Pediatric regimens for adolescent and young adults

Country	Regimen	EFS/DFS	Reference
USA	DFCI	72	[104]
Spain	PETHEMA ALL-96	60	[103]
France	GRAALL-2003	58	[105]
Netherlands/Belgium	HOVON 70	66	[101]

and this was accomplished by the ALL-96 protocol. Among 81 patients aged 15–30 years, the CR rate was 98%, and 6-year EFS and OS were 61% and 69%, respectively, with no differences between adolescents and young adults [103].

- *Dana-Farber Cancer Institute (DFCI) ALL Regimen*

  This trial assessed the feasibility of treating adult patients aged 18–50 years with the DFCI Pediatric ALL Consortium regimen. Eighty-five percent of patients achieved a CR after 1 month of intensive induction therapy. The 4-year DFS and 4-year OS were 69% and 67%, respectively. They concluded that a pediatric-like treatment strategy for young adults is feasible, is associated with tolerable toxicity, and results in improved outcomes compared with historical regimens in young adult patients with ALL [104].

- *Group for Research on Adult Acute Lymphoblastic Leukemia (GRAALL)-2003 and GRAALL-2005 Regimen*

  The aim of GRAALL-2003 study was to test a pediatric-inspired treatment in adult patients up to the age of 60 years. In this trial, the CR rate was 94%. EFS and OS rates were 55% and 60%, respectively. In a subgroup analysis, patients ≥45 years had a similar incidence of relapse (30% vs. 32%) but significantly higher rates of chemotherapy-related deaths (23% vs. 5%) and deaths during first CR (22% vs. 5%) as compared with patients ≤45 years which makes this regimen better suited for the AYA population [105]. This was the basis for the C10403 trial including patients up to the age of 40 years.

  In an update on their data, the GRAALL-2005 was aimed to determine the upper age limit for treatment tolerability of a pediatric-inspired protocol of hyperfractionated cyclophosphamide (hyper-C) dose intensification in 787 patients. Randomization to the hyper-C arm vs. a standard dose of cyclophosphamide did not increase the CR rate or prolong EFS or OS. Overall, patients <55 years of age were able to tolerate this intensive pediatric-derived treatment [106].

- *C10403 Regimen*

  To address the feasibility and efficacy of using a pediatric regimen for AYA patients administered by adult treatment teams, a prospective study, C10403, was performed. The treatment arm employed interim maintenance with escalating doses of MTX (without leucovorin rescue) followed by asparaginase (Capizzi MTX) as in the PC arm of the Children's Oncology Group (COG) study AALL0232 [25]. From 2007 to 2012, 318 patients with median age 24 years (range: 17–39 years) were enrolled. Median EFS was 78.1 months, more than double the historical control of 30 months. Three-year EFS was 59% and 3-year OS was 73%. Thus, use of a pediatric regimen for AYAs up to age 40 was found to be feasible and effective, resulting in improved survival rates compared with historical controls [107].

  In all of the above studies, the upper age limit varied from 40 to 59 years, but a higher chemotherapy-related toxicity was observed with increasing age. Thus, young adults benefit from pediatric-inspired approaches but the upper age limit of applicability should be determined by individual protocols.

Clinical Case II (Continued)

The patient completes induction chemotherapy according to the C10403 protocol without significant complications. Bone marrow biopsy on day 28 demonstrates CR with no detectable MRD by MFC. At this stage, a decision was made not to proceed to HSCT. He continues therapy as per protocol. Following intensive post-remission consolidation, he moves on to starting maintenance therapy. At this time, he unfortunately loses his job and the associated health insurance. He is unable to bear the cost of medications and does not refill them. With multidisciplinary support for his socioeconomic situation, he is able to complete treatment.

Hematopoietic Stem Cell Transplant

The MRC UKALLXII/ECOG E2993 [63] was the largest prospective study of 1484 patients evaluating the role of allogeneic HSCT in first remission. Specific to AYAs, this trial enrolled 234 patients <20 years old and 301 patients 20–29 years old. A significant OS benefit in favor of allogeneic HSCT was seen only in those with standard-risk disease (62% vs. 52%; $P = 0.02$), defined as <35 years of age with no adverse biological features. The 5-year OS for patients aged 15–29 years was 45%.

Although these results suggest that allogeneic HSCT in first remission may be superior in young adults without high-risk features, the principal limitation of these studies was the use of adult treatment regimens in treating AYA patients. Hence, the comparison of 422 patients (18–50 years) reported to the Center for International Blood and Marrow Transplant Research (CIBMTR) with 108 age-matched patients who received a DFCI pediatric-inspired regimen showed no difference of 4-year relapse rates (24% vs. 23%). Due to a high treatment-related mortality in allogeneic HSCT (37% vs. 6%, $P < 0.0001$), the 4-year OS was significantly better in non-transplanted patients (45% vs. 73%, $P < 0.0001$) [108]. Similarly, another retrospective study evaluated the CALGB 10403 regimen for post-remission therapy in 295 AYAs compared to a contemporary matched cohort of 217 AYAs undergoing allogeneic HSCT in first remission reported to the CIBMTR. The pediatric-inspired chemotherapy regimen was found to be superior in terms of OS, DFS, and non-relapse mortality [109].

Thus, in the current era of excellent outcomes in AYAs treated with intensified pediatric-based regimens, HSCT should be reserved for patients determined to be high risk based on molecular aberrations and MRD evaluation.

Psychosocial Support

Non-adherence to treatment regimens and missed appointments are a significant challenge in AYAs seen in up to 65% patients [110]. This is due to complex and prolonged regimens administered outpatient. The diagnosis and treatment at a young age also has a significant impact on psychosocial functioning. Fear about prognosis, loss of independence, treatment-related toxicities, and financial issues can negatively impact quality of life. These patients are thus optimally treated in a supportive outpatient setting with a multidisciplinary approach unique to this patient population.

Clinical Case III

A 28-year-old man presents with a mediastinal mass and dyspnea on exertion. At presentation, CBC is as follows: WBC 50×10^9/L, hemoglobin 6.5 g/dL, and platelets 11×10^9/L. A bone marrow aspirate/biopsy shows 60% blasts positive for CD2, CD5, CD17, cytoplasmic CD3, CD10, weak CD4, and TdT, diagnostic of T-ALL. Cytogenetics are normal and cerebrospinal fluid examination is negative. He is treated with a combination of standard chemotherapy with nelarabine according to the COG AALL0434 protocol.

Risk Stratification

Factors that have been reported to increase the risk of relapse in patients with T-ALL include age, CNS involvement, an initial WBC count $>100 \times 10^9$, a complex karyotype, CD13 expression, and CD1a-negativity. However these have been inconsistent across studies [111]. Karyotypic abnormalities are present in most patients with T-ALL, but there are no recurrent disease defining abnormalities. Recurrent gene mutations associated with prognosis have been identified in T-ALL. *NOTCH* gene mutations are present in 60% of cases [112] and *FBXW7* in 15% of cases [113]. These mutations are associated with a favorable prognosis, while mutations in *NRAS*, *KRAS*, or *PTEN* are associated with a higher incidence of relapse [114]. Similar to B-ALL, MRD is the most important prognostic factor in T-ALL as well [115]. Early T-cell precursor (ETP) ALL was recognized as a new provisional entity in the 2016 update to the World Health Organization classification of acute leukemia [116]. It comprises 15% of T-ALL and has a distinct biology. It has stem cell-like features and is associated with chemotherapy resistance. It requires intensified therapy with consideration of allogeneic HSCT particularly in patients with persistent MRD [117, 118].

Upfront Treatment

Childhood T-cell ALL is considered high risk with an inferior prognosis, and these patients are now treated in the high-risk arms of pediatric protocols with improved outcomes. In contrast, adult T-ALL has similar outcomes to B-ALL. In the

UKALLXII/ECOG 2993, the rate of CR for T-ALL and B-ALL was equivalent (94% vs. 93%; P = 0.5), and there was a trend toward improved 5-year OS in the patients with T-ALL (48% vs. 42%; P = 0.07). Similar results have been reported in other studies as well [5, 32, 34, 35, 111]. Hence, adult T-ALL patients are generally treated with the same regimens as those used for B-ALL. However, enhanced understanding of T-lineage biology and prognostic features has impacted the approach to treatment of T-ALL.

A vital aspect is the recognition of improved outcomes in young adults treated with pediatric regimens. These regimens heavily use asparaginase as compared to adult regimens and can explain the favorable outcomes [119]. The commonly used hyper-CVAD regimen does not incorporate asparaginase and may not be adequate for T-ALL treatment [120, 121]. Another important consideration is that T-ALL patients are more likely to have CNS involvement at presentation than B-ALL (9.6% vs. 4.4%; P = 0.001). Patients with CNS disease at diagnosis have inferior 5-year OS (42% vs. 29%) due to an increased risk of both systemic and CNS relapse [41]. Pediatric trials have demonstrated improved EFS in T-ALL when high-dose MTX is added as an intensification phase [122], and, hence, most T-ALL protocols have adopted high-dose MTX in addition to intrathecal chemotherapy. Additionally, the incorporation of dexamethasone (instead of prednisone) in frontline regimens has also been reported to decrease the risk of relapse in T-ALL [123].

Decision-making after remission requires an assessment of prognostic factors to determine whether to continue consolidation/maintenance chemotherapy or to consider allogeneic HSCT. Among the T-ALL patients in the UKALLXII/ECOG 2993, having a sibling donor halved the chance of relapse (25% vs. 51%; P < 0.0001) but modestly increased non-relapse mortality (22% vs. 12%; P = 0.06). Allogeneic HSCT is thus an effective therapy and can be considered for adult patients with high-risk T-ALL [111].

Nelarabine (nel) is a prodrug converted in vivo to ara-GTP especially in T cells. The COG AALL0434 [124] evaluated the safety and efficacy of nel when incorporated into COG augmented BFM (ABFM) chemotherapy in newly diagnosed T-ALL pediatric and young adult patients (1–30 years). The 4-year DFS for nel vs. no nel was 88.9 vs. 83.3% (P = 0.0332). Among patients randomized to escalating dose MTX (CMTX), the 4-year DFS was 92.2% vs. 89.8% (P = 0.3825), and for those randomized to high-dose MTX, 4-year DFS was 86.2% vs. 78% (P = 0.024) for nel vs. no nel. Overall toxicity and neurotoxicity were acceptable and not significantly different between all arms. The outcomes observed on this trial were markedly superior to any trial for children and young adults with T-ALL, and most groups have incorporated this as a new standard of care.

Recently, a phase II study of nel combined with hyper-CVAD in 67 adult patients (18–78 years) revealed [125] that it is safe and effective upfront, but compared to hyper-CVAD alone, there was no survival benefit with the addition of nel. The reason nel did not improve outcomes in adults could be the late incorporation of nel and the exclusion of asparaginase in the hyper-CVAD regimen.

Relapsed/Refractory Treatment

The goal in T-ALL is to prevent relapse through optimization of de novo therapy since treatment of relapsed disease is challenging and the salvage rates are dismal. Unlike B-ALL, where several novel agents have been approved for relapsed/refractory disease, there is a paucity of options beyond nelarabine and chemotherapy.

Nelarabine In October 2005, the FDA granted approval to nelarabine for relapsed/refractory T-ALL based on two phase II trials, one in pediatric and the other in adult patients. In the pediatric trial of 39 patients, 13% had a CR and 23% had a CRi. The adult trial of 28 patients demonstrated a CR in 18% and CR/CRi in 21% patients [126, 127].

Investigational Agents

New treatments for T-cell ALL are critically needed [128]. Gamma secretase is required for NOTCH1 signaling, and gamma secretase inhibitors are being developed. Ruxolitinib or other JAK/STAT pathway inhibitors may be an option especially for ETP-ALL. The BCL-2 inhibitor venetoclax is being investigated. T-ALL expresses CD30 and brentuximab could be used, while daratumumab, a mAb to CD38, has shown efficacy in preclinical trials [129]. A CD7-targeted CAR-T cell without self-destruction has also been developed. OBI-3424 is a highly selective prodrug that is converted by aldo-keto reductase family 1 member C3 (AKR1C3) to a potent DNA-alkylating agent and is under study as well [118]. These are discussed in a separate chapter.

Conclusion

The approach to management of ALL is one of the most complex and intensive strategies in cancer. The cure rates and survival outcomes for patients with ALL have improved dramatically over the past several decades primarily among children. Improvements are largely due to advances in the understanding of the molecular biology and pathogenesis of the disease, incorporation of risk-adapted therapy, advent of new targeted agents, and the use of allogeneic HSCT. However, survival rates for adult patients remain inadequate and are especially guarded in older patients at approximately 20%. The approval and discovery of more effective and targeted therapies for ALL and moving novel therapies in the upfront setting will hopefully improve the outcomes for these patients.

Conflicts of Interest Shimoli V. Barot declares no conflicts of interest. Anjali S. Advani: honoraria, Pfizer; consulting/research funding, Amgen; consulting, GlycoMimetics; research support, MacroGenics, AbbVie, Pfizer, GlycoMimetics

References

1. Hunger SP, Lu X, Devidas M, et al. Improved survival for children and adolescents with acute lymphoblastic leukemia between 1990 and 2005: a report from the Children's Oncology Group. J Clin Oncol. 2012; https://doi.org/10.1200/JCO.2011.37.8018.
2. Jabbour E, O'Brien S, Konopleva M, Kantarjian H. New insights into the pathophysiology and therapy of adult acute lymphoblastic leukemia. Cancer. 2015; https://doi.org/10.1002/cncr.29383.
3. Fielding AK, Richards SM, Chopra R, et al. Outcome of 609 adults after relapse of acute lymphoblastic leukemia (ALL); an MRC UKALL12/ECOG 2993 study. Blood. 2007; https://doi.org/10.1182/blood-2006-05-018192.
4. Siegel SE, Stock W, Johnson RH, et al. Pediatric-inspired treatment regimens for adolescents and young adults with Philadelphia chromosome–negative acute lymphoblastic leukemia: a review. JAMA Oncol. 2018; https://doi.org/10.1001/jamaoncol.2017.5305.
5. Rowe JM, Buck G, Burnett AK, et al. Induction therapy for adults with acute lymphoblastic leukemia: results of more than 1500 patients from the international ALL trial: MRC UKALL XII/ECOG E2993. Blood. 2005; https://doi.org/10.1182/blood-2005-04-1623.
6. Wetzler M, Dodge RK, Mrózek K, et al. Prospective karyotype analysis in adult acute lymphoblastic leukemia: the Cancer and Leukemia Group B experience. Blood. 1999; https://doi.org/10.1182/blood.V93.11.3983.
7. Moorman AV, Harrison CJ, Buck GAN, et al. Karyotype is an independent prognostic factor in adult acute lymphoblastic leukemia (ALL): analysis of cytogenetic data from patients treated on the Medical Research Council (MRC) UKALLXII/Eastern Cooperative Oncology Group (ECOG) 2993 trial. Blood. 2007; https://doi.org/10.1182/blood-2006-10-051912.
8. Cytogenetic abnormalities in adult acute lymphoblastic leukemia: correlations with hematologic findings outcome. A Collaborative Study of the Group Francais de Cytogenetique Hematologique [published erratum appears in Blood 1996 Oct 1;88(7):2818]. *Blood.* 1996. https://doi.org/10.1182/blood.v87.8.3135.bloodjournal8783135.
9. Mancini M, Scappaticci D, Cimino G, et al. A comprehensive genetic classification of adult acute lymphoblastic leukemia (ALL): analysis of the GIMEMA 0496 protocol. Blood. 2005; https://doi.org/10.1182/blood-2004-07-2922.
10. Pullarkat V, Slovak ML, Kopecky KJ, Forman SJ, Appelbaum FR. Impact of cytogenetics on the outcome of adult acute lymphoblastic leukemia: results of Southwest Oncology Group 9400 study. Blood. 2008; https://doi.org/10.1182/blood-2007-10-116186.
11. Gleißner B, Gökbuget N, Bartram CR, et al. Leading prognostic relevance of the BCR-ABL translocation in adult acute B-lineage lymphoblastic leukemia: a prospective study of the German Multicenter Trial Group and confirmed polymerase chain reaction analysis. Blood. 2002; https://doi.org/10.1182/blood.V99.5.1536.
12. Den Boer ML, van Slegtenhorst M, De Menezes RX, et al. A subtype of childhood acute lymphoblastic leukaemia with poor treatment outcome: a genome-wide classification study. Lancet Oncol. 2009; https://doi.org/10.1016/S1470-2045(08)70339-5.
13. Mullighan CG, Su X, Zhang J, et al. Deletion of IKZF1 and prognosis in acute lymphoblastic leukemia. N Engl J Med. 2009; https://doi.org/10.1056/NEJMoa0808253.
14. Hoelzer D, Bassan R, Dombret H, et al. Acute lymphoblastic leukaemia in adult patients: ESMO clinical practice guidelines for diagnosis, treatment and follow-up. Ann Oncol. 2016; https://doi.org/10.1093/annonc/mdw025.
15. Roberts KG, Morin RD, Zhang J, et al. Genetic alterations activating kinase and cytokine receptor signaling in high-risk acute lymphoblastic leukemia. Cancer Cell. 2012; https://doi.org/10.1016/j.ccr.2012.06.005.
16. Roberts KG, Li Y, Payne-Turner D, et al. Targetable kinase-activating lesions in Ph-like acute lymphoblastic leukemia. N Engl J Med. 2014; https://doi.org/10.1056/NEJMoa1403088.

17. Roberts KG, Gu Z, Payne-Turner D, et al. High frequency and poor outcome of Philadelphia chromosome-like acute lymphoblastic leukemia in adults. J Clin Oncol. 2017; https://doi.org/10.1200/JCO.2016.69.0073.
18. Jain N, Roberts KG, Jabbour E, et al. Ph-like acute lymphoblastic leukemia: a high-risk subtype in adults. Blood. 2017; https://doi.org/10.1182/blood-2016-07-726588.
19. Hunger SP, Mullighan CG. Redefining ALL classification: toward detecting high-risk ALL and implementing precision medicine. Blood. 2015; https://doi.org/10.1182/blood-2015-02-580043.
20. Roberts KG. The biology of Philadelphia chromosome-like ALL. Best Pract Res Clin Haematol. 2017; https://doi.org/10.1016/j.beha.2017.07.003.
21. Gottlieb AJ, Weinberg V, Ellison RR, et al. Efficacy of daunorubicin in the therapy of adult acute lymphocytic leukemia: a prospective randomized trial by cancer and leukemia. Blood. 1984; https://doi.org/10.1182/blood.v64.1.267.bloodjournal641267.
22. Bostrom BC, Sensel MR, Sather HN, et al. Dexamethasone versus prednisone and daily oral versus weekly intravenous mercaptopurine for patients with standard-risk acute lymphoblastic leukemia: a report from the Children's Cancer Group. Blood. 2003; https://doi.org/10.1182/blood-2002-08-2454.
23. Mitchell CD, Richards SM, Kinsey SE, Lilleyman J, Vora A, Eden TOB. Benefit of dexamethasone compared with prednisolone for childhood acute lymphoblastic leukaemia: results of the UK Medical Research Council ALL97 randomized trial. Br J Haematol. 2005; https://doi.org/10.1111/j.1365-2141.2005.05509.x.
24. Pui CH. Central nervous system disease in acute lymphoblastic leukemia: prophylaxis and treatment. Hematology Am Soc Hematol Educ Program. 2006; https://doi.org/10.1182/asheducation-2006.1.142.
25. Larsen EC, Devidas M, Chen S, et al. Dexamethasone and high-dose methotrexate improve outcome for children and young adults with high-risk B-acute lymphoblastic leukemia: a report from Children's Oncology Group study AALL0232. J Clin Oncol. 2016; https://doi.org/10.1200/JCO.2015.62.4544.
26. Hunger SP. Glucocorticoid selection for pediatric ALL. Blood. 2016; https://doi.org/10.1182/blood-2016-02-701664.
27. Clavell LA, Gelber RD, Cohen HJ, et al. Four-agent induction and intensive asparaginase therapy for treatment of childhood acute lymphoblastic leukemia. N Engl J Med. 1986; https://doi.org/10.1056/NEJM198609113151101.
28. Wetzler M, Sanford BL, Kurtzberg J, et al. Effective asparagine depletion with pegylated asparaginase results in improved outcomes in adult acute lymphoblastic leukemia: Cancer and Leukemia Group B study 9511. Blood. 2007; https://doi.org/10.1182/blood-2006-09-045351.
29. Annino L, Vegna ML, Camera A, et al. Treatment of adult acute lymphoblastic leukemia (ALL): long-term follow-up of the GIMEMA ALL 0288 randomized study. Blood. 2002; https://doi.org/10.1182/blood.V99.3.863.
30. Larson RA, Dodge RK, Burns CP, et al. A five-drug remission induction regimen with intensive consolidation for adults with acute lymphoblastic leukemia: Cancer and Leukemia Group B study 8811. Blood. 1995; https://doi.org/10.1182/blood.v85.8.2025.bloodjournal8582025.
31. Pui CH, Cheng C, Leung W, et al. Extended follow-up of long-term survivors of childhood acute lymphoblastic leukemia. N Engl J Med. 2003; https://doi.org/10.1056/NEJMoa035091.
32. Larson RA, Dodge RK, Linker CA, et al. A randomized controlled trial of filgrastim during remission induction and consolidation chemotherapy for adults with acute lymphoblastic leukemia: CALGB study 9111. Blood. 1998;
33. Stock W, Johnson JL, Stone RM, et al. Dose intensification of daunorubicin and cytarabine during treatment of adult acute lymphoblastic leukemia: results of Cancer and Leukemia Group B study 19802. Cancer. 2013; https://doi.org/10.1002/cncr.27617.
34. Kantarjian H, Thomas D, O'Brien S, et al. Long-term follow-up results of hyperfractionated cyclophosphamide, vincristine, doxorubicin, and dexamethasone (Hyper-CVAD), a dose-intensive regimen, in adult acute lymphocytic leukemia. Cancer. 2004; https://doi.org/10.1002/cncr.20668.

35. Kantarjian HM, O'Brien S, Smith TL, et al. Results of treatment with hyper-CVAD, a dose-intensive regimen, in adult acute lymphocytic leukemia. J Clin Oncol. 2000; https://doi.org/10.1200/jco.2000.18.3.547.
36. Hunault-Berger M, Leguay T, Thomas X, et al. A randomized study of pegylated liposomal doxorubicin versus continuous-infusion doxorubicin in elderly patients with acute lymphoblastic leukemia: the GRAALL-SA1 study. Haematologica. 2011; https://doi.org/10.3324/haematol.2010.027862.
37. Goekbuget N, Beck J, Brueggemann M, et al. Moderate intensive chemotherapy including CNS-prophylaxis with liposomal cytarabine is feasible and effective in older patients with Ph-negative acute lymphoblastic leukemia (ALL): results of a prospective trial from the German Multicenter Study Group for Adult ALL (GMALL). Blood. 2012; https://doi.org/10.1182/blood.v120.21.1493.1493.
38. Ribera JM, García O, Oriol A, et al. Feasibility and results of subtype-oriented protocols in older adults and fit elderly patients with acute lymphoblastic leukemia: results of three prospective parallel trials from the PETHEMA group. Leuk Res. 2016; https://doi.org/10.1016/j.leukres.2015.11.012.
39. Poch Martell M, Atenafu EG, Minden MD, et al. Treatment of elderly patients with acute lymphoblastic leukaemia using a paediatric-based protocol. Br J Haematol. 2013; https://doi.org/10.1111/bjh.12561.
40. Bleyer WA, Poplack DG. Prophylaxis and treatment of leukemia in the central nervous system and other sanctuaries. Semin Oncol. 1985; https://doi.org/10.5555/uri:pii:0093775485900065.
41. Lazarus HM, Richards SM, Chopra R, et al. Central nervous system involvement in adult acute lymphoblastic leukemia at diagnosis: results from the international ALL trial MRC UKALL XII/ECOG E2993. Blood. 2006; https://doi.org/10.1182/blood-2005-11-4666.
42. Reman O, Pigneux A, Huguet F, et al. Central nervous system involvement in adult acute lymphoblastic leukemia at diagnosis and/or at first relapse: results from the GET-LALA group. Leuk Res. 2008; https://doi.org/10.1016/j.leukres.2008.04.011.
43. Omura GA, Moffitt S, Vogler WR, Salter MM. Combination chemotherapy of adult acute lymphoblastic leukemia with randomized central nervous system prophylaxis. Blood. 1980; https://doi.org/10.1182/blood.v55.2.199.bloodjournal552199.
44. Jabbour E, Thomas D, Cortes J, Kantarjian HM, O'Brien S. Central nervous system prophylaxis in adults with acute lymphoblastic leukemia: current and emerging therapies. Cancer. 2010; https://doi.org/10.1002/cncr.25008.
45. Sancho JM, Ribera JM, Oriol A, et al. Central nervous system recurrence in adult patients with acute lymphoblastic leukemia: frequency and prognosis in 467 patients without cranial irradiation for prophylaxis. Cancer. 2006; https://doi.org/10.1002/cncr.21948.
46. Cortes J, O'Brien SM, Pierce S, Keating MJ, Freireich EJ, Kantarjian HM. The value of high-dose systemic chemotherapy and intrathecal therapy for central nervous system prophylaxis in different risk groups of adult acute lymphoblastic leukemia. Blood. 1995; https://doi.org/10.1182/blood.v86.6.2091.bloodjournal8662091.
47. Pui CH, Mahmoud HH, Rivera GK, et al. Early intensification of intrathecal chemotherapy virtually eliminates central nervous system relapse in children with acute lymphoblastic leukemia. Blood. 1998; https://doi.org/10.1182/blood.v92.2.411.414k34_411_415.
48. Dekker AW, van't Veer MB, Sizoo W, et al. Intensive postremission chemotherapy without maintenance therapy in adults with acute lymphoblastic leukemia. Dutch Hemato-Oncology Research Group. J Clin Oncol. 1997;15(2):476–82.
49. Storring JM, Minden MD, Kao S, et al. Treatment of adults with BCR-ABL negative acute lymphoblastic leukaemia with a modified paediatric regimen. Br J Haematol. 2009; https://doi.org/10.1111/j.1365-2141.2009.07712.x.
50. Maury S, Chevret S, Thomas X, et al. Rituximab in B-lineage adult acute lymphoblastic leukemia. N Engl J Med. 2016; https://doi.org/10.1056/NEJMoa1605085.
51. Thomas DA, O'Brien S, Faderl S, et al. Chemoimmunotherapy with a modified hyper-CVAD and rituximab regimen improves outcome in de novo Philadelphia chromosome – negative precursor B-lineage acute lymphoblastic leukemia. J Clin Oncol. 2010; https://doi.org/10.1200/JCO.2009.26.9456.

52. Hoelzer D, Gökbuget N. Chemoimmunotherapy in acute lymphoblastic leukemia. Blood Rev. 2012; https://doi.org/10.1016/j.blre.2011.08.001.
53. Maiti A, Kantarjian HM, Ravandi F, et al. Updated results of frontline ofatumumab-hyper-CVAD in adults with CD20+ acute lymphoblastic leukemia. J Clin Oncol. 2017; https://doi.org/10.1200/jco.2017.35.15_suppl.7033.
54. Bazarbachi AH, Yilmaz M, Ravandi F, et al. A phase 2 study of hyper-CVAD plus ofatumumab as frontline therapy in CD20+ acute lymphoblastic leukemia (ALL): updated results. J Clin Oncol. 2018; https://doi.org/10.1200/jco.2018.36.15_suppl.7041.
55. Awasthi A, Ayello J, Van de Ven C, et al. Obinutuzumab (GA101) compared to rituximab significantly enhances cell death and antibody-dependent cytotoxicity and improves overall survival against CD20+ rituximab-sensitive/-resistant Burkitt lymphoma (BL) and precursor B-acute lymphoblastic leukaemia. Br J Haematol. 2015; https://doi.org/10.1111/bjh.13764.
56. Gökbuget N, Kneba M, Raff T, et al. Adult patients with acute lymphoblastic leukemia and molecular failure display a poor prognosis and are candidates for stem cell transplantation and targeted therapies. Blood. 2012; https://doi.org/10.1182/blood-2011-09-377713.
57. Berry DA, Zhou S, Higley H, et al. Association of minimal residual disease with clinical outcome in pediatric and adult acute lymphoblastic leukemia: a meta-analysis. JAMA Oncol. 2017; https://doi.org/10.1001/jamaoncol.2017.0580.
58. Bassan R, Brüggemann M, Radcliffe HS, Hartfield E, Kreuzbauer G, Wetten S. A systematic literature review and metaanalysis of minimal residual disease as a prognostic indicator in adult B-cell acute lymphoblastic leukemia. Haematologica. 2019; https://doi.org/10.3324/haematol.2018.201053.
59. Hefazi M, Litzow MR. Recent advances in the biology and treatment of B-cell acute lymphoblastic leukemia. Blood Lymphat Cancer Targets Ther. 2018; https://doi.org/10.2147/blctt.s170351.
60. https://www.fda.gov/news-events/press-announcements/fda-authorizes-first-next-generation-sequencing-based-test-detect-very-low-levels-remaining-cancer
61. Raff T, Gökbuget N, Lüschen S, et al. Molecular relapse in adult standard-risk ALL patients detected by prospective MRD monitoring during and after maintenance treatment: data from the GMALL 06/99 and 07/03 trials. Blood. 2007; https://doi.org/10.1182/blood-2006-07-037093.
62. Thomas X, Boiron JM, Huguet F, et al. Outcome of treatment in adults with acute lymphoblastic leukemia: analysis of the LALA-94 trial. J Clin Oncol. 2004; https://doi.org/10.1200/JCO.2004.10.050.
63. Goldstone AH, Richards SM, Lazarus HM, et al. In adults with standard-risk acute lymphoblastic leukemia, the greatest benefit is achieved from a matched sibling allogeneic transplantation in first complete remission, and an autologous transplantation is less effective than conventional consolidation/maintenance chemotherapy in all patients: final results of the International ALL Trial (MRC UKALL XII/ECOG E2993). Blood. 2008; https://doi.org/10.1182/blood-2007-10-116582.
64. Ram R, Gafter-Gvili A, Vidal L, et al. Management of adult patients with acute lymphoblastic leukemia in first complete remission: systematic review and meta-analysis. Cancer. 2010; https://doi.org/10.1002/cncr.25136.
65. Gupta V, Richards S, Rowe J. Allogeneic, but not autologous, hematopoietic cell transplantation improves survival only among younger adults with acute lymphoblastic leukemia in first remission: an individual patient data meta-analysis. Blood. 2013; https://doi.org/10.1182/blood-2012-07-445098.
66. Terwilliger T, Abdul-Hay M. Acute lymphoblastic leukemia: a comprehensive review and 2017 update. Blood Cancer J. 2017; https://doi.org/10.1038/bcj.2017.53.
67. O'Brien S, Schiller G, Lister J, et al. High-dose vincristine sulfate liposome injection for advanced, relapsed, and refractory adult Philadelphia chromosome-negative acute lymphoblastic leukemia. J Clin Oncol. 2013; https://doi.org/10.1200/JCO.2012.46.2309.

68. Jeha S, Gaynon PS, Razzouk BI, et al. Phase II study of clofarabine in pediatric patients with refractory or relapsed acute lymphoblastic leukemia. J Clin Oncol. 2006; https://doi.org/10.1200/JCO.2005.03.8554.
69. Kantarjian H, Gandhi V, Cortes J, et al. Phase 2 clinical and pharmacologic study of clofarabine in patients with refractory or relapsed acute leukemia. Blood. 2003; https://doi.org/10.1182/blood-2003-03-0925.
70. Advani AS, Gundacker HM, Sala-Torra O, et al. Southwest Oncology Group Study S0530: a phase 2 trial of clofarabine and cytarabine for relapsed or refractory acute lymphocytic leukaemia. Br J Haematol. 2010; https://doi.org/10.1111/j.1365-2141.2010.08387.x.
71. Bassan R, Fumagalli M, Chiaretti S, et al. Phase II trial with sequential clofarabine and cyclophosphamide for refractory and relapsed Philadelphia-negative adult acute lymphoblastic leukemia. Results of the GIMEMA LAL 1610 protocol. Leuk Lymphoma. 2019; https://doi.org/10.1080/10428194.2019.1639170.
72. Topp MS, Gökbuget N, Zugmaier G, et al. Phase II trial of the anti-CD19 bispecific T cell-engager blinatumomab shows hematologic and molecular remissions in patients with relapsed or refractory B-precursor acute lymphoblastic leukemia. J Clin Oncol. 2014; https://doi.org/10.1200/JCO.2014.56.3247.
73. Topp MS, Gökbuget N, Stein AS, et al. Safety and activity of blinatumomab for adult patients with relapsed or refractory B-precursor acute lymphoblastic leukaemia: a multicentre, single-arm, phase 2 study. Lancet Oncol. 2015; https://doi.org/10.1016/S1470 2045(14)71170-2.
74. Kantarjian H, Stein A, Gökbuget N, et al. Blinatumomab versus chemotherapy for advanced acute lymphoblastic leukemia. N Engl J Med. 2017; https://doi.org/10.1056/NEJMoa1609783.
75. Gökbuget N, Dombret H, Bonifacio M, et al. Blinatumomab for minimal residual disease in adults with B-cell precursor acute lymphoblastic leukemia. Blood. 2018; https://doi.org/10.1182/blood-2017-08-798322.
76. Tisagenlecleucel vs blinatumomab or inotuzumab for patients with relapsed/refractory B-cell precursor acute lymphoblastic leukemia. https://ClinicalTrials.gov/show/NCT03628053
77. Blinatumomab added to prephase and consolidation therapy in precursor B-acute lymphoblastic leukemia in adults. https://ClinicalTrials.gov/show/NCT03541083
78. Sequential chemotherapy and blinatumomab to improve minimal residual disease response and survival in acute lymphoblastic leukemia. https://ClinicalTrials.gov/show/NCT03367299
79. Blinatumomab and pembrolizumab for adults with relapsed/refractory B-cell acute lymphoblastic leukemia with high marrow lymphoblasts. https://ClinicalTrials.gov/show/NCT03160079
80. Blinatumomab in treating patients with B-cell acute lymphoblastic leukemia with minimal residual disease. https://ClinicalTrials.gov/show/NCT02458014
81. Combination chemotherapy with or without blinatumomab in treating patients with newly diagnosed BCR-ABL-negative B lineage acute lymphoblastic leukemia. https://ClinicalTrials.gov/show/NCT02003222
82. DiJoseph JF, Armellino DC, Boghaert ER, et al. Antibody-targeted chemotherapy with CMC-544: a CD22-targeted immunoconjugate of calicheamicin for the treatment of B-lymphoid malignancies. Blood. 2004; https://doi.org/10.1182/blood-2003-07-2466.
83. Kantarjian HM, DeAngelo DJ, Stelljes M, et al. Inotuzumab ozogamicin versus standard of care in relapsed or refractory acute lymphoblastic leukemia: final report and long-term survival follow-up from the randomized, phase 3 INO-VATE study. Cancer. 2019; https://doi.org/10.1002/cncr.32116.
84. Kantarjian HM, DeAngelo DJ, Stelljes M, et al. Inotuzumab ozogamicin versus standard therapy for acute lymphoblastic leukemia. N Engl J Med. 2016; https://doi.org/10.1056/NEJMoa1509277.
85. Inotuzumab ozogamicin and vincristine sulfate liposome in treating patients with relapsed or refractory CD22+ B-cell acute lymphoblastic leukemia. https://ClinicalTrials.gov/show/NCT03851081

86. Inotuzumab ozogamicin and conventional chemotherapy in patients aged 56 years and older with ALL. https://ClinicalTrials.gov/show/NCT03460522
87. Inotuzumab ozogamicin in treating patients with B-cell acute lymphocytic leukemia with positive minimal residual disease. https://ClinicalTrials.gov/show/NCT03441061
88. Inotuzumab ozogamicin and frontline chemotherapy in treating young adults with newly diagnosed B acute lymphoblastic leukemia. https://ClinicalTrials.gov/show/NCT03150693
89. Kantarjian HM, DeAngelo DJ, Advani AS, et al. Hepatic adverse event profile of inotuzumab ozogamicin in adult patients with relapsed or refractory acute lymphoblastic leukaemia: results from the open-label, randomised, phase 3 INO-VATE study. Lancet Haematol. 2017; https://doi.org/10.1016/S2352-3026(17)30103-5.
90. Maude SL, Laetsch TW, Buechner J, et al. Tisagenlecleucel in children and young adults with B-cell lymphoblastic leukemia. N Engl J Med. 2018; https://doi.org/10.1056/NEJMoa1709866.
91. Shah NN, Fry TJ. Mechanisms of resistance to CAR T cell therapy. Nat Rev Clin Oncol. 2019; https://doi.org/10.1038/s41571-019-0184-6.
92. Park JH, Rivière I, Gonen M, et al. Long-term follow-up of CD19 CAR therapy in acute lymphoblastic leukemia. N Engl J Med. 2018; https://doi.org/10.1056/NEJMoa1709919.
93. Maude SL, Frey N, Shaw PA, et al. Chimeric antigen receptor T cells for sustained remissions in leukemia. N Engl J Med. 2014; https://doi.org/10.1056/NEJMoa1407222.
94. Le RQ, Li L, Yuan W, et al. FDA approval summary: tocilizumab for treatment of chimeric antigen receptor T cell-induced severe or life-threatening cytokine release syndrome. Oncologist. 2018; https://doi.org/10.1634/theoncologist.2018-0028.
95. Lacayo NJ, Pullarkat VA, Stock W, et al. Safety and efficacy of venetoclax in combination with navitoclax in adult and pediatric relapsed/refractory acute lymphoblastic leukemia and lymphoblastic lymphoma. Blood. 2019;134(Supplement_1):285. https://doi.org/10.1182/blood-2019-126977.
96. Ribeiro RC, Abromowitch M, Raimondi SC, Murphy SB, Behm F, Williams DL. Clinical and biologic hallmarks of the Philadelphia chromosome in childhood acute lymphoblastic leukemia. Blood. 1987; https://doi.org/10.1182/blood.v70.4.948.bloodjournal704948.
97. Harrison CJ, Moorman AV, Barber KE, et al. Interphase molecular cytogenetic screening for chromosomal abnormalities of prognostic significance in childhood acute lymphoblastic leukaemia: a UK Cancer Cytogenetics Group Study. Br J Haematol. 2005; https://doi.org/10.1111/j.1365-2141.2005.05497.x.
98. Roberts KG. Genetics and prognosis of ALL in children vs adults. Hematology. 2018; https://doi.org/10.1182/asheducation-2018.1.137.
99. Stock W, La M, Sanford B, et al. What determines the outcomes for adolescents and young adults with acute lymphoblastic leukemia treated on cooperative group protocols? A comparison of Children's Cancer Group and Cancer and Leukemia Group B studies. Blood. 2008; https://doi.org/10.1182/blood-2008-01-130237.
100. Boissel N, Auclerc MF, Lhéritier V, et al. Should adolescents with acute lymphoblastic leukemia be treated as old children or young adults? Comparison of the French FRALLE-93 and LALA-94 trials. J Clin Oncol. 2003; https://doi.org/10.1200/JCO.2003.02.053.
101. Rijneveld AW, Van Der Holt B, Daenen SMGJ, et al. Intensified chemotherapy inspired by a pediatric regimen combined with allogeneic transplantation in adult patients with acute lymphoblastic leukemia up to the age of 40. Leukemia. 2011; https://doi.org/10.1038/leu.2011.141.
102. Gökbuget N, Beck J, Brandt K, et al. Significant improvement of outcome in adolescents and young adults (AYAs) aged 15–35 years with acute lymphoblastic leukemia (ALL) with a pediatric derived adult ALL protocol; results of 1529 AYAs in 2 consecutive trials of the German Multicenter Study Group for Adult ALL (GMALL). Blood. 2013; https://doi.org/10.1182/blood.v122.21.839.839.
103. Ribera JM, Oriol A, Sanz MA, et al. Comparison of the results of the treatment of adolescents and young adults with standard-risk acute lymphoblastic leukemia with the programa Español

de tratamiento en hematología pediatric-based protocol ALL-96. J Clin Oncol. 2008; https://doi.org/10.1200/JCO.2007.13.7265.
104. DeAngelo DJ, Stevenson KE, Dahlberg SE, et al. Long-term outcome of a pediatric-inspired regimen used for adults aged 18–50 years with newly diagnosed acute lymphoblastic leukemia. Leukemia. 2015; https://doi.org/10.1038/leu.2014.229.
105. Huguet F, Leguay T, Raffoux E, et al. Pediatric-inspired therapy in adults with Philadelphia chromosome-negative acute lymphoblastic leukemia: the GRAALL-2003 study. J Clin Oncol. 2009; https://doi.org/10.1200/JCO.2008.18.6916.
106. Huguet F, Chevret S, Leguay T, et al. Intensified therapy of acute lymphoblastic leukemia in adults: report of the randomized GRAALL-2005 clinical trial. J Clin Oncol. 2018; https://doi.org/10.1200/JCO.2017.76.8192.
107. Stock W, Luger SM, Advani AS, et al. A pediatric regimen for older adolescents and young adults with acute lymphoblastic leukemia: results of CALGB 10403. Blood. 2019; https://doi.org/10.1182/blood-2018-10-881961.
108. Seftel MD, Neuberg D, Zhang MJ, et al. Pediatric-inspired therapy compared to allografting for Philadelphia chromosome-negative adult ALL in first complete remission. Am J Hematol. 2016; https://doi.org/10.1002/ajh.24285.
109. Wieduwilt MJ, Stock W, Advani AS, et al. Superior survival with post-remission pediatric-inspired chemotherapy compared to myeloablative allogeneic hematopoietic cell transplantation in adolescents and young adults with Ph-negative acute lymphoblastic leukemia in first complete remission: comparison of CALGB 10403 to patients reported to the CIBMTR. Blood. 2019;134(Supplement_1):261. https://doi.org/10.1182/blood-2019-128560.
110. Kondryn HJ, Edmondson CL, Hill J, Eden TOB. Treatment non-adherence in teenage and young adult patients with cancer. Lancet Oncol. 2011; https://doi.org/10.1016/S1470-2045(10)70069-3.
111. Marks DI, Paietta EM, Moorman AV, et al. T-cell acute lymphoblastic leukemia in adults: clinical features, immunophenotype, cytogenetics, and outcome from the large randomized prospective trial (UKALL XII/ECOG 2993). Blood. 2009; https://doi.org/10.1182/blood-2009-08-231217.
112. Weng AP, Ferrando AA, Lee W, et al. Activating mutations of NOTCH1 in human T cell acute lymphoblastic leukemia. Science (80-). 2004; https://doi.org/10.1126/science.1102160.
113. Yeh CH, Bellon M, Pancewicz-Wojtkiewicz J, Nicot C. Oncogenic mutations in the FBXW7 gene of adult T-cell leukemia patients. Proc Natl Acad Sci U S A. 2016; https://doi.org/10.1073/pnas.1601537113.
114. Mansour MR, Sulis ML, Duke V, et al. Prognostic implications of NOTCH1 and FBXW7 mutations in adults with T-cell acute lymphoblastic leukemia treated on the MRC UKALLXII/ECOG E2993 protocol. J Clin Oncol. 2009; https://doi.org/10.1200/JCO.2009.22.0996.
115. Schrappe M, Valsecchi MG, Bartram CR, et al. Late MRD response determines relapse risk overall and in subsets of childhood T-cell ALL: results of the AIEOP-BFM-ALL 2000 study. Blood. 2011; https://doi.org/10.1182/blood-2011-03-338707.
116. Coustan-Smith E, Mullighan CG, Onciu M, et al. Early T-cell precursor leukaemia: a subtype of very high-risk acute lymphoblastic leukaemia. Lancet Oncol. 2009; https://doi.org/10.1016/S1470-2045(08)70314-0.
117. Genescà E, Morgades M, Montesinos P, et al. Unique clinico-biological, genetic and prognostic features of adult early T cell precursor acute lymphoblastic leukemia. Haematologica. 2019; https://doi.org/10.3324/haematol.2019.225078.
118. Luskin MR, DeAngelo DJ. T-cell acute lymphoblastic leukemia: current approach and future directions. Adv Cell Gene Ther. 2019; https://doi.org/10.1002/acg2.70.
119. Amylon MD, Shuster J, Pullen J, et al. Intensive high-dose asparaginase consolidation improves survival for pediatric patients with T cell acute lymphoblastic leukemia and advanced stage lymphoblastic lymphoma: a Pediatric Oncology Group study. Leukemia. 1999; https://doi.org/10.1038/sj.leu.2401310.

120. Kota VK, Hathaway AR, Shah BD, et al. Poor outcomes with hyper CVAD induction for T-cell lymphoblastic leukemia/lymphoma. Blood. 2015; https://doi.org/10.1182/blood.v126.23.3762.3762.
121. Kozlowski P, Åström M, Ahlberg L, et al. High relapse rate of T cell acute lymphoblastic leukemia in adults treated with Hyper-CVAD chemotherapy in Sweden. Eur J Haematol. 2014; https://doi.org/10.1111/ejh.12269.
122. Asselin BL, Devidas M, Wang C, et al. Effectiveness of high-dose methotrexate in T-cell lymphoblastic leukemia and advanced-stage lymphoblastic lymphoma: a randomized study by the Children's Oncology Group (POG 9404). Blood. 2011; https://doi.org/10.1182/blood-2010-06-292615.
123. Möricke A, Zimmermann M, Valsecchi MG, et al. Dexamethasone vs prednisone in induction treatment of pediatric ALL: results of the randomized trial AIEOP-BFM ALL 2000. Blood. 2016; https://doi.org/10.1182/blood-2015-09-670729.
124. Dunsmore KP, Winter S, Devidas M, et al. COG AALL0434: a randomized trial testing nelarabine in newly diagnosed t-cell malignancy. J Clin Oncol. 2018; https://doi.org/10.1200/jco.2018.36.15_suppl.10500.
125. Abaza Y, Kantarjian HM, Faderl S, et al. Hyper-CVAD plus nelarabine in newly diagnosed adult T-cell acute lymphoblastic leukemia and T-lymphoblastic lymphoma. Am J Hematol. 2018; https://doi.org/10.1002/ajh.24947.
126. Berg SL, Blaney SM, Devidas M, et al. Phase II study of nelarabine (compound 506U78) in children and young adults with refractory T-cell malignancies: a report from the Children's Oncology Group. J Clin Oncol. 2005; https://doi.org/10.1200/JCO.2005.03.426.
127. Cohen MH, Johnson JR, Justice R, Pazdur R. FDA drug approval summary: nelarabine (Arranon®) for the treatment of T-cell lymphoblastic leukemia/lymphoma. Oncologist. 2008; https://doi.org/10.1634/theoncologist.2006-0017.
128. Durinck K, Goossens S, Peirs S, et al. Novel biological insights in T-cell acute lymphoblastic leukemia. Exp Hematol. 2015; https://doi.org/10.1016/j.exphem.2015.05.017.
129. Bride KL, Vincent TL, Im SY, et al. Preclinical efficacy of daratumumab in T-cell acute lymphoblastic leukemia. Blood. 2018; https://doi.org/10.1182/blood-2017-07-794214.
130. Zhang X, Rastogi P, Shah B, Zhang L. B lymphoblastic leukemia/lymphoma: new insights into genetics, molecular aberrations, subclassification and targeted therapy. Oncotarget. 2017;8(39):66728–41. https://doi.org/10.18632/oncotarget.19271.
131. Labar B, Suciu S, Zittoun R, et al. Allogeneic stem cell transplantation in acute lymphoblastic leukemia and non-Hodgkin's lymphoma for patients $\geq$ 50 years old in first complete remission: results of the EORTC ALL-3 trial. Haematologica. 2004;
132. Gokbuget N, Hoelzer D, Arnold R, et al. Treatment of adult all according to protocols of the German Multicenter Study Group for Adult ALL (GMALL). Hematol Oncol Clin North Am. 2000; https://doi.org/10.1016/S0889-8588(05)70188-X.
133. Takeuchi J, Kyo T, Naito K, et al. Induction therapy by frequent administration of doxorubicin with four other drugs, followed by intensive consolidation and maintenance therapy for adult acute lymphoblastic leukemia: the JALSG-ALL93 study. Leukemia. 2002; https://doi.org/10.1038/sj.leu.2402526.
134. Thiebaut A, Vernant JP, Degos L, et al. Adult acute lymphocytic leukemia study testing chemotherapy and autologous and allogeneic transplantation: a follow-up report of the French protocol LALA 87. Hematol Oncol Clin North Am. 2000; https://doi.org/10.1016/S0889-8588(05)70190-8.
135. Linker C, Damon L, Ries C, Navarro W. Intensified and shortened cyclical chemotherapy for adult acute lymphoblastic leukemia. J Clin Oncol. 2002; https://doi.org/10.1200/JCO.2002.07.116.
136. Ramanujachar R, Richards S, Hann I, et al. Adolescents with acute lymphoblastic leukaemia: outcome on UK national paediatric (ALL97) and adult (UKALLXII/E2993) trials. Pediatr Blood Cancer. 2007; https://doi.org/10.1002/pbc.20749.

137. Usvasalo A, Räty R, Knuutila S, et al. Acute lymphoblastic leukemia in adolescents and young adults in Finland. Haematologica. 2008; https://doi.org/10.3324/haematol.12466.
138. de Bont JM, van der Holt B, Dekker AW, van der Does-van den Berg A, Sonneveld R, Pieters R. Significant difference in outcome for adolescents with acute lymphoblastic leukemia treated on pediatric vs adult protocols in the Netherlands [1]. Leukemia. 2004; https://doi.org/10.1038/sj.leu.2403538.
139. Testi AM, Valsecchi MG, Conter V, et al. Difference in outcome of adolescents with acute lymphoblastic leukemia (ALL) enrolled in pediatric (AIEOP) and adult (GIMEMA) protocols. Blood. 2004; https://doi.org/10.1182/blood.v104.11.1954.1954.
140. Moorman AV. New and emerging prognostic and predictive genetic biomarkers in B-cell precursor acute lymphoblastic leukemia. Haematologica. 2016;101(4):407–16. https://doi.org/10.3324/haematol.2015.141101.
141. Wei G, Wang J, Huang H, et al. Novel immunotherapies for adult patients with B-lineage acute lymphoblastic leukemia. J Hematol Oncol. 2017;10:150. https://doi.org/10.1186/s13045-017-0516-x.

Chapter 6
Acute Lymphoblastic Leukemia in Infants: A Distinctive, High-Risk Subtype of Childhood Acute Lymphoblastic Leukemia

Erin H. Breese, Rishi S. Kotecha, and Erin M. Guest

Introduction

Infant acute lymphoblastic leukemia (ALL), defined as ALL diagnosed prior to the first birthday, is a rare, aggressive cancer with a poor prognosis. In the United States, the incidence of ALL in infants is 1.9 cases per 100,000 or about 80 to 100 infants diagnosed each year [1]. Infant ALL is slightly more common among females compared to males (F:M ratio 1.4:1), and approximately 20% of cases are diagnosed in the first 3 months of life [1–4]. Infant ALL is a high-risk subtype of childhood ALL, associated with an event-free survival (EFS) of 45% [2–6]. Whereas many subsets of children with ALL have seen improvements over time, overall survival for infants with ALL has remained poor (Fig. 6.1) [7]. Additional unfavorable prognostic features in infants include very young age (age less than 3 or 6 months at diagnosis has each been used in clinical trials to define higher-risk cohorts),

E. H. Breese
Department of Pediatrics, University of Cincinnati College of Medicine, Division of Oncology, Cancer and Blood Diseases Institute, Cincinnati Children's Hospital Medical Center, Cincinnati, OH, USA
e-mail: erin.breese@cchmc.org

R. S. Kotecha
Department of Clinical Haematology, Oncology, Blood and Marrow Transplantation, Perth Children's Hospital, Perth, WA, Australia

Leukaemia Translational Research Laboratory, Telethon Kids Cancer Centre, Telethon Kids Institute, University of Western Australia, Perth, WA, Australia

Curtin Medical School, Curtin University, Perth, WA, Australia
e-mail: rishi.kotecha@health.wa.gov.au

E. M. Guest (✉)
University of Missouri-Kansas City, Division of Pediatric Hematology/Oncology/Blood and Marrow Transplantation, Children's Mercy Kansas City, Kansas City, MO, USA
e-mail: eguest@cmh.edu

M. R. Litzow, E. A. Raetz (eds.), *Clinical Management of Acute Lymphoblastic Leukemia*, https://doi.org/10.1007/978-3-030-85147-7_6

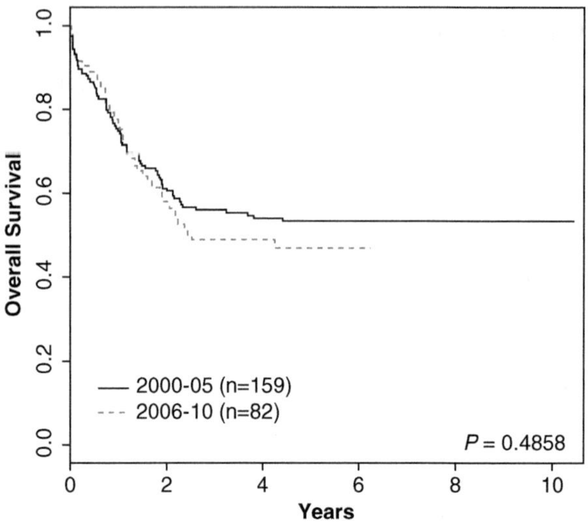

Fig. 6.1 Overall survival for infants with acute lymphoblastic leukemia. Data includes infants enrolled in frontline Children's Oncology Group clinical trials from 2000 to 2005 and 2006 to 2010

hyperleukocytosis with white blood cell (WBC) count greater than 300,000/μL at diagnosis, poor response to prednisone during the first week of induction therapy, presence of *KMT2A* (formerly *MLL*) gene rearrangement (*KMT2A*-r), and persistence of minimal residual disease (MRD) in the bone marrow following induction chemotherapy [2–6, 8–12]. Of these factors, the principal defining biological feature is presence of *KMT2A*-r. The EFS of infants with *KMT2A*-r ALL is significantly inferior compared to infants without *KMT2A*-r (36–66% vs. 74–93%) [2–6, 13]. Treatments with very intensive chemotherapy, with or without allogeneic hematopoietic stem cell transplantation (HSCT), have been unsuccessful in improving the poor outcomes of infants with *KMT2A*-r ALL, and modern clinical trials are focused on delivering novel targeted therapies in an effort to improve outcome for these high-risk infants.

In this chapter, we examine the unique biological features of infant ALL that make it challenging to cure with current available therapies. We review the design and outcomes of prior clinical trials and discuss treatment strategies that are currently in development.

Biological Features

In the late 1980s/early 1990s, scientists identified abnormalities of chromosome band 11q23 as key recurring cytogenetic features in hematological malignancies, including ALL and acute myeloid leukemia (AML) [14]. Alterations of 11q23 were associated with secondary leukemias in patients whose previous therapy included topoisomerase II inhibitors, as well as in infants less than 1 year of age with acute leukemia [15, 16]. Chromosomal translocations at this locus were found to disrupt the human trithorax gene (*HRX*) and resulted in expression of a chimeric protein containing the DNA binding domain of HRX fused to various translocation protein partners [17]. A subsequent review of 96 infants with ALL treated on Pediatric Oncology Group (POG) protocols demonstrated that 81% had molecular evidence of a *HRX* (subsequently renamed *MLL* or *KMT2A*) rearrangement [18]. These cases were associated with younger age at diagnosis, higher WBC count at diagnosis, and poor prognosis.

Extensive characterization of infant ALL has demonstrated *KMT2A*-r as a clear oncogenic driver. While 94 distinct direct translocation partner genes have been identified, the vast majority of infant ALL cases are characterized by *KMT2A*-r involving the *AFF1* (49%), *MLLT1* (22%), *MLLT3* (16%), and *MLLT10* (6%) genes [19]. Most of these rearrangements occur between exon 9 and intron 11 in the major breakpoint cluster region of the *KMT2A* gene and result in a fusion transcript which encodes for the N-terminus of the MLL protein (MLL-N), fused in frame with its translocation partner. The MLL-N contains key functional domains including a domain for binding Menin, AT-hook motifs (DNA-binding domains), two speckled nuclear localization domains, and two repression domains [20]. The wild-type MLL protein is proteolytically cleaved into the N-terminal fragment and the C-terminal fragment, which then associate within a multiprotein complex that regulates chromatin modification and gene expression, specifically in genes involved in embryogenesis, hematopoiesis, and stem cell function [20].

Early studies exploring the mechanisms of leukemic transformation in infant ALL have postulated that the *KMT2A* translocation is the sentinel event in *KMT2A*-r infant leukemia and is sufficient to act as the sole driver for leukemic transformation. *KMT2A*-r infant ALL has a nearly 100% concordance rate in monozygotic twins with evidence of a shared molecularly identical clone confirming an *in utero* origin [21]. The short latency of *KMT2A*-r leukemia, occurring within the first year of life for infants and within 2 years for those that develop therapy-related secondary *KMT2A*-r leukemia, also suggests the translocation event may be sufficient for leukemic transformation. Our understanding of the molecular drivers of leukemogenesis has been advanced by recent insights revealed through the application of next-generation sequencing. Infant ALL with *KMT2A*-r is notable for an extremely low frequency of somatic mutations (1.3 non-silent mutations per case in the dominant clone) [22–24]. The most frequent co-occurring mutations can be found within the tyrosine kinase-PI3K-RAS signaling pathways [22, 24]. *RAS* family mutations are often subclonal and demonstrate a heterogeneous pattern of clonal evolution [25]. *RAS* pathway mutations have been associated with a high WBC at diagnosis and glucocorticoid resistance and confer a proliferative advantage [25]. Additionally, while activating mutations in *FLT3* are not commonly seen, expression profiling has demonstrated significant upregulation of *FLT3* gene expression in *KMT2A*-r infant ALL, with high-level gene expression of the wild-type protein associated with phosphorylation and activation of the protein [20]. Furthermore, abnormal DNA methylation is a striking feature of infant ALL blasts with *KMT2A*-r and provides a potential target for epigenetic therapies [26–30].

Leukemias with *KMT2A*-r are notable for their high-level expression of *HOX* cluster genes and the HOX cofactor *MEIS1* [31, 32]. These genes are normally expressed in hematopoietic stem cells and progenitors, with decreasing expression as cells differentiate [33]. Recruitment of the MLL fusion protein (MLL-FP) to loci of target genes is facilitated by the interaction with the polymerase-associated factor complex (PAFc) and the trimolecular complex comprising MLL, Menin, and the chromatin-binding protein lens epithelium-derived growth factor (LEDGF), which have been found to be critical for MLL-FP-mediated leukemic transformation [34]. The MLL-FP recruits components of the super elongation complex (SEC), which includes MLL fusion partners (AFF1, AFF4, AF9, and ENL); the elongation factors ELL2, ELL3, EAF1, and EAF2; and the positive transcription elongation factor b (P-TEFb), which promotes transcriptional elongation through phosphorylation of RNA polymerase II. The AF9 and ENL fusion partners also form components of the DotCom complex, which includes AF10 and AF17, and the H3K79 methyltransferase, DOT1L. Recruitment of DOT1L to target genes by corresponding MLL-FPs can further promote transcriptional activation, with increased levels of H3K79 methylation found at MLL-FP targeted genomic loci such as *HOXA9* and *MEIS1* (Fig. 6.2) [35, 36]. Importantly, constitutive expression of *HOXA9 ex vivo* results in immortalization of hematopoietic progenitors [37]. Similarly, constitutive activation leads to stem cell-like properties found in *KMT2A*-r leukemias and is required for their survival.

Given the relatively simple genetic background of *KMT2A*-r leukemia, it has been an attractive model to explore mechanisms of leukemogenesis. Mouse models have demonstrated that differences in *KMT2A* fusion partner, cell of origin, timing of expression, and the microenvironment can influence the resulting immunophenotype (B-ALL, AML, T-ALL, or mixed phenotype acute leukemia) and latency of leukemia development [38]. Early models of *KMT2A-MLLT3*-driven leukemia demonstrated a strong bias toward myeloid disease. In these models, expression of the fusion transcript in primitive long-term hematopoietic stem cells resulted in shorter latency and more resistance to chemotherapy than those derived from differentiated granulocyte-macrophage progenitors [39]. This suggests that the chemotherapy-resistant disease seen in infant ALL may be related to a more primitive cell of origin. Subsequent studies expressing the *KMT2A-MLLT3* fusion in fetal liver cells revealed the potential for lymphoid leukemia, and newer models using genetic engineering to express the *KMT2A-MLLT3* or *KMT2A-MLLT1* oncogenes from the endogenous *KMT2A* locus in cord blood-derived CD34+ cells led to ALL, AML, and mixed lineage leukemias (*KMT2A-MLLT3*) and ALL (*KMT2A-MLLT1*) in xenografts, demonstrating the potential plasticity of these leukemias based on cell of origin and the microenvironment [40, 41]. While *KMT2A-AFF1*-driven leukemia models have proven more challenging to develop, a recent model using a human/murine cDNA hybrid fusion transcript for *KMT2A-Aff1* resulted in a pro-B ALL that more accurately recapitulates the immunophenotype and molecular features of human *KMT2A-AFF1* ALL [42]. Additionally, a recently identified CD10-negative Pre-Pro-B-cell progenitor found in fetal liver and fetal

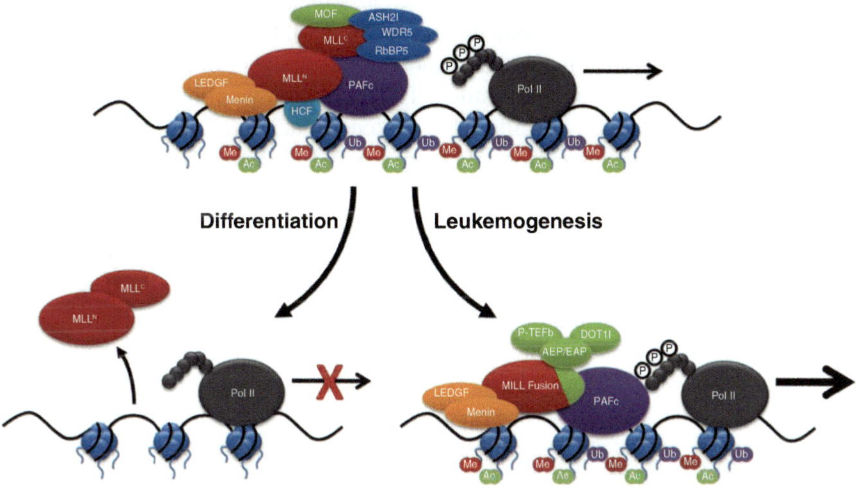

Fig. 6.2 MLL complex proteins during normal and malignant hematopoiesis. MLL interacts with a variety of protein complexes in hematopoietic stem and progenitor cells to promote transcription of critical target genes like *HOXA9* and *MEIS1*. The PAF complex (PAFc) associates with RNA polymerase II (Pol II) and recruits the RAD6/BRE1 E2/E3 ubiquitin ligase, which promotes mono-ubiquitination of histone H2B (Ub). H2B mono-ubiquitination is a histone mark associated with transcriptional activation. PAFc, along with Menin/LEDGF, recruits the MLL complex to target genes which delivers H3K4 (Me) methyltransferase activity and promotes gene transcription. MLL associates with the HAT MOF, which promotes further gene transcription through histone H4K16 acetylation (Ac). During hematopoietic differentiation, MLL is not recruited to target genes in part due to decreased transcription of PAFc. Insufficient recruitment of MLL leads to decreased expression of target genes. Chromosomal translocations involving *KMT2A (MLL)* generate MLL fusion proteins that can recruit transcriptional activation complexes dependent on the fusion partner. These complexes involve the recruitment of pTEFb, which is required to phosphorylate the RNA Pol II C-terminal domain, which promotes transcriptional elongation. The H3K79 methyltransferase DOT1l is also recruited to some MLL fusion proteins, which can further promote transcriptional activation. (Image and edited caption reprinted with permission [36])

bone marrow may serve as a potential cell of origin and provide additional insight into the unique biology found in infant leukemia [43].

Treatment

Treatment for infants with ALL has evolved significantly over time [44]. Infants were initially treated by individual study groups on childhood ALL protocols. The unfavorable prognosis carried by infants diagnosed at less than 1 year of age led to risk adaptation within childhood ALL studies, with stratification of infants to high-risk regimens. Combined analysis of infants enrolled on successive childhood ALL protocols led to the identification of several independent risk factors associated with an inferior outcome, including presence of *KMT2A*-r, hyperleukocytosis at presentation, absence of CD10 antigen, age less than 6 months at diagnosis, and poor response to initial prednisone therapy [9, 45, 46]. Outcomes of infants treated on childhood ALL protocols remained poor, and the number of infants recruited by each individual study group was limited. This limitation was pivotal in stimulating the development of infant-specific ALL protocols facilitated by collaboration of study groups. The outcomes for infant-specific ALL studies are summarized in Table 6.1.

The first US-based infant-specific ALL trials were conducted by the Children's Cancer Group (CCG-107 and CCG-1883) and the Pediatric Oncology Group (POG 8493 and POG 9107). Compared to infants treated on childhood ALL protocols, these studies introduced the concept of delivering intensified therapy to infants, demonstrating a progressive, modest improvement in survival; however outcomes remained poor with marrow relapse being the primary cause of treatment failure [12, 47, 48]. The CCG studies successfully replaced cranial radiotherapy with intrathecal and high-dose systemic therapy as an effective strategy for central

Table 6.1 Summary of published results for infant-specific collaborative group acute lymphoblastic leukemia protocols

Group	Study	Year	Number analyzed	RI rate (%)	5-year EFS (%)	5-year OS (%)	5-year EFS *KMT2A*-R (%)	5-year EFS non-*KMT2A*-R (%)	References
CCG	CCG-107	1984–1988	98	87.8	32.6	42.8	–	–	[12, 48]
	CCG-1883	1989–1993	135	94.1	37.6	50.2	–	–	
	CCG-1953	1996–2000	115	82.5	43.2	46.8	33.6	60.3	[48, 49]
POG	POG 8493	1984–1990	84	89.3	25.0	31.6	–	–	[47]
	POG 9107	1991–1993	47	89.4	31.9	40.2	–	–	
	POG 9407 (cohorts 1 + 2)	1996–2000	68	–	47.0	53.0	–	–	[51]
COG	P9407 (cohort 3)	2001–2006	141	91.8	42.3	52.9	35.5	69.7	[4]
UK CLWP	Infant 87	1987–1999	40	92.5	22.5[a]	30.0[a]	–	–	[54, 55]
	Infant 92		86	94.2	29.0[a]	42.5[a]	–	–	
Interfant	Interfant-99	1999–2005	478	93.9	46.5[a]	53.8[a]	36.4[b]	74.5[b]	[2, 3]
	Interfant-06	2006–2016	651	92.9	46.1[a]	58.2[a]	36.4[a]	73.9[a]	[2]
JILSG	MLL96	1995–1998	55	94.1	50.9	60.5	38.6	95.5	[57]
	MLL98	1998–2001	47						
JPLSG	MLL03	2004–2009	62	67.7	43.2[b]	67.2[b]	43.2[b]	–	[6]
	MLL-10	2011–2015	90	91.1	70.9	85.0	66.2	93.3	[13]

CCG Children's Cancer Group, *COG* Children's Oncology Group, *EFS* event-free survival, *JILSG* Japan Infant Leukemia Study Group, *JPLSG* Japanese Pediatric Leukemia/Lymphoma Study Group, *OS* overall survival, *POG* Pediatric Oncology Group, *RI* remission induction, *UK CLWP* United Kingdom Childhood Leukemia Working Party (UK CLWP studies included 9 patients between 12 and 18 months of age with biological features of infant ALL)

[a]6-year EFS and OS

[b]4-year EFS and OS

nervous system (CNS) prophylaxis, whereas the POG studies were able to demonstrate low rates of isolated CNS relapse with triple intrathecal therapy. The subsequent parallel POG 9407 (cohorts 1 and 2) and CCG-1953 protocols implemented further early treatment intensification, which led to a reduction in relapse rate; however this was countered by excessive treatment-related morbidity and mortality [48–51]. When CCG and POG merged to form the Children's Oncology Group (COG), amendments were made to P9407, and cohort 3 received a short infusion of daunorubicin rather than continuous infusion and prednisone rather than dexamethasone [51]. Despite a reduction in the rate of early deaths compared to preceding cohorts, cohort 3 experienced a high rate of relapse, resulting in relatively unchanged outcomes. Independent factors associated with an inferior outcome included age ≤90 days at diagnosis, hyperleukocytosis at presentation, and presence of *KMT2A*-r [4]. The successor COG study, AALL0631, also required an initial amendment to reduce the intensity of induction therapy due to excessive toxicity [52]. COG AALL0631 was pivotal in being the first study to demonstrate the safety and feasibility of adding a novel targeted therapy to post-induction chemotherapy for infants with *KMT2A*-r ALL. Although addition of the FLT3 inhibitor, lestaurtinib, did not improve overall outcomes, benefit was shown for a subset of patients who achieved potent pharmacodynamic inhibition of FLT3 and whose leukemia cells were sensitive to *ex vivo* FLT3 inhibition, highlighting the need for identification and selection of infants with ALL that may be sensitive to novel agents in future studies [5, 53]. This study also demonstrated that flow cytometry-based MRD, detected at a level of ≥0.01% in the bone marrow, is a powerful predictor of EFS for infants with *KMT2A*-r ALL [8]. The COG AALL15P1 pilot study has recently completed accrual and aims to test the tolerability and biologic activity of adding 5-day cycles of azacitidine, a demethylating agent, prior to each block of chemotherapy following induction (NCT02828358). St Jude Children's Research Hospital is also conducting a pilot trial, testing the safety of bortezomib, a proteasome inhibitor, and vorinostat, a histone deacetylase inhibitor, on a chemotherapy backbone (NCT02553460).

The first infant-specific studies conducted by the United Kingdom Childhood Leukemia Working Party, Infant 87 and Infant 92, drew similar conclusions to the early CCG and POG studies, identifying significant treatment-related toxicity and high relapse rates despite delivering increased therapeutic intensity [54, 55]. The Interfant Study Group subsequently formed in 1999 and currently comprises of over 20 international and national study groups. The first trial of the Interfant Study Group, Interfant-99, employed a hybrid treatment schedule, composed of elements used in the treatment of both ALL and AML. No additional benefit was seen for infants who were randomized to a late intensification course [3]. This study was notably the first in infants to identify the prognostic impact of detectable MRD in the bone marrow following induction and consolidation [11]. A significantly higher relapse rate was identified for congenital ALL, defined as diagnosis in the first month of life [10]. The outcome for infants who relapsed on Interfant-99 was dismal with 3-year overall survival of 20.9% for all patients and 24.9% for those treated with curative intent [56]. The subsequent study, Interfant-06, showed no benefit of early post-induction intensification with myeloid compared to lymphoid-based chemotherapy for *KMT2A*-r infant ALL and no improvement in overall outcome compared to Interfant-99 [2]. Both studies affirmed the presence of *KMT2A*-r, age less than 6 months at diagnosis, and poor response to initial prednisone therapy as independent adverse prognostic factors for outcome, with hyperleukocytosis at presentation also identified as an adverse prognostic factor on Interfant-06 [2, 3]. The Interfant Study Group has recently completed accrual for a pilot study testing the feasibility, safety, and efficacy of adding one post-induction course of the monoclonal antibody blinatumomab, a bi-specific T-cell engager, to the standard Interfant-06 chemotherapy backbone for infants with *KMT2A*-r ALL (EudraCT 2016-004674-17).

In Japan, allogeneic HSCT has historically been the standard approach for treating infants with *KMT2A*-r ALL. Two consecutive protocols, MLL96 and MLL98, scheduled HSCT following induction and three courses of post-remission intensification. These studies identified a high proportion of relapses between first complete remission and HSCT, indicating the need for more effective post-remission therapy [57]. Infants with relapsed/refractory disease fared poorly with 5-year overall survival of 25.6%, with failure to achieve remission after salvage therapy independently identified as a poor prognostic factor [58]. The MLL03 study conducted by the Japanese Pediatric Leukemia/Lymphoma Study Group (JPLSG) built on findings of the preceding studies with the aim of early phase HSCT, within 4 months of initial induction. Although this strategy was able to effectively prevent early relapse and enabled patients to receive HSCT, there was a low overall complete remission rate and a substantial number of infants relapsed following HSCT, highlighting the limited efficacy of HSCT for treatment of infants with *KMT2A*-r ALL [6]. As such, the subsequent JPLSG MLL-10 study risk stratified infants to spare HSCT in non-high-risk patients and introduced early intensification of therapy with the inclusion of high-dose cytarabine within an early consolidation phase following induction, leading to significantly improved outcomes. Clearance of MRD at the end of the early consolidation phase was confirmed as an independent prognostic factor for favorable outcome [13].

The indications for use of allogeneic HSCT for treatment of infants with ALL remain unresolved. Findings are limited by the absence of a randomized study comparing HSCT to chemotherapy alone, and analysis of prior studies is subject to selection bias of higher-risk infants for HSCT. All study groups have demonstrated that infants without *KMT2A*-r have acceptable outcomes using an intensive chemotherapy approach without requiring HSCT [2–4, 13, 49, 57]. For *KMT2A*-r infants, the COG demonstrated no difference in outcome between those that received HSCT compared to those that received chemotherapy alone [59]. The Interfant-99 study was able to demonstrate benefit for HSCT; however this was restricted to a high-risk subgroup of *KMT2A*-r infants who were less than 6 months of age at diagnosis and either had a poor prednisone response or hyperleukocytosis at diagnosis [60]. The JPLSG MLL-10 study achieved good outcomes by limiting HSCT to high-risk *KMT2A*-r infants who were less than 6 months of age at diagnosis or had CNS involvement [13]. Given these findings, HSCT is reserved for a high-risk subset of infants with *KMT2A*-r ALL on Interfant and JPLSG studies and is omitted from COG protocols. Given the emergence of novel therapies and increasing recognition of late effects in survivors of infant leukemia following HSCT, this treatment modality is likely to be utilized even less frequently in the future [57, 61].

Future Directions

Novel strategies are desperately needed for the treatment of infant ALL with *KMT2A*-r. Preclinical models have generated evidence for several potential drug targets, including inhibition of DOT1L, FLT3, DNA methyltransferase, histone deacetylase, BCL-2, and the Menin-MLL interaction. Molecularly targeted therapy with DOT1L inhibition did not produce the desired results in a clinical trial of relapsed *KMT2A*-r leukemia in adults, but different DOT1L inhibitors remain under investigation in preclinical studies [62, 63]. As discussed, FLT3 inhibition may have failed to improve overall outcomes in COG AALL0631, but could be beneficial for a select cohort of infants with *KMT2A*-r ALL whose leukemic blasts display *in vitro* sensitivity to FLT3 inhibition [5, 53]. A small molecule inhibitor of the Menin-MLL interaction has entered a first-in-human trial (NCT04065399) after showing marked activity in *KMT2A*-r preclinical models, including infant ALL, and may be feasible to investigate in infants in the near future [64]. Currently, the COG is developing a phase 2 trial of venetoclax, a BCL-2 inhibitor, in combination with chemotherapy for the treatment of infants with *KMT2A*-r ALL. BCL-2 inhibition has shown activity against *KMT2A*-r ALL in preclinical models, and venetoclax has been identified as a promising therapeutic agent for *KMT2A*-r infant ALL [65–67].

Immunotherapy is likely to form an important component of future clinical trials for infant ALL. Immunotherapy has led to remarkable improvements in outcomes in the treatment of relapsed childhood ALL, but its applicability to infant ALL remains unclear [68–71]. Chimeric antigen receptor T-cell (CAR T-cell) therapy, either autologous or off-the-shelf, is available to infants at relapse in some countries, although the efficacy of CAR T-cell therapy in infants is not yet known [72, 73]. CAR T-cell therapy is an attractive alternative to upfront chemotherapy for infants with ALL, but is not without potential challenges. These challenges may include inability to harvest sufficient T-cells, exhaustion of T-cells following chemotherapy, and the potential for lineage switch to myeloid leukemia at relapse [74]. The results of early CAR T-cell studies in infants with relapsed or refractory ALL and the results of the Interfant Study Group's pilot blinatumomab trial in upfront therapy will be very informative to the development of future treatment approaches. Further investigation of anti-CD22 therapy with inotuzumab ozogamicin may also be warranted, following promising findings from a retrospective study in a small cohort of infants and young children with relapsed or refractory ALL [75].

Conclusion

Infant ALL remains a high-risk subtype of childhood ALL, with no major advances in therapy nor improvements in outcome over several decades. This can be attributed, at least in part, to the characteristic chemotherapy refractory nature of *KMT2A*-r infant ALL. A number of novel treatment strategies have shown strong preclinical evidence of efficacy. Any therapy that successfully targets *KMT2A*-r has the potential to result in a major breakthrough for this disease. The international infant ALL research community is actively collaborating to discover molecular targets, test agents in preclinical models, and implement clinical trials, with the primary aim to prioritize improvements in outcome for infants with ALL.

References

1. Howlander N, Noone AM, Krapcho M, Miller D, Brest A, Yu M, et al., editors. SEER Cancer Statistics Review, 1975–2016. Bethesda: National Cancer Institute. https://seer.cancer.gov/csr/1975_2016 based on November 2018 SEER data submission, posted to the SEER web site, April 2019.
2. Pieters R, De Lorenzo P, Ancliffe P, Aversa LA, Brethon B, Biondi A, et al. Outcome of infants younger than 1 year with acute lymphoblastic leukemia treated with the Interfant-06 protocol: results from an international phase III randomized study. J Clin Oncol. 2019;37(25):2246–56.
3. Pieters R, Schrappe M, De Lorenzo P, Hann I, De Rossi G, Felice M, et al. A treatment protocol for infants younger than 1 year with acute lymphoblastic leukaemia (Interfant-99): an observational study and a multicentre randomised trial. Lancet. 2007;370(9583):240–50.
4. Dreyer ZE, Hilden JM, Jones TL, Devidas M, Winick NJ, Willman CL, et al. Intensified chemotherapy without SCT in infant ALL: results from COG P9407 (cohort 3). Pediatr Blood Cancer. 2015;62(3):419–26.
5. Brown P, Kairalla J, Wang C, Dreyer Z, Salzer W, Sorenson M, et al. Addition of FLT3 inhibitor lestaurtinib to post-induction chemotherapy does not improve outcomes in MLL-rearranged infant acute lymphoblastic leukemia (ALL): AALL0631, a Children's Oncology Group study. Pediatr Blood Cancer. 2016;63(S3):S5–S321.
6. Koh K, Tomizawa D, Moriya Saito A, Watanabe T, Miyamura T, Hirayama M, et al. Early use of allogeneic hematopoietic stem cell transplantation for infants with MLL gene-rearrangement-positive acute lymphoblastic leukemia. Leukemia. 2015;29(2):290–6.
7. Raetz E, Lu X, Devidas M, Loh M, Winick N, Carroll W, et al. Continued improvements in overall survival (OS) in children with newly diagnosed acute lymphoblastic leukemia (ALL): a Children's Oncology Group (COG) report. Pediatr Blood Cancer. 2018;65(S1):e27057.
8. Brown P, Kairalla J, Hilden J, Dreyer Z, Carroll A, Heerema NA, et al. Minimal residual disease (MRD) predicts outcomes in KMT2A-rearranged but not KMT2A-wild type infant acute lymphoblastic leukemia (ALL): AALL0631, a Children's Oncology Group study. Pediatr Blood Cancer. 2019;66(S4):e27989.
9. Dordelmann M, Reiter A, Borkhardt A, Ludwig WD, Gotz N, Viehmann S, et al. Prednisone response is the strongest predictor of treatment outcome in infant acute lymphoblastic leukemia. Blood. 1999;94(4):1209–17.
10. van der Linden MH, Valsecchi MG, De Lorenzo P, Moricke A, Janka G, Leblanc TM, et al. Outcome of congenital acute lymphoblastic leukemia treated on the Interfant-99 protocol. Blood. 2009;114(18):3764–8.

11. Van der Velden VH, Corral L, Valsecchi MG, Jansen MW, De Lorenzo P, Cazzaniga G, et al. Prognostic significance of minimal residual disease in infants with acute lymphoblastic leukemia treated within the Interfant-99 protocol. Leukemia. 2009;23(6):1073–9.
12. Reaman GH, Sposto R, Sensel MG, Lange BJ, Feusner JH, Heerema NA, et al. Treatment outcome and prognostic factors for infants with acute lymphoblastic leukemia treated on two consecutive trials of the Children's Cancer Group. J Clin Oncol. 1999;17(2):445–55.
13. Tomizawa D, Miyamura T, Imamura T, Watanabe T, Moriya Saito A, Ogawa A, et al. A risk-stratified therapy for infants with acute lymphoblastic leukemia: a report from the JPLSG MLL-10 trial. Blood. 2020;136(16):1813–23.
14. Heim S, Mitelman F. Cancer Cytogenetics. Alan R Liss; New York 1987.
15. Kaneko Y, Shikano T, Maseki N, Sakurai M, Sakurai M, Takeda T, et al. Clinical characteristics of infant acute leukemia with or without 11q23 translocations. Leukemia. 1988;2(10):672–6.
16. Pui CH, Ribeiro RC, Hancock ML, Rivera GK, Evans WE, Raimondi SC, et al. Acute myeloid leukemia in children treated with epipodophyllotoxins for acute lymphoblastic leukemia. N Engl J Med. 1991;325(24):1682–7.
17. Tkachuk DC, Kohler S, Cleary ML. Involvement of a homolog of Drosophila trithorax by 11q23 chromosomal translocations in acute leukemias. Cell. 1992;71(4):691–700.
18. Rubnitz JE, Link MP, Shuster JJ, Carroll AJ, Hakami N, Frankel LS, et al. Frequency and prognostic significance of HRX rearrangements in infant acute lymphoblastic leukemia: a Pediatric Oncology Group study. Blood. 1994;84(2):570–3.
19. Meyer C, Burmeister T, Groger D, Tsaur G, Fechina L, Renneville A, et al. The MLL recombinome of acute leukemias in 2017. Leukemia. 2018;32(2):273–84.
20. Winters AC, Bernt KM. MLL-rearranged leukemias - an update on science and clinical approaches. Front Pediatr. 2017;5:4.
21. Greaves MF, Maia AT, Wiemels JL, Ford AM. Leukemia in twins: lessons in natural history. Blood. 2003;102(7):2321–33.
22. Andersson AK, Ma J, Wang J, Chen X, Gedman AL, Dang J, et al. The landscape of somatic mutations in infant MLL-rearranged acute lymphoblastic leukemias. Nat Genet. 2015;47(4):330–7.
23. Kostadinov R, Farooqi M, Yoo B, Farrow E, Kelley S, Gibson M, et al. Landscape of somatic mutations and gene expression changes in relapsed infant MLL-rearranged acute lymphoblastic leukemia. Blood. 2016;128(22):1735.
24. Agraz-Doblas A, Bueno C, Bashford-Rogers R, Roy A, Schneider P, Bardini M, et al. Unraveling the cellular origin and clinical prognostic markers of infant B-cell acute lymphoblastic leukemia using genome-wide analysis. Haematologica. 2019;104(6):1176–88.
25. Mansur MB, Ford AM, Emerenciano M. The role of RAS mutations in MLL-rearranged leukaemia: a path to intervention? Biochim Biophys Acta Rev Cancer. 2017;1868(2):521–6.
26. Schafer E, Irizarry R, Negi S, McIntyre E, Small D, Figueroa ME, et al. Promoter hypermethylation in MLL-r infant acute lymphoblastic leukemia: biology and therapeutic targeting. Blood. 2010;115(23):4798–809.
27. Stumpel DJ, Schneider P, van Roon EH, Boer JM, de Lorenzo P, Valsecchi MG, et al. Specific promoter methylation identifies different subgroups of MLL-rearranged infant acute lymphoblastic leukemia, influences clinical outcome, and provides therapeutic options. Blood. 2009;114(27):5490–8.
28. Stumpel DJ, Schneider P, van Roon EH, Pieters R, Stam RW. Absence of global hypomethylation in promoter hypermethylated Mixed Lineage Leukaemia-rearranged infant acute lymphoblastic leukaemia. Eur J Cancer. 2013;49(1):175–84.
29. Stumpel DJ, Schotte D, Lange-Turenhout EA, Schneider P, Seslija L, de Menezes RX, et al. Hypermethylation of specific microRNA genes in MLL-rearranged infant acute lymphoblastic leukemia: major matters at a micro scale. Leukemia. 2011;25(3):429–39.
30. Bergmann AK, Castellano G, Alten J, Ammerpohl O, Kolarova J, Nordlund J, et al. DNA methylation profiling of pediatric B-cell lymphoblastic leukemia with KMT2A rearrangement identifies hypomethylation at enhancer sites. Pediatr Blood Cancer. 2017;64(3):e26251.

31. Yokoyama A. Transcriptional activation by MLL fusion proteins in leukemogenesis. Exp Hematol. 2017;46:21–30.
32. Armstrong SA, Golub TR, Korsmeyer SJ. MLL-rearranged leukemias: insights from gene expression profiling. Semin Hematol. 2003;40(4):268–73.
33. Collins CT, Hess JL. Deregulation of the HOXA9/MEIS1 axis in acute leukemia. Curr Opin Hematol. 2016;23(4):354–61.
34. Chan AKN, Chen CW. Rewiring the epigenetic networks in MLL-rearranged leukemias: epigenetic dysregulation and pharmacological interventions. Front Cell Dev Biol. 2019;7:81.
35. Ballabio E, Milne TA. Epigenetic control of gene expression in leukemogenesis: cooperation between wild type MLL and MLL fusion proteins. Mol Cell Oncol. 2014;1(2):e955330.
36. Muntean AG, Hess JL. The pathogenesis of mixed lineage leukemia. Annu Rev Pathol. 2012;7:283–301.
37. Schnabel CA, Jacobs Y, Cleary ML. HoxA9-mediated immortalization of myeloid progenitors requires functional interactions with TALE cofactors Pbx and Meis. Oncogene. 2000;19(5):608–16.
38. Milne TA. Mouse models of MLL leukemia: recapitulating the human disease. Blood. 2017;129(16):2217–23.
39. Stavropoulou V, Kaspar S, Brault L, Sanders MA, Juge S, Morettini S, et al. MLL-AF9 expression in hematopoietic stem cells drives a highly invasive AML expressing EMT-related genes linked to poor outcome. Cancer Cell. 2016;30(1):43–58.
40. Chen W, O'Sullivan MG, Hudson W, Kersey J. Modeling human infant MLL leukemia in mice: leukemia from fetal liver differs from that originating in postnatal marrow. Blood. 2011;117(12):3474–5.
41. Buechele C, Breese EH, Schneidawind D, Lin CH, Jeong J, Duque-Afonso J, et al. MLL leukemia induction by genome editing of human CD34+ hematopoietic cells. Blood. 2015;126(14):1683–94.
42. Lin S, Luo RT, Ptasinska A, Kerry J, Assi SA, Wunderlich M, et al. Instructive role of MLL-fusion proteins revealed by a model of t(4;11) pro-B acute lymphoblastic leukemia. Cancer Cell. 2016;30(5):737–49.
43. O'Byrne S, Elliott N, Rice S, Buck G, Fordham N, Garnett C, et al. Discovery of a CD10-negative B-progenitor in human fetal life identifies unique ontogeny-related developmental programs. Blood. 2019;134(13):1059–71.
44. Kotecha RS, Gottardo NG, Kees UR, Cole CH. The evolution of clinical trials for infant acute lymphoblastic leukemia. Blood Cancer J. 2014;4:e200.
45. Pui CH, Behm FG, Downing JR, Hancock ML, Shurtleff SA, Ribeiro RC, et al. 11q23/MLL rearrangement confers a poor prognosis in infants with acute lymphoblastic leukemia. J Clin Oncol. 1994;12(5):909–15.
46. Silverman LB, McLean TW, Gelber RD, Donnelly MJ, Gilliland DG, Tarbell NJ, et al. Intensified therapy for infants with acute lymphoblastic leukemia: results from the Dana-Farber Cancer Institute Consortium. Cancer. 1997;80(12):2285–95.
47. Salzer WL, Devidas M, Carroll WL, Winick N, Pullen J, Hunger SP, et al. Long-term results of the Pediatric Oncology Group studies for childhood acute lymphoblastic leukemia 1984-2001: a report from the Children's Oncology Group. Leukemia. 2010;24(2):355–70.
48. Gaynon PS, Angiolillo AL, Carroll WL, Nachman JB, Trigg ME, Sather HN, et al. Long-term results of the Children's Cancer Group studies for childhood acute lymphoblastic leukemia 1983-2002: a Children's Oncology Group Report. Leukemia. 2010;24(2):285–97.
49. Hilden JM, Dinndorf PA, Meerbaum SO, Sather H, Villaluna D, Heerema NA, et al. Analysis of prognostic factors of acute lymphoblastic leukemia in infants: report on CCG 1953 from the Children's Oncology Group. Blood. 2006;108(2):441–51.
50. Salzer W, Dinndorf P, Dreyer Z, Hilden J, Reaman GH. Analysis of infectious complications in infants with acute lymphoblastic leukemia treated on the Children's Cancer Group protocol 1953: a report from the Children's Oncology Group. J Pediatr Hematol Oncol. 2009;31(6):398–405.

51. Salzer WL, Jones TL, Devidas M, Hilden JM, Winick N, Hunger S, et al. Modifications to induction therapy decrease risk of early death in infants with acute lymphoblastic leukemia treated on Children's Oncology Group P9407. Pediatr Blood Cancer. 2012;59(5):834–9.
52. Salzer WL, Jones TL, Devidas M, Dreyer ZE, Gore L, Winick NJ, et al. Decreased induction morbidity and mortality following modification to induction therapy in infants with acute lymphoblastic leukemia enrolled on AALL0631: a report from the Children's Oncology Group. Pediatr Blood Cancer. 2015;62(3):414–8.
53. Brown PA, Kairalla J, Hilden JM, Dreyer ZE, Carroll AJ, Heerema NA, et al. FLT3 inhibitor correlative laboratory assays impact outcomes in KMT2A-rearranged infant acute lymphoblastic leukemia (ALL) patients treated with lestaurtinib: AALL0631, a Children's Oncology Group study. Blood. 2019;134(Supplement_1):1293.
54. Chessells JM, Eden OB, Bailey CC, Lilleyman JS, Richards SM. Acute lymphoblastic leukaemia in infancy: experience in MRC UKALL trials. Report from the Medical Research Council Working Party on Childhood Leukaemia. Leukemia. 1994;8(8):1275–9.
55. Chessells JM, Harrison CJ, Watson SL, Vora AJ, Richards SM, Medical Research Council Working Party on Childhood Leukaemia. Treatment of infants with lymphoblastic leukaemia: results of the UK Infant Protocols 1987-1999. Br J Haematol. 2002;117(2):306–14.
56. Driessen EM, de Lorenzo P, Campbell M, Felice M, Ferster A, Hann I, et al. Outcome of relapsed infant acute lymphoblastic leukemia treated on the Interfant-99 protocol. Leukemia. 2016;30(5):1184–7.
57. Tomizawa D, Koh K, Sato T, Kinukawa N, Morimoto A, Isoyama K, et al. Outcome of risk-based therapy for infant acute lymphoblastic leukemia with or without an MLL gene rearrangement, with emphasis on late effects: a final report of two consecutive studies, MLL96 and MLL98, of the Japan Infant Leukemia Study Group. Leukemia. 2007;21(11):2258–63.
58. Tomizawa D, Koh K, Hirayama M, Miyamura T, Hatanaka M, Saikawa Y, et al. Outcome of recurrent or refractory acute lymphoblastic leukemia in infants with MLL gene rearrangements: a report from the Japan Infant Leukemia Study Group. Pediatr Blood Cancer. 2009;52(7):808–13.
59. Dreyer ZE, Dinndorf PA, Camitta B, Sather H, La MK, Devidas M, et al. Analysis of the role of hematopoietic stem-cell transplantation in infants with acute lymphoblastic leukemia in first remission and MLL gene rearrangements: a report from the Children's Oncology Group. J Clin Oncol. 2011;29(2):214–22.
60. Mann G, Attarbaschi A, Schrappe M, De Lorenzo P, Peters C, Hann I, et al. Improved outcome with hematopoietic stem cell transplantation in a poor prognostic subgroup of infants with mixed-lineage-leukemia (MLL)-rearranged acute lymphoblastic leukemia: results from the Interfant-99 study. Blood. 2010;116(15):2644–50.
61. Aoki Y, Hayakawa A, Koike K, Tauchi H, Ishii E, Koh K, et al. Late effects in survivors of infant acute lymphoblastic leukemia from the 3 consecutive Japanese nationwide clinical trials. Blood. 2019;134(Supplement_1):4559.
62. Daigle SR, Olhava EJ, Therkelsen CA, Basavapathruni A, Jin L, Boriack-Sjodin PA, et al. Potent inhibition of DOT1L as treatment of MLL-fusion leukemia. Blood. 2013;122(6):1017–25.
63. Stein EM, Garcia-Manero G, Rizzieri DA, Tibes R, Berdeja JG, Savona MR, et al. The DOT1L inhibitor pinometostat reduces H3K79 methylation and has modest clinical activity in adult acute leukemia. Blood. 2018;131(24):2661–9.
64. Krivtsov AV, Evans K, Gadrey JY, Eschle BK, Hatton C, Uckelmann HJ, et al. A Menin-MLL inhibitor induces specific chromatin changes and eradicates disease in models of MLL-rearranged leukemia. Cancer Cell. 2019;36(6):660–73.e11.
65. Urtishak KA, Edwards AY, Wang LS, Hudome A, Robinson BW, Barrett JS, et al. Potent obatoclax cytotoxicity and activation of triple death mode killing across infant acute lymphoblastic leukemia. Blood. 2013;121(14):2689–703.
66. Suryani S, Carol H, Chonghaile TN, Frismantas V, Sarmah C, High L, et al. Cell and molecular determinants of in vivo efficacy of the BH3 mimetic ABT-263 against pediatric acute lymphoblastic leukemia xenografts. Clin Cancer Res. 2014;20(17):4520–31.

67. Khaw SL, Suryani S, Evans K, Richmond J, Robbins A, Kurmasheva RT, et al. Venetoclax responses of pediatric ALL xenografts reveal sensitivity of MLL-rearranged leukemia. Blood. 2016;128(10):1382–95.
68. Locatelli F, Zugmaier G, Rizzari C, Morris JD, Gruhn B, Klingebiel T, et al. Effect of blinatumomab vs chemotherapy on event-free survival among children with high-risk first relapse B-cell acute lymphoblastic leukemia: a randomized clinical trial. JAMA. 2021;325(9):843–54.
69. Brown PA, Ji L, Xu X, Devidas M, Hogan LE, Borowitz MJ, et al. Effect of postreinduction therapy consolidation with blinatumomab vs chemotherapy on disease-free survival in children, adolescents and young adults with first relapse of B-cell acute lymphoblastic leukemia: a randomized clinical trial. JAMA. 2021;325(9):833–42.
70. Maude SL, Laetsch TW, Buechner J, Rives S, Boyer M, Bittencourt H, et al. Tisagenlecleucel in children and young adults with B-cell lymphoblastic leukemia. N Engl J Med. 2018;378(5):439–48.
71. Clesham K, Rao V, Bartram J, Ancliff P, Ghorashian S, O'Connor D, et al. Blinatumomab for infant acute lymphoblastic leukemia. Blood. 2020;135(17):1501–4.
72. Qasim W, Zhan H, Samarasinghe S, Adams S, Amrolia P, Stafford S, et al. Molecular remission of infant B-ALL after infusion of universal TALEN gene-edited CAR T cells. Sci Transl Med. 2017;9(374):eaaj2013.
73. Annesley C, Summers C, Pulsipher MA, Wayne AS, Rivers J, Lamble AJ, et al. Clinical experience of CAR T cell immunotherapy for relapsed and refractory infant ALL demonstrates feasibility and favorable responses. Blood. 2019;134(Supplement_1):3869.
74. Gardner R, Wu D, Cherian S, Fang M, Hanafi LA, Finney O, et al. Acquisition of a CD19-negative myeloid phenotype allows immune escape of MLL-rearranged B-ALL from CD19 CAR-T-cell therapy. Blood. 2016;127(20):2406–10.
75. Brivio E, Chantrain CF, Gruber TA, Thano A, Rialland F, Contet A, et al. Inotuzumab ozogamicin in infants and young children with relapsed or refractory acute lymphoblastic leukaemia: a case series. Br J Haematol. 2021;193(6):1172–7.

Chapter 7
Treatment of Elderly Patients with Acute Lymphoblastic Leukemia

Marc Schwartz and Matthew Wieduwilt

Introduction

Epidemiology and Outcomes in Older ALL

In the United States in 2019, acute lymphoblastic leukemia (ALL) represented 0.3% of new cancer cases or approximately 6000 cases, with a median age at diagnosis of 16 years old. Approximately half of these cases occurred in the pediatric/adolescent population (<20 years old). While 21.7% of new ALL cases from 2012 to 2016 in the United States occurred in patients aged 55 years or older, 52.2% of all deaths related to ALL occurred in this older age group [1]. The age definition for the term "older adult" is heterogeneously defined, and in this chapter it will refer to adults 55–65 years of age and older consistent with previous reviews on this topic [2].

Long-term survival for ALL in both the pediatric and adolescent/young adult (AYA) populations has improved dramatically over the last five decades in large part due to high rates of participation in large randomized cooperative group trials and possibly adoption of pediatric-inspired chemotherapy regimens in AYAs [3–4]. Improvements in survival for older adults have been minimal, however, with long-term survival rates still less than 20% [5–7]. Poor outcomes in older adults are attributed in part to poor tolerance of intensive chemotherapeutic regimens resulting in high rates of induction mortality and death in remission. Comorbidity scores such as the Charlson Comorbidity Index (CCI) and Hematopoietic cell transplant

M. Schwartz (✉)
Division of Hematology, University of Colorado, Aurora, CO, USA
e-mail: marc.schwartz@cuanschutz.edu

M. Wieduwilt
University of Oklahoma, Stephenson Cancer Center,
Oklahoma City, OK, USA

M. R. Litzow, E. A. Raetz (eds.), *Clinical Management of Acute Lymphoblastic Leukemia*, https://doi.org/10.1007/978-3-030-85147-7_7

comorbidity index (HCT-CI) predict early death rates with induction chemotherapy in ALL and may be routinely assessed in older adults when making decisions about initial therapy [8].

Biology of ALL in Older Adults

ALL in older adults has distinct cytogenetic and molecular features compared to the pediatric and AYA populations [9–12]. Phenotypically, the vast majority of ALL in older adults is B-lineage ALL, while T-lineage ALL is rare [11–12]. Philadelphia chromosome (Ph)-positive ALL is characterized by the t(9;22)(q34;q11) translocation that creates an activated fusion protein between BCR and the tyrosine kinase ABL1 (BCR-ABL1). The incidence of Ph-positive ALL increases with age and has been reported to occur in 25–50% of older patients in different series [11–14]. Since the development of highly effective BCR-ABL1 tyrosine kinase inhibitors (TKIs), Ph positivity is not a consistent risk factor for poor survival as in the past in older adults and may confer better survival than Ph-negative ALL [13–14]. Philadelphia chromosome-like (Ph-like) ALL is characterized by a gene expression profile similar to Ph + ALL but without the BCR-ABL1 fusion. Ph-like ALL is typically associated with other kinase-activating alterations including CRLF2 rearrangements often in association with activating JAK protein mutations, ABL class fusions, and JAK2, CSF3R, or EPOR rearrangements [16]. The incidence of Ph-like ALL increases with age with a peak in younger adults (21–39 years old) and incidence of approximately 20–25% in older adults and is associated with poor responses to conventional chemotherapy [17–19]. In addition, KMT2A (MLL) alterations confer a poor prognosis and are more common in adult ALL accounting for approximately 8% of cases. Other genetic aberrations associated with poor outcomes that have been found to be enriched in older adults include t(14;18)(q32;q21), low hypodiploidy (31–39 chromosomes), complex karyotype, TP53 mutations, and Ikaros (IKZF1) deletions [11–12, 15, 20–23]. T-cell ALL is uncommon in older adults and the genetics in older ALL is not well characterized. In T-cell ALL or lymphoblastic lymphoma patients in general, activating mutations in NOTCH1 and mutations in FBXW7, a regulator of NOTCH1 degradation, are present in approximately 60% and 15% of cases, respectively [24–28]. Mutations in NOTCH1 and FBXW7 have been associated with a favorable early treatment response and better prognosis in some studies [29–33]. Therapy-related ALL (t-ALL) is a recently recognized entity defined by previous exposure to genotoxic therapy (chemotherapy or radiation) and is reported to comprise ~3–9% of adult ALL with median age at onset of 55–61 years. t-ALL cases are enriched for KMT2A rearrangements and MDS-like abnormalities such as monosomal karyotypes. Compared to ALL without history of genotoxic therapy exposure, t-ALL is associated with worse prognosis although this may be overcome with allogeneic HCT [34–35].

Treatment of Ph-Negative ALL in Older Adults

Curative-intent therapy for older adults with Ph-negative B-cell and T-cell ALL has historically entailed treatment with "adult" chemotherapy regimens that include high doses of myelosuppressive agents including an anthracycline often with cyclophosphamide together with vincristine, corticosteroids, and intrathecal therapy. Asparaginase, a cornerstone of treatment in younger patients, is not routinely given to older patients given high levels of toxicity in older adults. Older adults treated with these "adult" regimens have higher rates of infection and induction mortality, greater requirements for chemotherapy dose reductions or holds, and worse long-term survival compared to younger adults [36–38]. Lower-intensity "elderly" chemotherapy protocols are more tolerable in older adults, but long-term survival is about 20–30% due to high rates of relapse [39–43].

Compared to adult ALL regimens, pediatric-inspired regimens contain higher cumulative doses of the non-myelosuppressive agents including asparaginase, vincristine, and corticosteroids, as well as intensified CNS prophylaxis and lower cumulative doses of myelosuppressive drugs. Treatment of younger adults with intensive, asparaginase-containing, pediatric-style regimens results in long-term cure rates of 50–70%, an improvement over historical results achieved with "adult" regimens for this age group [4, 44]. The tolerability of pediatric-inspired regimens decreases significantly around 40–55 years of age where the benefit of the pediatric approach appears to be similar to less toxic regimens. This is due in part to increased asparaginase-related toxicity, which manifests as higher induction mortality and a high incidence of hepatotoxicity, thrombosis, pancreatitis, and hyperglycemia with increasing age [45–48]. In an ongoing phase II trial testing a pediatric-inspired regimen with two doses of pegylated asparaginase at 1000 U/m^2 given during induction for adults aged 25–65 years, induction death occurred in 18% of the first 90 patients treated and was associated with age (>40 vs ≤40 years old; OR = 18.5, $p = 0.01$), prompting investigators to amend the protocol such that a single dose of pegylated asparaginase at 1000 U/m^2 will be administered for adults >40 years of age [49]. The Dana Farber consortium showed the feasibility of giving older adults >50 years of age a low dose of pegylated asparaginase (500 U/m^2) during induction; however higher doses that were initially administered (2000 U/m^2 or 1500 U/m^2) in this phase II protocol resulted in unacceptable rates of severe hepatotoxicity [50]. Other groups have shown that age-adapted pediatric-inspired protocols are feasible in older adults and may result in improved outcomes compared with less intensive regimens [51, 52]. Due to the small number of patients on clinical trials, little data exists to help guide different treatment for T-cell ALL, relative to B-cell ALL, in elderly patients. T-cell ALL in the elderly is typically managed with regimens used in Ph-negative B-cell ALL, and reported outcomes seem similar. An analysis of 100 older patients aged 55–65 years treated on UK ALLXII/E2993 demonstrated similar 5-year EFS between B-cell and T-cell ALL patients [38].

As we have reached or exceeded the limits of chemotherapy tolerability in older adults, the development and approval in the relapsed/refractory ALL setting of highly active targeted therapies with manageable toxicities holds promise to extend more effective and safer treatment options to older patients with newly diagnosed Ph-negative B-cell ALL. Inotuzumab ozogamicin is a CD22-targeted antibody-drug conjugate that when internalized in B-lymphoblasts releases ozogamicin inside the cell leading to DNA damage and cell death. In a phase III study in adults aged 18–79 years with relapsed or refractory B-cell ALL, inotuzumab ozogamicin achieved a high CR rate of 74% versus 31% with standard chemotherapy ($P < 0.0001$) [53]. Blinatumomab is a CD19-targeted bi-functional T-cell engaging antibody that directs a patient's own T-cells to cells expressing CD19 leading to cytotoxic T-cell activation and targeted killing of B-lymphoblasts and normal B-cells. In a phase III study of blinatumomab in adults with relapsed or refractory B-cell ALL, the overall CR rate was 44% versus 25% with chemotherapy ($P < 0.001$) with an MRD negativity rate of 76% versus 48% with chemotherapy. Therapy discontinuation occurred in 12% of blinatumomab patients, 4% for neurologic toxicity and 1% for cytokine release syndrome [54].

Numerous promising approaches are being explored with these two drugs in frontline treatment of adult B-cell ALL. A number of large studies are evaluating inotuzumab ozogamicin in the frontline setting for adults with B-cell ALL either combined with chemotherapy (EWALL-INO, NCT03249870; MD Anderson 2010-0991, NCT01371630; ALL 001, NCT03962465), given as blocks of inotuzumab ozogamicin alone before or between blocks of cytotoxic chemotherapy (GMALL INITIAL-1, NCT03460522; Alliance 041501, NCT03150693; ALLTogether1, NCT04307576), or in sequence before blinatumomab (Alliance 041703, NCT03739814). The combination of inotuzumab ozogamicin with hyper-fractionated cyclophosphamide, vincristine, and dexamethasone (miniHyperCVD) with or without subsequent blinatumomab is being explored in older adults with Ph-negative B-cell ALL at MD Anderson (NCT01371630). In a propensity score analysis comparing the regimen with historical hyperCVAD-treated patients, early results show a high overall CR rate of 98% versus 88%, and induction mortality of 0% versus 8%, respectively. Comparing survival for inotuzumab ozogamicin with miniHyperCVD to hyperCVAD, 3-year overall survivals were 63% and 34% ($P = 0.004$), and 3-year event-free survivals were 64% and 34% ($P = 0.003$), respectively [55]. Although randomized studies and longer follow-up are needed, the results to date support the concept that less intense therapy incorporating inotuzumab ozogamicin and/or blinatumomab may improve outcomes for older patients with Ph-negative ALL.

Blinatumomab is also being actively studied as part of frontline therapy in adults, including older adults, fit for intensive chemotherapy (ECOG 1910, NCT02003222; GRAALL-QUEST, NCT03709719; LAL2317, NCT03367299; HOVON146ALL, NCT03541083), and results of these studies are eagerly awaited. Even less toxic approaches, foregoing traditional cytotoxic chemotherapy in induction altogether, are being pursued for older and less fit patients in the front line including blinatumomab alone followed by POMP (mercaptopurine, vincristine, methotrexate, prednisone) maintenance (SWOG 1318, NCT02143414) and inotuzumab ozogamicin followed by blinatumomab without maintenance (Alliance 041703, NCT03739814).

A preliminary report of SWOG 1318 reported outcomes of 29 older patients with a median age of 75 years (range 66–84 years) with newly diagnosed Ph-negative B-cell ALL. The overall complete response rate was 66% with an MRD negativity rate of 92%. Frontline blinatumomab was very well tolerated with no deaths in induction (through day 28), one case of grade 3 cytokine-release syndrome, and one case of grade 3 neurotoxicity. With 1-year median follow-up, DFS and OS were 65% and 56%, respectively [56].

Currently there is no single standard of care chemotherapy regimen for older adults with untreated Ph-negative ALL although the experience with intensive adult-type or pediatric-based chemotherapy regimens suggests that these regimens result in excessive toxicity and poor outcomes in most older adults. On the other hand, age-adapted regimens may be appropriate for a select group of very fit older patients. When available, enrollment on clinical trials, especially those trials pursuing less toxic regimens with promising efficacy, is recommended for all older adults with ALL. See Table 7.1 for the summary of selected regimens and Table 7.2 for novel regimens.

Treatment of Ph-Positive ALL in Older Adults

Prior to the advent of BCR-ABL1 targeted TKIs, older adults with Ph-positive ALL had 5-year survival rates of approximately 10%. This was attributable to intrinsic chemotherapy resistance of Ph-positive ALL, high induction death rates in older adults, and ineligibility for myeloablative allogeneic HCT [57]. With an excellent single-agent activity and safety profile, tyrosine kinase inhibitors (TKIs) have become cornerstones of the management of all patients with Ph-positive disease, and their incorporation into frontline regimens has allowed for de-escalation of cytotoxic therapies in induction. The addition of imatinib to a standard intensive chemotherapy backbone in adults with Ph + ALL improved outcomes, in large part by facilitating allogeneic HCT [58, 59]. In a prospective trial of imatinib added to the hyperCVAD backbone in adults with Ph + ALL, 5-year survival was 43% but was significantly worse for adults aged >60 years compared to ≤60 (median OS 16.4 vs 87.2 months) [60].

The second-generation TKIs dasatinib and nilotinib appear superior to imatinib due to activity against a wider spectrum of BCR-ABL1 kinase domain mutations that confer resistance to imatinib and, in the case of dasatinib, penetration into the central nervous system [61, 62]. A prospective trial of dasatinib plus hyperCVAD in 72 adults with a median age of 55 (range 21–80; n = 46/70 age ≥60) reported an impressive 5-year survival of 52% [63]. A multicenter SWOG-led study evaluated dasatinib with hyperCVAD followed by allogeneic HCT for patients up to 60 years old with a matched donor. In a landmark analysis, survival at 3 years was superior in those receiving allogeneic HCT vs those who continued on dasatinib with hyper-CVAD alone (HR 0.35, 95% CI 0.12–0.97, P = 0.037) supporting an ongoing important role for allogeneic HCT when using second-generation TKI-based

Table 7.1 Selected regimens and outcomes for older adults treated with chemotherapy for ALL

Study	*N*	Median age, years (range)	Ph	T-cell, %	Induction	Post-remission (all include maintenance)	CR rate, %	Induction mortality, %	Overall survival
PETHEMA ALL-96 [37]	33 (≥55 yo) 239 (<55 yo)	65 (56–77)		17 (≥55 yo) 33 (<55 yo)	DNR, VCR, PDN, CPM, L-ASP	C1: 6MP, HDMTX, VM26, AraC C2: DNR, VCR, DEX, CPM, L-ASP	58 (≥55 yo)	36 (≥55 yo)	39% (2 y, ≥55 yo)
MDACC [16]	122 (≥60 yo) 409 (<60 yo)	NR	+/−	NA	CPM, VCR, DOX, DEX	HDMTX + araC x4 alternating with CPM, VCR, DOX, DEX x3	84 (≥60 yo) 92 (<60 yo)	10 (≥60 yo) 2 (<60 yo)	20% (5 y, ≥60 yo) 48% (5 y, <60 yo)
UKALL12/ E2993 [18]	100 (55–65 yo) 1814 (14–54 yo)	NR	+/−	14 (55–65 yo) 19 (14-54 yo)	1: DNR, VCR, L-ASP, PDN 2: CPM, araC, 6MP	INT: HDMTX + ASP x3 CONS: alloHCT, autoHCT, or chemo	73 (≥55 yo) 93 (<55 yo)	18 (≥55 yo) 4 (<55 yo)	21% (5 y, ≥55 yo) 41% (5 y, all)
GRAALL-SA1 [21]	60	NR (55–80)	–	12	1: DOX (Arm A) or PEG-DOX (Arm B), VCR,DEX 2: DOX or PEG-DOX, VCR, DEX, CPM	VCR + DOX (Arm A) or PEG-DOX (Arm B) x2 alternating with CPM, araC, 6MP x2	82 (overall) 90 (arm A) 72 (arm B)	7 (arm A) 10 (arm B)	10 mo (median, both arms) 35% (2 y, Arm A) 24% (2 y, Arm B)
GMALL [20]	268	67 (55–85)	–	15	1: DEX, VCR, IDA 2: CPM, araC	IDMTX + L-ASP x3 alternating with araC x2, then re-induction with CPM, VCR, IDA, araC	76	14	23% (5 y)
ALLOLD07 [19]	56	66 (56–79)	–	NA	1: DEX, VCR, IDA 2: CPM, araC	IDMTX + L-ASP x3 alternating with araC x3	74	13	12.4 mo (median)

DFCI [25]	30	58 (51–72)	+/–	3	DOX, VCR, PDN, PEG-ASP	CONS1: clofarabine, PDN, PEG-ASP CNS: DOX, VCR, DEX, 6MP, PEG-ASP CONS2: DOX, VCR, DEX, 6MP, PEG-ASP x 8 cycles	67	3	52% (2 y, CR1)
GRAALL-2005 [28]	93 (55–60 yo) 787 (18–60 yo)	36 (18–60)	+/–	33 (all ages)	VCR, DNR, L-ASP, CPM Salvage: IDA, araC	CONS1: araC, DEX, L-ASP (block I); VCR, MTX, L-ASP, 6MP (block II); MTX, CPM, VP16 (block III) CONS2: same as CONS1 LI: PDN, VCR, L-ASP, CPM (early CR) or IDA, araC (late CR)	80 (≥55 yo) 92 (all ages)	18 (≥55 yo) 6 (all ages)	27.4% (5 y, ≥55 yo) 58.5% (5 y, all)

Abbreviations: *Ph* Philadelphia chromosome, *N* number of patients, *CR* complete response, *NA* not reported/available, *y* years, *yo* years old, *CPM* cyclophosphamide, *VCR* vincristine, *DOX* doxorubicin, *DEX* dexamethasone, *HDMTX* high-dose methotrexate, *IDMTX* intermediate-dose methotrexate, *araC* cytarabine, *DNR* daunorubicin, *L-ASP* native *e. coli* L-asparaginase, *PEG-DOX* pegylated doxorubicin, *6MP* 6-mercaptopurine, *IDA* idarubicin, *PDN* prednisone, *PEG-asp* pegylated asparaginase, *MDACC* MD Anderson Cancer Center, *GRAALL* Group for Research on Adult Acute Lymphoblastic Leukemia, *GMALL* German Multicenter ALL, *DFCI* Dana Farber Cancer Institute

Table 7.2 Selected ongoing frontline studies of novel agents for older adults with ALL

Study	NCT Identifier	Phase	Ph	Age (years)	Treatment
SWOG 1318	NCT02143414	II	–	≥65	Blinatumomab followed by POMP maintenance
Alliance 041703	NCT03739814	II	–	≥60	Inotuzumab ozogamicin followed by blinatumomab
MDACC	NCT01371630	II	–	≥65	Inotuzumab ozogamicin + low intensity chemo +/– blinatumomab, followed by POMP maintenance
EWALL-INO	NCT03249870	II	–	≥55	Inotuzumab ozogamicin + low intensity chemo
ECOG 1910	NCT02003222	III	–	30–70	Modified ECOG2993 chemotherapy → MRD- after intensification randomized to blinatumomab blocks versus no blinatumomab in consolidation
HOVON146ALL	NCT03541083	II	–	18–70	Chemotherapy with 3 cycles of blinatumomab given during prephase, consolidation, and prior to alloHCT or maintenance
GIMEMA	NCT02744768	II	+	≥18	Dasatinib + prednisone followed by blinatumomab
SWOG 1318	NCT02143414	II	+	≥65	Dasatinib + prednisone followed by blinatumomab
MDACC	NCT03263572	II	+	≥60	Ponatinib + blinatumomab

Abbreviations: *Ph* Philadelphia chromosome, *SWOG* Southwest Oncology Group, *POMP* mercaptopurine, vincristine, methotrexate, prednisone, *Alliance* Alliance for Clinical Trials in Oncology, *MDACC* MD Anderson Cancer Center, *EWALL* European ALL Working Group, *ECOG* Eastern Cooperative Oncology Group, *MRD* minimal residual disease, *HOVON* Dutch-Belgian Hemato-Oncology Cooperative Group, *GIMEMA* Gruppo Italiano Malattie EMatologiche dell'Adulto

regimens [59]. CALGB 10701 used dasatinib plus dexamethasone induction in adults ≥18 years, with patients age 18–70 years undergoing reduced-intensity conditioning (RIC) allogeneic HCT in remission if they had a HLA-matched donor and autologous HCT if they did not. Patients >70 years of age or unable to undergo HCT received maintenance chemotherapy. The 3-year survival was 55% for the entire group, with those who underwent protocol-specified allogeneic HCT, autologous HCT, or chemo having 3-year survivals of 75%, 71%, and 55%, respectively [62]. Multiple studies have shown excellent results with autologous HCT in Ph-positive B-cell ALL with long-term survival similar between allogeneic and autologous HCTs [64–66]. Although haploidentical HCT may now be expanding donor options for patients, autologous HCT may still be considered for some older, fit patients.

Ponatinib, a third-generation TKI, may have an advantage over both imatinib and second-generation TKIs due to its activity against the BCR-ABL1 T315I resistance mutation present in approximately 75% of Ph + ALL cases relapsing on or after dasatinib-based therapy [62, 67]. A prospective trial of ponatinib plus hyperCVAD in adults with median age 46 years (range 21–80 year; $n = 20/86$ age ≥60) reported

3-month complete molecular response (CMR) rate of 74% and 3-year survival of 78%. Due to high incidence of cardiovascular events, several dose modifications of ponatinib were made. A final dosing scheme of 45 mg days 1–14 during induction, 30 mg daily continuously starting with the second cycle, and then 15 mg daily once a CMR was achieved appeared to be safer [68, 69]. In adults aged 27–85 years with Ph-positive ALL, ponatinib 45 mg oral daily plus corticosteroids has been shown to be safe and effective with CR rate at 6 weeks of 95%, a marrow CMR rate at 24 weeks of 46%, and a 1-year OS of 88%. One patient died of complications possibly related to ponatinib [70]. Although initial results are promising, longer follow-up is needed in all ponatinib studies to understand the curative potential and potential late toxicities of ponatinib-based regimens.

Lower-intensity approaches in older adults with Ph + ALL involving a TKI in combination with corticosteroids alone or low-intensity chemotherapy do not compromise hematologic remission rates compared to intensive approaches and should therefore be offered to older and less fit adults [62, 67, 71–75]. Remission rates with these approaches are 95–100% with almost no induction deaths. Optimal post-remission therapy after TKI with corticosteroid or low-intensity chemotherapy induction aiming to eliminate TKI-resistant clones is not well defined, although allogeneic HCT appears to provide the most durable remissions but with consequent transplant-related morbidity and mortality [62, 67]. Whether TKIs in combination with intensive chemotherapy provide an advantage over lower-intensity approaches for fit older adults with Ph + ALL is unclear, although at least one study showed no difference in survival in adults up to age 60 treated with a low- versus high-intensity chemotherapy combination plus imatinib [72]. For many older patients, there is poor tolerability of allogeneic HCT and intensive chemotherapy leaving them with few effective options for post-remission therapy as relapse rates with maintenance TKI alone are high, at least with first- and second-generation TKIs. The ongoing D ALBA study (NCT02744768) treated 63 patients age 24 82 years with Ph positive ALL with dasatinib and prednisone followed by 2–5 courses of blinatumomab. In a 2019 presentation of interim results, investigators reported 12-month OS and DFS of 94% and 88%, respectively [76]. Two US cooperative group studies are studying TKI with corticosteroid induction follow by blinatumomab and TKI in older patients unfit (SWOG1318, age 65 years and older) or fit (ECOG-ACRIN 9181, age 18–70 years) for allogeneic HCT. Results of these ongoing studies may transform therapy for both older and younger Ph-positive ALL.

Achievement of a complete molecular response (CMR), defined as absence of detectable BCR-ABL1 transcripts by quantitative PCR testing with sensitivity of 0.001–0.01% at 3 months into treatment, has been shown to be a significant predictor of overall survival with TKI-based regimens, regardless of the specific TKI used [77]. Treatment with ponatinib-based regimens has been shown to produce high rates of early CMR and low relapse rates which may also predict excellent long-term outcomes even without allogeneic HCT [68, 69]. In this respect, ponatinib may be the most effective TKI for all adults with Ph-positive ALL, principally by overcoming the ABL1 T315I TKI resistance mutation, although data from prospective randomized comparisons with second-generation TKI- or imatinib-based regimens are lacking. See Table 7.3 for a summary of TKI-based regimens and Table 7.2 for ongoing studies.

Relapsed or Refractory ALL in Older Adults

Relapsed or refractory (R/R) ALL historically has been associated with dismal prognosis regardless of age, with allogeneic HCT offering a chance for long-term remission in a minority of adults [78, 79]. The landscape of therapies for adults with R/R ALL has recently expanded however with approval of the novel agents blinatumomab and inotuzumab ozogamicin (InO). In a randomized phase 3 trial, adults with R/R Ph-negative ALL treated with blinatumomab had a higher complete response (CR) rate (33.6% vs 15.7%, $p < 0.001$) and better event-free survival (EFS)

Table 7.3 Frontline TKI-based regimens for older adults with Ph + ALL

Study	Year	Regimen	*N*	Median age, years (range)	CR rate (%)	IM (%)	Overall survival
LAL0201-B [75]	2007	Imatinib + prednisone	29	69 (61–83)	100	0	20 mo (median)
MDACC [40]	2015	Imatinib + hyperCVAD	54 (all pts) 16 (>60 yo)	51 (17–84)	93	2	43% (5 yr, all pts) 14% (5 yr, age > 60)
LAL1205 [46]	2011	Dasatinib + prednisone	53	53.6 (24–77)	100	0	69.2% (20 mos)
MDACC [43]	2015	Dasatinib + hyperCVAD	72	55 (21–80)	96	4	52% (5 yr)
EWALL-Ph01 [53]	2016	Dasatinib, vincristine, dexamethasone	91	69	96	4	36% (5 yr)
CALGB 10701 [42]	2018	Dasatinib + dexamethasone induction then alloHCT, autoHCT, or chemotherapy	64	60 (22–87)	97	0	55% (3 yr)
Korean [80]	2015	Nilotinib + multi-agent chemotherapy	90	47 (17–77)	91	9	72% (2 yr)
EWALL-Ph02 [54]	2018	Nilotinib, vincristine, dexamethasone	72	65.5	94	1.3	47 (4 yr)
LAL 1811 [50]	2017	Ponatinib + prednisone	42	68 (27–85)	95	2.3	87.5% (1 yr)
MDACC [48]	2019	Ponatinib + hyperCVAD	86	46 (21–80)	100	0	78% (3 yr)

Abbreviations: *N* number of patients, *CR* complete response, *IM* induction mortality, *mo* months, *MDACC* MD Anderson Cancer Center, *hyperCVAD* hyperfractionated cyclophosphamide, vincristine, adriamycin, dexamethasone, *yo* years old, *yr* year, *pts* patients, *EWALL* European ALL Working Group, *CALGB* Cancer and Leukemia Group B, *alloHCT* allogeneic hematopoietic cell transplant, *autoHCT* autologous hematopoietic cell transplant

(HR 0.55, $p < 0.001$) and overall survival (median 7.7 vs 4.0 mo; HR 0.71, $p = 0.01$) [53]. Blinatumomab also has activity in R/R Ph + ALL, as demonstrated by a 36% CR/CRh rate (including four of ten patients with the T315I mutation) in a phase II trial of adults who were refractory to or intolerant of at least one second- or later-generation TKI [80]. Blinatumomab was also approved for adults with persistent minimal residual disease (MRD) based on results of a phase 2 single-arm study, which showed that treatment with up to four cycles of blinatumomab converted 88% of MRD positive ($\geq 10^{-3}$) to MRD negative, which was associated with higher RFS and OS compared to those who remained MRD positive (38.8 vs 12.5 months) [81]. Two distinct toxicities observed with blinatumomab are cytokine release syndrome (CRS) and neurotoxicity. CRS is mediated by increased levels of cytokines related to activated cytotoxic T-cells. The precise mechanism of neurotoxicity with blinatumomab is not known; however prior neurologic events are a risk factor [82]. In a comparison of older (≥65 years) versus younger adults (<65 years) enrolled on two phase II studies of blinatumomab in R/R ALL, incidence of all ≥grade 3 adverse event (AEs) was similar between age groups (86% vs 80%) except for ≥grade 3 neurologic AEs which occurred with greater frequency among older adults (28% vs 13%) [83].

Inotuzumab ozogamicin is an antibody-drug conjugate (ADC) consisting of an anti-CD22 humanized monoclonal antibody bound to the alkylating agent calicheamicin (ozogamicin). In the latest follow-up of the randomized phase III trial of inotuzumab ozogamicin versus standard chemotherapy for adults aged ≥18 years of age with relapsed or refractory ALL, patients who received inotuzumab ozogamicin had better rates of complete response or complete response with incomplete count recovery (CR/CRi) (73.8% vs 30.9%, $p < 0.0001$) and longer 2-year survival (22.8% vs 10%; HR 0.75, $p = 0.0105$) [53]. Hepatic toxicity including veno-occlusive disease/sinusoidal obstruction syndrome (VOD) has been observed with inotuzumab ozogamicin with a VOD risk of 14%. The risk for developing VOD is increased when allogeneic HCT is performed after inotuzumab ozogamicin. In a subgroup analysis of the phase 3 trial comparing outcomes in older (≥55 yo) versus younger (<55 yo) adults, older patients who proceeded to alloHCT after InO had higher rate of VOD (41% vs 17%) [84]. Limiting inotuzumab ozogamicin to two cycles and avoiding double-alkylator conditioning therapy may lessen the risk of VOD after HCT [85].

Compared to B-cell ALL, development of targeted therapies for T-cell ALL has been slower. Nelarabine is a purine analog and pro-drug of 9-β-D-arabinofuranosylguanine (ara-G) with selective activity for T-cell ALL (Shewach, Ullmna) [86, 87]. Two phase II clinical trials have addressed the activity of nelarabine monotherapy in relapsed or refractory T-cell ALL or lymphoblastic lymphoma (LBL). CALGB 19801 studied single agent nelarabine in 39 patients with a median age of 34 years (range 16–66 years) with relapsed T-cell ALL or LBL including 6 patients over the age of 50. The CR rate was 31% with a median DFS and OS of 20 weeks [88]. A second study by the GMALL treated 126 patients with a median age of 33 years (range 18–81 years) with R/R T-cell ALL or LBL with nelarabine monotherapy. Sixteen patients were 56 years of age or older. The cumulative CR and PR rates were 36% and 10%, respectively. Median overall survival was 6 months with a 3-year survival of 12%. Long-term survival was seen in patients undergoing allogeneic HCT in CR [89]. Myelosuppression is common with nelarabine, and neurotoxicity, principally peripheral sensory neuropathy but also grade 3–4 CNS toxicity in 3–4% of patients, is a significant side effect. The safety and efficacy of nelarbine have not been well studied in the older population, but it is an appropriate treatment choice for older patients with R/R T-cell ALL or LBL [88, 89].

For older adults with R/R Ph-negative B-cell ALL, either blinatumomab or inotuzumab ozogamicin is an appropriate option with the goal of achieving MRD-negative CR which should be followed by allogeneic HCT (for those who are HCT candidates), though caution regarding HCT after inotuzumab ozogamicin must be emphasized given the elevated risk for developing VOD. For older adults with Ph-negative B-cell ALL who have persistent MRD after initial therapy and are HCT candidates, blinatumomab followed by allogeneic HCT may be appropriate. For R/R T-cell ALL, nelarabine is a uniquely active agent appropriate for older patients either for disease control or ideally as a bridge to allogeneic HCT. See Table 7.4 for a summary of novel therapies for R/R ALL.

Allogeneic HCT for Older Adults with ALL

In several donor vs. no-donor comparisons of myeloablative allogeneic HCT in adults with ALL in CR1, the benefit of allogeneic HCT was established in terms of increasing long-term leukemia-free survival (LFS) rates to 45–75% versus 30–40% with chemotherapy alone [90, 91]. A landmark meta-analysis of donor vs no-donor trials showed that MAC allogeneic HCT in CR1 provided a survival benefit for adults <35 years of age (OR = 0.79, $p = 0.0003$), but not for adults ≥35 years of age (OR = 1.01, $p = 0.9$). In the older group, excessive transplant-related mortality negated the potential benefit of reduced relapse [92]. In recent years, indications for allogeneic HCT in ALL have shifted, mainly due to the recognition that residual disease below the minimal CR threshold (MRD) after induction is the strongest independent risk factor for relapse regardless of specific MRD assay, timing of assessment, or level of detection [93, 94]. Several groups have demonstrated a disease-free survival benefit for HCT in CR1 for adults with Ph-negative ALL who have detectable MRD after induction, while in contrast those without detectable MRD did not benefit from HCT [93–95]. As such, more effective frontline therapies may obviate the need for allogeneic HCT for the large majority of patients with Ph-negative ALL in first remission. For patients with Ph-positive ALL, HCT in CR1 allogeneic HCT has traditionally been recommended although there is emerging data to suggest that patients who achieve an early complete molecular response may have excellent long-term outcomes even without HCT [63, 77].

Reduced intensity conditioning (RIC) regimens allow for an HCT-mediated graft-versus-leukemia effect with potentially less toxicity in older adults with comorbidities or poor fitness. The largest outcomes series was reported by the

Table 7.4 Novel therapies for adults with relapsed/refractory ALL

Study	Agent	Eligibility	*N*	Age (years)	Response rate	MRD –ve	AlloHCT rate	Overall survival
TOWER [34]	Blinatumomab	R/R Ph- B-cell ALL	271	41 (18–80)	34% (CR) 44% (CR/CRh/CRi)	76%	24%	7.7 mo (median)
ALCANTARA [60]	Blinatumomab	R/R Ph + ALL (failing second or later generation TKI)	45	55 (23–78)	36% (CR/CRh)	88%	25%	7.1 mo (median)
INO-VATE [33]	Inotuzumab ozogamicin	R/R B-cell ALL	164	47 (18–78)	74% (CR/CRi)	71%	48%	7.7 mo (median)
MSKCC [77]	19-28z CAR T cells	R/R B-cell ALL	53	44 (23–74)	83% (CR)	47%	39%	12.9 mo (median)
KTE-X19 [78]	CAR T	R/R B-cell ALL	45	46 (18–77)	68% (CR/CRi)	73%	NR	NR
U Wash [79]	CAR T	R/R B-cell ALL	53	39 (20–76)	85% (CR)	85%	40%	20 mo (median, MRD -ve CR) 5 mo (median, no response)

Abbreviations: *N* number of patients, *MRD –ve* minimal residual disease negative, *AlloHCT* allogeneic hematopoietic cell transplant, *R/R* relapsed or refractory, *Ph-* Philadelphia chromosome negative, *ALL* acute lymphoblastic leukemia, *CR* complete response, *CRh* CR with partial hematologic recovery, *CRi* CR with incomplete count recovery, *mo* months, *Ph+* Philadelphia chromosome positive, *MSKCC* Memorial Sloan Kettering Cancer Center, *CAR T* chimeric antigen receptor modified T-cells, *NR* not reported, *U Wash* University of Washington

CIBMTR, in which 273 adults aged 55 years or older undergoing RIC allogeneic HCT between 2001 and 2012 had a 3-year NRM, CIR, and OS of 25%, 47%, and 38%, respectively [96]. Other reported comparisons of MAC versus RIC in adults with ALL have not demonstrated inferiority of RIC although these were small studies [97–101]. For fit older patients, RIC allogeneic HCT remains a treatment option although high rates of NRM and relapse are expected based on available data and the superiority of RIC allogeneic HCT over chemotherapy alone has yet to be convincingly demonstrated in the older population.

Future Directions in the Management of Older Adults with ALL

Given the marked single-agent activity of blinatumomab and InO in R/R ALL and their tolerable safety profile in older adults, several active protocols are evaluating these agents in the frontline setting in older adults with ALL either as monotherapies, given together in sequence, or given in combination with chemotherapy or TKIs. A summary of these ongoing trials is listed in Table 7.4. The key relevant questions to be addressed in these trials are the following:

1. Is the optimal use of blinatumomab in the frontline setting with induction, as prophylactic therapy in case of MRD persistence after induction, or as a routine component of post-remission therapy?
2. What is the best intensity and schedule of chemotherapy in combination with inotuzumab ozogamicin?
3. Is a cytotoxic chemotherapy-free approach to induction feasible in older adults with inotuzumab ozogamicin and blinatumomab given sequentially?
4. What are the toxicities when combining novel agents with chemotherapy or TKIs?

Anti-CD19 chimeric antigen receptor modified T-cells (CAR-T) are being evaluated for adults with R/R B-ALL. Available results from these early phase trials suggest a high rate of MRD-negative remissions; however relapses are common even with consolidative allogeneic HCT [102–104]. The major relevant questions for anti-CD19 CAR-T will be its relative safety, efficacy, and feasibility compared to blinatumomab or inotuzumab ozogamicin given alone or in combination.

Acknowledgement The authors declare no competing financial interests.

References

1. National Cancer Institute: Cancer Stat Facts: Leukemia: Acute lymphocytic leukemia (ALL). https://seer.cancer.gov/statfacts/html/alyl.html.

2. Gokbuget N. Treatment of older patients with acute lymphoblastic leukaemia. Drugs Aging. 2018;35(1):11–26.
3. Pui CH, Yang JJ, Hunger SP, Pieters R, Schrappe M, Biondi A, et al. Childhood acute lymphoblastic leukemia: progress through collaboration. J Clin Oncol. 2015;33(27):2938–48.
4. Muffly L, Curran E. Pediatric-inspired protocols in adult acute lymphoblastic leukemia: are the results bearing fruit? Hematology. 2019;2019(1):17–23.
5. Lennmyr E, Karlsson K, Ahlberg L, Garelius H, Hulegardh E, Izarra AS, et al. Survival in adult acute lymphoblastic leukaemia (ALL): a report from the Swedish ALL registry. Eur J Haematol. 2019;103(2):88–98.
6. Geyer MB, Hsu M, Devlin SM, Tallman MS, Douer D, Park JH. Overall survival among older US adults with ALL remains low despite modest improvement since 1980: SEER analysis. Blood. 2017;129(13):1878–81.
7. Dinmohamed AG, Szabo A, van der Mark M, Visser O, Sonneveld P, Cornelissen JJ, et al. Improved survival in adult patients with acute lymphoblastic leukemia in the Netherlands: a population-based study on treatment, trial participation and survival. Leukemia. 2016;30(2):310–7.
8. Wermann WK, Viardot A, Kayser S, Alakel N, Elmaagacli A, Faul C, et al. Comorbidities are frequent in older patients with de novo acute lymphoblastic leukemia (all) and correlate with induction mortality: analysis of more than 1200 patients from GMALL data bases. Blood. 2018;132(Supplement 1):660.
9. Iacobucci I, Mullighan CG. Genetic basis of acute lymphoblastic leukemia. J Clin Oncol. 2017;35(9):975–83.
10. Roberts KG. Genetics and prognosis of ALL in children vs adults. Hematology. 2018;2018(1):137–45.
11. Chiaretti S, Vitale A, Cazzaniga G, Orlando SM, Silvestri D, Fazi P, et al. Clinico-biological features of 5202 patients with acute lymphoblastic leukemia enrolled in the Italian AIEOP and GIMEMA protocols and stratified in age cohorts. Haematologica. 2013;98(11):1702–10.
12. Moorman AV, Chilton L, Wilkinson J, Ensor HM, Bown N, Proctor SJ. A population-based cytogenetic study of adults with acute lymphoblastic leukemia. Blood. 2010;115(2):206–14.
13. Byun JM, Koh Y, Shin DY, Kim I, Yoon SS, Lee JO, et al. BCR-ABL translocation as a favorable prognostic factor in elderly patients with acute lymphoblastic leukemia in the era of potent tyrosine kinase inhibitors. Haematologica. 2017;102(5):e187–e90.
14. Kozlowski P, Lennmyr E, Ahlberg L, Bernell P, Hulegardh E, Karbach H, et al. Age but not Philadelphia positivity impairs outcome in older/elderly patients with acute lymphoblastic leukemia in Sweden. Eur J Haematol. 2017;99(2):141–9.
15. Fedullo AL, Messina M, Elia L, Piciocchi A, Gianfelici V, Lauretti A, et al. Prognostic implications of additional genomic lesions in adult Philadelphia chromosome-positive acute lymphoblastic leukemia. Haematologica. 2019;104(2):312–8.
16. Roberts KG, Li Y, Payne-Turner D, Harvey RC, Yang YL, Pei D, et al. Targetable kinase-activating lesions in Ph-like acute lymphoblastic leukemia. N Engl J Med. 2014;371(11):1005–15.
17. Roberts KG, Gu Z, Payne-Turner D, McCastlain K, Harvey RC, Chen IM, et al. High frequency and poor outcome of Philadelphia chromosome-like acute lymphoblastic leukemia in adults. J Clin Oncol. 2017;35(4):394–401.
18. Tasian SK, Hurtz C, Wertheim GB, Bailey NG, Lim MS, Harvey RC, et al. High incidence of Philadelphia chromosome-like acute lymphoblastic leukemia in older adults with B-ALL. Leukemia. 2017;31(4):981–4.
19. Jain N, Roberts KG, Jabbour E, Patel K, Eterovic AK, Chen K, et al. Ph-like acute lymphoblastic leukemia: a high-risk subtype in adults. Blood. 2017;129(5):572–81.
20. Ribera J, Granada I, Morgades M, Vives S, Genesca E, Gonzalez C, et al. The poor prognosis of low hypodiploidy in adults with B-cell precursor acute lymphoblastic leukaemia is restricted to older adults and elderly patients. Br J Haematol. 2019;186(2):263–8.

21. Holmfeldt L, Wei L, Diaz-Flores E, Walsh M, Zhang J, Ding L, et al. The genomic landscape of hypodiploid acute lymphoblastic leukemia. Nat Genet. 2013;45(3):242–52.
22. Stengel A, Schnittger S, Weissmann S, Kuznia S, Kern W, Kohlmann A, et al. TP53 mutations occur in 15.7% of ALL and are associated with MYC-rearrangement, low hypodiploidy, and a poor prognosis. Blood. 2014;124(2):251–8.
23. Ribera J, Morgades M, Zamora L, Montesinos P, Gomez Segui I, Pratcorona M, et al. Prognostic significance of copy number alterations in adolescent and adult patients with precursor B acute lymphoblastic leukemia enrolled in PETHEMA protocols. Cancer. 2015;121(21):3809–17.
24. Litzow MR, Ferrando AA. How I treat T-cell acute lymphoblastic leukemia in adults. Blood. 2015;126(7):833–41.
25. Weng AP, Ferrando AA, Lee W, et al. Activating mutations of NOTCH1 in human T cell acute lymphoblastic leukemia. Science. 2004;306(5694):269–71.
26. Malyukova A, Dohda T, von der Lehr N, et al. The tumor suppressor gene hCDC4 is frequently mutated in human T-cell acute lymphoblastic leukemia with functional consequences for Notch signaling. Cancer Res. 2007;67(12):5611–6.
27. Thompson BJ, Buonamici S, Sulis ML, et al. The SCFFBW7 ubiquitin ligase complex as a tumor suppressor in T cell leukemia. J Exp Med. 2007;204(8):1825–35.
28. O'Neil J, Grim J, Strack P, et al. FBW7 mutations in leukemic cells mediate NOTCH pathway activation and resistance to gamma-secretase inhibitors. J Exp Med. 2007;204(8):1813–24.
29. Breit S, Stanulla M, Flohr T, et al. Activating NOTCH1 mutations predict favorable early treatment response and long-term outcome in childhood precursor T-cell lymphoblastic leukemia. Blood. 2006;108(4):1151–7.
30. Asnafi V, Buzyn A, Le Noir S, et al. NOTCH1/ FBXW7 mutation identifies a large subgroup with favorable outcome in adult T-cell acute lymphoblastic leukemia (T-ALL): a Group for Research on Adult Acute Lymphoblastic Leukemia (GRAALL) study. Blood. 2009;113(17):3918–24.
31. Clappier E, Collette S, Grardel N, et al.; EORTC- CLG.NOTCH1 and FBXW7 mutations have a favorable impact on early response to treatment, but not on outcome, in children with T-cell acute lymphoblastic leukemia (T-ALL) treated on EORTC trials 58881 and 58951. Leukemia. 2010;24(12):2023–31.
32. Mansour MR, Sulis ML, Duke V, et al. Prognostic implications of NOTCH1 and FBXW7 mutations in adults with T-cell acute lymphoblastic leukemia treated on the MRC UKALLXII/ ECOG E2993 protocol. J Clin Oncol. 2009;27(26):4352–6.
33. Zuurbier L, Homminga I, Calvert V, et al. NOTCH1 and/or FBXW7 mutations predict for initial good prednisone response but not for improved outcome in pediatric T-cell acute lymphoblastic leukemia patients treated on DCOG or COALL protocols. Leukemia. 2010;24(12):2014–22.
34. Aldoss I, Stiller T, Tsai NC, Song JY, Cao T, Bandara NA, et al. Therapy-related acute lymphoblastic leukemia has distinct clinical and cytogenetic features compared to de novo acute lymphoblastic leukemia, but outcomes are comparable in transplanted patients. Haematologica. 2018;103(10):1662–8.
35. Saygin C, Kishtagari A, Cassaday RD, Reizine N, Yurkiewicz I, Liedtke M, et al. Therapy-related acute lymphoblastic leukemia is a distinct entity with adverse genetic features and clinical outcomes. Blood Adv. 2019;3(24):4228–37.
36. O'Brien S, Thomas DA, Ravandi F, Faderl S, Pierce S, Kantarjian H. Results of the hyperfractionated cyclophosphamide, vincristine, doxorubicin, and dexamethasone regimen in elderly patients with acute lymphocytic leukemia. Cancer. 2008;113(8):2097–101.
37. Sancho JM, Ribera JM, Xicoy B, Morgades M, Oriol A, Tormo M, et al. Results of the PETHEMA ALL-96 trial in elderly patients with Philadelphia chromosome-negative acute lymphoblastic leukemia. Eur J Haematol. 2007;78(2):102–10.

38. Sive JI, Buck G, Fielding A, Lazarus HM, Litzow MR, Luger S, et al. Outcomes in older adults with acute lymphoblastic leukaemia (ALL): results from the international MRC UKALL XII/ECOG2993 trial. Br J Haematol. 2012;157(4):463–71.
39. Ribera JM, Garcia O, Oriol A, Gil C, Montesinos P, Bernal T, et al. Feasibility and results of subtype-oriented protocols in older adults and fit elderly patients with acute lymphoblastic leukemia: results of three prospective parallel trials from the PETHEMA group. Leuk Res. 2016;41:12–20.
40. Goekbuget N, Beck J, Brueggemann M, Burmeister T, Buss EC, Frickhofen N, et al. Moderate intensive chemotherapy including CNS-prophylaxis with liposomal cytarabine is feasible and effective in older patients with Ph-negative acute lymphoblastic leukemia (ALL): results of a prospective trial from the German Multicenter Study Group for Adult ALL (GMALL). Blood. 2012;120(21):1493.
41. Hunault-Berger M, Leguay T, Thomas X, Legrand O, Huguet F, Bonmati C, et al. A randomized study of pegylated liposomal doxorubicin versus continuous-infusion doxorubicin in elderly patients with acute lymphoblastic leukemia: the GRAALL-SA1 study. Haematologica. 2011;96(2):245–52.
42. Goekbuget N, Leguay T, Hunault M, Al-Nawakil C, Chevallier P, Dombret H, et al. First European chemotherapy schedule for elderly patients with acute lymphoblastic leukemia: promising remission rate and feasible moderate dose intensity consolidation. Blood. 2008;112(11):304.
43. Schwartz P, Hunault-Berger M, Chevallier PL, et al. French results with the EWALL chemotherapy backbone in older patients with Philadelphia chromosome negative acute lymphoblastic leukemia: a GRAALL report. Haematologica. 2013;98:463. (abstr S1124)
44. Stock W, Luger SM, Advani AS, Yin J, Harvey RC, Mullighan CG, et al. A pediatric regimen for older adolescents and young adults with acute lymphoblastic leukemia: results of CALGB 10403. Blood. 2019;133(14):1548–59.
45. Huguet F, Leguay T, Raffoux E, Thomas X, Beldjord K, Delabesse E, et al. Pediatric-inspired therapy in adults with Philadelphia chromosome-negative acute lymphoblastic leukemia: the GRAALL-2003 study. J Clin Oncol. 2009;27(6):911–8.
46. Huguet F, Chevret S, Leguay T, Thomas X, Boissel N, Escoffre-Barbe M, et al. Intensified therapy of acute lymphoblastic leukemia in adults: report of the randomized GRAALL-2005 clinical trial. J Clin Oncol. 2018;36(24):2514–23.
47. Kao S, Xu W, Gupta V, Minden M, Schuh A, Schimmer AD, et al. Outcome of patients age 60 and over with acute lymphoblastic leukemia (ALL) treated with a modified pediatric protocol. Blood. 2008;112(11):3962.
48. Ribera JM, Garcia O, Gil C, Mercadal S, Garcia-Cadenas I, Montesinos P, et al. Comparison of intensive, pediatric-inspired therapy with non-intensive therapy in older adults aged 55-65 years with Philadelphia chromosome-negative acute lymphoblastic leukemia. Leuk Res. 2018;68:79–84.
49. Patel B, Kirkwood AA, Dey A, Marks DI, McMillan AK, Menne TF, et al. Pegylated-asparaginase during induction therapy for adult acute lymphoblastic leukaemia: toxicity data from the UKALL14 trial. Leukemia. 2017;31(1):58–64.
50. Fathi AT, DeAngelo DJ, Stevenson KE, Kolitz JE, Asch JD, Amrein PC, et al. Phase 2 study of intensified chemotherapy and allogeneic hematopoietic stem cell transplantation for older patients with acute lymphoblastic leukemia. Cancer. 2016;122(15):2379–88.
51. Gros FX, Dumas P-Y, Forcade E, Calmettes C, Robles M, Servant V, et al. Improved outcome with a pediatric-inspired regimen for Philadelphia-negative acute lymphoblastic leukemia in the elderly. Blood. 2017;130(Supplement 1):2560.
52. Gros FX, Dumas P-Y, Forcade E, Calmettes C, Robles M, Servant V, et al. Feasibility and outcome of late intensification with native l-asparaginase for acute lymphoblastic leukemia in the elderly: a single center experience. Blood. 2017;130(Supplement 1):1296.
53. Kantarjian HM, DeAngelo DJ, Stelljes M, Liedtke M, Stock W, Gokbuget N, et al. Inotuzumab ozogamicin versus standard of care in relapsed or refractory acute lymphoblastic leukemia:

final report and long-term survival follow-up from the randomized, phase 3 INO-VATE study. Cancer. 2019;125(14):2474–87.
54. Kantarjian H, Stein A, Gökbuget N, Fielding AK, Schuh AC, Ribera J-M, et al. Blinatumomab versus chemotherapy for advanced acute lymphoblastic leukemia. N Engl J Med. 2017;376(9):836–47.
55. Jabbour EJ, Sasaki K, Ravandi F, et al. Inotuzumab ozogamicin in combination with low-intensity chemotherapy (mini-HCVD) with or without blinatumomab versus standard intensive chemotherapy (HCVAD) as frontline therapy for older patients with Philadelphia chromosome-negative acute lymphoblastic leukemia: a propensity score analysis. Cancer. 2019;125:2579–86.
56. Advani AS, Moseley A, O'Dwyer KM, et al. Results of SWOG 1318: a Phase 2 trial of blinatumomab followed by Pomp (prednisone, vincristine, methotrexate, 6-mercaptopurine) maintenance in elderly patients with newly diagnosed Philadelphia chromosome negative B-cell acute lymphoblastic leukemia. Blood. 2018;132(Supplement 1):33.
57. Wieduwilt MJ. How should we treat older adults with Ph+ adult ALL and what novel approaches are being investigated? Best Pract Res Clin Haematol. 2017;30(3):201–11.
58. Fielding AK, Rowe JM, Buck G, Foroni L, Gerrard G, Litzow MR, et al. UKALLXII/ECOG2993: addition of imatinib to a standard treatment regimen enhances long-term outcomes in Philadelphia positive acute lymphoblastic leukemia. Blood. 2014;123(6):843–50.
59. Ravandi F, Othus M, O'Brien SM, et al. US Intergroup study of chemotherapy plus dasatinib and allogeneic stem cell transplant in Philadelphia chromosome positive ALL. Blood Adv. 2016;1:250–9.
60. Daver N, Thomas D, Ravandi F, Cortes J, Garris R, Jabbour E, et al. Final report of a phase II study of imatinib mesylate with hyper-CVAD for the front-line treatment of adult patients with Philadelphia chromosome-positive acute lymphoblastic leukemia. Haematologica. 2015;100(5):653–61.
61. Porkka K, Koskenvesa P, Lundán T, Rimpiläinen J, Mustjoki S, et al. Dasatinib crosses the blood-brain barrier and is an efficient therapy for central nervous system Philadelphia chromosome-positive leukemia. Blood. 2008;112(4):1005–12.
62. Wieduwilt MJ, Yin J, Wetzler M, Uy GL, Powell BL, Kolitz JE, et al. A phase II study of dasatinib and dexamethasone as primary therapy followed by transplantation for adults with newly diagnosed Ph/BCR-ABL1-positive acute lymphoblastic leukemia (Ph+ ALL): final results of Alliance/CALGB Study 10701. Blood. 2018;132(Supplement 1):309.
63. Ravandi F, O'Brien SM, Cortes JE, Thomas DM, Garris R, Faderl S, et al. Long-term follow-up of a phase 2 study of chemotherapy plus dasatinib for the initial treatment of patients with Philadelphia chromosome-positive acute lymphoblastic leukemia. Cancer. 2015;121(23):4158–64.
64. Bassan R, Rossi G, Pogliani EM, et al. Chemotherapy-phased imatinib pulses improve long-term outcome of patients with Philadelphia chromosome-positive acute lymphoblastic leukemia: Northern Italy Leukemia Group Protocol 09/00. J Clin Oncol. 2010;28:3644–52.
65. Wetzler M, Watson D, Stock W, et al. Autologous transplantation for Philadelphia chromosome-positive acute lymphoblastic leukemia achieves outcomes similar to allogeneic transplantation: results of CALGB Study 10001 (Alliance). Haematologica. 2014;99:111–5.
66. Chalandon Y, Thomas X, Hayette S, et al. Randomized study of reduced-intensity chemotherapy combined with imatinib in adults with Ph-positive acute lymphoblastic leukemia. Blood. 2015;125:3711–9.
67. Foa R, Vitale A, Vignetti M, Meloni G, Guarini A, De Propris MS, et al. Dasatinib as first-line treatment for adult patients with Philadelphia chromosome-positive acute lymphoblastic leukemia. Blood. 2011;118(25):6521–8.
68. Jabbour E, Short NJ, Ravandi F, Huang X, Daver N, DiNardo CD, et al. Combination of hyper-CVAD with ponatinib as first-line therapy for patients with Philadelphia chromosome-positive acute lymphoblastic leukaemia: long-term follow-up of a single-centre, phase 2 study. Lancet Haematol. 2018;5(12):e618–e27.

69. Short NJ, Kantarjian HM, Ravandi F, Huang X, Daver NG, DiNardo CD, et al. Long-term safety and efficacy of hyper-CVAD plus ponatinib as frontline therapy for adults with Philadelphia chromosome-positive acute lymphoblastic leukemia. Blood. 2019;134(Supplement_1):283.
70. Martinelli G, Piciocchi A, Papayannidis C, Paolini S, Robustelli V, Soverini S, et al. First report of the Gimema LAL1811 Phase II prospective study of the combination of steroids with ponatinib as frontline therapy of elderly or unfit patients with Philadelphia chromosome-positive acute lymphoblastic leukemia. Blood. 2017;130(Supplement 1):99.
71. Ottmann OG, Wassmann B, Pfeifer H, Giagounidis A, Stelljes M, Duhrsen U, et al. Imatinib compared with chemotherapy as front-line treatment of elderly patients with Philadelphia chromosome-positive acute lymphoblastic leukemia (Ph+ALL). Cancer. 2007;109(10):2068–76.
72. Chalandon Y, Thomas X, Hayette S, Cayuela J-M, Abbal C, Huguet F, et al. Randomized study of reduced-intensity chemotherapy combined with imatinib in adults with Ph-positive acute lymphoblastic leukemia. Blood. 2015;125(24):3711–9.
73. Rousselot P, Coudé MM, Gokbuget N, Gambacorti Passerini C, Hayette S, Cayuela J-M, et al. Dasatinib and low-intensity chemotherapy in elderly patients with Philadelphia chromosome–positive ALL. Blood. 2016;128(6):774–82.
74. Ottmann OG, Pfeifer H, Cayuela J-M, Spiekermann K, Jung W, Beck J, et al. Nilotinib (Tasigna®) and low intensity chemotherapy for first-line treatment of elderly patients with BCR-ABL1-positive acute lymphoblastic leukemia: final results of a prospective multicenter trial (EWALL-PH02). Blood. 2018;132(Supplement 1):31.
75. Vignetti M, Fazi P, Cimino G, Martinelli G, Di Raimondo F, Ferrara F, et al. Imatinib plus steroids induces complete remissions and prolonged survival in elderly Philadelphia chromosome–positive patients with acute lymphoblastic leukemia without additional chemotherapy: results of the Gruppo Italiano Malattie Ematologiche dell'Adulto (GIMEMA) LAL0201-B protocol. Blood. 2007;109(9):3676–8.
76. Chiaretti S, Bassan R, Vitale A, Elia L, Piciocchi A, et al. Dasatinib-Blinatumomab combination for the front-line treatment of adult Ph+ ALL patients. Updated results of the Gimema LAL2116 D-Alba trial. Blood. 2019;134(Supplement_1):740.
77. Short NJ, Jabbour E, Sasaki K, Patel K, O'Brien SM, Cortes JE, et al. Impact of complete molecular response on survival in patients with Philadelphia chromosome-positive acute lymphoblastic leukemia. Blood. 2016;128(4):504–7.
78. Thomas DA, Kantarjian H, Smith TL, Koller C, Cortes J, O'Brien S, et al. Primary refractory and relapsed adult acute lymphoblastic leukemia: characteristics, treatment results, and prognosis with salvage therapy. Cancer. 1999;86(7):1216–30.
79. Gokbuget N, Stanze D, Beck J, Diedrich H, Horst HA, Huttmann A, et al. Outcome of relapsed adult lymphoblastic leukemia depends on response to salvage chemotherapy, prognostic factors, and performance of stem cell transplantation. Blood. 2012;120(10):2032–41.
80. Martinelli G, Boissel N, Chevallier P, et al. Complete hematologic and molecular response in adult patients with relapsed/refractory Philadelphia chromosome-positive b-precursor acute lymphoblastic leukemia following treatment with blinatumomab: results from a phase II, single-arm, multicenter study. J Clin Oncol. 2017;35(16):1795–802.
81. Gokbuget N, Dombret H, Bonifacio M, Reichle A, Graux C, Faul C, et al. Blinatumomab for minimal residual disease in adults with B-cell precursor acute lymphoblastic leukemia. Blood. 2018;131(14):1522–31.
82. Jain T, Litzow MR. Management of toxicities associated with novel immunotherapy agents in acute lymphoblastic leukemia. Ther Adv Hematol. 2020;11:2040620719899897.
83. Kantarjian HM, Stein AS, Bargou RC, Grande Garcia C, Larson RA, Stelljes M, et al. Blinatumomab treatment of older adults with relapsed/refractory B-precursor acute lymphoblastic leukemia: results from 2 phase 2 studies. Cancer. 2016;122(14):2178–85.
84. Jabbour EJ, DeAngelo DJ, Stelljes M, Stock W, Liedtke M, Gokbuget N, et al. Efficacy and safety analysis by age cohort of inotuzumab ozogamicin in patients with relapsed or refractory acute lymphoblastic leukemia enrolled in INO-VATE. Cancer. 2018;124(8):1722–32.

85. Kebriaei P, Cutler C, de Lima M, et al. Management of important adverse events associated with inotuzumab ozogamicin: expert panel review. Bone Marrow Transplant. 2018;53(4):449–56.
86. Shewach DS, Mitchell BS. Differential metabolism of 9-beta-D-arabinofuranosylguanine in human leukemic cells. Cancer Res. 1989;49(23):6498–502.
87. Ullman B, Martin DW Jr. Specific cytotoxicity of arabinosylguanine toward cultured T lymphoblasts. J Clin Invest. 1984;74(3):951–5.
88. DeAngelo DJ, Yu D, Johnson JL, et al. Nelarabine induces complete remissions in adults with relapsed or refractory T-lineage acute lymphoblastic leukemia or lymphoblastic lymphoma: Cancer and Leukemia Group B study 19801. Blood. 2007;109(12):5136–42.
89. Gokbuget N, Basara N, Baurmann H, et al. High single-drug activity of nelarabine in relapsed T-lymphoblastic leukemia/lymphoma offers curative option with subsequent stem cell transplantation. Blood. 2011;118(13):3504–11.
90. Thomas X, Boiron JM, Huguet F, Dombret H, Bradstock K, Vey N, et al. Outcome of treatment in adults with acute lymphoblastic leukemia: analysis of the LALA-94 trial. J Clin Oncol. 2004;22(20):4075–86.
91. Goldstone AH, Richards SM, Lazarus HM, Tallman MS, Buck G, Fielding AK, et al. In adults with standard-risk acute lymphoblastic leukemia, the greatest benefit is achieved from a matched sibling allogeneic transplantation in first complete remission, and an autologous transplantation is less effective than conventional consolidation/maintenance chemotherapy in all patients: final results of the International ALL Trial (MRC UKALL XII/ECOG E2993). Blood. 2008;111(4):1827–33.
92. Gupta V, Richards S, Rowe J. Allogeneic, but not autologous, hematopoietic cell transplantation improves survival only among younger adults with acute lymphoblastic leukemia in first remission: an individual patient data meta-analysis. Blood. 2013;121(2):339–50.
93. Bassan R, Bruggemann M, Radcliffe HS, Hartfield E, Kreuzbauer G, Wetten S. A systematic literature review and meta-analysis of minimal residual disease as a prognostic indicator in adult B-cell acute lymphoblastic leukemia. Haematologica. 2019;104(10):2028–39.
94. Gokbuget N, Kneba M, Raff T, Trautmann H, Bartram CR, Arnold R, et al. Adult patients with acute lymphoblastic leukemia and molecular failure display a poor prognosis and are candidates for stem cell transplantation and targeted therapies. Blood. 2012;120(9):1868–76.
95. Dhedin N, Huynh A, Maury S, Tabrizi R, Beldjord K, Asnafi V, et al. Role of allogeneic stem cell transplantation in adult patients with Ph-negative acute lymphoblastic leukemia. Blood. 2015;125(16):2486–96.
96. Ribera J-M, Morgades M, Ciudad J, Barba P, Martino R, Montesinos P, et al. Post-remission treatment with chemotherapy or allogeneic hematopoietic stem cell transplantation (alloHSCT) of High-Risk (HR) Philadelphia Chromosome-Negative (Ph-neg) adult acute lymphoblastic leukemia (ALL) according to minimal residual disease (MRD). Preliminary results of the Pethema ALL-HR-11 trial. Blood. 2015;126(23):1333.
97. Rosko A, Wang HL, de Lima M, Sandmaier B, Khoury HJ, Artz A, et al. Reduced intensity conditioned allograft yields favorable survival for older adults with B-cell acute lymphoblastic leukemia. Am J Hematol. 2017;92(1):42–9.
98. Roth-Guepin G, Canaani J, Ruggeri A, Labopin M, Finke J, Cornelissen JJ, et al. Allogeneic stem cell transplantation in acute lymphoblastic leukemia patients older than 60 years: a survey from the acute leukemia working party of EBMT. Oncotarget. 2017;8(68):112972–9.
99. Mohty M, Labopin M, Volin L, Gratwohl A, Socie G, Esteve J, et al. Reduced-intensity versus conventional myeloablative conditioning allogeneic stem cell transplantation for patients with acute lymphoblastic leukemia: a retrospective study from the European Group for Blood and Marrow Transplantation. Blood. 2010;116(22):4439–43.
100. Bachanova V, Marks DI, Zhang MJ, Wang H, de Lima M, Aljurf MD, et al. Ph+ ALL patients in first complete remission have similar survival after reduced intensity and myeloablative allogeneic transplantation: impact of tyrosine kinase inhibitor and minimal residual disease. Leukemia. 2014;28(3):658–65.

101. Yoon JH, Min GJ, Park SS, Jeon YW, Lee SE, Cho BS, et al. Minimal residual disease-based long-term efficacy of reduced-intensity conditioning versus myeloablative conditioning for adult Philadelphia-positive acute lymphoblastic leukemia. Cancer. 2019;125(6):873–83.
102. Park JH, Riviere I, Gonen M, et al. Long-term follow-up of CD19 CAR therapy in acute lymphoblastic leukemia. N Engl J Med. 2018;378(5):449–59.
103. Shah BD, Bishop MR, Oluwole OO, et al. End of phase I results of ZUMA-3, a phase 1/2 study of KTE-X19, anti-CD19 chimeric antigen receptor (CAR) T cell therapy, in adult patients (pts) with relapsed/refractory (R/R) acute lymphoblastic leukemia (ALL). J Clin Oncol. 2019;37(15_suppl):7006.
104. Hay KA, Gauthier J, Hirayama AV, et al. Factors associated with durable EFS in adult B-cell ALL patients achieving MRD-negative CR after CD19 CAR T-cell therapy. Blood. 2019;133(15):1652–63.

Chapter 8
Treatment of Childhood Philadelphia Chromosome-Positive Acute Lymphoblastic Leukemia

Melissa A. Burns and Lewis B. Silverman

Introduction

The Philadelphia chromosome, t(9;22)(q34;q11), is present in approximately 5% of children with acute lymphoblastic leukemia (ALL) and leads to production of a BCR-ABL1 fusion protein with constitutive tyrosine kinase activity [1]. It is more common in older children, with an incidence rising to nearly 25% in young adults, and is associated with a higher white blood cell (WBC) count at diagnosis compared to other ALL subtypes [1]. Historically, ALL harboring the t(9;22) chromosomal translocation (Ph+ ALL) has been associated with a poor prognosis and was previously considered an indication for hematopoietic stem cell transplant (HSCT) in first complete remission (CR1). However, with introduction of tyrosine kinase inhibitors (TKI) targeting BCR-ABL1 (Table 8.1), such as imatinib [2–4] and

Table 8.1 Summary of clinically available BCR-ABL1 tyrosine kinase inhibitors

TKI	Tested as single agent in children	Tested in combination with chemotherapy in children	CNS penetrant	Active against T315I resistance mutation
Imatinib	Yes	Yes	No	No
Dasatinib	Yes	Yes	Yes	No
Nilotinib	Yes	No	No	No
Ponatinib	Open phase I/II trial (NCT03934372)	Open phase I/II trial (NCT04501614)	No	Yes

M. A. Burns · L. B. Silverman (✉)
Department of Pediatric Oncology, Dana-Farber Cancer Institute, Harvard Medical School, Boston, MA, USA
e-mail: Melissa_Burns@dfci.harvard.edu; Lewis_Silverman@dfci.harvard.edu

M. R. Litzow, E. A. Raetz (eds.), *Clinical Management of Acute Lymphoblastic Leukemia*, https://doi.org/10.1007/978-3-030-85147-7_8

dasatinib [5–7], outcomes for this subset of ALL have improved and have transformed treatment for these children.

Treatment of Newly Diagnosed Pediatric Philadelphia-Positive Acute Lymphoblastic Leukemia

Treatment in the Pre-Tyrosine Kinase Era

Prior to the introduction of TKIs in the early 2000s, allogeneic HSCT in CR1 was considered standard of care; however, despite this intensified treatment approach, the outcome for Ph+ ALL was inferior to other subtypes of childhood ALL. In a retrospective study of 326 children with Ph+ ALL treated between 1986 and 1996 from 10 cooperative groups or institutions in the Unites States and Europe, the 5-year event-free survival (EFS) was 28%, and the 5-year overall survival (OS) was 40% [8]. The frequency of induction failure (18%) and relapse for those achieving remission (54%) in this cohort was significantly higher than in other contemporaneously treated pediatric ALL patients [8–13]. For those who achieved complete remission, treatment with an HLA-matched related donor HSCT was associated with a more favorable outcome, with 5-year disease-free survival (DFS) of 65% following HSCT versus 25% for those treated with chemotherapy alone and a 5-year OS of 72% versus 42%, respectively. This advantage, however, was not seen for other donor types, including matched unrelated donors owing to the high incidence of transplant-associated mortality in this group [8].

A follow-up retrospective review of 610 children with Ph+ ALL treated between 1995 and 2005 demonstrated similarly poor outcomes with a 7-year EFS of 32% and OS of 44.9% [14]. As in the earlier study, HSCT in CR1 was associated with a better outcome; the risk of relapse at 5 years was reduced by nearly two-thirds with a hazard ratio (HR) of 0.32 (95% CI 0.2–0.52) for HSCT compared with chemotherapy alone, and the 5-year DFS was superior (43% for HSCT versus 34% for chemotherapy alone, $p = 0.049$) [14]. Overall, this study showed only modest improvement in outcomes during the 1995–2005 era; importantly, OS for Ph+ ALL patients treated in the pre-TKI era remained poor at less than 50%, significantly worse than that for non-Ph+ ALL.

Imatinib Combined with Chemotherapy

The introduction of imatinib, a TKI targeting the BCR-ABL1 fusion protein, in the early 2000s resulted in a transformation of treatment for pediatric Ph+ ALL. Initial studies of imatinib, conducted in adult patients with chronic myeloid leukemia, demonstrated potent antileukemic activity and favorable tolerability [15]. This work led to early phase trials in children with relapsed/refractory Ph+ ALL; the activity of single-agent imatinib was demonstrated, but responses were short-lived [16], providing the rationale to test this agent in combination with cytotoxic chemotherapy in children with newly diagnosed Ph+ ALL.

One of the first studies to test the combination of TKI with chemotherapy was Children's Oncology Group (COG) AALL0031, which enrolled children and adolescents with newly diagnosed Ph+ ALL between 2002 and 2006. On this study, patients were treated with an intensive chemotherapy backbone and received imatinib 340 mg/m^2/day at first discontinuously to ascertain the safety of the combination [17]. The 50 patients enrolled on the last cohort of the study, cohort 5, received continuously dosed imatinib combined with the intensive cytotoxic chemotherapy backbone. All children with a matched related donor were allocated to HSCT after the first two consolidation blocks. The 3-year EFS for all children in cohort 5 was 80.5%, significantly higher than the EFS of 40.9% for historical controls [8]. Of the 50 children treated with continuous imatinib in cohort 5, 25 received chemotherapy only, 21 were allocated for matched sibling donor HSCT, and 11 subjects received an unrelated or mismatched donor HSCT. Importantly, there was no difference in 5-year DFS for children enrolled to cohort 5 (continuous imatinib) treated with chemotherapy alone (70%) versus those who underwent HSCT in CR1 from either related donor (65%) or unrelated donor (59%) (Fig. 8.1) [18]. While the number of patients treated without HSCT was small, this trial provided the first evidence that HSCT in CR1 may not be a necessary component of therapy for all children with Ph+ ALL who receive a TKI along with chemotherapy as initial treatment.

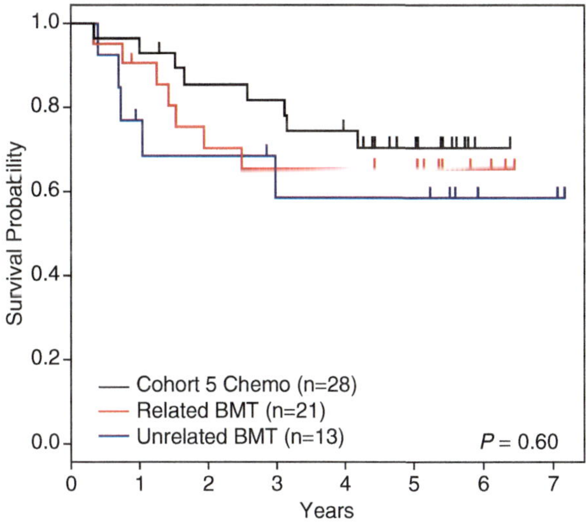

Fig. 8.1 Long-term follow-up of children treated on COG AALL0031. Comparison of outcomes on COG AALL0031 demonstrated no difference in 5-year disease-free survival for children in Cohort 5 treated with chemotherapy plus imatinib compared to children in all cohorts who proceeded to a hematopoietic stem cell transplant (HSCT) from either a related donor or unrelated donor HSCT. Children who did not achieve complete remission by the end of consolidation block 2 were excluded from the analysis. (Adapted from Schultz, K.R., et al. *Leukemia* 2014 Jul;28(7):1467–71, with permission [18])

At the same time that COG AALL0031 was being conducted, the European intergroup study of postinduction treatment for Philadelphia chromosome-positive ALL (EsPhALL) enrolled children with newly diagnosed Ph+ ALL between 2004 and 2009 on a randomized clinical trial designed to test whether outcome was improved when imatinib was added to a high-risk Berlin-Frankfurt-Münster (BFM) chemotherapy regimen [19]. Following induction therapy, patients were stratified as good risk or poor risk based on peripheral blood response to a prednisone prophase and marrow response at the end of multiagent induction; patients classified as good risk were randomized to receive chemotherapy alone or chemotherapy plus discontinuously dosed imatinib at 300 mg/m^2/day. Poor risk patients were directly assigned to receive imatinib. HSCT in CR1 was recommended for all poor risk patients and for good risk patients with a matched sibling donor. In total, 178 children were enrolled and classified as good risk. Interpretation of this study is limited because of the high non-compliance rate with randomized assignment in good risk patients (nearly 30% assigned to the chemotherapy-alone arm received imatinib) and early closure before reaching goal accrual when favorable results of COG AALL0031 (on which patients received continuous dosing of imatinib) became known. As a result, the study was not sufficiently powered to answer the primary study question. Nevertheless, the EsPhALL2004 study demonstrated the safety and efficacy of imatinib on a BFM high-risk backbone. The overall DFS of patients treated on this trial appeared to be better than historic controls, and when analyzed as-treated (and not by intent-to-treat), good risk patients who received imatinib had a superior DFS (5-year DFS rate was 77% for patients who received imatinib and 55% for patients who did not receive imatinib, $p = 0.02$). Of note, 80% of patients on the EsPhALL study, including 77% of good risk patients, underwent HSCT in CR1; thus no conclusion could be drawn regarding the role of HSCT over chemotherapy alone.

Following the early closure of EsPhALL2004, the EsPhALL group opened a successor trial, EsPhALL2010, on which imatinib was given continuously rather than discontinuously; notably, imatinib was started mid-induction rather than after the completion of induction. HSCT in CR1 was initially recommended for good risk patients with a matched sibling donor or poor risk patients with any available donor; however, beginning in 2012, indications for HSCT were limited to only those patients with high minimal residual disease (MRD) ($\geq 5 \times 10^{-4}$) at the end of the consolidation or with detectable MRD at any level after the third high-risk block, regardless of initial risk classification or available donor type. Of the 155 patients enrolled on the study, morphologic CR was attained in 97% of participants ($N = 151$), which was significantly higher than the CR rate on the predecessor EsPhALL trial (78%), suggesting that earlier administration of imatinib improved induction response. The 5-year EFS and OS rates were similar between the EsPhALL2010 trial (57% and 71.8%, respectively) and the initial EsPhALL trial, even though significantly fewer patients received HSCT in first CR on the latter trial (38% of patients on EsPhALL2010), providing evidence that the previous strategy of transplanting most Ph+ ALL patients in CR1 was not associated with a survival advantage. Of note, a relatively high rate of treatment-related mortality was observed on the EsPhALL2010 trial (~15% of patients), primarily from infection during intensive chemotherapy blocks.

Based on the high rates of treatment-related mortality observed when imatinib is combined with intensive chemotherapy regimens, the COG and EsPhALL groups are currently conducting a joint, international trial (EsPhALL2017/COG AALL1631), the goal of which is to minimize short- and long-term toxicities while maintaining or improving cure rates. All patients on the trial receive imatinib beginning at day 15 of induction. Standard-risk (SR) patients, defined as those with low MRD ($<5 \times 10^{-4}$ at the end of the second block of chemotherapy at about week 12 of treatment), are randomized to receive one of two chemotherapy backbones, the EsPhALL backbone (considered the standard treatment) or a less intensive backbone similar to what non-Ph+ high-risk (HR) ALL patients receive on COG trials [20, 21]. HR patients, defined by slow response at a single timepoint (MRD $\geq 5 \times 10^{-4}$ after 10–12 weeks of therapy), are treated initially on the EsPhALL backbone but are allocated to allogeneic HSCT; for these patients, the study aims to determine the feasibility of administering post-HSCT imatinib.

Dasatinib Combined with Chemotherapy

Dasatinib is a second-generation TKI with more potent in vitro inhibition of ABL kinase and better CNS penetration than imatinib; it has also been shown to be active in patients with imatinib resistance [6, 7, 22, 23]. Based on these potential advantages, COG conducted a trial (AALL0622) on which dasatinib was administered on the same intensive chemotherapy backbone used in the AALL0031 imatinib trial; however, unlike AALL0031, on which all non-transplanted Ph+ ALL patients received cranial radiation, only CNS-3 patients were irradiated on AAL0622. On the AALL0622 trial, dasatinib was started at day 15 of the induction phase with the hope of achieving more rapid early response. The study included two cohorts, cohort 1 received discontinuous dasatinib administration, and cohort 2, which opened once cohort 1 was found to be safe and tolerable, received continuously dosed dasatinib. Patients were stratified as HR if they had MRD $\geq 1\%$ at end- induction or $\geq 0.01\%$ at end of the second consolidation cycle; all other patients were classified as SR. HSCT was recommended for all HR patients and for SR patients who had a matched sibling donor. In total, 39 eligible patients were treated in cohort 1 and 21 in cohort 2. CR was achieved after induction in 98% of patients, significantly higher than rate of end-induction CR on COG AALL0031 ($p = 0.01$) [17, 24], indicating that adding TKI mid-induction leads to better early response rates, consistent with the results of the EsPhALL2010 trial. Additionally, 59% of AALL0622 versus 25% of AALL0031 patients had MRD <0.01% at the end of induction ($P < 0.001$). Frequency of adverse events was similar between the two trials, suggesting that dasatinib was not associated with excess toxicity. The 5-year DFS was 68% for AALL0031 (imatinib) and 60% for AALL0622 (dasatinib), and the 5-year OS was 81% and 86%, respectively, suggesting that there was no significant difference between the two TKIs in preventing relapses or leading to long-term cures. Despite its superior CNS penetration, dasatinib did not completely abrogate the risk of CNS relapse: for non-irradiated patients on AALL0622, the 5-year cumulative incidence (CI) of CNS relapse (isolated or combined) was 15%.

In 2012, COG and EsPhALL opened a joint, single-arm, international phase 2 study of dasatinib combined with the EsPhALL chemotherapy backbone (based on AIEOP-BFM HR ALL regimen), enrolling 106 eligible patients. Long-term results from the trial are still pending, although preliminary data suggests that EFS and OS appear to be similar to previous COG and EsPhALL Ph+ ALL trials [18, 19, 24–26].

On the CCCG-ALL-2015 Ph+ ALL trial conducted by the Chinese Children's Cancer Group, pediatric Ph+ ALL patients were randomized to receive either imatinib or dasatinib added to a modified St. Jude Total XV/XVI backbone. The dose of imatinib on the trial (300 mg/m²/day) was lower than that used on COG trials, while the dose of dasatinib (80 mg/m²/day) was higher than the dose on the COG AALL0622 trial (60 mg/m²/day). The 4-year EFS and OS rates were 71% and 88.4%, respectively, on the dasatinib arm, compared with 48.9% and 69.2% on the imatinib arm [27]. However, caution is needed in interpreting these results given the relatively short follow-up (26.4 months) and the fact that outcome of patients who received imatinib on this trial was markedly inferior to imatinib-treated patients on previous pediatric Ph+ ALL trials conducted by COG and EsPhALL. Nonetheless, the preliminary favorable outcome of the dasatinib arm suggests that there may be advantages to using the higher dose of dasatinib; confirmation of this finding awaits longer follow-up.

Other TKIs

Other ABL-class TKIs, including nilotinib [28] and ponatinib [29], are commonly used for adult Ph+ ALL; however, their safety profile in combination with chemotherapy for children with Ph+ ALL has not been established. Therefore, they should not be considered as first-line agents in this disease but may be beneficial in relapsed cases with resistance to imatinib or dasatinib. Early phase pediatric trials of ponatinib, administered alone and in conjunction with chemotherapy, are ongoing. While results from the PACE study in adults with Ph+ ALL are promising [30], the safety and efficacy of this TKI in children remain unknown.

HSCT in First Complete Remission

Prior to introduction of TKIs, HSCT in CR1 was considered standard of care for pediatric Ph+ ALL. With the introduction of TKIs, however, a smaller percentage of patients have been allocated to HSCT in CR1 on successive clinical trials performed over the last two decades, with similar rates of long-term EFS and OS (Table 8.2). In fact, on COG AALL0622, the trial with the highest long-term OS, only 32% of patients received HSCT in CR1. On that trial, salvage post-relapse was reasonably

Table 8.2 Summary of clinical trials of TKI in combination with cytotoxic chemotherapy for childhood Ph+ ALL

Trial	Years open	Chemotherapy backbone	TKI	Indications for HSCT (% HSCT)	EFS	OS
COG AALL0031 [17, 18]	2002–2006	AALL0031	Imatinib	HLA MSD (Cohort 5 only 43%[a])	5-year 58%	5-year 70%
EsPhALL2004 [19, 35]	2004–2009	HR BFM	Imatinib	Poor Risk[b] or Good Risk with MSD (77%)	5-year 60.3%	5-year 71.5%
COG AALL 0622 [24]	2008–2012	AALL0031	Dasatinib	HR[c] or SR with MSD (32%)	5-year 60%	5-year 86%
EsPhALL2010 [26]	2010–2014	HR BFM	Imatinib	High MRD[d] (38%)	5-year 57%	5-year 71.8%
COG AALL 1122 [25]	2012–2014	HR BFM	Dasatinib	High MRD[e] (14%)	TBD	TBD
CCCG-ALL-2015 [27]	2015–2018	Modified St Jude Total XV/XVI	Imatinib	High MRD[f] (4%)	4-year 48.9%	4-year 69.2%
			Dasatinib	High MRD[f] (1%)	4-year 71%	4-year 88.4%
COG AALL 1631	2017–ongoing	HR: HR BFM SR: HR BFM versus AALL0232	Imatinib	High MRD[d] (TBD)	TBD	TBD

HLA human leukocyte antigen, *HSCT* hematopoietic stem cell transplant, *MSD* matched sibling donor, *TKI* tyrosine kinase inhibitor, *TBD* to be determined

[a]13 of 44 patients in cohort 5 had an available MSD and proceeded to HSCT on study. Of the remaining 31 patients, 6 were removed from study treatment and proceeded to HSCT with an alternative donor

[b]Poor early response (Leukemic blat count ≥1000 cells/μl following 7-day steroid prophase or >25% marrow blasts at day 15 of induction) or failure to achieve complete remission (<5% marrow blasts) at end induction

[c]M2/M3 marrow, MRD ≥1% at end of Induction or MRD ≥0.01% at end of consolidation block 2

[d]High MRD defined as $\geq 5 \times 10^{-4}$ at timepoint 2, ~10–12 weeks following initiation of treatment

[e]High MRD defined as $\geq 5 \times 10^{-4}$ at timepoint 2, ~10–12 weeks following initiation of treatment, or any detectable level of MRD at timepoint 3, end of third consolidation block

[f]High MRD defined as ≥1% at end induction (timepoint 1)

favorable in those who were treated initially without HSCT in CR1 (5-year EFS of 60% and 5-year OS of 88%), indicating that the strategy of reserving HSCT for post-relapse treatment (rather than in CR1) leads to favorable overall survival while sparing the majority of patients the long-term risks associated with HSCT.

For those patients who are treated with HSCT in CR1, an unresolved question is whether post-HSCT TKI is beneficial. Several studies of adult patients with Ph+ ALL transplanted in CR1 have suggested that post-HSCT TKI administration is associated with more favorable DFS [31–33]. However, there are few reports of this treatment strategy in pediatric Ph+ ALL patients. On COG AALL0031, the only pediatric study to date that has prospectively collected information on the use of post-HSCT TKI, 21 pediatric patients who underwent matched sibling donor HSCT received post-HSCT imatinib beginning 4–6 months after HSCT and remained on TKI for a total duration of 6 months. While this study demonstrated feasibility and safety of administering imatinib post-HSCT, there was no significant benefit to 3-year EFS when compared to a historical control group [17, 34]. It is important to note that this analysis is limited by small sample size, low starting dose of imatinib, and the relatively late and short duration of exposure to imatinib. Further studies are necessary to determine the role of post-HSCT TKI in children with Ph+ ALL; this question is being addressed in the currently accruing international EsPhALL2017/COG AALL1631 trial.

Prognostic Factors in Pediatric Ph+ ALL

Due to the rarity of the diagnosis of pediatric Ph+ ALL, identification of prognostic factors in this population has been limited by the small sample size of most clinical trials; however, some studies have identified potentially significant prognostic factors, which could be used to define risk groups and stratify therapy.

Age and Presenting Leukocyte Count

There are conflicting data regarding the prognostic impact of age and presenting leukocyte count in pediatric Ph+ ALL. In a retrospective review of 610 children with Ph+ ALL treated between 1995 and 2005 without TKI, both age and leukocyte count had prognostic significance on DFS, with the best outcome observed in Ph+ ALL patients presenting with NCI SR features (age <10 years and WBC <50,000/μL) and the worst outcome in those with presenting leukocyte counts >100,000/μL, regardless of age [14]. Conversely, on the COG AALL0031 study (on which all patients received imatinib), NCI risk group (defined by age and presenting leukocyte count) lacked prognostic significance [17].

Data from two consecutive EsPhALL trials has identified elevated leukocyte count as a significant predictor of outcome. On the EsPhALL2004 trial (randomized comparison of imatinib versus no imatinib), a cox regression model including risk group (defined by prednisone prophase response), age, and presenting leukocyte count identified only presenting leukocyte count as an independent risk factor of outcome; when the same analysis was restricted to patients who had received imatinib, results were essentially unchanged [35]. Similarly, on the EsPhALL2010 trial (in which all patients received continuously dosed imatinib), cox regression analysis including risk group, age, and leukocyte count identified presenting leukocyte count ≥100,000/μL as the only independent risk factor predicting inferior EFS [26].

In fact, when the analysis was repeated on a subgroup of patients with evaluable end-consolidation MRD (at week 12 of treatment), presenting leukocyte count ≥100,000/μL retained independent prognostic significance, but MRD did not [26].

Early Morphologic Response

In the pre-TKI era, slow early response to chemotherapy, as assessed by peripheral blood absolute blast count after a 7-day prophase and/or morphology of marrow obtained in the midst of multiagent remission induction, was shown to be associated with adverse outcome in pediatric Ph+ ALL [14]. Slow early response by either of these measures was more frequent in Ph+ ALL patients than in other children with ALL; in multivariable analyses, prednisone poor response and slow early marrow response were associated with inferior DFS and OS [14]. Based on this finding, slow early morphologic response was the only factor used to allocate patients to the HR group on the EsPhALL2004 and 2010 trials [19, 26].

Minimal Residual Disease (MRD)

Detection of MRD is a key prognostic determinant in childhood ALL and has been incorporated into risk stratification of contemporary ALL treatment protocols [21, 36–40]. However, there are more limited data regarding the prognostic significance of MRD in Ph+ ALL patients. In the EsPhALL2004 study, MRD was measured at the end of induction (TP1) and the IB phase (TP2) using quantitative real-time PCR to detect immunoglobulin and T-cell receptor gene rearrangements (*Ig/TCR* PCR), with a cut-off of $\geq 5 \times 10^{-4}$ used to define high MRD. MRD non-detectability at end induction (TP1), observed in only 9 of 90 evaluable patients, was associated with a favorable prognosis (none of the 9 patients relapsed); however, there was no significant difference in cumulative incidence of relapse between children with low but detectable MRD and those with high MRD at TP1 [41]. Achievement of negative MRD at TP2 (observed in 14 of 64 patients without negative MRD at TP1) was also associated with a relatively favorable outcome, with a 5-year cumulative incidence of relapse (CIR) of 14.3% [19, 41].

Conversely, on COG AALL0031, end-induction MRD did not predict outcome in cohort 5 patients (who received continuous imatinib beginning after the induction phase); 3-year EFS was similar for patients with high versus low MRD using a 0.01% cut-off, as assessed by flow cytometry [17]. On the subsequent COG AALL0622 trial (utilizing dasatinib), patients were risk stratified on the basis of MRD (assessed by flow cytometry); those with MRD ≥1% at end induction or ≥0.01% after two intensive consolidation cycles were considered HR and allocated to HSCT; all other patients were classified as SR [24]. There was no difference in

EFS ($p = 0.84$) or OS ($p = 0.8$) by risk group; however, given that patients with high MRD were classified as HR and thus received more intensive therapy (with nearly all children proceeding to HSCT in CR1) than those with low MRD (the majority of whom did not proceed to HSCT), interpretation of the prognostic significance of MRD based on these results is not possible.

In addition to flow cytometry and *Ig/TCR* PCR, another method to assess MRD in Ph+ ALL is quantitative RT-PCR (RQ-PCR) of *BCR-ABL1* transcript expression. On the EsPhALL2004 study, the overall concordance rate between *BCR-ABL1* PCR and *Ig/TCR* PCR was 69% [41]. In general, *BCR-ABL1* PCR values tended to be higher than those obtained by *Ig/TCR* PCR; however, similar to *Ig/TCR* PCR, *BCR-ABL1* PCR negativity at TP1 or TP2 was associated with a low risk of relapse. In another study, MRD was assessed in 48 patients using a DNA-based assay to measure *BCR-ABL1* genomic copies rather than the standard *BCR-ABL1* RQ-PCR, which measures transcript expression [42]. In that study, nearly 20% of patients with a p190 fusion and 12.5% of patients with the p210 fusion had at least a log-fold higher level of disease when assessed by *BCR-ABL1* genomic rearrangement compared with *Ig/TCR* PCR. When comparing MRD results between the two assays, there was no significant difference in outcome between patients with concordant and discordant MRD, although patient numbers are small. Of note, *BCR-ABL1* fusion was identified in non-blast myeloid cells, B-cells, and T-cells in four patients with discordant *BCR-ABL1* and *Ig/TCR* MRD results but not in seven patients with concordant results, suggesting that, at least in some cases with discordant results, patients may have chronic myeloid leukemia (CML)-like biology with *BCR-ABL1* occurring in a stem cell or multipotent progenitor cell. Larger studies are necessary to confirm this provocative finding and to determine its impact on outcome.

IKZF1 Deletions

Alterations of the *IKZF1* gene are observed in approximately 15% of patients with Ph-negative B-ALL but are more frequent in those who are Ph+ [24]. In the Ph-negative cases, *IKZF1* deletions have been shown to have independent adverse prognostic significance [37]. There are limited data regarding the prognostic significance of *IKZF1* gene aberrations in pediatric Ph+ ALL. In a retrospective study of 191 patients treated between 1995 and 2010, *IKZF1* deletions (found in 66% of the tested cohort) were associated with significantly worse DFS and OS [43]. However, in a subset analysis including only patients treated on the initial EsPhALL trial (most of whom received imatinib), the trend toward inferior outcome with *IKZF1* deletions did not achieve statistical significance. In another retrospective analysis that included 44 patients treated on COG AALL0622 with available samples, *IKZF1* deletions were identified in 56% of the study cohort and were significantly associated with inferior 5-year EFS and OS [24].

Treatment of Relapsed Philadelphia Chromosome-Positive Acute Lymphoblastic Leukemia

Despite overall improvement in outcome since TKIs have been incorporated into frontline therapy, relapse is not infrequent in pediatric Ph+ ALL. However, salvage rates post-relapse are relatively favorable, particularly for those who were not treated with HSCT in CR1 [24]. At present, the standard treatment for a child with relapsed Ph+ ALL includes reinduction with combination chemotherapy plus continuous TKI followed by HSCT with a total body irradiation (TBI)-based regimen. Given the potential for emergence of TKI resistance mutations, resistance testing should be sent at the time of relapse; however, preliminary data suggest that resistance mutations are uncommon in most children with relapsed Ph+ ALL, and therefore re-treatment with imatinib or dasatinib appears to be effective. For children who relapse after HSCT, curative options include a second transplant if CR has been achieved or more novel therapies, including CAR T-cell directed therapy [44], or other immunotherapeutic approaches combined with TKI [45].

Summary

The introduction of TKI, notably imatinib and dasatinib, to combination chemotherapy has led to improvement in outcomes for children with Ph+ ALL and has changed the standard of care for this HR subgroup. Clinical trials conducted over the last two decades have demonstrated that HSCT in CR1 no longer is necessary to cure the majority of children with Ph+ ALL. Current international efforts are now aimed at reducing acute and long-term toxicities while maintaining or improving cure rates for these children and identifying novel prognostic factors to improve risk stratification. Future studies will need to explore whether the incorporation of novel treatment strategies, including immunotherapeutic therapies and alternative BCR-ABL1-targeted therapies, such as asciminib, an allosteric inhibitor [46], can further improve outcomes for this HR patient subset.

References

1. Childhood Acute Lymphoblastic Leukemia Treatment (PDQ(R)): Health Professional Version. PDQ Cancer Information Summaries. Bethesda; 2002.
2. Druker BJ, Sawyers CL, Kantarjian H, Resta DJ, Reese SF, Ford JM, et al. Activity of a specific inhibitor of the BCR-ABL tyrosine kinase in the blast crisis of chronic myeloid leukemia and acute lymphoblastic leukemia with the Philadelphia chromosome. N Engl J Med. 2001;344(14):1038–42.
3. Mauro MJ, O'Dwyer M, Heinrich MC, Druker BJ. STI571: a paradigm of new agents for cancer therapeutics. J Clin Oncol. 2002;20(1):325–34.

4. Savage DG, Antman KH. Imatinib mesylate--a new oral targeted therapy. N Engl J Med. 2002;346(9):683–93.
5. Carter TA, Wodicka LM, Shah NP, Velasco AM, Fabian MA, Treiber DK, et al. Inhibition of drug-resistant mutants of ABL, KIT, and EGF receptor kinases. Proc Natl Acad Sci U S A. 2005;102(31):11011–6.
6. Shah NP, Tran C, Lee FY, Chen P, Norris D, Sawyers CL. Overriding imatinib resistance with a novel ABL kinase inhibitor. Science. 2004;305(5682):399–401.
7. O'Hare T, Walters DK, Stoffregen EP, Jia T, Manley PW, Mestan J, et al. In vitro activity of Bcr-Abl inhibitors AMN107 and BMS-354825 against clinically relevant imatinib-resistant Abl kinase domain mutants. Cancer Res. 2005;65(11):4500–5.
8. Arico M, Valsecchi MG, Camitta B, Schrappe M, Chessells J, Baruchel A, et al. Outcome of treatment in children with Philadelphia chromosome-positive acute lymphoblastic leukemia. N Engl J Med. 2000;342(14):998–1006.
9. Silverman LB, Gelber RD, Young ML, Dalton VK, Barr RD, Sallan SE. Induction failure in acute lymphoblastic leukemia of childhood. Cancer. 1999;85(6):1395–404.
10. Conter V, Arico M, Valsecchi MG, Rizzari C, Testi A, Miniero R, et al. Intensive BFM chemotherapy for childhood ALL: interim analysis of the AIEOP-ALL 91 study. Associazione Italiana Ematologia Oncologia Pediatrica. Haematologica. 1998;83(9):791–9.
11. Conter V, Arico M, Valsecchi MG, Rizzari C, Testi AM, Messina C, et al. Extended intrathecal methotrexate may replace cranial irradiation for prevention of CNS relapse in children with intermediate-risk acute lymphoblastic leukemia treated with Berlin-Frankfurt-Munster-based intensive chemotherapy. The Associazione Italiana di Ematologia ed Oncologia Pediatrica. J Clin Oncol. 1995;13(10):2497–502.
12. Schrappe M, Reiter A, Sauter S, Ludwig WD, Wormann B, Harbott J, et al. [Concept and interim result of the ALL-BFM 90 therapy study in treatment of acute lymphoblastic leukemia in children and adolescents: the significance of initial therapy response in blood and bone marrow]. Klin Padiatr. 1994;206(4):208–21.
13. Pui CH, Evans WE. Acute lymphoblastic leukemia. N Engl J Med. 1998;339(9):605–15.
14. Arico M, Schrappe M, Hunger SP, Carroll WL, Conter V, Galimberti S, et al. Clinical outcome of children with newly diagnosed Philadelphia chromosome-positive acute lymphoblastic leukemia treated between 1995 and 2005. J Clin Oncol. 2010;28(31):4755–61.
15. O'Brien SG, Guilhot F, Larson RA, Gathmann I, Baccarani M, Cervantes F, et al. Imatinib compared with interferon and low-dose cytarabine for newly diagnosed chronic-phase chronic myeloid leukemia. N Engl J Med. 2003;348(11):994–1004.
16. Champagne MA, Capdeville R, Krailo M, Qu W, Peng B, Rosamilia M, et al. Imatinib mesylate (STI571) for treatment of children with Philadelphia chromosome-positive leukemia: results from a Children's Oncology Group phase 1 study. Blood. 2004;104(9):2655–60.
17. Schultz KR, Bowman WP, Aledo A, Slayton WB, Sather H, Devidas M, et al. Improved early event-free survival with imatinib in Philadelphia chromosome-positive acute lymphoblastic leukemia: a children's oncology group study. J Clin Oncol. 2009;27(31):5175–81.
18. Schultz KR, Carroll A, Heerema NA, Bowman WP, Aledo A, Slayton WB, et al. Long-term follow-up of imatinib in pediatric Philadelphia chromosome-positive acute lymphoblastic leukemia: Children's Oncology Group study AALL0031. Leukemia. 2014;28(7):1467–71.
19. Biondi A, Schrappe M, De Lorenzo P, Castor A, Lucchini G, Gandemer V, et al. Imatinib after induction for treatment of children and adolescents with Philadelphia-chromosome-positive acute lymphoblastic leukaemia (EsPhALL): a randomised, open-label, intergroup study. Lancet Oncol. 2012;13(9):936–45.
20. Larsen EC, Devidas M, Chen S, Salzer WL, Raetz EA, Loh ML, et al. Dexamethasone and high-dose methotrexate improve outcome for children and young adults with high-risk B-acute lymphoblastic leukemia: a report from Children's Oncology Group Study AALL0232. J Clin Oncol. 2016;34(20):2380–8.
21. Borowitz MJ, Wood BL, Devidas M, Loh ML, Raetz EA, Salzer WL, et al. Prognostic significance of minimal residual disease in high risk B-ALL: a report from Children's Oncology Group study AALL0232. Blood. 2015;126(8):964–71.

22. Lombardo LJ, Lee FY, Chen P, Norris D, Barrish JC, Behnia K, et al. Discovery of N-(2-chloro-6-methyl- phenyl)-2-(6-(4-(2-hydroxyethyl)- piperazin-1-yl)-2-methylpyrimidin-4-ylamino)thiazole-5-carboxamide (BMS-354825), a dual Src/Abl kinase inhibitor with potent antitumor activity in preclinical assays. J Med Chem. 2004;47(27):6658–61.
23. Tokarski JS, Newitt JA, Chang CY, Cheng JD, Wittekind M, Kiefer SE, et al. The structure of dasatinib (BMS-354825) bound to activated ABL kinase domain elucidates its inhibitory activity against imatinib-resistant ABL mutants. Cancer Res. 2006;66(11):5790–7.
24. Slayton WB, Schultz KR, Kairalla JA, Devidas M, Mi X, Pulsipher MA, et al. Dasatinib plus intensive chemotherapy in children, adolescents, and young adults with Philadelphia chromosome-positive acute lymphoblastic leukemia: results of Children's Oncology Group Trial AALL0622. J Clin Oncol. 2018;36(22):2306–14.
25. Hunger SP, Saha V, Devidas M, Grazia Valsecchi M, Gastier Foster J, Cazzaniga G, et al. CA180-372: an international collaborative phase 2 trial of dasatinib and chemotherapy in pediatric patients with newly diagnosed Philadelphia chromosome positive acute lymphoblastic leukemia (Ph+ ALL). Blood. 2017;130(Supplement 1):98.
26. Biondi A, Gandemer V, De Lorenzo P, Cario G, Campbell M, Castor A, et al. Imatinib treatment of paediatric Philadelphia chromosome-positive acute lymphoblastic leukaemia (EsPhALL2010): a prospective, intergroup, open-label, single-arm clinical trial. Lancet Haematol. 2018;5(12):e641–e52.
27. Shen S, Chen X, Cai J, Yu J, Gao J, Hu S, et al. Effect of dasatinib vs imatinib in the treatment of pediatric Philadelphia chromosome-positive acute lymphoblastic leukemia: a randomized clinical trial. JAMA Oncol. 2020;6(3):358–66.
28. Kim DY, Joo YD, Lim SN, Kim SD, Lee JH, Lee JH, et al. Nilotinib combined with multiagent chemotherapy for newly diagnosed Philadelphia-positive acute lymphoblastic leukemia. Blood. 2015;126(6):746–56.
29. Jabbour E, Kantarjian H, Ravandi F, Thomas D, Huang X, Faderl S, et al. Combination of hyper-CVAD with ponatinib as first-line therapy for patients with Philadelphia chromosome-positive acute lymphoblastic leukaemia: a single-centre, phase 2 study. Lancet Oncol. 2015;16(15):1547–55.
30. Cortes JE, Kim DW, Pinilla-Ibarz J, le Coutre P, Paquette R, Chuah C, et al. A phase 2 trial of ponatinib in Philadelphia chromosome-positive leukemias. N Engl J Med. 2013;369(19):1783–96.
31. Nishiwaki S, Miyamura K, Kato C, Terakura S, Ohashi K, Sakamaki H, et al. Impact of post-transplant imatinib administration on Philadelphia chromosome-positive acute lymphoblastic leukaemia. Anticancer Res. 2010;30(6):2415–8.
32. Brissot E, Labopin M, Beckers MM, Socie G, Rambaldi A, Volin L, et al. Tyrosine kinase inhibitors improve long-term outcome of allogeneic hematopoietic stem cell transplantation for adult patients with Philadelphia chromosome positive acute lymphoblastic leukemia. Haematologica. 2015;100(3):392–9.
33. Kebriaei P, Saliba R, Rondon G, Chiattone A, Luthra R, Anderlini P, et al. Long-term follow-up of allogeneic hematopoietic stem cell transplantation for patients with Philadelphia chromosome-positive acute lymphoblastic leukemia: impact of tyrosine kinase inhibitors on treatment outcomes. Biol Blood Marrow Transplant. 2012;18(4):584–92.
34. Satwani P, Sather H, Ozkaynak F, Heerema NA, Schultz KR, Sanders J, et al. Allogeneic bone marrow transplantation in first remission for children with ultra-high-risk features of acute lymphoblastic leukemia: a children's oncology group study report. Biol Blood Marrow Transplant. 2007;13(2):218–27.
35. Biondi A, Cario G, De Lorenzo P, Castor A, Conter V, Leoni V, et al. Long-term follow up of pediatric Philadelphia positive acute lymphoblastic leukemia treated with the EsPhALL2004 study: high white blood cell count at diagnosis is the strongest prognostic factor. Haematologica. 2019;104(1):e13–e6.
36. Borowitz MJ, Devidas M, Hunger SP, Bowman WP, Carroll AJ, Carroll WL, et al. Clinical significance of minimal residual disease in childhood acute lymphoblastic leukemia and

its relationship to other prognostic factors: a Children's Oncology Group study. Blood. 2008;111(12):5477–85.
37. Vrooman LM, Blonquist TM, Harris MH, Stevenson KE, Place AE, Hunt SK, et al. Refining risk classification in childhood B acute lymphoblastic leukemia: results of DFCI ALL Consortium Protocol 05-001. Blood Adv. 2018;2(12):1449–58.
38. Berry DA, Zhou S, Higley H, Mukundan L, Fu S, Reaman GH, et al. Association of minimal residual disease with clinical outcome in pediatric and adult acute lymphoblastic leukemia: a meta-analysis. JAMA Oncol. 2017;3(7):e170580.
39. Schrappe M, Valsecchi MG, Bartram CR, Schrauder A, Panzer-Grumayer R, Moricke A, et al. Late MRD response determines relapse risk overall and in subsets of childhood T-cell ALL: results of the AIEOP-BFM-ALL 2000 study. Blood. 2011;118(8):2077–84.
40. Conter V, Bartram CR, Valsecchi MG, Schrauder A, Panzer-Grumayer R, Moricke A, et al. Molecular response to treatment redefines all prognostic factors in children and adolescents with B-cell precursor acute lymphoblastic leukemia: results in 3184 patients of the AIEOP-BFM ALL 2000 study. Blood. 2010;115(16):3206–14.
41. Cazzaniga G, De Lorenzo P, Alten J, Rottgers S, Hancock J, Saha V, et al. Predictive value of minimal residual disease in Philadelphia-chromosome-positive acute lymphoblastic leukemia treated with imatinib in the European intergroup study of post-induction treatment of Philadelphia-chromosome-positive acute lymphoblastic leukemia, based on immunoglobulin/T-cell receptor and BCR/ABL1 methodologies. Haematologica. 2018;103(1):107–15.
42. Hovorkova L, Zaliova M, Venn NC, Bleckmann K, Trkova M, Potuckova E, et al. Monitoring of childhood ALL using BCR-ABL1 genomic breakpoints identifies a subgroup with CML-like biology. Blood. 2017;129(20):2771–81.
43. van der Veer A, Zaliova M, Mottadelli F, De Lorenzo P, Te Kronnie G, Harrison CJ, et al. IKZF1 status as a prognostic feature in BCR-ABL1-positive childhood ALL. Blood. 2014;123(11):1691–8.
44. Maude SL, Laetsch TW, Buechner J, Rives S, Boyer M, Bittencourt H, et al. Tisagenlecleucel in children and young adults with B-cell lymphoblastic leukemia. N Engl J Med. 2018;378(5):439–48.
45. Maino E, Sancetta R, Viero P, Imbergamo S, Scattolin AM, Vespignani M, et al. Current and future management of Ph/BCR-ABL positive ALL. Expert Rev Anticancer Ther. 2014;14(6):723–40.
46. Schoepfer J, Jahnke W, Berellini G, Buonamici S, Cotesta S, Cowan-Jacob SW, et al. Discovery of asciminib (ABL001), an allosteric inhibitor of the tyrosine kinase activity of BCR-ABL1. J Med Chem. 2018;61(18):8120–35.

Chapter 9
Treatment of Adult Philadelphia Chromosome-Positive Acute Lymphoblastic Leukemia

Oliver G. Ottmann

Introduction

The translocation t(9;22)(q34;q11) is identified in approximately 25% of adults with B-cell precursor ALL and is the single most frequent cytogenetic abnormality in adult ALL, referred to as Philadelphia-positive (Ph+) ALL. Juxtaposition of the BCR gene on chromosome 22 and the ABL1 gene on chromosome 9 results in a BCR-ABL1 fusion gene and a chimeric oncoprotein that leads to constitutive activation of the ABL1 tyrosine kinase and downstream signalling cascades. Its frequency increases with age with up to 50% of cases in patients older than 60 years [1]. Up to two decades ago, Ph+ ALL was the most lethal subtype of acute lymphoblastic leukemia in adults, characterized by an older median age at diagnosis, lower complete remission, and high relapse rates even with intensive induction and consolidation chemotherapy. Allogeneic stem cell transplantation (HSCT) was the only realistic curative option but could be realized in only a minority of patients, who were subsequently at high risk of transplant-related mortality, morbidity, and relapse.

The dismal prognosis of this disease changed profoundly with recognition of the key leukemogenic role of the chimeric BCR-ABL1 oncoprotein and its deregulated tyrosine kinase activity and the advent of BCR-ABL1-directed tyrosine kinase inhibitors (TKI). Imatinib was the first TKI to be evaluated in Ph+ ALL, and its impact on prognosis has been attributed to the higher proportion of patients undergoing HSCT in CR1 and lower levels of disease at the time of transplant [2]. Clinical trials evaluating the more potent second- and third-generation TKI dasatinib, nilotinib, and ponatinib in the first-line setting have indicated they may improve patient outcome even without HSCT, although no randomized comparison of TKI has yet been reported in the adult population. A clinical trial directly comparing imatinib

O. G. Ottmann (✉)
Division of Cancer and Genetics, School of Medicine, Cardiff University, Cardiff, UK
e-mail: OttmannO@Cardiff.ac.uk

M. R. Litzow, E. A. Raetz (eds.), *Clinical Management of Acute Lymphoblastic Leukemia*, https://doi.org/10.1007/978-3-030-85147-7_9

and ponatinib in conjunction with the same chemotherapy backbone is currently ongoing (EWALL-PH03; ClinicalTrials.gov Identifier: NCT04688983). Swedish ALL Registry data collected between 2007 and 2015 demonstrate that the use of TKI coincided with an improvement of the prognosis of Ph+ ALL in adults up to 65 years of age on par with or superior to that of Ph-negative ALL. In this real-life setting, 5-year survival in patients 18–45 y was 64%, in patients 46–65 y 56%, and in patients >65 y 18% [3].

Optimal management of patients with Ph+ ALL is complex and requires considerable attention to detail concerning choice and scheduling of TKI, appropriate use of chemotherapy, the indication for allogeneic HSCT, and monitoring of minimal residual disease. The underlying therapeutic principles, controversies, remaining challenges, and recent developments in treatment of Ph+ ALL in adults are the focus of this chapter.

Clinical Features and Diagnosis

Initial clinical presentation of Ph+ ALL is typical of acute B-cell precursor (BCP) ALL in general, with clinical manifestations of anemia, thrombocytopenia, and neutropenia. Dense infiltration of the bone marrow by lymphoblasts and a high WBC dominated by morphologically undifferentiated blast cells is usually but not invariably present, as is mild to moderate hepatosplenomegaly and lymphadenopathy. Clinical signs and symptoms of central nervous system involvement and other extramedullary involvement, e.g., of the skin, testes, and soft tissues, should be carefully ascertained. They are more frequent in Ph+ ALL but are not per se indicative of this subtype. A lumbar puncture (LP) is part of routine diagnostic workup for ALL but may be deferred for a few days in case of very high peripheral blast count to avoid contaminating the CSF by leukemic blasts. A LP should be performed in an atraumatic manner and always be accompanied by intrathecal prophylactic chemotherapy.

Immunophenotyping is essential to confirm the diagnosis of a morphologically suspected ALL, and coexpression of myeloid-associated antigens on otherwise typical lymphoblasts may raise initial suspicion of a BCR-ABL1-positive ALL, particularly in patients older than 50 years. Definitive diagnosis of Ph+ ALL requires cytogenetic and/or molecular genetic analyses, the results of which should be available within days. Conventional karyotyping to demonstrate the translocation t(9;22) as hallmark of Ph+ leukemia is considered mandatory by many hematologists, while others consider fluorescent in situ hybridization (FISH) sufficient. While FISH can be performed rapidly and is relatively inexpensive, cytogenetic analysis may reveal additional chromosomal aberrations (ACA) that have been shown to be prognostic of outcome but would be missed by FISH. More recently, next-generation sequencing (NGS) has become more widely used and may replace cytogenetics as a diagnostic tool.

In a patient with confirmed Ph+ ALL, RT-PCR analysis of BCR-ABL1 transcripts will identify which breakpoint is present, i.e., the $p190^{BCR\text{-}ABL1}$ isoform seen in about two-thirds of patients with Ph+ ALL or the $p210^{BCR\text{-}ABL1}$ breakpoint more typical of chronic myeloid leukemia (CML) in the remaining one-third. Lymphoid blast crisis of a previously undiagnosed CML as opposed to Ph+ ALL may be suggested by basophilia, an unexpectedly high platelet count or pronounced splenomegaly but is irrelevant from a clinical management point of view as both entities are treated identically. Identification of the correct BCR-ABL1 isoform is important for MRD monitoring by qRT-PCR assessment of BCR-ABL1 transcript levels. However, qRT-PCR is not acceptable as the sole diagnostic test for Ph+ ALL as atypical BCR-ABL1 transcripts may be missed. A diagnostic leukemic sample is also needed to identify clone-specific immunoglobulin and T-cell receptor gene rearrangements used for MRD analysis by PCR [4]. Determination of a leukemia-associated immunophenotype for MRD monitoring by flow cytometry requires an initial diagnostic sample, although this may not be needed when standardized MFC protocols developed by the EURO-MRD consortium are used [5]. HLA typing should be performed in all patients in whom allogeneic HSCT may be even remotely considered.

Assessment of laboratory parameters, virus serology, and cardiac, pulmonary, renal, and hepatic function follows essentially the same principles as for other acute leukemias. Cardiac risk factors and vascular status should be comprehensively assessed particularly if treatment with nilotinib or ponatinib is anticipated, with attention to the QT interval on ECG as some of the TKI may cause QT prolongation.

Conventional and Genetic Risk Factors

Although Ph+ ALL is considered a very high-risk subtype in adults, several additional parameters are indicative of a particularly poor prognosis despite optimal treatment. Age is inversely correlated with prognosis, and WBC >30/nl, additional chromosomal abnormalities, and supernumerary Ph chromosomes at diagnosis have been associated with inferior outcome [6–8]. Recurring genomic abnormalities in genes involved in B-cell development, e.g., IKZF1 and CDKN2A/B deletions, have been linked with less favorable outcome, and recent evidence indicates that the number of affected genes is prognostically relevant [9–13]. Data on the prognostic relevance of BCR-ABL1 isotype are likewise conflicting. Whereas the $p210^{BCR\text{-}ABL1}$ breakpoint has been associated with inferior OS and EFS [14], no impact on DFS was observed in a trial testing dasatinib monotherapy, despite a more rapid decrease of MRD levels in patients with the p190 isoform [15]. A meta-analysis to comprehensively assess the impact of BCR-ABL1 isoforms on the clinical outcomes of Ph+ ALL patients similarly suggested that p210 was associated with slightly inferior event-free survival (EFS) but not overall survival (OS), a finding possibly not valid in the setting of second- and third-generation TKI. Clinically, CNS involvement is also a harbinger of a higher risk of relapse and usually may precede systemic relapse.

Standard Treatment for Newly Diagnosed Ph+ ALL

As in all types of ALL, initial prephase therapy of approximately 5-day duration with corticosteroids and optional vincristine or low-dose cyclophosphamide is used for cytoreduction and to bridge the time to molecular confirmation of the diagnosis.

Supportive standard of care is not unique to Ph+ ALL. Comprehensive reviews including clinical management of adult and pediatric patients are provided in two recent publications [16, 17].

Induction Therapy

After demonstration of clinical activity in relapsed and refractory Ph+ ALL [18–21], imatinib and subsequently other BCR-ABL1 active TKIs were introduced into the front-line setting and are now an integral part of the treatment paradigm. Several key findings from initial clinical trials have had a major impact on determining the standard therapeutic approach, specifically (a) addition of TKI to chemotherapy regimens for ALL is largely well tolerated and increases the CR rate substantially, (b) earlier addition of imatinib to chemotherapy increases its efficacy and improves patient outcome in adults and children [22, 23], and (c) imatinib alone was superior to chemotherapy as induction therapy for newly diagnosed Ph+ ALL [24]. Consistently, all TKI-based induction regimens achieve CR rates of 90–100%, irrespective of age, performance status, or presence of other risk factors. TKI are started as soon as the diagnosis of Ph+ ALL has been established, usually within 5 days of initial presentation. Rigorous CNS-directed prophylaxis with intrathecal chemotherapy (methotrexate, cytosine arabinoside, and dexamethasone) is essential to minimize the elevated risk of CNS relapse. This is mandatory also with dasatinib, despite its unique ability among TKIs to cross the blood-brain barrier and reach therapeutic concentrations in the CSF [25]. CNS irradiation no longer plays a pivotal role in CNS-directed prophylaxis in most regimens for Ph+ ALL.

The high CR rate induced by TKI has led to a reevaluation of the role and intensity of chemotherapy during induction. This was conclusively addressed in a randomized trial by the GRAALL Cooperative Study Group which established that the combination of imatinib with a deintensified induction regimen was superior to the combination with intensive chemotherapy in terms of higher CR rate, less toxicity, and lower induction mortality, without adversely affecting long-term outcome [26]. Data from phase II trials with all BCR-ABL1-active TKI used for Ph+ ALL are consistent with these results [15, 24, 27]. Consequently, the concept of employing a

TKI alone or in conjunction with steroids and possibly vincristine has been widely adopted as induction therapy particularly for, but not limited to, elderly patients. Some regimens for younger patients have retained the combination of intensive chemotherapy with TKI during induction [28, 29]. The role of TKI dose during induction has not been rigorously examined. Adherence to a higher imatinib dose appears to be clinically superior as shown by a trial demonstrating that delivery of less than 90% of the planned dose of 800 mg imatinib per day was associated with higher probability of relapse and inferior survival even when followed by allogeneic HSCT [30]. Additional considerations of TKI usage and dose will be discussed in detail below.

Postremission Therapy

Preventing disease recurrence remains a considerable challenge and is not achieved by continuation of imatinib or a second-generation TKI alone or in combination with corticosteroids. In a trial with dasatinib as front-line therapy, all patients achieved CR, but the relapse rate was inversely correlated with the intensity of postremission therapy [15]. Most current regimens for fit patients therefore combine a TKI with intensive, possibly age-adapted consolidation chemotherapy or allocate patients to allogeneic HSCT. Usually one or two consolidation cycles are administered prior to transplantation to maintain the CR, reduce MRD levels, and provide additional CNS protection afforded by high-dose ara-C and MTX.

Postremission therapy for patients who do not undergo HSCT is administered most commonly as either a BFM-style regimen with different consolidation cycles, reinduction and prolonged maintenance, or the hyperCVAD regimen followed by maintenance [31–34]. TKI and chemotherapy are usually given concurrently; alternating schedules showed no advantage [23]. Overall tolerability is good, but the combination of asparaginase with TKI may aggravate toxicity and should probably be avoided. The aim of non-transplant therapy is to complete regimen-specified consolidation cycles combining TKI with chemotherapy followed by maintenance chemotherapy, e.g., the POMP regimen combined with a TKI until at least the end of year 2 of therapy. Thereafter, it is common practice to continue TKI indefinitely even if MRD remains undetectable, with switching to an alternative inhibitor in the event of TKI-associated toxicity or poor tolerability [28, 35–37].

Stem Cell Transplantation

Historically allogeneic stem cell transplantation (HSCT) has been considered the definite curative modality and arguably remains the therapeutic gold standard among transplant-eligible patients with Ph+ ALL against which other therapies are compared. The limitation of donor availability has been largely eliminated by larger donor registries and the option of alternative donor transplants [38, 39]. The time from diagnosis to HSCT nowadays ranges from 3 to 6 months. Because of substantial transplant-related mortality and morbidity caused by graft versus host disease and infections, the decision on whether to refer a patient for HSCT has become a matter for debate [40].

In adults, numerous trials of imatinib-based first-line therapy have shown significantly superior relapse-free survival and overall survival in patients who underwent allogeneic HSCT compared with non-transplanted patients [2, 23, 26, 36, 41–44]. Similar results were obtained in studies with dasatinib and nilotinib, suggesting superiority of HSCT even when compared with the more potent second-generation TKI [29, 45, 46]. However, the anti-leukemic efficacy of HSCT is partially negated by the high transplant-related mortality ranging from 20% to 40% in ALL and an often debilitating morbidity caused by GvHD and prolonged immunosuppression. No comparative data are available demonstrating that initial therapy with a second- or third-generation TKI is superior to imatinib in patients subsequently undergoing allogeneic HSCT. Age, performance status, comorbidities, and tolerability of initial therapy are used to assess the patient's transplant risk, with the Sorror score being a widely used instrument [47]. Disease status at transplant (CR1 vs. ≥CR2; CR vs. active disease), MRD (negative vs. positive), and pre-HSCT treatment strategy (TKI plus chemotherapy vs. TKI plus steroids) were found to be predictive of overall and relapse-free survival after HSCT in a large registry study conducted by the Italian GITMO [48]. Because the often high TRM in ALL may counterbalance the superior anti-leukemic efficacy of allogeneic HSCT, there is an ongoing debate whether patients with a good molecular response may be considered for not being transplanted in CR1 [49]. In one of the largest prospective studies published to date, allogeneic transplantation was associated with a significant benefit in relapse-free survival overall, but not in patients achieving major molecular response (MMolR, defined as a BCR-ABL1/ABL ratio of <0.1% in the bone marrow) who had a comparable outcome with or without allogeneic transplantation [26]. In a retrospective analysis comparing TKI plus chemotherapy with HSCT as postremission therapy, patients proceeding to allo-HCT fared better than those receiving imatinib with chemotherapy alone, but in a low-risk cohort defined by good MRD response and low WBC at diagnosis, there was no significant difference in CIR, DFS, and OS between the transplant and nontransplant cohorts [50]. A similar pattern was observed in a Korean study with the second-generation TKI nilotinib, in which no survival benefit with alloHSCT was noted among the subset of patients achieving CMR [45]. While some data suggest a lack of additional benefit of allo-HCT in patients with deep molecular responses to second-generation TKI plus chemotherapy, the limitations of existing studies highlight the need for a randomized study to conclusively define the role of allo-HCT in patients with a good molecular response [51].

Conditioning Regimens The high TRM following myeloablative conditioning for ALL and increasing ability to achieve pre-transplant MRD negativity with TKI-based therapy has prompted interest in the use of reduced-intensity conditioning (RIC) regimens. In several non-randomized trials, long-term outcome of patients with Ph+ ALL following RIC- and MAC-based HSCT was similar, although patients in the RIC cohorts tended to be older with higher transplant risk [52–54]. In a study of patients aged 50 years or more who were MRD-negative at HSCT after receiving TKI before transplant, overall mortality, relapse, and non-relapse mortality were not significantly increased with RIC compared with MAC. However, RIC was associated with superior overall survival due to a lower incidence of non-relapse mortality in patients with a poor performance status or a high HCT comorbidity index [52]. Long-term outcomes with RIC and MAC HSCT were also shown to be comparable in another study of patients transplanted in CR1 after TKI-based chemotherapy [54].

The relevance of MRD status for outcome in relation to conditioning intensity was highlighted in a trial comparing adult patients with Ph+ ALL in CR1 who received RIC or MAC. With patients matched for age, donor type, and year of HCT, 1-year TRM was significantly lower with RIC than MAC (13% vs 36%), while the 3-year relapse rate was higher with RIC (49% vs. 28%), resulting in similar overall survival (RIC 39% vs MAC 35%). MRD positivity before HSCT was associated with higher risk of relapse with RIC vs MAC. Conversely, patients achieving MRD negativity following pre-HSCT TKI had significantly superior OS (55%) with RIC HSCT compared with a similar MRD population after MAC (55% vs. 33%) [53]. The overall conclusion from the available, non-randomized studies is that RIC is a valid alternative for Ph+ ALL patients ineligible for MAC, preferably with an MRD-negative status at the time of HSCT.

Autologous SCT

Historically ASCT has had no role in treatment of Ph+ ALL due to an excessively high relapse rate. Recognition that pre-ASCT MRD levels were prognostic of outcome [55] and that front-line therapy with TKI resulted in deeper molecular responses prompted the EBMT to conduct a retrospective analysis which suggested that the availability of TKI coincided with improved outcome following ASCT for Ph+ ALL [56]. A subsequent retrospective comparison of myeloablative allogeneic HSCT with ASCT for adults with Ph+ ALL in first molecular remission performed between 2007 and 2014 revealed nearly identical overall survival at 2 years after ASCT, MSD-HSCT, and URD-HSCT. The higher relapse rate following ASCT was offset by lower NRM. Total body irradiation-based regimens were associated with reduced risk of relapse and overall mortality [57]. A prospective phase II trial in which patients were non-randomly assigned to receive allogeneic ($n = 15$) or autologous ($n = 19$) SCT likewise suggested that both approaches can result in similar DFS and OS and supported the notion that depth of molecular response is an important determinant of outcome following ASCT [58]. These data indicate that ASCT may be an alternative option in patients considered to be ineligible for allogeneic HSCT, provided they are in molecular remission. Additional evidence for the potential utility of ASCT stems from a prospective GRAAPH-2005 trial demonstrating that in patients who achieved a major molecular response (BCR-ABL1/ABL1 ratio $\leq 0.1\%$), OS and RFS were identical following ASCT and allogenic HSCT

[26]. In view of uncertainties concerning impact of different TKI, their continuation after ASCT, and the criteria for molecular remission, a randomized comparison of these treatment modalities should be awaited before routinely adopting ASCT as therapy for Ph+ ALL.

TKI as Post-Transplant Maintenance

Relapse accounts for about half of treatment failures after HSCT and subsequent therapies are often unsuccessful. The role of TKI administration after transplantation has been evaluated in two large retrospective analyses and several small, mostly single-arm prospective trials, indicating that use of imatinib after HSCT is associated with a lower relapse rate and better outcome compared with historic controls [59, 60]. Second-generation TKI and ponatinib have been used in a considerably smaller number of patients, but their administration after HSCT appears to be safe [61, 62]. The only randomized clinical trials addressing post-transplant TKI demonstrated excellent and virtually identical long-term survival with both prophylactic and pre-emptive, MRD-triggered administration of imatinib [63]. Thus, one of these two approaches should be considered standard in the post-transplant setting [64]. MRD should be monitored frequently, preference given to BM as source of material, and close attention paid to the assay sensitivity. Tolerability of all TKI after HSCT is worse than in non-transplanted patients, but recommendations on the duration of TKI maintenance after HSCT range from 1 to over 2 years if possible [63–65]. Proposed algorithms for use of TKI in the post-transplant setting for Ph+ ALL are summarized in a position paper by the EBMT [64] and a comprehensive review of published data [60].

Minimal Residual Disease

The concept of quantitating low-level measurable (minimal) residual disease as a prognostic marker and guide to therapy in ALL is well established and applies equally to the Ph+ ALL subtype. Three different methodologies are commonly used, qRT-PCR for BCR-ABL1 transcripts, PCR analysis of clonal immunoglobulin (Ig) and T cell receptor (TCR) gene rearrangements, and multicolor flow cytometry (MFC) [66–70]. Results obtained with these methods correlate, but sensitivity, complexity, assay variability, and costs differ considerably, making it impossible to equate results across platforms and often laboratories. Thus, while MRD is an accepted surrogate marker for efficacy of treatment and correlates with outcome, managing individual patients with Ph+ ALL is critically dependent on correct interpretation of MRD results, the intricacies of which are often underappreciated. Ig/TCR PCR is the most standardized methodology and is relatively expensive and complex, necessitating identification of clonal markers at diagnosis and expertise in data analysis. It is the preferred methodology in the pediatric setting, whereas experience with CML has made qRT-PCR for BCR-ABL1 transcripts the most widely used technique in adult patients. Interlaboratory variability with qRT-PCR can be substantial, and guidelines for standardizing methodology, interpretation, and reporting of results are essential. Importantly, it has been recognized that in a small proportion of patients, these two methods yield discrepant results, most commonly with negative MRD by Ig/TCR combined with detection of BCR-ABL1 transcripts by qRT-PCR, although the inverse has also been observed [71]. The biology underlying this discrepancy and the clinical implications remain to be defined, but parallel use of both methodologies has been adopted in current clinical trials.

Flow cytometry is the method for monitoring MRD most commonly used in the USA but less frequently in Europe. Efforts to standardize MFC for MRD analysis in ALL are ongoing [70].

From a practical point of view, bone marrow is the preferred source of material for MRD testing with an approximately 1–3 log greater sensitivity than with peripheral blood. This and other important technical aspects of MRD analysis have recently been reviewed [66]. Clinically meaningful analysis requires a sufficiently large quantitative range of each individual assay, and this information should be provided with each test result. Failure to comply with this may lead to reporting MRD results as negative merely because of inadequate sensitivity of the assay, with potentially profound clinical consequences. MRD monitoring in Ph+ ALL is initiated after induction and continued after consolidation cycles and is thus performed earlier and more frequently than customary for CML. The decline in MRD levels typically is most pronounced during the first 3 months of treatment; it is uncertain whether the kinetics of MRD response are prognostic of outcome as suggested by two Korean studies [72, 73]. Results may be reported as log decrease from starting values, as copy numbers or ratio of leukemic to control transcripts. Details of MRD monitoring are provided in several excellent reviews [66] and are beyond the scope of this chapter, but the key message is that correct clinical interpretation requires attention to these technical details.

The goal of therapy is to achieve the lowest possible levels of MRD, ideally below the level of detectability within the first few months of treatment. MRD early during therapy, i.e., after induction, is most informative in terms of a likely poor outcome if levels remain high, whereas low MRD at later time points is prognostic of a favorable long-term prognosis. For an individual patient, the clinical implications of low or even negative MRD differ profoundly from those in CML, as non-transplanted patients even with low or undetectable MRD face a probability of relapse-free survival of up to 50% [26].

MRD monitoring provides not only prognostic information but is the basis for deciding whether to continue planned therapy or switch to alternative treatment to prevent relapse. Clinical intervention based on detectable MRD rather than morphologic evidence of relapse has been demonstrated to be superior for blinatumomab treatment of patients with ALL including Ph+ ALL, leading to FDA and EMA approval of blinatumomab initially for MRD positive Ph negative and more recently Ph+ ALL [74]. The concept of molecular failure or molecular relapse as indication for initiating or switching therapy in Ph+ ALL is supported by clinical trials and is not applicable only to blinatumomab. The depth of response to therapy as determined by quantitative assessment of MRD at the time of HSCT is increasingly being recognized as an important predictor of outcome and parameter informing transplant decisions [48].

Kinase Domain Mutations

Resistance to TKI therapy is most frequently associated with point mutations in the tyrosine kinase domain (KD) of BCR-ABL1. Such mutations may pre-date the start of TKI treatment but are not identified by routine methodologies for mutational analysis. However, rising levels of BCR-ABL transcripts should prompt mutation analysis [75]. The spectrum of clinically relevant mutations appears to be more restricted than in CML and depends on the TKI used, largely in line with the degree of kinase inhibition determined by preclinical in vitro assays. Whereas mutations in the p-loop of the BCR-ABL1 KD predominate with imatinib-based therapy, this shifts to a greater frequency of the T315I gatekeeper mutation with dasatinib and nilotinib. Approximately two-thirds of patients with Ph+ ALL who relapsed while receiving dasatinib as front-line therapy harbored the T315I mutation. The only currently approved TKI with activity against T315I is ponatinib, which also potently inhibits the other types of mutations associated with TKI resistance. Clinical activity against TKD mutations has also been demonstrated in a trial using the bispecific T-cell engager blinatumomab in conjunction with dasatinib as front-line therapy for Ph+ ALL [76]. Testing for BCR-ABL1 KD mutations is therefore mandatory when clinical relapse occurs and should be used to determine which TKI to switch to [75]. In the absence of mutation data, ponatinib has the greatest chance of inhibiting the malignant clone. Because of the limited sensitivity of Sanger sequencing which requires a variant allele frequency (VAF) of about 20%, NGS has become the method of choice for mutation testing, providing a sensitivity of 1–5% [75]. Using even more sensitive techniques, low-level KD mutations have been identified in TKI-naïve patients at diagnosis and to give rise to relapse, with at times very rapid growth kinetics [9, 37, 77]. As the clinical implications of preexisting low-level mutations have not been prospectively evaluated, mutational testing at diagnosis is not yet part of routine patient management but is recommended by a position paper on NGS sequencing for Ph+ ALL [75].

Selecting the Best TKI

Based on results of in vitro kinase assays, second- and third-generation TKI (dasatinib, nilotinib, and ponatinib) have the theoretical advantage of greater potency than imatinib in suppressing BCR-ABL1 kinase activity. Conversely, selectivity in terms of kinase inhibition is greatest for imatinib and nilotinib, whereas dasatinib and even more so ponatinib are multi-kinase inhibitors that suppress activity of a broad range of kinases. These include SRC family kinases (SFK) which have been suggested to contribute to leukemogenesis, although their clinical relevance in Ph+ ALL remains uncertain. The kinase inhibition profiles appear to co-determine TKI-specific toxicities.

Most trials conducted to date involve imatinib-based regimens, and in some countries imatinib is the only TKI approved and available for front-line therapy. Clinical criteria for selecting TKI are based primarily on efficacy and safety data from relatively small, single-arm phase 2 trials and historical controls given the lack of comparative randomized trials. The only exception is a recent randomized study comparing dasatinib with imatinib in the context of intensive chemotherapy in pediatric and adolescent patients up to 18 years of age showing that dasatinib given at 80 mg/m2 per day was more effective than imatinib at 300 mg/m2 per day in improving event-free and overall survival [78]. In contrast, long-term follow-up of two consecutive studies evaluating the hyperCVAD regimen together with either imatinib or dasatinib showed no significant difference in remission duration, RFS, or OS [79]. An overview of clinical trials using imatinib or the second- and third-generation TKI as front-line therapy for adult patients is provided in Table 9.1.

Dasatinib is the only BCR-ABL1-active TKI that reaches therapeutic levels in the CSF, providing a theoretical rationale for its preferential use in patients with CNS involvement [25, 80]. It is common practice to combine dasatinib with intrathecal chemotherapy in patients with active CNS disease until complete blast cell clearance from the CSF has been achieved, following the same treatment principles as for patients with Ph-negative ALL.

The main vulnerability of TKIs is the emergence of KD mutations as a principal mechanism of resistance, and the spectrum of KD mutations that confer resistance differs among TKIs. While all successor compounds to imatinib have broader activity against most KD mutations [81], all currently approved TKIs except for ponatinib display a shared vulnerability in the form of the T315I gatekeeper mutation, which has emerged as the most prevalent mutation associated with relapse on dasatinib-based therapy. Conceptually, TKI resistance should therefore occur less frequently with ponatinib, although resistance due to compound mutations has been described [82].

The only published experience with ponatinib as front-line treatment for Ph+ ALL to date has been in combination with hyperCVAD. In this single-arm phase 2 trial, the initial starting dose of ponatinib was reduced from 45 mg orally daily to 30 mg to reduce the incidence of arterial occlusive events, with further reduction to 15 mg once a complete molecular response defined as absence of quantifiable BCR-ABL1 transcripts was achieved [28]. All patients achieved CR and 83% a complete molecular response, with 5-year CR duration and OS rates of 83% and 71%, respectively, superior to historical controls. In a post hoc 6-month landmark analysis, whether or not patients underwent allogeneic HSCT had no impact on survival (Fig. 9.1) [83]. Likewise, a propensity score analysis showed that treatment with

Table 9.1 Prospective trials of second- and third-generation TKI in first-line therapy for Ph+ ALL

TKI	Treatment regimen	*N*	Age	CR rate	Molecular response	Allogeneic HSCT rate	RFS/EFS	Survival	Ref.
Dasatinib									
70 mg BID	Prednisone	53	54 [24–77]		15% (d 85)	42%	22% (20 mos.)	31% (20 mos.)	[15]
50 mg BID/100 mg QD 100 mg QD-70 mg QD	HyperCVAD	72	55 [21–80]	96%	65% (overall)	17%	44% (5y)	46% (5y)	[35]
50 mg BID/100 mg QD 70 mg QD	HyperCVAD	97	44 [20–60]	88%	–	42%	62% (3y)	69% (3y)	[29]
140 mg QD; >70y: 100 mg QD	Low-intensity EWALL backbone	71	69 [55–83]		24% (consolidation)	10%	28% (5y)	36% (5y)	[37]
140 mg QD	Corticosteroids	63	54 [24–82]	98%	60% (2 cycles blinatumomab consolidation	38%	88% (18 mos. med. FU)	95% (18 mos. med. FU)	[76]
Nilotinib									
400 mg BID	Intensive chemotherapy	90	47 [17–71]	91%	77% (3 mo)	63%	72% (2y)	72% (2y)	[45]
400 mg BID	Low-intensity EWALL backbone	72	66 [55–85]	94%	58% $<10^{-4}$ (consolidation)	33%	42% (4y)	47% (4y)	[100]
Ponatinib									
45–30-15 mg QD	HyperCVAD	76	47 [IQR 39–61]	98%			70% (3y)		[28]

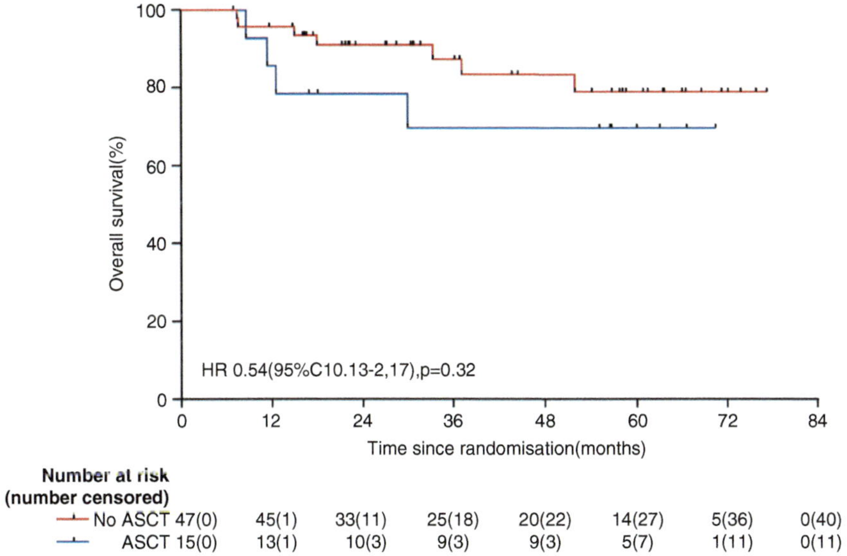

Fig. 9.1 Survival of patients receiving hyperCVAD in combination with ponatinib as first-line therapy for Ph+ ALL. Kaplan-Meier curves with and without censoring for allogeneic HSCT. Median follow-up is 66 months (interquartile range 22–63 months). (With permission from [28])

HCVAD plus ponatinib was associated with longer EFS and OS compared with treatment with HCVAD plus dasatinib [84].

Tolerability and safety profiles of the TKI used to treat Ph+ ALL differ and may influence the choice of drug, but toxicity is usually manageable. Imatinib is associated with gastrointestinal discomfort and facial edema but has no major toxicity concerns. Pleural and pericardial effusions are seen with dasatinib requiring dose interruption and modification. Nilotinib and ponatinib may cause amylase and lipase elevations and clinically symptomatic pancreatitis, particularly in patients with a history of pancreatitis. Reports of cardiovascular AEs with nilotinib and particularly ponatinib and of pulmonary arterial hypertension with dasatinib have raised concerns about long-term sequelae of drugs that may be administered for decades [85]. The cardiovascular ischemic as well as embolic or thrombotic peripheral vascular events associated with ponatinib and nilotinib necessitate a thorough evaluation of the patients' cardiovascular status and disease history before commencing with TKI therapy. Factors associated with increased risk of cardiovascular occlusion events include older age; higher dose; history of myocardial infarction or prior vascular events; prior history of ischemia, hypertension, diabetes, or hyperlipidemia; and ponatinib dose [86]. Experience in CML and Ph+ ALL suggests that patients are generally not able to tolerate 45 mg long term and that dose reduction to 30 mg during initial therapy for Ph+ ALL largely mitigates arterial occlusive events without compromising efficacy [28]. Further reduction to 15 mg in patients achieving complete molecular response has been reported to be feasible, but lower doses are not recommended as blood concentrations are below those found to completely suppress the emergence of BCR-ABL mutations in preclinical studies [28, 87]. In patients at high risk of experiencing cardiovascular events, management includes normalization of blood pressure, blood glucose, and lipids by pharmacologic and lifestyle intervention and monitoring [88].

Combining TKI with Immunooncology Agents

The need to improve the remission duration achieved with TKI alone and minimize the toxicity of chemotherapy has led to evaluation of approaches combining TKI with immunotherapy. Extremely promising results were achieved in a trial conducted by the GIMEMA in which an 85-day induction period with dasatinib and corticosteroids was followed by up to five cycles of blinatumomab added to dasatinib [76]. By the end of dasatinib induction on day 85, a CR was achieved in 98% of the 63 enrolled patients, and 29% had a molecular response, which increased to 60% after two cycles of blinatumomab. Overall and disease-free survival was 95% and 88%, respectively, at a median follow-up of 18 months and with approximately 40% of patients undergoing allogeneic HSCT. ABL1 mutations detected in six patients with MRD were cleared by blinatumomab. This concept of largely chemotherapy-free (except for intrathecal prophylaxis) first-line therapy for Ph+ ALL is being tested in a randomized trial of elderly patients in which one of three treatment arms combines ponatinib with blinatumomab from the start of induction therapy (EWALL-PH03; NCT04688983). A randomized phase III trial of steroids plus either dasatinib or ponatinib (investigator's choice) with chemotherapy or blinatumomab as induction for adult patients up to 75 years with newly diagnosed Ph+ ALL is also enrolling patients (EA9181; NCT04530565). Another still ongoing, non-randomized parallel group phase 2 trial is examining blinatumomab and combination chemotherapy or dasatinib, prednisone, and blinatumomab in treating older patients with acute lymphoblastic leukemia, including Ph+ ALL (SWOG 1318, NCT02143414) (Fig. 9.2).

Salvage Therapy

Relapse remains the main cause of treatment failure in patients with Ph+ ALL and carries a dismal prognosis, particularly if relapse occurs within 18 months of initial CR or after HSCT [89–91]. Most patients with recurrent Ph+ ALL will have received one or more prior TKI and developed resistance, so testing for BCR-ABL1 KD mutations is mandatory. These results inform the choice of TKI, but response rates are low even with an appropriate inhibitor. Single-agent second- and third-generation TKI induced a hematologic response in 16–46% of patients with recurring Ph+ ALL [19–21, 92, 93], and median overall survival was short. Despite ponatinib being

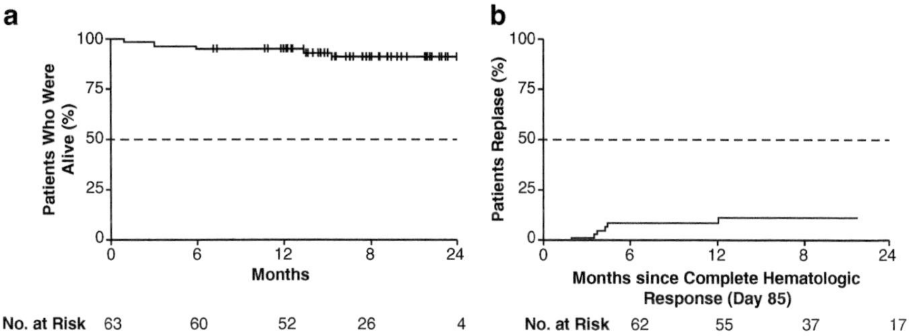

Fig. 9.2 Survival and cumulative incidence of relapse in patients with Ph+ ALL receiving dasatinib and blinatumomab as first-line therapy. Shown are the percentages of all patients with overall survival (Panel A) and relapse (Panel B). Tick marks indicate censored data. (With permission from [76])

active against the threonine-to-isoleucine mutation at position 315, median PFS and OS with ponatinib monotherapy of 32 heavily pretreated patients including 22 with a T315I mutation were only 3 months and 8 months, respectively [87]. These results were largely duplicated in a retrospective observational study (OPAL) of ponatinib salvage therapy in a real-life setting, demonstrating an acceptable safety profile and encouraging CR rate but poor overall outcome even in patients proceeding to allogeneic HSCT [94].

The focus of novel treatment approaches for relapsed or refractory (R/R) Ph+ ALL has therefore shifted to immunotherapeutic strategies including antibody drug conjugates, T-cell engaging antibodies (BiTEs), and chimeric antigen receptor T-cells (CART). A retrospective analysis of the subset of patients with R/R Ph+ ALL enrolled in the phase 3 (INO-VATE) study of inotuzumab ozogamicin (InO) showed higher CR and molecular remission rates and longer PFS with InO compared with standard of care but no benefit in median OS, despite a considerably higher rate of allogeneic HSCT [95, 96]. In the only study examining the bispecific T-cell engager (BiTE) blinatumomab as single agent exclusively in R/R Ph+ ALL (ALCANTARA), 36% of patients achieved CR/CRh during the first two cycles, including four of ten patients with the T315I mutation [97]. While most patients in CR also reached molecular CR (88%), only 16% of the patients underwent HSCT, and median relapse-free survival and overall survival were 6.7 and 7.1 months, respectively.

Considering the uncertain response and short response duration of single-agent therapy, current treatment approaches are focusing on combination therapies such as TKI combined with chemotherapy or immunotherapy. In a retrospective analysis of a chemotherapy-free approach combining blinatumomab with ponatinib in 26 relapsed/refractory Ph+ ALL patients, all but 1 achieved complete morphologic remission, and 23 achieved a complete molecular response; the median overall (OS) and event-free (EFS) survivals were 20 and 15.3 months, respectively. Despite some reversible neurotoxicity and cytokine release syndrome, tolerability was viewed as favorable and efficacy encouraging, warranting prospective evaluation [98].

Chimeric antigen receptor (CAR) T-lymphocytes engineered to express receptors targeting the B-cell antigen CD19 are approved for the treatment of children and young adults with relapsed and refractory ALL. CD19 CAR T-cell therapy has shown encouraging response and outcome data including in a small number ($n = 16$) of patients with Ph+ ALL [99]. Because cytokine release syndrome (CRS) and neurotoxicity are encountered in a clinically significant proportion of patients, the role of CART cell therapy in Ph+ ALL remains to be determined, including where in the treatment course it is best positioned, whether it may replace HSCT, and whether it should precede or follow immunotherapy.

Apart from the addition of BCR-ABL1-directed TKI, available modalities are the same as or other B-lineage ALL for which more extensive data are available than for Ph+ ALL, and experience with immunotherapy for Ph-negative BCP-ALL studies can largely be extrapolated to Ph+ ALL, as discussed in Chaps. 12 and 14. In view of the short survival with current salvage regimens, it is paramount to prevent overt disease recurrence. The therapeutic approach to molecular or hematologic relapse is determined by prior therapy, duration of previous CR, eligibility for and expected time to allogeneic HSCT, performance status, and comorbidities.

Summary and Conclusions

With the availability of TKI as first-line therapy for Ph+ ALL, the initial goals of treatment have shifted from achieving a complete remission to inducing a deep molecular response while simultaneously minimizing the toxicity of induction therapy. In fit patients, allogeneic HSCT remains the standard postremission therapy against which new therapies have to be compared, but the benefit of HSCT in patients with a good molecular response is increasingly being questioned. Studies combining potent second- and third-generation TKI with other classes of targeted therapies, most notably immunotherapeutic agents such as blinatumomab, increase the molecular response rate and may lead to a paradigm change in which cytotoxic chemotherapy is no longer required. Monitoring of residual disease throughout therapy provides critical, therapeutically actionable information with molecular persistence or molecular relapse as clear indications for therapeutic intervention. Hematologic relapse has unfortunately retained its dismal prognosis and should be prevented at all cost. Further improvements in first-line treatment based on targeted and immunotherapeutic strategies utilizing antibody-based or cellular therapies will have the greatest impact on prognosis,

References

1. Burmeister T, Schwartz S, Bartram CR, Gokbuget N, Hoelzer D, Thiel E, et al. Patients' age and BCR-ABL frequency in adult B-precursor ALL: a retrospective analysis from the GMALL study group. Blood. 2008;112(3):918–9.

2. Fielding AK, Rowe JM, Buck G, Foroni L, Gerrard G, Litzow MR, et al. UKALLXII/ECOG2993: addition of imatinib to a standard treatment regimen enhances long-term outcomes in Philadelphia positive acute lymphoblastic leukemia. Blood. 2014;123(6):843–50.
3. Lennmyr E, Karlsson K, Ahlberg L, Garelius H, Hulegardh E, Izarra AS, et al. Survival in adult acute lymphoblastic leukaemia (ALL): a report from the Swedish ALL Registry. Eur J Haematol. 2019;103(2):88–98.
4. Szczepanski T, Beishuizen A, Pongers-Willemse MJ, Hahlen K, Van Wering ER, Wijkhuijs AJ, et al. Cross-lineage T cell receptor gene rearrangements occur in more than ninety percent of childhood precursor-B acute lymphoblastic leukemias: alternative PCR targets for detection of minimal residual disease. Leukemia. 1999;13(2):196–205.
5. Theunissen P, Mejstrikova E, Sedek L, van der Sluijs-Gelling AJ, Gaipa G, Bartels M, et al. Standardized flow cytometry for highly sensitive MRD measurements in B-cell acute lymphoblastic leukemia. Blood. 2017;129(3):347–57.
6. Aldoss I, Stiller T, Cao TM, Palmer JM, Thomas SH, Forman SJ, et al. Impact of additional cytogenetic abnormalities in adults with Philadelphia chromosome-positive acute lymphoblastic leukemia undergoing allogeneic hematopoietic cell transplantation. Biol Blood Marrow Transplant. 2015;21(7):1326–9.
7. Seol CA, Cho YU, Jang S, Park CJ, Lee JH, Lee JH, et al. Prognostic significance of recurrent additional chromosomal abnormalities in adult patients with Philadelphia chromosome-positive acute lymphoblastic leukemia. Cancer Genet. 2017;216-217:29–36.
8. Short NJ, Kantarjian HM, Sasaki K, Ravandi F, Ko H, Cameron Yin C, et al. Poor outcomes associated with +der(22)t(9;22) and −9/9p in patients with Philadelphia chromosome-positive acute lymphoblastic leukemia receiving chemotherapy plus a tyrosine kinase inhibitor. Am J Hematol. 2017;92(3):238–43.
9. Pfeifer H, Lange T, Wystub S, Wassmann B, Maier J, Binckebanck A, et al. Prevalence and dynamics of bcr-abl kinase domain mutations during imatinib treatment differ in patients with newly diagnosed and recurrent bcr-abl positive acute lymphoblastic leukemia. Leukemia. 2012;26(7):1475–81.
10. Martinelli G, Iacobucci I, Storlazzi CT, Vignetti M, Paoloni F, Cilloni D, et al. IKZF1 (Ikaros) deletions in BCR-ABL1-positive acute lymphoblastic leukemia are associated with short disease-free survival and high rate of cumulative incidence of relapse: a GIMEMA AL WP report. J Clin Oncol. 2009;27(31):5202–7.
11. Mullighan CG. The genomic landscape of acute lymphoblastic leukemia in children and young adults. Hematology Am Soc Hematol Educ Program. 2014;2014(1):174–80.
12. Mullighan CG, Miller CB, Radtke I, Phillips LA, Dalton J, Ma J, et al. BCR-ABL1 lymphoblastic leukaemia is characterized by the deletion of Ikaros. Nature. 2008;453(7191):110–4.
13. van der Veer A, Zaliova M, Mottadelli F, De Lorenzo P, Te Kronnie G, Harrison CJ, et al. IKZF1 status as a prognostic feature in BCR-ABL1-positive childhood ALL. Blood. 2014;123(11):1691–8.
14. Jing Y, Chen H, Liu M, Zhou M, Guo Y, Gao C, et al. Susceptibility of Ph-positive all to TKI therapy associated with Bcr-Abl rearrangement patterns: a retrospective analysis. PLoS One. 2014;9(11):e110431.
15. Foa R, Vitale A, Vignetti M, Meloni G, Guarini A, De Propris MS, et al. Dasatinib as first-line treatment for adult patients with Philadelphia chromosome-positive acute lymphoblastic leukemia. Blood. 2011;118(25):6521–8.
16. Cook J, Litzow M. Advances in supportive care for acute lymphoblastic leukemia. Curr Hematol Malig Rep. 2020;15(4):276–93.
17. Brown P, Inaba H, Annesley C, Beck J, Colace S, Dallas M, et al. Pediatric acute lymphoblastic Leukemia, version 2.2020, NCCN clinical practice guidelines in oncology. J Natl Compr Cancer Netw. 2020;18(1):81–112.
18. Druker BJ, Sawyers CL, Kantarjian H, Resta DJ, Reese SF, Ford JM, et al. Activity of a specific inhibitor of the BCR-ABL tyrosine kinase in the blast crisis of chronic myeloid leukemia and acute lymphoblastic leukemia with the Philadelphia chromosome. N Engl J Med. 2001;344(14):1038–42.

19. Ottmann O, Dombret H, Martinelli G, Simonsson B, Guilhot F, Larson RA, et al. Dasatinib induces rapid hematologic and cytogenetic responses in adult patients with Philadelphia chromosome positive acute lymphoblastic leukemia with resistance or intolerance to imatinib: interim results of a phase 2 study. Blood. 2007;110(7):2309–15.
20. Ottmann OG, Druker BJ, Sawyers CL, Goldman JM, Reiffers J, Silver RT, et al. A phase 2 study of imatinib in patients with relapsed or refractory Philadelphia chromosome-positive acute lymphoid leukemias. Blood. 2002;100(6):1965–71.
21. Ottmann OG, Larson RA, Kantarjian HM, le Coutre PD, Baccarani M, Hochhaus A, et al. Phase II study of nilotinib in patients with relapsed or refractory Philadelphia chromosome--positive acute lymphoblastic leukemia. Leukemia. 2013;27(6):1411–3.
22. Schultz KR, Bowman WP, Aledo A, Slayton WB, Sather H, Devidas M, et al. Improved early event-free survival with imatinib in Philadelphia chromosome-positive acute lymphoblastic leukemia: a children's oncology group study. J Clin Oncol. 2009;27(31):5175–81.
23. Wassmann B, Pfeifer H, Goekbuget N, Beelen DW, Beck J, Stelljes M, et al. Alternating versus concurrent schedules of imatinib and chemotherapy as front-line therapy for Philadelphia-positive acute lymphoblastic leukemia (Ph+ ALL). Blood. 2006;108(5):1469–77.
24. Ottmann OG, Wassmann B, Pfeifer H, Giagounidis A, Stelljes M, Duhrsen U, et al. Imatinib compared with chemotherapy as front-line treatment of elderly patients with Philadelphia chromosome-positive acute lymphoblastic leukemia (Ph+ALL). Cancer. 2007;109(10):2068–76.
25. Porkka K, Koskenvesa P, Lundan T, Rimpilainen J, Mustjoki S, Smykla R, et al. Dasatinib crosses the blood-brain barrier and is an efficient therapy for central nervous system Philadelphia chromosome-positive leukemia. Blood. 2008;112(4):1005–12.
26. Chalandon Y, Thomas X, Hayette S, Cayuela JM, Abbal C, Huguet F, et al. Randomized study of reduced-intensity chemotherapy combined with imatinib in adults with Ph-positive acute lymphoblastic leukemia. Blood. 2015;125(24):3711–9.
27. Chiaretti S. Should treatment of Philadelphia chromosome-positive acute lymphoblastic leukemia be intensive? Intensive treatment is not necessary, at least in induction. Clin Adv Hematol Oncol. 2016;14(11):892–6.
28. Jabbour E, Short NJ, Ravandi F, Huang X, Daver N, DiNardo CD, et al. Combination of hyper-CVAD with ponatinib as first-line therapy for patients with Philadelphia chromosome-positive acute lymphoblastic leukaemia: long-term follow-up of a single-centre, phase 2 study. Lancet Haematol. 2018;5(12):e618–e27.
29. Ravandi F, Othus M, O'Brien SM, Forman SJ, Ha CS, Wong JYC, et al. US intergroup study of chemotherapy plus dasatinib and allogeneic stem cell transplant in Philadelphia chromosome positive ALL. Blood Adv. 2016;1(3):250–9.
30. Lim SN, Joo YD, Lee KH, Kim DY, Lee JH, Lee JH, et al. Long-term follow-up of imatinib plus combination chemotherapy in patients with newly diagnosed Philadelphia chromosome-positive acute lymphoblastic leukemia. Am J Hematol. 2015;90(11):1013–20.
31. Abou Dalle I, Jabbour E, Short NJ, Ravandi F. Treatment of Philadelphia chromosome-positive acute lymphoblastic leukemia. Curr Treat Options in Oncol. 2019;20(1):4.
32. Bleckmann K, Schrappe M. Advances in therapy for Philadelphia-positive acute lymphoblastic leukaemia of childhood and adolescence. Br J Haematol. 2016;172(6):855–69.
33. Carobolante F, Chiaretti S, Skert C, Bassan R. Practical guidance for the management of acute lymphoblastic leukemia in the adolescent and young adult population. Ther Adv Hematol. 2020;11:2040620720903531.
34. Ravandi F. Current management of Philadelphia chromosome positive ALL and the role of stem cell transplantation. Hematology Am Soc Hematol Educ Program. 2017;2017(1):22–7.
35. Ravandi F, O'Brien SM, Cortes JE, Thomas DM, Garris R, Faderl S, et al. Long-term follow-up of a phase 2 study of chemotherapy plus dasatinib for the initial treatment of patients with Philadelphia chromosome-positive acute lymphoblastic leukemia. Cancer. 2015;121(23):4158–64.

36. Thomas DA, Faderl S, Cortes J, O'Brien S, Giles FJ, Kornblau SM, et al. Treatment of Philadelphia chromosome-positive acute lymphocytic leukemia with hyper-CVAD and imatinib mesylate. Blood. 2004;103(12):4396–407.
37. Rousselot P, Coude MM, Gokbuget N, Gambacorti Passerini C, Hayette S, Cayuela JM, et al. Dasatinib and low-intensity chemotherapy in elderly patients with Philadelphia chromosome-positive ALL. Blood. 2016;128(6):774–82.
38. Gao L, Zhang C, Gao L, Liu Y, Su Y, Wang S, et al. Favorable outcome of haploidentical hematopoietic stem cell transplantation in Philadelphia chromosome-positive acute lymphoblastic leukemia: a multicenter study in Southwest China. J Hematol Oncol. 2015;8:90.
39. Xue YJ, Suo P, Huang XJ, Lu AD, Wang Y, Zuo YX, et al. Superior survival of unmanipulated haploidentical haematopoietic stem cell transplantation compared with intensive chemotherapy as post-remission treatment for children with very high-risk Philadelphia chromosome negative B-cell acute lymphoblastic leukaemia in first complete remission. Br J Haematol. 2020;188(5):757–67.
40. Litzow MR. Allogeneic transplantation for patients with Philadelphia chromosome positive acute lymphoblastic leukemia: is it imperative in the tyrosine kinase inhibitor era? Best Pract Res Clin Haematol. 2018;31(4):357–60.
41. Bassan R, Rossi G, Pogliani EM, Di Bona E, Angelucci E, Cavattoni I, et al. Chemotherapy-phased imatinib pulses improve long-term outcome of adult patients with Philadelphia chromosome-positive acute lymphoblastic leukemia: Northern Italy Leukemia Group protocol 09/00. J Clin Oncol. 2010;28(22):3644–52.
42. de Labarthe A, Rousselot P, Huguet-Rigal F, Delabesse E, Witz F, Maury S, et al. Imatinib combined with induction or consolidation chemotherapy in patients with de novo Philadelphia chromosome-positive acute lymphoblastic leukemia: results of the GRAAPH-2003 study. Blood. 2007;109(4):1408–13.
43. Ribera JM, Oriol A, Gonzalez M, Vidriales B, Brunet S, Esteve J, et al. Concurrent intensive chemotherapy and imatinib before and after stem cell transplantation in newly diagnosed Philadelphia chromosome-positive acute lymphoblastic leukemia. Final results of the CSTIBES02 trial. Haematologica. 2010;95(1):87–95.
44. Yanada M, Naoe T. Imatinib combined chemotherapy for Philadelphia chromosome-positive acute lymphoblastic leukemia: major challenges in current practice. Leuk Lymphoma. 2006;47(9):1747–53.
45. Kim DY, Joo YD, Lim SN, Kim SD, Lee JH, Lee JH, et al. Nilotinib combined with multiagent chemotherapy for newly diagnosed Philadelphia-positive acute lymphoblastic leukemia. Blood. 2015;126(6):746–56.
46. Liu B, Wang Y, Zhou C, Wei H, Lin D, Li W, et al. Nilotinib combined with multi-agent chemotherapy in newly diagnosed Philadelphia chromosome-positive acute lymphoblastic leukemia: a single-center prospective study with long-term follow-up. Ann Hematol. 2019;98(3):633–45.
47. Sorror ML, Sandmaier BM, Storer BE, Maris MB, Baron F, Maloney DG, et al. Comorbidity and disease status based risk stratification of outcomes among patients with acute myeloid leukemia or myelodysplasia receiving allogeneic hematopoietic cell transplantation. J Clin Oncol. 2007;25(27):4246–54.
48. Candoni A, Rambaldi A, Fanin R, Velardi A, Arcese W, Ciceri F, et al. Outcome of allogeneic hematopoietic stem cell transplantation in adult patients with Philadelphia chromosome-positive acute lymphoblastic leukemia in the era of tyrosine kinase inhibitors: a registry-based study of the Italian blood and marrow transplantation society (GITMO). Biol Blood Marrow Transplant. 2019;25(12):2388–97.
49. Litzow MR, Fielding AK, Luger SM, Paietta E, Ofran Y, Rowe JM, et al. The evolving role of chemotherapy and hematopoietic cell transplants in Ph-positive acute lymphoblastic leukemia in adults. Bone Marrow Transplant. 2017;52(12):1592–8.
50. Wang J, Jiang Q, Xu LP, Zhang XH, Chen H, Qin YZ, et al. Allogeneic stem cell transplantation versus tyrosine kinase inhibitors combined with chemotherapy in patients with

Philadelphia chromosome-positive acute lymphoblastic leukemia. Biol Blood Marrow Transplant. 2018;24(4):741–50.
51. Wieduwilt MJ. In the era of BCR-ABL1 inhibitors, are we closing the survival gap between allogeneic hematopoietic cell transplantation and chemotherapy for Philadelphia chromosome-positive acute lymphoblastic leukemia in first complete remission? Biol Blood Marrow Transplant. 2018;24(4):637–8.
52. Akahoshi Y, Nishiwaki S, Arai Y, Harada K, Najima Y, Kanda Y, et al. Reduced-intensity conditioning is a reasonable alternative for Philadelphia chromosome-positive acute lymphoblastic leukemia among elderly patients who have achieved negative minimal residual disease: a report from the Adult Acute Lymphoblastic Leukemia Working Group of the JSHCT. Bone Marrow Transplant. 2020;55(7):1317–25.
53. Bachanova V, Marks DI, Zhang MJ, Wang H, de Lima M, Aljurf MD, et al. Ph+ ALL patients in first complete remission have similar survival after reduced intensity and myeloablative allogeneic transplantation: impact of tyrosine kinase inhibitor and minimal residual disease. Leukemia. 2014;28(3):658–65.
54. Yoon JH, Min GJ, Park SS, Jeon YW, Lee SE, Cho BS, et al. Minimal residual disease-based long-term efficacy of reduced-intensity conditioning versus myeloablative conditioning for adult Philadelphia-positive acute lymphoblastic leukemia. Cancer. 2019;125(6):873–83.
55. Giebel S, Stella-Holowiecka B, Krawczyk-Kulis M, Gokbuget N, Hoelzer D, Doubek M, et al. Status of minimal residual disease determines outcome of autologous hematopoietic SCT in adult ALL. Bone Marrow Transplant. 2010;45(6):1095–101.
56. Giebel S, Labopin M, Gorin NC, Caillot D, Leguay T, Schaap N, et al. Improving results of autologous stem cell transplantation for Philadelphia-positive acute lymphoblastic leukaemia in the era of tyrosine kinase inhibitors: a report from the Acute Leukaemia Working Party of the European Group for Blood and Marrow Transplantation. Eur J Cancer. 2014;50(2):411–7.
57. Giebel S, Labopin M, Potter M, Poire X, Sengeloev H, Socie G, et al. Comparable results of autologous and allogeneic haematopoietic stem cell transplantation for adults with Philadelphia-positive acute lymphoblastic leukaemia in first complete molecular remission: an analysis by the Acute Leukemia Working Party of the EBMT. Eur J Cancer. 2018;96:73–81.
58. Wetzler M, Watson D, Stock W, Koval G, Mulkey FA, Hoke EE, et al. Autologous transplantation for Philadelphia chromosome-positive acute lymphoblastic leukemia achieves outcomes similar to allogeneic transplantation: results of CALGB study 10001 (Alliance). Haematologica. 2014;99(1):111–5.
59. Brissot E, Labopin M, Beckers MM, Socie G, Rambaldi A, Volin L, et al. Tyrosine kinase inhibitors improve long-term outcome of allogeneic hematopoietic stem cell transplantation for adult patients with Philadelphia chromosome positive acute lymphoblastic leukemia. Haematologica. 2015;100(3):392–9.
60. Warraich Z, Tenneti P, Thai T, Hubben A, Amin H, McBride A, et al. Relapse prevention with tyrosine kinase inhibitors after allogeneic transplantation for Philadelphia chromosome-positive acute lymphoblast leukemia: a systematic review. Biol Blood Marrow Transplant. 2020;26(3):e55–64.
61. Liu H, Xuan L, Lin R, Deng L, Fan Z, Nie D, et al. A new pre-emptive TKIs strategy for preventing relapse based on BCR/ABL monitoring for Ph+ALL undergoing allo-HCT: a prospective clinical cohort study. Leukemia. 2020;35(7):2054–63.
62. Nanno S, Matsumoto K, Nakamae M, Okamura H, Nishimoto M, Hirose A, et al. Effect of prophylactic post-transplant ponatinib administration on outcomes in patients with Philadelphia chromosome-positive acute lymphoblastic leukemia. Clin Lymphoma Myeloma Leuk. 2020;20(12):813–9 e1.
63. Pfeifer H, Wassmann B, Bethge W, Dengler J, Bornhauser M, Stadler M, et al. Randomized comparison of prophylactic and minimal residual disease-triggered imatinib after allogeneic stem cell transplantation for BCR-ABL1-positive acute lymphoblastic leukemia. Leukemia. 2013;27(6):1254–62.

64. Giebel S, Czyz A, Ottmann O, Baron F, Brissot E, Ciceri F, et al. Use of tyrosine kinase inhibitors to prevent relapse after allogeneic hematopoietic stem cell transplantation for patients with Philadelphia chromosome-positive acute lymphoblastic leukemia: a position statement of the Acute Leukemia Working Party of the European Society for Blood and Marrow Transplantation. Cancer. 2016;122(19):2941–51.
65. Saini N, Marin D, Ledesma C, Delgado R, Rondon G, Popat UR, et al. Impact of TKIs post-allogeneic hematopoietic cell transplantation in Philadelphia chromosome-positive ALL. Blood. 2020;136(15):1786–9.
66. Bruggemann M, Kotrova M. Minimal residual disease in adult ALL: technical aspects and implications for correct clinical interpretation. Blood Adv. 2017;1(25):2456–66.
67. Bruggemann M, Schrauder A, Raff T, Pfeifer H, Dworzak M, Ottmann OG, et al. Standardized MRD quantification in European ALL trials: proceedings of the Second International Symposium on MRD assessment in Kiel, Germany, 18-20 September 2008. Leukemia. 2010;24(3):521–35.
68. van der Velden VH, Cazzaniga G, Schrauder A, Hancock J, Bader P, Panzer-Grumayer ER, et al. Analysis of minimal residual disease by Ig/TCR gene rearrangements: guidelines for interpretation of real-time quantitative PCR data. Leukemia. 2007;21(4):604–11.
69. van Dongen JJ, Macintyre EA, Gabert JA, Delabesse E, Rossi V, Saglio G, et al. Standardized RT-PCR analysis of fusion gene transcripts from chromosome aberrations in acute leukemia for detection of minimal residual disease. Report of the BIOMED-1 Concerted Action: investigation of minimal residual disease in acute leukemia. Leukemia. 1999;13(12):1901–28.
70. van Dongen JJ, van der Velden VH, Bruggemann M, Orfao A. Minimal residual disease diagnostics in acute lymphoblastic leukemia: need for sensitive, fast, and standardized technologies. Blood. 2015;125(26):3996–4009.
71. Nagel I, Bartels M, Duell J, Oberg HH, Ussat S, Bruckmueller H, et al. Hematopoietic stem cell involvement in BCR-ABL1-positive ALL as a potential mechanism of resistance to blinatumomab therapy. Blood. 2017;130(18):2027–31.
72. Lee S, Kim DW, Cho BS, Yoon JH, Shin SH, Yahng SA, et al. Impact of minimal residual disease kinetics during imatinib-based treatment on transplantation outcome in Philadelphia chromosome-positive acute lymphoblastic leukemia. Leukemia. 2012;26(11):2367–74.
73. Yoon JH, Yhim HY, Kwak JY, Ahn JS, Yang DH, Lee JJ, et al. Minimal residual disease-based effect and long-term outcome of first-line dasatinib combined with chemotherapy for adult Philadelphia chromosome-positive acute lymphoblastic leukemia. Ann Oncol. 2016;27(6):1081–8.
74. Gokbuget N, Dombret H, Bonifacio M, Reichle A, Graux C, Faul C, et al. Blinatumomab for minimal residual disease in adults with B-cell precursor acute lymphoblastic leukemia. Blood. 2018;131(14):1522–31.
75. Soverini S, Albano F, Bassan R, Fabbiano F, Ferrara F, Foa R, et al. Next-generation sequencing for BCR-ABL1 kinase domain mutations in adult patients with Philadelphia chromosome-positive acute lymphoblastic leukemia: a position paper. Cancer Med. 2020;9(9):2960–70.
76. Foa R, Bassan R, Vitale A, Elia L, Piciocchi A, Puzzolo MC, et al. Dasatinib-Blinatumomab for Ph-positive acute lymphoblastic leukemia in adults. N Engl J Med. 2020;383(17):1613–23.
77. Pfeifer H, Wassmann B, Pavlova A, Wunderle L, Oldenburg J, Binckebanck A, et al. Kinase domain mutations of BCR-ABL frequently precede imatinib-based therapy and give rise to relapse in patients with de novo Philadelphia-positive acute lymphoblastic leukemia (Ph+ ALL). Blood. 2007;110(2):727–34.
78. Shen S, Chen X, Cai J, Yu J, Gao J, Hu S, et al. Effect of dasatinib vs imatinib in the treatment of pediatric Philadelphia chromosome-positive acute lymphoblastic leukemia: a randomized clinical trial. JAMA Oncol. 2020;6(3):358–66.
79. Ravandi F, Jorgensen JL, Thomas DA, O'Brien S, Garris R, Faderl S, et al. Detection of MRD may predict the outcome of patients with Philadelphia chromosome-positive ALL treated with tyrosine kinase inhibitors plus chemotherapy. Blood. 2013;122(7):1214–21.

80. Pfeifer H, Wassmann B, Hofmann WK, Komor M, Scheuring U, Bruck P, et al. Risk and prognosis of central nervous system leukemia in patients with Philadelphia chromosome-positive acute leukemias treated with imatinib mesylate. Clin Cancer Res. 2003;9(13):4674–81.
81. Hantschel O, Rix U, Superti-Furga G. Target spectrum of the BCR-ABL inhibitors imatinib, nilotinib and dasatinib. Leuk Lymphoma. 2008;49(4):615–9.
82. Zabriskie MS, Eide CA, Tantravahi SK, Vellore NA, Estrada J, Nicolini FE, et al. BCR-ABL1 compound mutations combining key kinase domain positions confer clinical resistance to ponatinib in Ph chromosome-positive leukemia. Cancer Cell. 2014;26(3):428–42.
83. Jabbour E, Kantarjian H, Ravandi F, Thomas D, Huang X, Faderl S, et al. Combination of hyper-CVAD with ponatinib as first-line therapy for patients with Philadelphia chromosome-positive acute lymphoblastic leukaemia: a single-centre, phase 2 study. Lancet Oncol. 2015;16(15):1547–55.
84. Sasaki K, Jabbour EJ, Ravandi F, Short NJ, Thomas DA, Garcia-Manero G, et al. Hyper-CVAD plus ponatinib versus hyper-CVAD plus dasatinib as frontline therapy for patients with Philadelphia chromosome-positive acute lymphoblastic leukemia: a propensity score analysis. Cancer. 2016;122(23):3650–6.
85. Moslehi JJ, Deininger M. Tyrosine kinase inhibitor-associated cardiovascular toxicity in chronic myeloid leukemia. J Clin Oncol. 2015;33(35):4210–8.
86. Dorer DJ, Knickerbocker RK, Baccarani M, Cortes JE, Hochhaus A, Talpaz M, et al. Impact of dose intensity of ponatinib on selected adverse events: multivariate analyses from a pooled population of clinical trial patients. Leuk Res. 2016;48:84–91.
87. Cortes JE, Kantarjian H, Shah NP, Bixby D, Mauro MJ, Flinn I, et al. Ponatinib in refractory Philadelphia chromosome-positive leukemias. N Engl J Med. 2012;367(22):2075–88.
88. Cortes J. How to manage CML patients with comorbidities. Hematology Am Soc Hematol Educ Program. 2020;2020(1):237–42.
89. Ishida Y, Terasako K, Oshima K, Sakamoto K, Ashizawa M, Sato M, et al. Dasatinib followed by second allogeneic hematopoietic stem cell transplantation for relapse of Philadelphia chromosome-positive acute lymphoblastic leukemia after the first transplantation. Int J Hematol. 2010;92(3):542–6.
90. Fielding AK. Current treatment of Philadelphia chromosome-positive acute lymphoblastic leukemia. Hematology Am Soc Hematol Educ Program. 2011;2011:231–7.
91. Tavernier E, Boiron JM, Huguet F, Bradstock K, Vey N, Kovacsovics T, et al. Outcome of treatment after first relapse in adults with acute lymphoblastic leukemia initially treated by the LALA-94 trial. Leukemia. 2007;21(9):1907–14.
92. Cortes JE, Kim DW, Pinilla-Ibarz J, le Coutre P, Paquette R, Chuah C, et al. A phase 2 trial of ponatinib in Philadelphia chromosome-positive leukemias. N Engl J Med. 2013;369(19):1783–96.
93. Kantarjian H, Giles F, Wunderle L, Bhalla K, O'Brien S, Wassmann B, et al. Nilotinib in imatinib-resistant CML and Philadelphia chromosome-positive ALL. N Engl J Med. 2006;354(24):2542–51.
94. Tavitian S, Uzunov M, Berard E, Bouscary D, Thomas X, Raffoux E, et al. Ponatinib-based therapy in adults with relapsed or refractory Philadelphia chromosome-positive acute lymphoblastic leukemia: results of the real-life OPAL study. Leuk Lymphoma. 2020;61(9):2161–7.
95. Stock W, Martinelli G, Stelljes M, DJ DA, Gokbuget N, Advani AS, et al. Efficacy of inotuzumab ozogamicin in patients with Philadelphia chromosome-positive relapsed/refractory acute lymphoblastic leukemia. Cancer. 2021;127(6):905–13.
96. Kantarjian HM, DeAngelo DJ, Stelljes M, Martinelli G, Liedtke M, Stock W, et al. Inotuzumab ozogamicin versus standard therapy for acute lymphoblastic leukemia. N Engl J Med. 2016;375(8):740–53.
97. Martinelli G, Boissel N, Chevallier P, Ottmann O, Gokbuget N, Topp MS, et al. Complete hematologic and molecular response in adult patients with relapsed/refractory Philadelphia chromosome-positive B-precursor acute lymphoblastic leukemia following treatment

with blinatumomab: results from a phase II, single-arm, multicenter study. J Clin Oncol. 2017;35(16):1795–802.
98. Couturier MA, Thomas X, Raffoux E, Huguet F, Berthon C, Simand C, et al. Blinatumomab + ponatinib for relapsed/refractory Philadelphia chromosome-positive acute lymphoblastic leukemia in adults. Leuk Lymphoma. 2020:1–10.
99. Park JH, Riviere I, Gonen M, Wang X, Senechal B, Curran KJ, et al. Long-term follow-up of CD19 CAR therapy in acute lymphoblastic leukemia. N Engl J Med. 2018;378(5):449–59.
100. Ottmann OG, Pfeifer H, Cayuela JM, Spiekermann K, Jung W, Beck J, et al. Nilotinib (Tasigna®) and low intensity chemotherapy for first-line treatment of elderly patients with BCR-ABL1-positive acute lymphoblastic leukemia: final results of a prospective multicenter trial (EWALL-PH02). Blood. 2018;132

Chapter 10
Treatment of Ph-Like Acute Lymphoblastic Leukemia

Thai Hoa Tran and Sarah K Tasian

Definition of Ph-Like ALL

Ph-like ALL was originally identified in 2009 via gene expression profiling by two independent groups using different gene classifiers. Researchers in the Children's Oncology Group (COG), St. Jude Children's Research Hospital (SJCRH), and University of New Mexico (UNM) via the National Cancer Institute (NCI) TARGET initiative (https://ocg.cancer.gov/programs/target/projects/acute-lymphoblastic-leukemia) utilized Affymetrix gene expression microarray data to identify 257 gene probe sets that defined a distinct gene expression signature of both Ph+ ALL and Ph-like ALL [1], while the Dutch Children's Oncology Group led by den Boer and colleagues at Erasmus Medical Center used hierarchical clustering of 110 probe sets to predict 6 major pediatric ALL subtypes (T-cell ALL, *ETV6-RUNX1*, *KMT2A*-rearranged, *TCF3-PBX1*, *BCR-ABL1*, and high hyperdiploid) [2]. Despite sharing only nine common probe sets of seven genes (*CCND2*, *SH3BP5*, *ABL1*, *SOCS2*, *DUSP6*, *LST1*, and *EGFL7*), both gene classifiers identified a subset of HR B-ALL patients with poor survival who had frequent deletions of B-cell development genes, such as the transcription factor *IKZF1* [4]. These assays and additional advances in RNA sequencing were further able to define new genetic alterations deregulating

T. H. Tran
Division of Pediatric Hematology-Oncology, Charles-Bruneau Cancer Center, CHU Sainte-Justine, Montreal, QC, Canada

Department of Pediatrics, University of Montreal, Montreal, QC, Canada

S. K. Tasian (✉)
Division of Oncology and Center for Childhood Cancer Research, Children's Hospital of Philadelphia, Philadelphia, PA, USA

Department of Pediatrics, Perelman School of Medicine at the University of Pennsylvania and Abramson Cancer Center, Philadelphia, PA, USA
e-mail: tasians@chop.edu

M. R. Litzow, E. A. Raetz (eds.), *Clinical Management of Acute Lymphoblastic Leukemia*, https://doi.org/10.1007/978-3-030-85147-7_10

tyrosine kinase or cytokine receptor genes in Ph-like ALL, including *CRLF2*, *ABL1*, *PDGFRB*, and *JAK2* [5]. The COG/SJCRH/UNM group subsequently developed the first clinically validated Ph-like ALL screening assay, which measures the expression of 8 or 15 genes in a 384-well low-density array (LDA) microfluidic card to detect the Ph-like ALL signature. This clinical assay is now capable of results return within 24–48 h of sample submission [6]. The LDA card is currently being used by the COG and other consortia to screen all patients with newly diagnosed HR B-ALL for the Ph-like signature and to allocate those with LDA positivity for further downstream testing to identify specific Ph-like-associated genetic alterations [7]. It should be emphasized that the most clinically relevant endpoint in patients with Ph-like ALL remains identification of such oncogenic translocations and mutations that activate kinase signaling and may be therapeutically targeted.

Biology and Genomic Landscape of Ph-Like ALL

In their 2014 landmark paper, Roberts and colleagues described the genomic landscape of Ph-like ALL via a comprehensive genomic analysis of 154 children and young adults with HR B-ALL [8]. The unifying molecular hallmark of Ph-like ALL resides in the heterogeneous spectrum of genetic alterations activating cytokine receptor genes and kinase signaling pathways [8]. These alterations can be subdivided into four distinct genomically defined subsets based upon their underlying kinase-activating lesions, (1) alterations in JAK-STAT pathway genes (predominantly *CRLF2*, *JAK2*, *EPOR*, *IL7R*, *SH2B3*), (2) ABL class alterations (*ABL1*, *ABL2*, *CSF1R*, *PDGFRA*, and *PDGFRB*), (3) uncommon Ras pathway mutations (*NRAS*, *KRAS*, *NF1*, *PTPN11*, *CBL*), and (4) rare kinase fusions (*NTRK3*, *PTK2B*, *BLNK*, *LYN*), and are described in greater detail below (Table 10.1, Fig. 10.1) [8, 9]. While *CRLF2* (*cytokine receptor-like factor 2*) rearrangements also occur with lower frequency in children with standard-risk (SR) B-ALL [3, 10, 11] and in >50% of trisomy 21/Down syndrome (DS)-associated B-ALL [12, 13] (and may or may not have the associated Ph-like gene expression signature), other Ph-like ALL-associated kinase fusions have only extremely rarely been discovered in patients with SR disease.

Deletions of *IKZF1* and other lymphoid transcription factor genes occur commonly in Ph-like ALL, as has been similarly seen in Ph+ ALL [8, 14–17]. *IKZF1* encodes the zinc-finger DNA-binding Ikaros, a transcription factor essential for B-cell lymphoid development. Its alteration results in acquired stem cell-like properties, aberrant bone marrow stromal adhesion, and chemotherapy resistance [18–20]. The most common type of *IKZF1* alteration is intragenic focal deletion of exons 4–7, which results in the dominant-negative Ik6 isoform [20]. In one study, *IKZF1* alterations were detected in 68% of Ph-like ALL compared to 16% of non-Ph-like ALL cases [8]. Inferior clinical outcomes in patients with *IKZF1*-deleted Ph-like ALL have also been reported [8, 21]. Recent studies from European consortia have further described inferior outcomes of patients with the new *IKZF1*^{plus}

Table 10.1 Repertoire of Ph-like ALL kinase rearrangements, therapeutic targets, and potential clinical trials

Ph-like genetic subgroups	3′ kinase genes	5′ fusion partner genes	Kinase inhibitors	Clinical trials
JAK-STAT pathway alterations	*CRLF2*	*CSF2RA, IGH, P2RY8*	Ruxolitinib	NCT02420717 (MDACC)
	JAK2	*ATF7IP, BCR, EBF1, ETV6, GOLGA5, HMBOX1, OFD1, PAX5, PCM1, PPFIBP1, RFX3, SMU1, SNX29, SSBP2, STRN3, TERF2, TPR, USP25, ZBTB46, ZNF274, ZNF340*	Ruxolitinib	NCT02723994 (COG AALL1521)
	EPOR	*IGH, IGK, LAIR1, THADA*	Ruxolitinib	NCT03117751 (SJCRH Total XVII)
	TSLP	*IQGAP2*	Ruxolitinib	NCT03571321 (University of Chicago)
	IL2RB	*MYH9*	Ruxolitinib	
ABL class alterations	*ABL1*	*CENPC, ETV6, FOXP1, LSM14A, NUP153, NUP214, RANBP2, RCSD1, SFPQ, SHIP1, SNX1, SNX2, SPTNA1, ZMIZ1*	Dasatinib	NCT01406756 (COG AALL1131)
	ABL2	*PAG1, RCSD1, ZC3HAV1*	Dasatinib	NCT02143414 (SWOG S1318)
	CSF1R	*MEF2D, SSBP2, TBL1XR1*	Dasatinib	NCT02420717 (MDACC)
	PDGFRA	*FIP1L1*	Dasatinib	NCT03007147 (COG AALL1631)
	PDGFRB	*ATF7IP, EBF1, ETV6, NUMA1, SNX29, SSBP2, TNIP1, ZEB2, ZMYND8, ZNF608*	Dasatinib	NCT03117751 (SJCRH Total XVII)
	LYN	*GATAD2A, NCOR1*	Dasatinib	
Other kinases	*NTRK3*	*ETV6*	Entrectinib	NCT03066661
			Larotrectinib	NCT03834961
	PTK2B	*KDM6A, STAG2, TMEM2*	FAK inhibitor	
	FGFR1	*BCR*	Ponatinib	
	FLT3	*ZMYM2*	FLT3 inhibitor	
	TYK2	*MYB, SMARCA4, ZNF340*	JAK1/3 inhibitor	
	BLNK	*DNTT*		
	CBL	*KANK1*		
	DGKH	*ZFAND3*		

COG Children's Oncology Group, SJCRH St. Jude Children's Research Hospital, *MDACC* MD Anderson Cancer Center, *SWOG* Southwestern Oncology Group

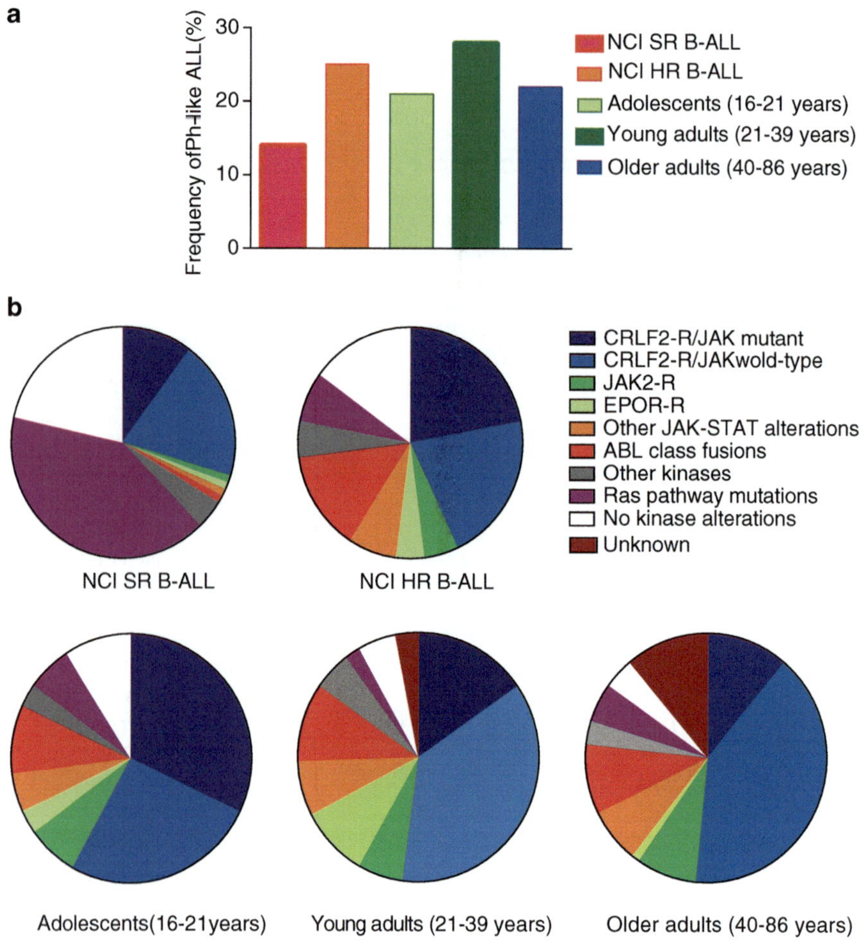

Fig. 10.1 Frequency of Ph-like ALL and genetic subtypes by age group. *NCI HR B-ALL* National Cancer Institute high-risk B-acute lymphoblastic leukemia, *NCI SR B-ALL* National Cancer Institute standard-risk B-acute lymphoblastic leukemia

molecular profile, which is defined by deletion of *IKZF1* co-occurring with one or more deletions in *PAX5*, *CDKN2A* (heterozygous or homozygous), *CDKN2B* (homozygous only), or the pseudoautosomal region 1 (PAR1) region of the sex chromosomes where *CRLF2* is located and in the absence of *ERG* deletion [22–25]. Stanulla and colleagues reported that the *IKZF1*^{plus} signature conferred the highest hazard ratio for relapse in multivariate analysis and could be incorporated in clinical decision algorithms to refine risk stratification in addition to MRD response [22]. The *IKZF1*^{plus} subgroup in these studies likely contains a high proportion of Ph-like ALL patients, as both populations share adverse clinical and biologic features of higher white blood cell (WBC) at diagnosis, poor prednisone response, positive minimal residual disease (MRD) after induction therapy, and higher frequency of the germline *GATA3* variant rs3824662 reported to predispose to developing Ph-like ALL [22–24, 26].

JAK-STAT Pathway Gene Alterations

Approximately half of children, adolescents, and adults with Ph-like ALL harbor *CRLF2* rearrangements [3, 27, 28], which leads to *CRLF2* overexpression and increased surface protein expression of the thymic stromal lymphopoietin receptor (TSLPR; encoded by *CRLF2*) detectable by flow cytometry [29]. *CRLF2* alterations occur via two major mechanisms: (1) focal deletion of PAR1 on chromosomes Xp22/Yp11 resulting in the *P2RY8-CRLF2* fusion or as (2) translocation to the immunoglobulin heavy chain enhancer region on chromosome 14, resulting in *IGH-CRLF2* rearrangement [12, 30]. Both rearrangements result in overexpression of full-length CRLF2, which heterodimerizes with the IL7R-alpha subunit to form the TSLPR involved in early B-cell development [31–33]. *P2RY8-CRLF2* fusions appear to occur more frequently in younger children and in those with DS-ALL [13], whereas *IGH-CRLF2* predominates among adolescents and young adults, particularly those of Hispanic ancestry [12, 30, 34, 35]. Rarely, activating *CRLF2* F232C point mutations, which typically coexist with *CRLF2* rearrangements, also lead to *CRLF2* deregulation [36]. Moreover, half of *CRLF2*-rearranged cases harbor concomitant *JAK2* or, less commonly, *JAK1* mutations. The most frequently occurring point mutation is *JAK2* R683G in the *JAK2* pseudokinase domain. *JAK1* V658F, which is analogous to the *JAK2* V617F mutation seen in adult myeloproliferative neoplasms, occurs much less frequently in *CRLF2*-rearranged Ph-like ALL [3, 8]. Sequence mutations in *IL7R* and *SH2B3* have also been identified in a small number of *CRLF2*-rearranged cases that lack concomitant JAK mutations [8, 37]. Uncommonly (~7% of patients), some children with detected *CRLF2* rearrangements leading to *CRLF2* overexpression (usually *P2RY8-CRLF2* fusions in children with SR B-ALL) do not have the Ph-like expression signature [37].

JAK2 and *EPOR* rearrangements are additional mutually exclusive JAK-STAT pathway alterations, each representing approximately 5–10% of Ph-like ALL cases [3, 8]. Some reports have noted an increased prevalence of *JAK2* fusions among the young adult population compared to children, ~15% vs 5%, respectively [6, 38]. *JAK2* is a promiscuous 3′ gene in Ph-like ALL with at least 19 different 5′ partner genes reported to date. All *JAK2* fusions are in-frame and disrupt the pseudokinase domain of JAK2, thus relieving from auto-inhibition of the kinase domain and resulting in constitutive activation of JAK-STAT signaling [5, 8, 9]. Four types of *EPOR* rearrangements have been described, each involving the juxtaposition of the *EPOR* gene to the enhancer region of immunoglobulin heavy (*IGH*) or κ (*IGK*) loci and leading to deregulated expression of a truncated form of *EPOR* that has been shown to drive Ph-like leukemogenesis and activated JAK/STAT signaling [39].

Insertion and truncation of *EPOR* into the upstream region of *LAIR1* or the *THADA* loci have also been reported in a very small number of patients [39]. As with *JAK2* fusions, prevalence of *EPOR* rearrangements rises with increasing age with peak prevalence among young adults [8, 39].

Additional mechanisms leading to JAK-STAT pathway activation beyond the aforementioned kinase or cytokine receptor-activating rearrangements implicate a diverse range of sequence mutations and copy number variations in genes such as *JAK1*, *JAK3*, *IL7R*, *SH2B3*, *IL2RB*, and *TYK2* [8]. These lesions collectively comprise 14% of children compared to 5% and 7.3% of adolescents and older adults, respectively [5, 8]. Although they lack a kinase-activating rearrangement, these cases often harbor chromosomal rearrangements expressing fusion oncoproteins involving transcription factor genes (*EBF1*, *PAX5*, *ETV6*) and/or epigenetic regulators (*CREBBP*, *SETD2*, *ASXL1*) that merit further study [5].

ABL Class Alterations

The second most clinically relevant subgroup of Ph-like ALL is ABL class alterations, which account for approximately 10% of cases [8, 27]. Prevalence peaks among children with NCI HR B-ALL at 17% and then decreases to about 10% in young and older adults [8, 27, 37]. ABL class rearrangements involve 3′ *ABL1*, *ABL2*, *CSF1R*, *PDGFRA*, or *PDGFRB* fusing with multiple 5′ partner genes. ABL class fusions exhibit sensitivity to ABL inhibitors, such as imatinib and dasatinib [3, 8, 9].

Ras Pathway Mutations

Approximately 4% of Ph-like ALL patients have activating mutations in Ras pathway genes, including *KRAS*, *NRAS*, *NF1*, *PTPN11*, and *CBL* [8]. Ras pathway mutations are usually subclonal and can occur as the sole detected anomaly or in conjunction with sentinel Ph-like translocations (e.g., *CRLF2*, ABL class, *JAK2*, or *EPOR* fusions) [8, 28]. Ras-activating mutations are also commonly found in hyperdiploid, hypodiploid, *KTM2A*-rearranged, and relapsed ALL and are also often subclonal [40–42]. It is not currently known whether these mutations are pathogenic drivers in childhood ALL.

Rare Kinase Fusions

Other rare fusions involving *NTRK3*, *BLNK*, *DGKH*, *LYN*, *FGFR1*, *PTK2B*, *FLT3*, or *TYK2* collectively account for 3% of Ph-like ALL [8, 37]. The *ETV6-NTRK3* fusion, which is present in various malignancies such as infantile fibrosarcoma and secretory breast carcinoma, can induce an aggressive ALL with in vitro and in vivo sensitivity to TRK inhibitors [43]. Functional modeling of other kinase fusions is important to determine their oncogenic role and identify novel therapeutic targets. As an example, *FGFR1* fusions may be targetable with ponatinib [44] or pazopanib [45] and *LYN* fusions (predicted to activate Src signaling) with dasatinib [46, 47].

Epidemiology and Clinical Picture of Ph-Like ALL

The prevalence of Ph-like ALL rises with increasing age and varies by gender, ethnicity, and NCI-defined risk groups. A recent meta-analysis of 15 studies reported that the pooled prevalence of Ph-like ALL across the age spectrum was 15.4% [48]. By age group, the Ph-like subtype comprised 15.6% of B-ALL cases in children 1 to 10 years old, 26.2% in adolescents aged 11 to 20 years old, 25.8% in young adults 21 to 40 years old, and 16.9% in adults older than 40 years [8, 27, 28, 48, 49]. Among children and adolescents with B-ALL, Ph-like ALL accounts for 13.6% of NCI SR cases and 22.4% of NCI HR cases [11, 37]. In comparison to Ph+ ALL, Ph-like ALL is three times more common in the pediatric age group [6]. Males are more commonly affected than females across the age spectrum with a male-to-female ratio of 1.5:1 among children and adults [8, 27]. Ph-like ALL also has a predilection for patients of Hispanic/Latino or Native American ethnicity, especially among those with *CRLF2* rearrangements. This phenomenon has been attributed in part to the increased prevalence of germline Ph-like ALL risk variant in *GATA3* (rs3824662) in Hispanic individuals with Native American genetic ancestry [26, 50, 51]. Furthermore, Ph-like ALL patients frequently have adverse clinical features with significantly higher rates of hyperleukocytosis at diagnosis, end-induction MRD positivity, and increased risk of treatment failure and relapse [8, 27, 34, 37, 49, 52]. The Ph-like ALL gene signature may confer an independent adverse risk factor, as shown in some multivariate analyses [27, 49, 53]. Patients harboring *PDGFRB*, *JAK2*, or *EPOR* fusions are notoriously associated with more aggressive disease course and frequent induction failure [8, 54–57].

The inferior survival of patients with Ph-like versus non-Ph-like ALL patients occurs across the age spectrum, and differential outcomes may exist within the heterogeneous Ph-like ALL subtypes based upon induction chemotherapy response. Children with NCI HR B-ALL and a retrospectively identified Ph-like expression signature treated on the COG AALL0232 phase 3 trial (NCT00075725) had a 5-year event-free survival (EFS) of 63% versus 86% ($p < 0.0001$) of those with non-Ph-like ALL [53]. Importantly, this inferior outcome was detected for patients with Ph-like ALL regardless of the randomized treatment arm assigned, which was in contrast to patients with non-Ph-like ALL with superiority of high-dose methotrexate versus dose-escalating Capizzi-style methotrexate in the first interim maintenance phase [53]. More recent analyses of children with NCI SR Ph-like ALL treated on the COG AALL0331 phase 3 trial (NCT00103285) [58] showed statistically inferior outcomes versus those with SR non-Ph-like ALL with 7-year EFS 82.4% and 90.7% ($p = 0.0022$). However, these patients appear to be salvageable at relapse with no difference in overall survival (OS) (93.2% vs 95.8%, $p = 0.14$) between the two groups [11]. In addition, recent data from the CALGB 10403 phase 2 trial (NCT00558519) also showed marked improvement in outcome for adolescents and young adults (AYA) less than 40 years of age when using a similarly intensive pediatric-inspired regimen, although outcomes for Ph-like ALL AYA patients in that trial remained unfavorable with estimated 3-year EFS of 42% compared to 69% ($p = 0.008$) for those with non-Ph-like ALL [59].

Clinical outcomes of patients with Ph-like ALL also worsen with increasing age. Four recent studies focused upon defining the incidence and characteristics of Ph-like ALL occurring in young and older adults with B-ALL. Among 49 adults with Ph-like ALL treated at the MD Anderson Cancer Center (MDACC), the 5-year OS was 23% for Ph-like ALL vs 59% (p = 0.006) for patients with non-Ph-like ALL [49]. Another study of 194 Ph-like ALL patients from 21 to 86 years old reported 5-year EFS for young adults (21–39 years old), adults (40–59 years), and older adults (60–86 years) of 40.4%, 29.8%, and 18.9%, respectively [27]. Two additional North American and German studies of adult Ph-like ALL cohorts confirmed the poor outcomes of this population [28, 34]. Ph-like ALL patients with concomitant *IKZF1* alterations may have further inferior outcomes compared to those without *IKZF1* alterations, although these analyses have been limited by small patient numbers [8, 21] (Table 10.2).

Diagnostic Modalities and Clinical Workflow Algorithms for Ph-Like ALL

The heterogeneous spectrum of kinase-activating alterations, cryptic nature of these genetic aberrations by conventional cytogenetic analysis, and complexity of required testing has rendered Ph-like ALL quite challenging to diagnose via clinical laboratory assays. Several cooperative oncology consortia have adopted different screening strategies largely based on the patient population size to be tested, development of more rapid next-generation sequencing platforms, and availability of therapeutic clinical trials [7].

Clinical diagnosis of Ph-like ALL has involved assessment of the pathognomonic gene expression signature (used by some, but not all, groups) and detection of targetable kinase-activating alterations. Gene expression profiling, the utilized discovery modality in initial European and North American studies [1, 2], is not readily available in the clinic and has now been largely replaced by the TaqMan LDA microfluidic card measuring the expression of 8- or 15-gene panels (*IGJ*, *SPATS2L*, *MUC4*, *CRLF2*, *CA6*, *NRXN3*, *BMPR1B*, *GPR110*, *CHN2*, *SEMA6A*, *PON2*, *SLC2A5*, *S100Z*, *TP53INP1*, *IFITM1*) now used by the COG to determine the Ph-like ALL signature [7, 53, 60]. An integrated score between 0 and 1 is generated from the 8- or 15-gene assay, with a predictive score ≥0.5 considered positive for the Ph-like gene signature [37]. Higher LDA score (e.g., >0.7) typically suggests an underlying kinase fusion [7]. This LDA-based approach has provided a rapid and cost-effective screening modality for some groups to identify patients with probable

Table 10.2 Prevalence, clinical features, and treatment outcomes of Ph-like ALL by different study groups

Study group	Study period	Patient population	Prevalence of Ph-like ALL n (%)	Median age at diagnosis (CI)	Median WBC at diagnosis (CI)	Male,%	Ph-like gene signature detection methods	Kinase alteration detection methods	Clinical trials	Treatment outcome	References
MDACC	2010–2012	Adult	n = 12, 22.6%	36 (20–57)	4.2 (1.0–29.3)	67	PAM	WGS	Inotuzumab monotherapy Phase 2 trials	1-year EFS: 33%	Jabbour et al. Blood 2019
		R/R						RNA-seq		1-year OS: 33%	
		B-ALL ($n = 53$)									
AIEOP-BFM	2000–2018	B-ALL ($n = 3854$)	ABL class ($n = 46$)	NA	NA	63	HC	FISH	Chemotherapy ($n = 33$)	5-year EFS: 49%	Cario et al. Haematologica 2019
								RT-PCR	Chemotherapy + TKI ($n = 13$)	5-year OS: 70%	
								CGH			
								RNA-seq			
FRALLE	NA	Pediatric and adults with B-ALL	ABL class ($n = 24$)	24 (5–72)	30 (4–570)	67	HC	FISH	Chemo + TKI ($n = 24$)	3-year EFS: 55%	Tanasi et al. Blood 2019
CAALL								RT-MLFA		3-year OS: 77%	
GRAALL								RQ-PCR			
EWALL								BP-PCR			
EORTC								RNA-seq			
CALGB	2007–2012	AYA	$n = 41$, 31.3%	NA	NA	NA	LDA	LDA for CRLF2 aberration	Pediatric-based chemotherapy	3-year EFS: 42%	Stock et al. Blood 2019
		B-ALL ($n = 131$)							Regimen CALGB 10403	3-year OS: 63%	

(continued)

Table 10.2 (continued)

Study group	Study period	Patient population	Prevalence of Ph-like ALL n (%)	Median age at diagnosis (CI)	Median WBC at diagnosis (CI)	Male,%	Ph-like gene signature detection methods	Kinase alteration detection methods	Clinical trials	Treatment outcome	References
COG	2006–2008	SR	*n* = 139, 13.6%	NA	15.9 ± 13.7	50	LDA	FISH	COG AALL0331 phase 3 for SR B-ALL	7-year EFS: 82%	Roberts et al. Blood 2018
		B-ALL (*n* = 1023)						RT-PCR		7-year OS: 93%	
								Sanger sequencing			
								RNA-seq			
CALGB	NA	Adult	*n* = 194, 24.3%	40 (21–86)	56.6 (0.2–434)	61	PAM	FISH	Multiple trials	5-year EFS: 22.5%	Roberts et al. J Clin Oncol 2017
ECOG		B-ALL (*n* = 798)					LDA	PCR		5-year OS:23.8%	
MDACC								Sanger sequencing			
NILG								RNA-seq			
PMCC											
SWOG											
City of Hope											
GMALL	1999–2005	Adult	*n* = 26, 13%	31 (16–59)	NA	74	PAM	FISH	Multiple trials	5-year DFS: 19%	Herold et al. Haematologica 2017
		B-ALL (*n* = 207)						Q-PCR		5-year OS: 22%	
								Sanger sequencing			

MDACC	2000–2012	Adult	$n = 49$, 33.1%	33.5 (15–71)	17 (1–603)	66	PAM	FISH	Chemotherapy (hyperCVAD or augmented BFM)	5-year OS: 23%	Jain et al. Blood 2017
		B-ALL ($n = 148$)					LDA	Targeted NGS			
University Pennsylvania	NA	Adult	$n = 18$, 20.2%	43 (19–63)	71.1 ± 31.8 (median = 28.6)	69	LDA	FISH	Multiple trials	Median survival: 1.6 years	Tasian et al. Leukemia 2017
University of Michigan		B-ALL ($n = 89$)						PCR			
								RT-PCR			
								Sanger sequencing			
								Archer FusionPlex			
JACLS	NA	Pediatric	$n = 29$, 8%	8.8 (1.9–16)	94.3 (0.6–420)	76	GSEA	Multiplex RT-PCR	Multiple trials	5-year EFS: 48.6%	Imamura et al. Blood Cancer J 2016
TCCSG		B-ALL ($n = 373$)						RNA-seq		5-year OS: 73.5%	
CCLSG											
KYCCSG											
HOVON	1993–2009	Adult	$n = 21$, 17%	25 (16–59)	NA	NA	HC	RT-PCR	Multiple trials	3-year EFS: ~25%	Boer et al. Haematologica 2015
		B-ALL ($n = 127$)									

(continued)

Table 10.2 (continued)

Study group	Study period	Patient population	Prevalence of Ph-like ALL *n* (%)	Median age at diagnosis (CI)	Median WBC at diagnosis (CI)	Male,%	Ph-like gene signature detection methods	Kinase alteration detection methods	Clinical trials	Treatment outcome	References
COG SJCRH ECOG CALGB MDACC	2000–2007	Children, AYA with B-ALL (*n* = 1725)	*n* = 264, 15.3%	NA	106	cHR: 62 A: 73 YA: 82	PAM	FISH RT-PCR WES RNA-seq WGS	Multiple trials	5-year EFS: 58% (cHR), 41% (A), 24% (YA) 5-year OS: 73% (cHR), 66% (ado), 26% (YA)	Roberts et al. NEJM 2014
SJCRH	2000–2007	Pediatric B-ALL (*n* = 344)	*n* = 40, 11.6%	5.3 (1.3–18.6)	7.1 (1.7–258.3)	68	PAM	FISH RT-PCR Sanger sequencing RNA-seq WGS	MRD-based risk intensification regimen	5-year EFS: 90% 5-year OS: 92.5%	Roberts et al. J Clin Oncol 2014
DCOG COALL	1994–2015	Pediatric B-ALL (*n* = 572)	*n* = 94, 16%	7	44.5	49	HC	FISH CRLF2 mRNA expression by microarray	Multiple trials	5-year CIR: 32%	van der Veer et al. Blood 2013

COG	2002–2011	HR B-ALL ($n = 572$)	$n = 81$, 14%	NA	NA	NA	PAM	Kinome sequencing	COG AALL0232 phase 3 trial for HR B-ALL	5-year EFS: 62.6%	Loh et al. Blood 2013
COG	2000–2003	Pediatric B-ALL ($n = 221$)	$n = 68$, 31%	NA	NA	NA	PAM	SNP PCR	COG P9906	5-year EFS: 26%	Mullighan et al. NEJM 2009
DCOG	1990–2004	Pediatric	$n = 30$, 19%	NA	NA	NA	HC	RT-PCR	Multiple trials	5-year DFS: 60% (COALL)	Den Boer et al. Lancet Oncol 2009
COALL		B-ALL ($n = 154$)								5-year DFS: 57% (DCOG)	

AIEOP-BFM Associazione Italiana di Ematologia e Oncologia Pediatrica and Berlin-Frankfurt-Münster cooperative groups, *AYA* adolescents and young adults, *BP-PCR* breakpoint-specific multiplex polymerase chain reaction, *CAALL* French Protocol for the Treatment of ALL in Children and Adolescents, *CALGB* Cancer and Leukemia Group B, *CCLSG* Children's Cancer and Leukemia Study Group, *CGH* comparative genomic hybridization, *cHR* childhood high-risk, *CIR* cumulative incidence of relapse, *COALL* Childhood Oncology Acute Lymphoblastic Leukemia, *COG* Children's Oncology Group, *CRLF2* cytokine receptor like factor 2, *DCOG* Dutch Childhood Oncology Group, *DFS* disease-free survival, *EFS* event-free survival, *ECOG* Eastern Cooperative Oncology Group, *EORTC* European Organisation for Research and Treatment of Cancer, *EWALL* European Working Group on Adult ALL, *FISH* fluorescence in situ hybridization, *FRALLE* French Group for Childhood ALL, *GMALL* German Multicenter Study Group for Adult ALL, *GRAALL* French-Swiss-Belgian Group for Research on Adult Acute Lymphoblastic Leukemia, *GSEA* gene-set enrichment analysis, *HC* hierarchical clustering, *HOVON* Hemato-Oncologie voor Volwassenen Nederland, *JACLS* Japanese Association of Childhood Leukemia Study, *KYCCSG* Kyushu-Yamaguchi Children's Cancer Study Group, *LDA* low-density array, *MDACC* MD Anderson Cancer Center, *MLPA* multiplex ligation-dependent probe amplification, *MRD* minimal residual disease, *NILG* Northern Italy Leukemia Group, *NA* not available, *OS* overall survival, *PAM* prediction analysis of microarrays, *PMCC* Princess Margaret Cancer Centre, *RNA-seq* RNA sequencing, *RQ-PCR* real-time quantitative polymerase chain reaction, *R/R B-ALL* relapsed/refractory B-acute lymphoblastic leukemia, *RT-PCR* reverse transcription-polymerase chain reaction, *SJCRH* St. Jude Children's Research Hospital, *SNP* single-nucleotide polymorphism, *SR* standard risk, *SWOG* Southwestern Oncology Group, *TCCSG* Tokyo Children's Cancer Study Group, *TKI* tyrosine kinase inhibitor, *WES* whole-exome sequencing, *WGS* whole-genome sequencing

Ph-like ALL (LDA-positive) who require further detailed genomic characterization to identify targetable kinase-activating alterations. Aside from direct detection of *CRLF2* overexpression and *P2RY8-CRLF2* fusions on the LDA card, this modality is intended only as a screening tool and does not detect other Ph-like kinase-activating lesions. The LDA card is also capable of identifying and "ruling out" patients with Ph+ ALL and *ETV6-RUNX1* ALL who do not require additional Ph-like testing [61].

To enable detection of kinase-activating alterations (the most clinically relevant endpoint in the Ph-like ALL diagnostic work-up), several commercial, research-level, and clinical next-generation sequencing (NGS) platforms have been developed and are replacing prior multiplexed clinical RT-PCR panels [7, 62, 63]. The ArcherDx FusionPlex Heme panel uses anchored multiplex PCR-based enrichment with the ability to detect novel fusions involving 87 genes associated with hematologic malignancies [7]. The FoundationOne Heme panel is a targeted combined DNA and RNA sequencing method capable of fusion and mutation detection in >400 cancer-related genes [64]. Of particular interest, transcriptomic/RNA sequencing (RNA-seq) represents a powerful tool for comprehensive fusion and mutation detection in addition to identifying the Ph-like GEP by hierarchical clustering [7] and is becoming more clinically available. Indeed, RNA-seq is the only single platform capable of fulfilling the two essential aspects of Ph-like ALL's diagnosis, but is currently not considered time- or cost-effective for routine analysis of all patients. Clinical fusion and NGS assays are relatively more cost-effective, but still require a relatively long turnaround time (between 2 and 4 weeks) prior to clinical result reporting.

More rapid testing assays using conventional methods such as fluorescence in situ hybridization (FISH) and flow cytometry still retain clinical relevance for the diagnosis of Ph-like ALL. For example, dual color break-apart FISH probes are now commercially available for the canonical Ph-like 3′ kinase genes *ABL1*, *ABL2*, *PDGFRB*, *CRLF2*, *JAK2*, and *EPOR* with results typically delivered within 48 h. Since the vast majority of these kinase fusions are exclusively seen with the Ph-like phenotype, an abnormal FISH result might be sufficient to start tyrosine kinase inhibitor (TKI) therapy while waiting for confirmatory molecular testing. The COG has expanded its routine FISH panel to include ABL class FISH probes in its HR B-ALL AALL1732 phase 3 trial (NCT03959085) and its Ph+ ALL AALL1631 phase 3 trial (NCT03007147) in order to facilitate earlier introduction of TKI during induction for patients with identified ABL class alterations. Increased flow cytometric staining of TSLPR also suggests underlying *CRLF2* rearrangement, which is known to occur in over half of Ph-like ALL cases [29]. Flow cytometry availability in most institutions' diagnostic laboratories and rapid result return within 24 h makes TSLPR immunophenotyping a compelling additional Ph-like screening assay.

In summary, successful identification of patients with Ph-like ALL will most likely benefit from a combined approach of cytogenetic, FISH, and molecular analysis via fusion and NGS testing given the known genetic heterogeneity of this leukemia subtype and ongoing new discovery. Pragmatic clinical screening algorithms

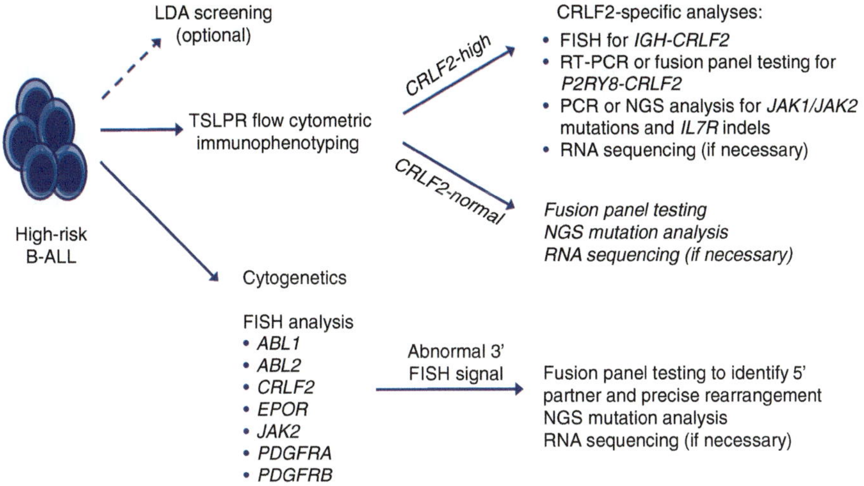

Fig. 10.2 Suggested clinical screening algorithm for Ph-like ALL. *CRLF2* cytokine receptor-like factor 2, *LDA* low-density array, *FISH* fluorescence in situ hybridization, *NGS* next-generation sequencing, *PCR* polymerase chain reaction, *RNA* ribonucleic acid, *RT-PCR* reverse transcription-polymerase chain reaction, *TSLPR* thymic stromal lymphopoietin receptor. (Adapted from Harvey & Tasian Blood Adv 2020)

will need to be personalized on one's available resources, patient volume, and clinical goals. A suggested diagnostic algorithm for Ph-like ALL is shown in Fig. 10.2 [7].

Precision Medicine Trials in Ph-Like ALL

Targeted Therapies

The recently characterized genomic landscape of Ph-like ALL has uncovered a myriad of kinase-activating alterations that expand the treatment paradigm of molecularly targeted therapies in ALL and leverage the success story of TKI incorporation for children and adults with Ph+ ALL [15, 65–68]. Despite their heterogeneity, Ph-like ALL-associated genetic alterations commonly converge to activate JAK-STAT, ABL, or Ras signaling pathways. Extensive in vitro and in vivo data have provided compelling evidence to incorporate relevant ABL/PDGFR- or JAK-directed TKIs in combination with chemotherapy to improve these patients' poor outcomes. The efficacy of such precision medicine approaches is currently being prospectively assessed in several clinical trials for children and adults with Ph-like ALL harboring ABL class alterations or JAK-STAT pathway gene lesions.

ABL class alterations phenocopy *BCR-ABL1* and exhibit exquisite sensitivity to imatinib and dasatinib in preclinical models [8, 9, 69]. There is increasing anecdotal evidence demonstrating that the addition of imatinib or dasatinib monotherapy or in combination with chemotherapy can induce remission in patients with relapsed/refractory ALL with ABL class alterations [8, 54–56, 70–72]. Based on this anecdotal experience in Ph-like ALL and the robust demonstration of safety and efficacy in children with Ph+ ALL, the COG AALL1131 phase 3 trial (NCT02883049) was amended in 2016 to add a dedicated treatment arm adding dasatinib to post-induction chemotherapy for Ph-like ALL patients with identified ABL class alterations. AALL1131 was closed to accrual in August 2019, and complete clinical results from this study are not yet available. The international phase 3 EsPhALL2017/COG AALL1631 trial (NCT03007147), which is randomizing two different chemotherapy backbones in combination with imatinib for children with Ph+ ALL, will extend eligibility to include patients with Ph-like ABL class fusions in 2020. The St. Jude Children's Research Hospital (SJCRH) Total Therapy XVII ALL (NCT03117751) protocol was activated in early 2017 and incorporates dasatinib beginning in induction therapy for those identified with an ABL class fusion by RNA-seq within 2 weeks of diagnosis [73]. An MDACC phase 2 trial for adults with relapsed/refractory Ph-like ALL and ABL class fusions (NCT02420717) also combined dasatinib with the intensive hyperCVAD chemotherapy backbone. Results have not yet been reported for these studies.

The largest class of Ph-like kinase-activating alterations constitutes those deregulating JAK-STAT signaling, making this pathway a major potential therapeutic vulnerability in Ph-like ALL, although JAK inhibitors have been less well studied in patients with ALL to date. Preclinical studies of engineered Ba/F3 cells and patient-derived xenograft (PDX) models harboring a diverse range of JAK-STAT pathway lesions (*CRLF2* rearrangements with or without *JAK* mutations, *JAK2* fusions, *EPOR* fusions, sequence mutations of *IL7R* and/or *SH2B3*) have shown in vitro and in vivo activity to different JAK inhibitors [8, 9, 29, 57, 69, 74–78]. Potent, but sometimes differential, preclinical activity of the JAK1/2 inhibitor ruxolitinib has been reported in Ph-like ALL models with *CRLF2* fusions or *JAK2* fusions, which may be influenced by the level of JAK pathway oncogene addiction or, potentially, by paradoxical JAK2 hyperphosphorylation with prolonged treatment [49, 74, 78]. Subsequent preclinical studies further demonstrated enhanced activity of combinatorial treatment with JAK and PI3K/mTOR inhibitors in Ph-like ALL cell lines and PDX models [75, 76]. Investigating dual pathway inhibition seems quite relevant for Ph-like ALL, as upregulation of alternative signaling pathways is a known mechanism of resistance to single-targeting agents [79, 80].

Based on these preclinical data, ruxolitinib is being assessed prospectively in several clinical trials for patients with JAK-STAT pathway-mutant Ph-like ALL. The COG AALL1521 phase 2 trial (NCT02723994) is investigating the efficacy of incorporating ruxolitinib with post-induction chemotherapy for children, adolescents, and young adults with HR Ph-like ALL harboring JAK-STAT pathway lesions [81]. In this study, patients are stratified into four different cohorts based on their underlying Ph-like genetic lesions and by end-induction MRD status to delineate potential differential efficacy for each subset. A soon-to-open phase 1 trial will also assess the safety and tolerability of ruxolitinib addition to chemotherapy specifically in a Ph-like ALL AYA population ages 18–39 years (NCT03571321). The two previously discussed SJRCH and MDACC trials also have a ruxolitinib treatment arm in combination with chemotherapy for patients with de novo or relapsed JAK-mutant Ph-like ALL, respectively.

The enriched prevalence of *IKZF1* deletions in Ph-like ALL opens up another potential therapeutic avenue for this HR patient population, although it is not yet known how these alterations might best be targeted. As above, *IKZF1* alterations are known to mediate aberrant stromal adhesion and therapy resistance in murine models of Ph+ ALL, and it is plausible that such effects could be reversed by retinoic acid compounds or focal adhesion kinase (FAK) inhibitors when combined with TKIs [18, 19].

Hematopoietic Stem Cell Transplantation

The role of hematopoietic stem cell transplantation (HSCT) in the care of patients with Ph-like ALL remains unclear in the TKI era [82]. Earlier data demonstrated definitive improvement in EFS and OS of children with Ph+ ALL with imatinib or dasatinib addition to chemotherapy, which also eliminated need for HSCT in most patients [15, 65, 83, 84]. Mirroring this Ph+ ALL experience, it is plausible that TKI addition to chemotherapy could be similarly successful for patients with ABL class Ph-like ALL.

A single-center study recently reported comparable outcomes between children with Ph-like ALL and non-Ph-like ALL (5-year EFS 90.0% vs 88.4%, $p = 0.41$, respectively) using MRD-directed therapy intensification for relevant patients [85]. Consequently, a significant higher proportion of patients with Ph-like ALL underwent HSCT in first remission due to end-induction MRD positivity [85], which is known to occur in two-thirds of children with Ph-like ALL [53]. These results demonstrate the therapeutic efficacy of HSCT in patients with Ph-like ALL and suggest that MRD is also an important outcome predictor in this patient population. Conversely, another single-center study reported that adult patients with Ph-like ALL fare comparably poorly even when they achieve post-remission MRD negativity (median OS for MRD+ group 23.0 months vs MRD-group 26.2 months; $p = 0.318$). Decisions for HSCT in first CR for adult patients may be challenged in the current era where pediatric-inspired chemotherapy regimens and access to front-line immunotherapy trials foster high hopes for inducing remission, deepening MRD response, and improving long-term survival [59, 86–89].

Antibody-Based and Cellular Immunotherapy

Major advances in immunotherapy during the past decade have revolutionized the landscape of relapsed leukemia therapy. The CD19xCD3 bispecific T-cell engager antibody blinatumomab, anti-CD22 antibody-drug conjugate inotuzumab ozogamicin, and CD19-redirected chimeric antigen receptor (CAR)-modified T-cell immunotherapy tisagenlecleucel have consecutively received FDA approval for patients with relapsed/refractory B-ALL based on several paradigm-shifting trials [88, 90–92]. Although the above trials did not specifically screen for the Ph-like ALL subtype, it is presumed that a reasonable proportion of these relapsed/refractory, heavily pretreated patients were Ph-like given their known high rates of chemoresistance and relapse. The randomized TOWER phase 3 trial (NCT02013167) showed that treatment with blinatumomab resulted in significantly higher remission rates and longer survival compared to standard chemotherapy among adults with relapsed/refractory Ph-negative B-ALL [88]. Subsequent results from the BLAST phase 2 trial (NCT01207388) demonstrated that the majority (78%) of MRD-positive adult B-ALL patients in first or later CR achieved a complete MRD response following one cycle of blinatumomab, which was associated with better outcomes than MRD non-responders [90]. Moreover, single-agent blinatumomab had strong anti-leukemic activity among adults with relapsed Ph+ ALL [93] and was associated with favorable treatment outcomes when compared to an external cohort receiving standard chemotherapy in a propensity score analysis [94]. The above data suggest that blinatumomab could be similarly efficacious in patients with Ph-like ALL. Favorable safety profiles and anti-leukemic activity with blinatumomab monotherapy were also observed in a heavily pre-treated relapsed/refractory pediatric B-ALL cohort [95, 96].

In a retrospective analysis of 53 adult patients with relapsed/refractory B-ALL treated with inotuzumab as salvage therapy, 12 patients identified as having the Ph-like subtype had an overall response rate (ORR) of 58%, including 3 with complete response (CR) (25%) and 4 with CR (33%) and partial hematologic recovery (CRh) [97]. Five of the seven (71%) Ph-like patients with inotuzumab-induced CR achieved MRD negativity [97]. Inotuzumab at the FDA-approved fractionated adult dosing of 1.8 mg/m^2 per cycle also induced impressive CR response rates among heavily pretreated children with relapsed/refractory B-ALL [98, 99]. In a retrospective study of 51 pediatric R/R B-ALL patients who received inotuzumab via a compassionate use program, the overall CR rate was 67%; 3 of 4 Ph-like ALL achieved CR/CR with incomplete count recovery (CRi), one of whom was MRD-negative [99].

Finally, anecdotal reports of CD19 chimeric antigen receptor (CAR) T-cell-induced remission in patients with relapsed/refractory Ph+ and Ph-like ALL have been reported [92]. The current COG AALL1721 phase 2 trial (NCT03876769) assessing the efficacy of tisagenlecleucel in patients with newly diagnosed HR B-ALL with end-consolidation MRD positivity excludes patients treated with kinase inhibitors, however, such as those Ph+ or Ph-like ALL. A planned phase 1 trial based upon promising preclinical data [100] will specifically investigate the clinical safety and preliminary efficacy of TSLPR-redirected CAR T-cell immunotherapy in children, adolescents, and young adults with *CRLF2*-rearranged/overexpressing leukemias, including Ph-like and Down syndrome-associated ALL.

A recent European trial combining blinatumomab and dasatinib has reported promising early results in adult patients with newly diagnosed Ph+ ALL, which is potentially translatable to ABL class Ph-like ALL [101]. Concerns have been raised with respect to potential antagonism of blinatumomab-dasatinib combination, as dasatinib has been shown to inhibit T-cell function and could potentially abrogate the desired anti-leukemic activity of blinatumomab that requires endogenous T-cell engagement [102]. Correlative functional assays that comprehensively assess potential immunomodulatory effects of dasatinib upon immune cells will provide critical data for future trial design.

Chemotherapy-sparing strategies are also being evaluated in clinical trials for older adults (≥65 years of age) with newly diagnosed Ph+ ALL or ABL class Ph-like ALL given their medical fragility and frequent inability to tolerate intensive chemotherapy. Small cases series previously reported anecdotal safety and efficacy of combining blinatumomab and dasatinib in small numbers of patients with relapsed/refractory Ph+ ALL or ABL class Ph-like ALL [70, 102–104]. The S1318 phase 2 trial (NCT02143414) is currently comparing the efficacy of blinatumomab with combination chemotherapy versus blinatumomab and dasatinib in older adults with ABL-driven leukemias. The D-ALBA phase 2 trial (NCT02744768) is also assessing rates of molecular remission after two cycles of blinatumomab and dasatinib consolidation therapy in adult patients with newly diagnosed Ph+ ALL. In an interim analysis, >50% of study patients achieved a molecular response at the primary endpoint with additional improvement to 80% MRD after four cycles [101] with 1-year disease-free and overall survival of 87.8% and 94.2%, respectively [101]. Longer-term follow-up is needed to confirm these early favorable results.

Conclusions and Future Perspectives

Ph-like ALL is now known to be a relatively prevalent subtype of B-ALL defined by its kinase activated gene expression signature and associated genetic alterations. Children and adults with Ph-like ALL have historically experienced high relapse rates and inferior clinical outcomes despite best-available conventional chemotherapy. Compelling evidence now exists from an extensive preclinical body of work for incorporation of relevant TKIs in combination with chemotherapy for these high-risk patients, although results from clinical trials testing these strategies are not yet known. Although Ph-like ALL is thrice as common than Ph+ ALL in children and adolescents, its genetic heterogeneity with >70 fusions identified to date [7] represents a limiting factor in designing appropriately statistically powered, randomized controlled trials to assess potential TKI efficacy within the major ABL class and CRLF2/JAK pathway-mutant subsets. As some patients with Ph-like ALL (particularly those with *EBF1-PDGFRB* or *JAK2* fusions) notoriously experience induction chemotherapy failure, future efforts must focus upon swift identification of these genetic alterations and TKI addition early in induction therapy. Such strategy has proven successful in children with Ph+ ALL with superior CR rates and MRD negativity with TKI addition mid-induction versus at the beginning of consolidation [15, 65]. Several immunotherapy modalities have now also demonstrated exciting efficacy in children with relapsed/refractory B-ALL. Ongoing and future clinical trials may help to elucidate the potential of such approaches (as monotherapy or combined with TKIs) more specifically in patients with Ph-like ALL.

International collaboration in designing the next generation of Ph-like ALL studies will expedite systematic study of novel treatment strategies that may improve clinical outcomes for this high-risk patient population [105]. Development and implementation of standardized clinical screening strategies among cooperative groups for rapid identification of patients with Ph-like ALL will also be essential for successful and efficient conduction of clinical trials. In parallel, future investigations in Ph-like ALL should also focus on investigating potential mechanisms of TKI resistance, as has been observed in patients with BCR-ABL1-driven chronic myeloid leukemia or Ph+ ALL with emergence of drug-resistant kinase domain mutations after long-term imatinib exposure [106–110]. Similar mutations have also been identified via in vitro saturation mutagenesis screens of Ph-like ALL with *EBF1-PDGFRB* fusions, and resistance mutations likely facilitating clinical relapse in patients with Ph-like ALL have now been reported [111, 112].

In summary, Ph-like ALL illustrates a paradigm of genomic discovery translation into targeted therapeutic approaches and presents an exciting opportunity for new precision medicine opportunities that aim to decrease relapse and improve long-term survival for patients with these high-risk leukemias across the age spectrum.

References

1. Mullighan CG, Su X, Zhang J, Radtke I, Phillips LA, Miller CB, et al. Deletion of IKZF1 and prognosis in acute lymphoblastic leukemia. N Engl J Med. 2009;360(5):470–80.
2. Den Boer ML, van Slegtenhorst M, De Menezes RX, Cheok MH, Buijs-Gladdines JG, Peters ST, et al. A subtype of childhood acute lymphoblastic leukaemia with poor treatment outcome: a genome-wide classification study. Lancet Oncol. 2009;10(2):125–34.
3. Tasian SK, Loh ML, Hunger SP. Philadelphia chromosome-like acute lymphoblastic leukemia. Blood. 2017;130(19):2064–72.
4. Boer JM, Marchante JR, Evans WE, Horstmann MA, Escherich G, Pieters R, et al. BCR-ABL1-like cases in pediatric acute lymphoblastic leukemia: a comparison between DCOG/Erasmus MC and COG/St. Jude signatures. Haematologica. 2015;100(9):e354–7.
5. Pui CH, Roberts KG, Yang JJ, Mullighan CG. Philadelphia chromosome-like acute lymphoblastic leukemia. Clin Lymphoma Myeloma Leuk. 2017;17(8):464–70.
6. Tran TH, Loh ML. Ph-like acute lymphoblastic leukemia. Hematology Am Soc Hematol Educ Program. 2016;2016(1):561–6.
7. Harvey RC, Tasian SK. Clinical diagnostics and treatment strategies for Philadelphia chromosome-like acute lymphoblastic leukemia. Blood Adv. 2020;4(1):218–28.
8. Roberts KG, Li Y, Payne-Turner D, Harvey RC, Yang YL, Pei D, et al. Targetable kinase-activating lesions in Ph-like acute lymphoblastic leukemia. N Engl J Med. 2014;371(11): 1005–15.
9. Roberts KG, Morin RD, Zhang J, Hirst M, Zhao Y, Su X, et al. Genetic alterations activating kinase and cytokine receptor signaling in high-risk acute lymphoblastic leukemia. Cancer Cell. 2012;22(2):153–66.
10. van der Veer A, Waanders E, Pieters R, Willemse ME, Van Reijmersdal SV, Russell LJ, et al. Independent prognostic value of BCR-ABL1-like signature and IKZF1 deletion, but not high CRLF2 expression, in children with B-cell precursor ALL. Blood. 2013;122(15):2622–9.

11. Roberts KG, Reshmi SC, Harvey RC, Chen IM, Patel K, Stonerock E, et al. Genomic and outcome analyses of Ph-like ALL in NCI standard-risk patients: a report from the Children's Oncology Group. Blood. 2018;132(8):815–24.
12. Russell LJ, Capasso M, Vater I, Akasaka T, Bernard OA, Calasanz MJ, et al. Deregulated expression of cytokine receptor gene, CRLF2, is involved in lymphoid transformation in B-cell precursor acute lymphoblastic leukemia. Blood. 2009;114(13):2688–98.
13. Hertzberg L, Vendramini E, Ganmore I, Cazzaniga G, Schmitz M, Chalker J, et al. Down syndrome acute lymphoblastic leukemia, a highly heterogeneous disease in which aberrant expression of CRLF2 is associated with mutated JAK2: a report from the International BFM Study Group. Blood. 2010;115(5):1006–17.
14. Mullighan CG, Miller CB, Radtke I, Phillips LA, Dalton J, Ma J, et al. BCR-ABL1 lymphoblastic leukaemia is characterized by the deletion of Ikaros. Nature. 2008;453(7191):110–4.
15. Slayton WB, Schultz KR, Kairalla JA, Devidas M, Mi X, Pulsipher MA, et al. Dasatinib plus intensive chemotherapy in children, adolescents, and young adults with Philadelphia chromosome-positive acute lymphoblastic leukemia: results of Children's Oncology Group Trial AALL0622. J Clin Oncol. 2018;36(22):2306–14.
16. van der Veer A, Zaliova M, Mottadelli F, De Lorenzo P, Te Kronnie G, Harrison CJ, et al. IKZF1 status as a prognostic feature in BCR-ABL1-positive childhood ALL. Blood. 2014;123(11):1691–8.
17. Martinelli G, Iacobucci I, Storlazzi CT, Vignetti M, Paoloni F, Cilloni D, et al. IKZF1 (Ikaros) deletions in BCR-ABL1-positive acute lymphoblastic leukemia are associated with short disease-free survival and high rate of cumulative incidence of relapse: a GIMEMA AL WP report. J Clin Oncol. 2009;27(31):5202–7.
18. Churchman ML, Mullighan CG. Ikaros: exploiting and targeting the hematopoietic stem cell niche in B-progenitor acute lymphoblastic leukemia. Exp Hematol. 2017;46:1–8.
19. Churchman ML, Low J, Qu C, Paietta EM, Kasper LH, Chang Y, et al. Efficacy of retinoids in IKZF1-mutated BCR-ABL1 acute lymphoblastic leukemia. Cancer Cell. 2015;28(3):343–56.
20. Vairy S, Tran TH. IKZF1 alterations in acute lymphoblastic leukemia: the good, the bad and the ugly. Blood Rev. 2020;44:100677.
21. Tran TH, Harris MH, Nguyen JV, Blonquist TM, Stevenson KE, Stonerock E, et al. Prognostic impact of kinase-activating fusions and IKZF1 deletions in pediatric high-risk B-lineage acute lymphoblastic leukemia. Blood Adv. 2018;2(5):529–33.
22. Stanulla M, Dagdan E, Zaliova M, Moricke A, Palmi C, Cazzaniga G, et al. IKZF1(plus) defines a new minimal residual disease-dependent very-poor prognostic profile in pediatric B-cell precursor acute lymphoblastic leukemia. J Clin Oncol. 2018;36(12):1240–9.
23. Steeghs EMP, Boer JM, Hoogkamer AQ, Boeree A, de Haas V, de Groot-Kruseman HA, et al. Copy number alterations in B-cell development genes, drug resistance, and clinical outcome in pediatric B-cell precursor acute lymphoblastic leukemia. Sci Rep. 2019;9(1):4634.
24. Zaliova M, Stuchly J, Winkowska L, Musilova A, Fiser K, Slamova M, et al. Genomic landscape of pediatric B-other acute lymphoblastic leukemia in a consecutive European cohort. Haematologica. 2019;104(7):1396–406.
25. Fedullo AL, Messina M, Elia L, Piciocchi A, Gianfelici V, Lauretti A, et al. Prognostic implications of additional genomic lesions in adult Philadelphia chromosome-positive acute lymphoblastic leukemia. Haematologica. 2019;104(2):312–8.
26. Perez-Andreu V, Roberts KG, Harvey RC, Yang W, Cheng C, Pei D, et al. Inherited GATA3 variants are associated with Ph-like childhood acute lymphoblastic leukemia and risk of relapse. Nat Genet. 2013;45(12):1494–8.
27. Roberts KG, Gu Z, Payne-Turner D, McCastlain K, Harvey RC, Chen IM, et al. High frequency and poor outcome of Philadelphia chromosome-like acute lymphoblastic leukemia in adults. J Clin Oncol. 2017;35(4):394–401.
28. Tasian SK, Hurtz C, Wertheim GB, Bailey NG, Lim MS, Harvey RC, et al. High incidence of Philadelphia chromosome-like acute lymphoblastic leukemia in older adults with B-ALL. Leukemia. 2017;31(4):981–4.

29. Tasian SK, Doral MY, Borowitz MJ, Wood BL, Chen IM, Harvey RC, et al. Aberrant STAT5 and PI3K/mTOR pathway signaling occurs in human CRLF2-rearranged B-precursor acute lymphoblastic leukemia. Blood. 2012;120(4):833–42.
30. Mullighan CG, Collins-Underwood JR, Phillips LA, Loudin MG, Liu W, Zhang J, et al. Rearrangement of CRLF2 in B-progenitor- and Down syndrome-associated acute lymphoblastic leukemia. Nat Genet. 2009;41(11):1243–6.
31. Scheeren FA, van Lent AU, Nagasawa M, Weijer K, Spits H, Legrand N, et al. Thymic stromal lymphopoietin induces early human B-cell proliferation and differentiation. Eur J Immunol. 2010;40(4):955–65.
32. Isaksen DE, Baumann H, Zhou B, Nivollet S, Farr AG, Levin SD, et al. Uncoupling of proliferation and Stat5 activation in thymic stromal lymphopoietin-mediated signal transduction. J Immunol. 2002;168(7):3288–94.
33. Isaksen DE, Baumann H, Trobridge PA, Farr AG, Levin SD, Ziegler SF. Requirement for stat5 in thymic stromal lymphopoietin-mediated signal transduction. J Immunol. 1999;163(11):5971–7.
34. Herold T, Schneider S, Metzeler KH, Neumann M, Hartmann L, Roberts KG, et al. Adults with Philadelphia chromosome-like acute lymphoblastic leukemia frequently have IGH-CRLF2 and JAK2 mutations, persistence of minimal residual disease and poor prognosis. Haematologica. 2017;102(1):130–8.
35. Moorman AV, Schwab C, Ensor HM, Russell LJ, Morrison H, Jones L, et al. IGH@ translocations, CRLF2 deregulation, and microdeletions in adolescents and adults with acute lymphoblastic leukemia. J Clin Oncol. 2012;30(25):3100–8.
36. Yoda A, Yoda Y, Chiaretti S, Bar-Natan M, Mani K, Rodig SJ, et al. Functional screening identifies CRLF2 in precursor B-cell acute lymphoblastic leukemia. Proc Natl Acad Sci U S A. 2010;107(1):252–7.
37. Reshmi SC, Harvey RC, Roberts KG, Stonerock E, Smith A, Jenkins H, et al. Targetable kinase gene fusions in high risk B-ALL: a study from the Children's Oncology Group. Blood. 2017;129(25):3352–61.
38. Roberts KG, Mullighan CG. Genomics in acute lymphoblastic leukaemia: insights and treatment implications. Nat Rev Clin Oncol. 2015;12(6):344–57.
39. Iacobucci I, Li Y, Roberts KG, Dobson SM, Kim JC, Payne-Turner D, et al. Truncating erythropoietin receptor rearrangements in acute lymphoblastic leukemia. Cancer Cell. 2016;29(2):186–200.
40. Wiemels JL, Kang M, Chang JS, Zheng L, Kouyoumji C, Zhang L, et al. Backtracking RAS mutations in high hyperdiploid childhood acute lymphoblastic leukemia. Blood Cells Mol Dis. 2010;45(3):186–91.
41. Holmfeldt L, Wei L, Diaz-Flores E, Walsh M, Zhang J, Ding L, et al. The genomic landscape of hypodiploid acute lymphoblastic leukemia. Nat Genet. 2013;45(3):242–52.
42. Irving J, Matheson E, Minto L, Blair H, Case M, Halsey C, et al. Ras pathway mutations are prevalent in relapsed childhood acute lymphoblastic leukemia and confer sensitivity to MEK inhibition. Blood. 2014;124(23):3420–30.
43. Roberts KG, Janke LJ, Zhao Y, Seth A, Ma J, Finkelstein D, et al. ETV6-NTRK3 induces aggressive acute lymphoblastic leukemia highly sensitive to selective TRK inhibition. Blood. 2018;132(8):861–5.
44. Brown LM, Bartolo RC, Davidson NM, Schmidt B, Brooks I, Challis J, et al. Targeted therapy and disease monitoring in CNTRL-FGFR1-driven leukaemia. Pediatr Blood Cancer. 2019;66(10):e27897.
45. Helsten T, Schwaederle M, Kurzrock R. Fibroblast growth factor receptor signaling in hereditary and neoplastic disease: biologic and clinical implications. Cancer Metastasis Rev. 2015;34(3):479–96.
46. Yano M, Imamura T, Asai D, Kiyokawa N, Nakabayashi K, Matsumoto K, et al. Identification of novel kinase fusion transcripts in paediatric B cell precursor acute lymphoblastic leukaemia with IKZF1 deletion. Br J Haematol. 2015;171(5):813–7.
47. Tanaka H, Takeuchi M, Takeda Y, Sakai S, Abe D, Ohwada C, et al. Identification of a novel TEL-Lyn fusion gene in primary myelofibrosis. Leukemia. 2010;24(1):197–200.

48. Owattanapanich W, Rujirachun P, Ungprasert P, Buaboonnam J, Techavichit P. Prevalence and clinical outcome of Philadelphia-like acute lymphoblastic leukemia: systematic review and meta-analysis. Clin Lymphoma Myeloma Leuk. 2020;20(1):e22–9.
49. Jain N, Roberts KG, Jabbour E, Patel K, Eterovic AK, Chen K, et al. Ph-like acute lymphoblastic leukemia: a high-risk subtype in adults. Blood. 2017;129(5):572–81.
50. Harvey RC, Mullighan CG, Chen IM, Wharton W, Mikhail FM, Carroll AJ, et al. Rearrangement of CRLF2 is associated with mutation of JAK kinases, alteration of IKZF1, Hispanic/Latino ethnicity, and a poor outcome in pediatric B-progenitor acute lymphoblastic leukemia. Blood. 2010;115(26):5312–21.
51. Madzio J, Pastorczak A, Sedek L, Braun M, Taha J, Wypyszczak K, et al. GATA3 germline variant is associated with CRLF2 expression and predicts outcome in pediatric B-cell precursor acute lymphoblastic leukemia. Genes Chromosomes Cancer. 2019;58(9):619–26.
52. Boer JM, Koenders JE, van der Holt B, Exalto C, Sanders MA, Cornelissen JJ, et al. Expression profiling of adult acute lymphoblastic leukemia identifies a BCR-ABL1-like subgroup characterized by high non-response and relapse rates. Haematologica. 2015;100(7):e261–4.
53. Loh ML, Zhang J, Harvey RC, Roberts K, Payne-Turner D, Kang H, et al. Tyrosine kinome sequencing of pediatric acute lymphoblastic leukemia: a report from the Children's Oncology Group TARGET Project. Blood. 2013;121(3):485–8.
54. Weston BW, Hayden MA, Roberts KG, Bowyer S, Hsu J, Fedoriw G, et al. Tyrosine kinase inhibitor therapy induces remission in a patient with refractory EBF1-PDGFRB-positive acute lymphoblastic leukemia. J Clin Oncol. 2013;31(25):e413–6.
55. Lengline E, Beldjord K, Dombret H, Soulier J, Boissel N, Clappier E. Successful tyrosine kinase inhibitor therapy in a refractory B-cell precursor acute lymphoblastic leukemia with EBF1-PDGFRB fusion. Haematologica. 2013;98(11):e146–8.
56. Schwab C, Ryan SL, Chilton L, Elliott A, Murray J, Richardson S, et al. EBF1-PDGFRB fusion in pediatric B-cell precursor acute lymphoblastic leukemia (BCP-ALL): genetic profile and clinical implications. Blood. 2016;127(18):2214–8.
57. Ding YY, Stern JW, Jubelirer TF, Wertheim GB, Li F, Chang F, et al. Clinical efficacy of ruxolitinib and chemotherapy in a child with Philadelphia chromosome-like acute lymphoblastic leukemia with GOLGA5-JAK2 fusion and induction failure. Haematologica. 2018;103(9):e427–31.
58. Maloney KW, Devidas M, Wang C, Mattano LA, Friedmann AM, Buckley P, et al. Outcome in children with standard-risk B-cell acute lymphoblastic leukemia: results of Children's Oncology Group Trial AALL0331. J Clin Oncol. 2020;38(6):602–12.
59. Stock W, Luger SM, Advani AS, Yin J, Harvey RC, Mullighan CG, et al. A pediatric regimen for older adolescents and young adults with acute lymphoblastic leukemia: results of CALGB 10403. Blood. 2019;133(14):1548–59.
60. Kang H, Chen IM, Wilson CS, Bedrick EJ, Harvey RC, Atlas SR, et al. Gene expression classifiers for relapse-free survival and minimal residual disease improve risk classification and outcome prediction in pediatric B-precursor acute lymphoblastic leukemia. Blood. 2010;115(7):1394–405.
61. Harvey RC, Tasian SK. Clinical diagnostics and treatment strategies for Philadelphia chromosome-like acute lymphoblastic leukemia. Blood Adv. 2020;4(1):218–28.
62. Surrey LF, MacFarland SP, Chang F, Cao K, Rathi KS, Akgumus GT, et al. Clinical utility of custom-designed NGS panel testing in pediatric tumors. Genome Med. 2019;11(1):32.
63. Chang F, Lin F, Cao K, Surrey LF, Aplenc R, Bagatell R, et al. Development and clinical validation of a large fusion gene panel for pediatric cancers. J Mol Diagn. 2019;21(5): 873–83.
64. He J, Abdel-Wahab O, Nahas MK, Wang K, Rampal RK, Intlekofer AM, et al. Integrated genomic DNA/RNA profiling of hematologic malignancies in the clinical setting. Blood. 2016;127(24):3004–14.
65. Schultz KR, Carroll A, Heerema NA, Bowman WP, Aledo A, Slayton WB, et al. Long-term follow-up of imatinib in pediatric Philadelphia chromosome-positive acute lymphoblastic leukemia: Children's Oncology Group study AALL0031. Leukemia. 2014;28(7): 1467–71.

66. Wassmann B, Pfeifer H, Goekbuget N, Beelen DW, Beck J, Stelljes M, et al. Alternating versus concurrent schedules of imatinib and chemotherapy as front-line therapy for Philadelphia-positive acute lymphoblastic leukemia (Ph+ ALL). Blood. 2006;108(5):1469–77.
67. Shen S, Chen X, Cai J, Yu J, Gao J, Hu S, et al. Effect of dasatinib vs imatinib in the treatment of pediatric Philadelphia chromosome-positive acute lymphoblastic leukemia: a randomized clinical trial. JAMA Oncol. 2020;6(3):358–66.
68. Lilly MB, Ottmann OG, Shah NP, Larson RA, Reiffers JJ, Ehninger G, et al. Dasatinib 140 mg once daily versus 70 mg twice daily in patients with Ph-positive acute lymphoblastic leukemia who failed imatinib: results from a phase 3 study. Am J Hematol. 2010;85(3):164–70.
69. Roberts KG, Yang YL, Payne-Turner D, Lin W, Files JK, Dickerson K, et al. Oncogenic role and therapeutic targeting of ABL-class and JAK-STAT activating kinase alterations in Ph-like ALL. Blood Adv. 2017;1(20):1657–71.
70. Tanasi I, Ba I, Sirvent N, Braun T, Cuccuini W, Ballerini P, et al. Efficacy of tyrosine kinase inhibitors in Ph-like acute lymphoblastic leukemia harboring ABL-class rearrangements. Blood. 2019;134(16):1351–5.
71. Kobayashi K, Miyagawa N, Mitsui K, Matsuoka M, Kojima Y, Takahashi H, et al. TKI dasatinib monotherapy for a patient with Ph-like ALL bearing ATF7IP/PDGFRB translocation. Pediatr Blood Cancer. 2015;62(6):1058–60.
72. Fazio F, Barberi W, Cazzaniga G, Fazio G, Messina M, Della Starza I, et al. Efficacy of imatinib and chemotherapy in a pediatric patient with Philadelphia-like acute lymphoblastic leukemia with Ebf1-Pdgfrb fusion transcript. Leuk Lymphoma. 2019:1–4.
73. Inaba H, Azzato EM, Mullighan CG. Integration of next-generation sequencing to treat acute lymphoblastic leukemia with targetable lesions: the St. Jude Children's Research Hospital approach. Front Pediatr. 2017;5:258.
74. Maude SL, Tasian SK, Vincent T, Hall JW, Sheen C, Roberts KG, et al. Targeting JAK1/2 and mTOR in murine xenograft models of Ph-like acute lymphoblastic leukemia. Blood. 2012;120(17):3510–8.
75. Tasian SK, Teachey DT, Li Y, Shen F, Harvey RC, Chen IM, et al. Potent efficacy of combined PI3K/mTOR and JAK or ABL inhibition in murine xenograft models of Ph-like acute lymphoblastic leukemia. Blood. 2017;129(2):177–87.
76. Zhang Q, Shi C, Han L, Jain N, Roberts KG, Ma H, et al. Inhibition of mTORC1/C2 signaling improves anti-leukemia efficacy of JAK/STAT blockade in CRLF2 rearranged and/or JAK driven Philadelphia chromosome-like acute B-cell lymphoblastic leukemia. Oncotarget. 2018;9(8):8027–41.
77. Khan M, Siddiqi R, Tran TH. Philadelphia chromosome-like acute lymphoblastic leukemia: a review of the genetic basis, clinical features, and therapeutic options. Semin Hematol. 2018;55(4):235–41.
78. Wu SC, Li LS, Kopp N, Montero J, Chapuy B, Yoda A, et al. Activity of the type II JAK2 inhibitor CHZ868 in B cell acute lymphoblastic leukemia. Cancer Cell. 2015;28(1):29–41.
79. Hurtz C, Tasian SK, Wertheim G, Astles R, Zebrowski A, Perl AE, et al. Adaptive reactivation of signaling pathways as a novel mechanism of resistance to JAK inhibitors in Ph-like ALL. Blood. 2016;128(22):755.
80. Gotesman M, Vo T-TT, Mallya S, Zhang Q, Shi C, Müschen M, et al. mTOR kinase inhibitors enhance efficacy of TKIs in preclinical models of Ph-like B-ALL. Blood. 2016;128(22):2763.
81. Tasian SK, Assad A, Hunter DS, Du Y, Loh ML. A phase 2 study of ruxolitinib with chemotherapy in children with Philadelphia chromosome-like acute lymphoblastic leukemia (INCB18424-269/AALL1521): dose-finding results from the part 1 safety phase. Blood. 2018;132(Supplement 1):555.
82. El Fakih R, Savani B, Mohty M, Aljurf M. Hematopoietic cell transplant consideration for Philadelphia chromosome-like acute lymphoblastic leukemia patients. Biol Blood Marrow Transplant. 2020;26(1):e16–20.
83. Schultz KR, Bowman WP, Aledo A, Slayton WB, Sather H, Devidas M, et al. Improved early event-free survival with imatinib in Philadelphia chromosome-positive acute lymphoblastic leukemia: a Children's Oncology Group Study. J Clin Oncol. 2009;27(31):5175–81.

84. Biondi A, Schrappe M, De Lorenzo P, Castor A, Lucchini G, Gandemer V, et al. Imatinib after induction for treatment of children and adolescents with Philadelphia-chromosome-positive acute lymphoblastic leukaemia (EsPhALL): a randomised, open-label, intergroup study. Lancet Oncol. 2012;13(9):936–45.
85. Roberts KG, Pei D, Campana D, Payne-Turner D, Li Y, Cheng C, et al. Outcomes of children with BCR-ABL1-like acute lymphoblastic leukemia treated with risk-directed therapy based on the levels of minimal residual disease. J Clin Oncol. 2014;32(27):3012–20.
86. Siegel SE, Stock W, Johnson RH, Advani A, Muffly L, Douer D, et al. Pediatric-inspired treatment regimens for adolescents and young adults with Philadelphia chromosome-negative acute lymphoblastic leukemia: a review. JAMA Oncol. 2018;4(5):725–34.
87. Kantarjian H, Ravandi F, Short NJ, Huang X, Jain N, Sasaki K, et al. Inotuzumab ozogamicin in combination with low-intensity chemotherapy for older patients with Philadelphia chromosome-negative acute lymphoblastic leukaemia: a single-arm, phase 2 study. Lancet Oncol. 2018;19(2):240–8.
88. Kantarjian H, Stein A, Gokbuget N, Fielding AK, Schuh AC, Ribera JM, et al. Blinatumomab versus chemotherapy for advanced acute lymphoblastic leukemia. N Engl J Med. 2017;376(9):836–47.
89. DeFilipp Z, Advani AS, Bachanova V, Cassaday RD, Deangelo DJ, Kebriaei P, et al. Hematopoietic cell transplantation in the treatment of adult acute lymphoblastic leukemia: updated 2019 evidence-based review from the American Society for Transplantation and Cellular Therapy. Biol Blood Marrow Transplant. 2019;25(11):2113–23.
90. Gokbuget N, Dombret H, Bonifacio M, Reichle A, Graux C, Faul C, et al. Blinatumomab for minimal residual disease in adults with B-cell precursor acute lymphoblastic leukemia. Blood. 2018;131(14):1522–31.
91. Kantarjian HM, DeAngelo DJ, Stelljes M, Martinelli G, Liedtke M, Stock W, et al. Inotuzumab ozogamicin versus standard therapy for acute lymphoblastic leukemia. N Engl J Med. 2016;375(8):740–53.
92. Maude SL, Laetsch TW, Buechner J, Rives S, Boyer M, Bittencourt H, et al. Tisagenlecleucel in children and young adults with B-cell lymphoblastic leukemia. N Engl J Med. 2018;378(5):439–48.
93. Martinelli G, Boissel N, Chevallier P, Ottmann O, Gokbuget N, Topp MS, et al. Complete hematologic and molecular response in adult patients with relapsed/refractory Philadelphia chromosome-positive B-precursor acute lymphoblastic leukemia following treatment with blinatumomab: results from a phase II, single-arm, multicenter study. J Clin Oncol. 2017;35(16):1795–802.
94. Rambaldi A, Ribera JM, Kantarjian HM, Dombret H, Ottmann OG, Stein AS, et al. Blinatumomab compared with standard of care for the treatment of adult patients with relapsed/refractory Philadelphia chromosome-positive B-precursor acute lymphoblastic leukemia. Cancer. 2020;126(2):304–10.
95. von Stackelberg A, Locatelli F, Zugmaier G, Handgretinger R, Trippett TM, Rizzari C, et al. Phase I/phase II study of blinatumomab in pediatric patients with relapsed/refractory acute lymphoblastic leukemia. J Clin Oncol. 2016;34(36):4381–9.
96. Gore L, Locatelli F, Zugmaier G, Handgretinger R, O'Brien MM, Bader P, et al. Survival after blinatumomab treatment in pediatric patients with relapsed/refractory B-cell precursor acute lymphoblastic leukemia. Blood Cancer J. 2018;8(9):80.
97. Jabbour E. Inotuzumab ozogamicin may overcome the impact of Philadelphia chromosome (Ph)-like phenotype in adult patients with relapsed/refractory ALL. Blood. 2019;134(Supplement_1):1641.
98. O'Brien MM, Ji L, Shah NN, Rheingold SR, Bhojwani D, Yi JS, et al. A phase 2 trial of inotuzumab ozogamicin (InO) in children and young adults with relapsed or refractory (R/R) CD22+ B-acute lymphoblastic leukemia (B-ALL): results from Children's Oncology Group Protocol AALL1621. Blood. 2019;134(Supplement 1):741.
99. Bhojwani D, Sposto R, Shah NN, Rodriguez V, Yuan C, Stetler-Stevenson M, et al. Inotuzumab ozogamicin in pediatric patients with relapsed/refractory acute lymphoblastic leukemia. Leukemia. 2019;33(4):884–92.

100. Qin H, Cho M, Haso W, Zhang L, Tasian SK, Oo HZ, et al. Eradication of B-ALL using chimeric antigen receptor-expressing T cells targeting the TSLPR oncoprotein. Blood. 2015;126(5):629–39.
101. Chiaretti S. Dasatinib-blinatumomab combination for the front-line treatment of adult Ph+ALL patients: updated results of the Gimema LAL2116 D-Alba trial. Blood. 2019;134(Supplement_1):740.
102. King AC, Pappacena JJ, Tallman MS, Park JH, Geyer MB. Blinatumomab administered concurrently with oral tyrosine kinase inhibitor therapy is a well-tolerated consolidation strategy and eradicates measurable residual disease in adults with Philadelphia chromosome positive acute lymphoblastic leukemia. Leuk Res. 2019;79:27–33.
103. Assi R, Kantarjian H, Short NJ, Daver N, Takahashi K, Garcia-Manero G, et al. Safety and efficacy of blinatumomab in combination with a tyrosine kinase inhibitor for the treatment of relapsed Philadelphia chromosome-positive leukemia. Clin Lymphoma Myeloma Leuk. 2017;17(12):897–901.
104. Petruzziello F, Giagnuolo G, Cazzaniga G, Beneduce G, Locatelli F, Stellato P, Fazio G, Mirabelli G, Menna G, Parasole R. Successful of chemo-free treatment with dasatinib and blinatumomab in a pediatric EBF1-PDGFRβ positive acute lymphoblastic leukemia. Blood. 2018;132(Suppl 1):5213.
105. Pui CH, Yang JJ, Hunger SP, Pieters R, Schrappe M, Biondi A, et al. Childhood acute lymphoblastic leukemia: progress through collaboration. J Clin Oncol. 2015;33(27):2938–48.
106. Shah NP, Sawyers CL. Mechanisms of resistance to STI571 in Philadelphia chromosome-associated leukemias. Oncogene. 2003;22(47):7389–95.
107. Soverini S, Branford S, Nicolini FE, Talpaz M, Deininger MW, Martinelli G, et al. Implications of BCR-ABL1 kinase domain-mediated resistance in chronic myeloid leukemia. Leuk Res. 2014;38(1):10–20.
108. Soverini S, Hochhaus A, Nicolini FE, Gruber F, Lange T, Saglio G, et al. BCR-ABL kinase domain mutation analysis in chronic myeloid leukemia patients treated with tyrosine kinase inhibitors: recommendations from an expert panel on behalf of European LeukemiaNet. Blood. 2011;118(5):1208–15.
109. Soverini S, Colarossi S, Gnani A, Rosti G, Castagnetti F, Poerio A, et al. Contribution of ABL kinase domain mutations to imatinib resistance in different subsets of Philadelphia-positive patients: by the GIMEMA Working Party on Chronic Myeloid Leukemia. Clin Cancer Res. 2006;12(24):7374–9.
110. Druker BJ. Circumventing resistance to kinase-inhibitor therapy. N Engl J Med. 2006;354(24):2594–6.
111. Yeung DT, Moulton DJ, Heatley SL, Nievergall E, Dang P, Braley J, et al. Relapse of BCR-ABL1-like ALL mediated by the ABL1 kinase domain mutation T315I following initial response to dasatinib treatment. Leukemia. 2015;29(1):230–2.
112. Zhang Y, Gao Y, Zhang H, Zhang J, He F, Hnizda A, et al. PDGFRB mutation and tyrosine kinase inhibitor resistance in Ph-like acute lymphoblastic leukemia. Blood. 2018;131(20):2256–61.

Chapter 11
Prophylaxis and Treatment of Central Nervous System (CNS) Acute Lymphoblastic Leukemia

Lauren D. Scherer and Eric S. Schafer

Introduction

Outcomes for acute lymphoblastic leukemia (ALL) have dramatically improved over the last several decades – particularly in children, but also in adults [1–5]. A critical component to this trend was the discovery in the 1970s of the central nervous system (CNS) as a sanctuary site for leukemic blasts that required targeted and anatomically directed therapy [6]. To date, it is unclear how leukemia cells enter the CNS, but hypotheses include translocation via the systemic circulation [7], direct extension from the bone marrow of the skull into the meninges via the bridging veins [8], entry of systemic leukemia cells via the choroid plexus, and direct invasion into the brain parenchyma via cranial capillaries (Fig. 11.1) [9]. Because systemically delivered chemotherapy generally has a diminished capacity to cross the blood-brain barrier (BBB) and accumulate in the cerebral spinal fluid (CSF), once present in the CNS, lymphoblasts are able to escape the full effects of drugs administered in this manner [10]. No matter how entry is achieved, presence of at least sub-microscopic leukemia in the CNS is likely present in the majority of patients at diagnosis, as evidenced by the fact that most CNS relapses occur in patients with no clinical or laboratory evidence of CNS leukemia at diagnosis [11] and early observations that more than 50% of ALL patients suffered CNS relapses prior to recognition of the need to treat the CNS compartment prophylactically [12, 13]. With the application of risk-directed, effective, systemic chemotherapy and prophylactic CNS-directed treatment including intrathecal chemotherapy, the rate of CNS relapse is now 5–6% [13–15]. Despite great advancements, the CNS is still the most common site of extramedullary relapse and remains an important cause of morbidity and mortality.

L. D. Scherer · E. S. Schafer (✉)
Baylor College of Medicine, Texas Children's Cancer and Hematology Centers, Houston, TX, USA
e-mail: ldschere@texaschildrens.org; esschafe@texaschildrens.org

M. R. Litzow, E. A. Raetz (eds.), *Clinical Management of Acute Lymphoblastic Leukemia*, https://doi.org/10.1007/978-3-030-85147-7_11

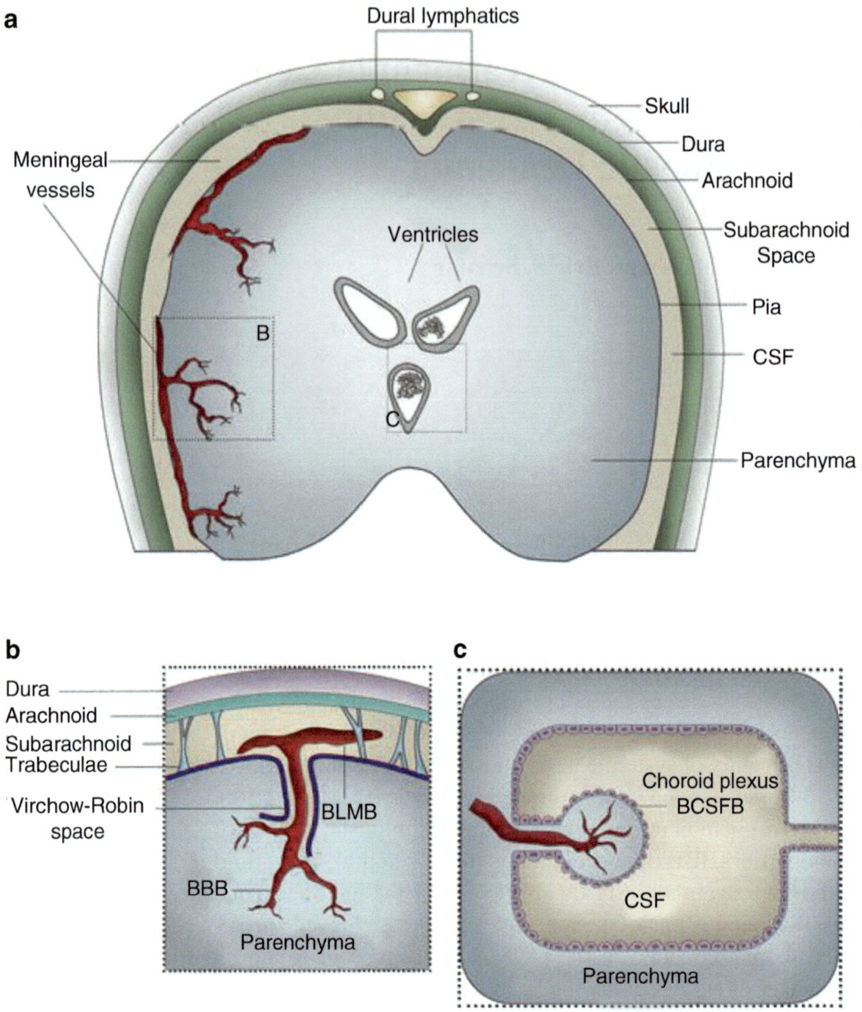

Fig. 11.1 (**a**) Schematic representation of the anatomical features of the CNS and possible entry routes for leukemic cells into the CNS. The meninges, which envelop the central nervous system (CNS), consist of the dura mater, the arachnoid mater, and the pia matter. The cerebrospinal fluid (CSF) is mainly produced by the choroid plexus (CPE) within the ventricles of the brain and circulates into the subarachnoid space located between the pia and the arachnoid membranes. Leukemic blasts may enter the CNS by passing through distinct barrier systems including the blood-brain barrier (BBB) in parenchymal microvessels, the blood-leptomeningeal barrier (BLMB) in meningeal microvessels, or the blood-CSF barrier (BCSFB) in the CPE. B, C: magnification of zone B, C, respectively (**b**, **c**). (From Firshman-Levy and Izraeli [10], with permission)

Diagnosis of CNS Disease in Patients with ALL

The treatment of ALL has become more precise and individualized based on current risk-stratification. Accurate diagnosis of CNS leukemia is crucial for determining risk and subsequent therapy. The gold standard to determine CNS involvement in ALL is by cerebrospinal fluid (CSF) cell count and cytology [14]. A sample of CSF is obtained from a diagnostic lumbar puncture (LP), and a cytospin slide is examined by light microscopy after Wright-Giemsa staining [16]. Cerebral spinal fluid cytology has been utilized and studied for well over 100 years; it is inexpensive and technically simple to process and promises rapid reporting of results [17]. However, it has some potentially significant limitations: cells in the CSF are scarce and if present degenerate rapidly ex vivo potentially confounding an accurate diagnosis which relies entirely on visual morphologic identification [17]. As a result, the sensitivity and specificity of CSF cytology to identify CNS leukemia have been questioned for decades. Early studies of conventional cytology have demonstrated false-negative rates up to 40% [18, 19], and so additional techniques have been developed and studied including terminal deoxynucleotide transferase staining, immunocytology, and flow cytometry [20–22]. In particular, flow cytometry, a technology known to increase leukemia minimal residual disease (MRD) sensitivity testing to 0.01%, has been shown to enhance CSF examination. One landmark study showed that, when compared to cytology, flow cytometry raised CNS leukemia diagnostic sensitivity from 73% to 96% and specificity from 94% to 97% [23]. Polymerase chain reaction (PCR), a technique which improves leukemic detection in the MRD setting by 1–2 logs over flow cytometry [24], is increasingly being used as a correlative study to cytology due to its improved sensitivity and ability to detect very low levels of blasts in the CSF [25, 26]. These enhanced modalities may be useful in patients with equivocal results by cytology and in particular may be useful in patients with CNS disease who are being monitored for lymphoblast clearance from CSF (lymphoblast residual disease), as morphological blast appearance may be altered with treatment [27, 28]. Due to differences in requirements for sample processing and standardization of interpreting results, technical complexity, and cost, these enhanced modalities should only be done in addition to gold standard cytology evaluation, rather than as a replacement. Magnetic resonance imaging (MRI) and computed tomography (CT) evaluations have shown to be predictive of leukemic infiltration in patients with neurologic symptoms [20, 29]. However, even with occult CNS disease, most patients are asymptomatic, and therefore imaging is not a preferred modality of diagnosing and staging CNS leukemia [30].

All ALL patients should receive an initial diagnostic LP. However, this procedure must be performed under optimal conditions in order to limit the risk of a traumatic lumber puncture (TLP) [31]. Traumatic lumbar punctures contaminated with red blood cells (RBCs) can make diagnosis and staging of CNS disease difficult. In addition, at the time of the initial LP, patients often have peripheral circulating leukemic blasts that can be introduced from the blood stream into the CNS during the procedure if the integrity of blood vessels is damaged by the penetrating spinal needle [32]. This is particularly concerning as some studies have reported an increased incidence of CNS relapse associated with TLP in the presence of peripheral blast cells [11, 33, 34]. For all newly diagnosed patients, the initial LP should be done by an experienced clinician after assurance that the patient has an adequate platelet count (>50,000/μL) and normal/near-normal coagulation tests (after product transfusions if necessary) to limit risk of bleeding [16]. In addition, most children will require some form of sedation to have optimal control of positioning and limit unanticipated patient movement [35]. In adults, LPs can be even more challenging given their baseline increased abdominal girth and higher incidence of obesity [36] which is known to increase risk of TLP [37]. In addition, adults can have other conditions making needle entry difficult such as spinal osteoarthritis [38]. In these cases LP by an interventional radiologist under fluoroscopy is less likely to result in a TLP [16].

Once the initial diagnostic LP is completed and cytology identifies presence or absence of lymphoblasts, CNS disease staging can be determined by cell count and number of blasts in the sample. In adult patients, diagnosis of CNS leukemia is made with at least 5 leukocytes/μL of CSF with leukemic blasts present or the presence of a cranial nerve palsy [39, 40]. In pediatric patients, any number of blasts in the sample of CSF has been associated with increased risk for CNS relapse in some acute leukemias [15, 41]. CNS risk stratification is therefore categorized into three groups including CNS1, indicating no identified CNS leukemia; CNS3, indicating overt CNS disease; and an intermediate category (CNS2) [42] (Table 11.1). There are some circumstances in which the diagnostic LP cannot be

Table 11.1 Classification of CNS leukemia at diagnosis

Classification		Cytology on cytospin	RBCs per μL	WBC per μL	Steinherz/Bleyer algorithm[a] result
CNS1		Negative	Any	Any	Not applicable
CNS2					
	2a	Positive	<10	<5	Negative
	2b	Positive	≥10	<5	Negative
	2c	Positive	≥10	≥5	Negative
CNS3					
	3a	Positive	<10	≥5	Positive
	3b	Positive	≥10	≥10	Positive
	3c	Defined by clinical signs of CNS leukemia (e.g., facial nerve palsy, brain/eye involvement)			

[a]Steinherz/Bleyer algorithm method of evaluating initial traumatic lumbar puncture:
If the patient has leukemic cells in the peripheral blood and the lumbar puncture is traumatic and contains ≥5 WBC/μL and blasts, the following algorithm should be used to distinguish between CNS2 and CNS3 disease (deemed positive if): (CSF WBC/CSF RBC) > [2x (peripheral blood WBC/peripheral blood RBC)]

Example of POSITIVE disease by Steinherz/Bleyer algorithm: CSF WBC = 60/μL; CSF RBC = 1500/μL; peripheral blood WBC 46,000/μL; peripheral blood RBC 3.0×10^6/μL (60/1500) = 0.04 > [2x(46,000/3.0×10^6)] = 0.015

performed safely due to severity of patient presentation and need to start patients on immediate systemic therapy. In other cases, patients have received steroids in a period just before ALL diagnosis for symptoms such as respiratory distress or lymphadenopathy. Under these circumstances patients often receive intensified CNS-directed therapy since partial pre-treatment of the CSF may obscure diagnostic results leading to falsely risk-stratifying patients to a lower CNS disease category [43, 44].

Risk-Stratified Treatment of CNS Disease

Presenting CNS status is used to determine risk stratification for CNS relapse and subsequent CNS-directed therapy. Approximately 5 to 10% of adults with ALL have CNS involvement at presentation, with increased involvement in patients with T-cell ALL versus B-cell ALL [45–47]. In comparison to adults, children have an increased overall incidence of CNS disease at presentation, although the immunophenotypic distribution is similar, with an increased proportion of children with T-cell ALL having CNS disease (CNS2 or CNS3) at presentation (30–35%) [48, 49] compared to B-cell ALL (10–15%) [42]. In a review of recent trials of pediatric patients with B-ALL from 2004 to 2010, the majority of patients were diagnosed as CNS1 disease (88.3%), with the remainder diagnosed with CNS2 disease (10.2%) and CNS3 disease (1.2%) [42]. In this study of over 8000 pediatric patients, those with CNS2 or CNS3 disease had inferior 5-year overall survival (OS) and event-free survival (EFS) compared to those with CNS1 disease (CNS1, 85% (±0.6%)/92.7% (±0.4%); CNS2, 76% (±2%)/86.8% (±1.6%); CNS3, 76% (±5%)/82.1% (±4.7%); $p < 0.001$ for both OS and EFS) and a significantly increased rate of CNS relapse (5.6% for CNS2, 5.1% for CNS3 – compared to a rate of 2% in CNS1 patients; $p < 0.001$). Among the CNS2 subcategories, there was no significant difference in EFS or OS or cumulative risk of relapse, suggesting that presence of lymphoblasts alone was independently associated with increased risk of CNS relapse [42]. Largely based on these data, most major pediatric oncology research consortia worldwide now intensify CNS targeted therapy for patients with diagnostically established CNS2 in addition to the long-standing intensification performed for patients with CNS3 disease [30, 50–53]. A similar recent review of pediatric T-ALL data demonstrated no difference in outcome between CNS1 and CNS2 patients, and therefore, those patients continue to be treated with equal attention paid to CNS prophylaxis [54–56]. In adults, factors associated with increased risk of CNS relapse, and thus consideration for increased CNS-directed therapy, include elevated lactate dehydrogenase levels (LDH), increased S-phase fraction, mature B-cell phenotype, T-cell phenotype, high diagnostic WBC counts, and overt CNS leukemia at diagnosis [14, 45, 57–62] (Table 11.2).

Table 11.2 Risk factors associated with CNS relapse in ALL

Leukemic blasts in CNS at diagnosis
High peripheral blood leukemia cell burden at diagnosis
T-cell phenotype
Leukemic cell genotypes
Pre-B ALL with *E2A-PBX1* fusion gene with t(1;19)
Hypodiploidy (< 45 chromosomes/leukemic cell)
KMT2A-rearrangement
Philadelphia chromosome t(9;22)
Host gene polymorphisms
Vitamin D receptor start site (high-risk ALL)
Thymidylate synthase (3/3) genotype (low-risk ALL)
Elevated lactate dehydrogenase (LDH) levels
Mature B-cell phenotype
Increased S-phase fraction of leukemia blasts

Methods of Initial CNS Prophylaxis and Treatment

For decades, pediatric protocols have focused on early and aggressive CNS-directed therapy, while adult protocols have been less CNS-focused [63, 64], which is now cited as a major potential factor in the traditional superiority of pediatric protocols in inducing long-term remissions over adult protocols [63, 64]. Adult and pediatric trials alike now incorporate early and aggressive prophylactic or treatment strategies for CNS disease that include BBB-crossing systemic and intrathecal chemotherapy and, in a decreasing number of circumstances, cranial radiation. In patients presenting with CNS disease, therapeutic strategies are intensified during the induction phase of chemotherapy before transitioning to prophylaxis once CNS disease has been controlled [14].

Cranial Radiation Therapy

Cranial radiation (CRT) has played a central role in the successful treatment of ALL since the CNS was discovered to be a sanctuary site [14]. The timing of CRT administration is based on potential interaction with systemic chemotherapy and therefore reserved for blocks of therapy with fewer CNS-directed agents or for treatment of patient symptoms, as radiation can rapidly improve nerve impingement and lead to salvage of function in cases of significant CNS disease [65]. When given, CRT is administered as fractionated doses to total 12 to 24 Gy depending on patient subgroup [50]. Adults may receive up to 24 Gy with minimal adverse effects [16]. However, in children, cranial or craniospinal radiation therapy is associated with a high risk of secondary neoplasms (21% at 20 years) [15], neurocognitive defects, multiple endocrinopathies, and higher mortality rate than the general population [66]. While there is a clear increase in effects with increased CRT doses, even at modern, reduced doses (12 to 18 Gy), children in long-term follow-up have demonstrated growth hormone deficiencies and poor emotional and cognitive quality of life [67]. Advances in BBB-crossing systemic therapies and intrathecally (IT) administered therapies have allowed for the reduction of CRT use. Today, use of CRT is reserved for only those patients at very high risk of CNS relapse [15], namely, those with occult CNS leukemia at diagnosis (CNS3 status), or as salvage therapy for those patients with CNS relapse [15]. Several recent pediatric protocols have demonstrated successful elimination of radiation in most patients, provided that intrathecal and systemic chemotherapy is appropriately intensified without compromising overall survival [65, 68–76].

Systemic Chemotherapy

Efforts to limit use of CRT in patients with ALL have been successful due to intensifying other methods of CNS-directed systemic and intrathecal chemotherapy. Development of effective systemic chemotherapy regimens relies on achieving and maintaining cytotoxic drug concentrations within the CNS. This includes the ability of the drug to cross the BBB, distribute within the brain parenchyma, and overcome mechanisms of transportation out of the CNS. Among systemic chemotherapeutic agents which can meet these criteria are corticosteroids, high-dose methotrexate (HDMTX), high-dose cytarabine, intensive asparaginase, and thiopurines. As such, these agents make up key pillars to modern ALL chemotherapy protocols.

Corticosteroids

Corticosteroids are an essential component of ALL treatment. For both pediatric and adult protocols, high-dose corticosteroids are used throughout the initial induction of remission phase of chemotherapy and in short courses (5–7 days) during consolidative and maintenance chemotherapy [14]. Dexamethasone and prednisone are most commonly used, but both adult and pediatric studies have demonstrated potential advantages of dexamethasone over prednisone for CNS control, due to the longer biological half-life of dexamethasone versus prednisone (>32 h vs 4 to 6 h, respectively) and lower protein binding property of dexamethasone that results in higher CNS bioavailability [77, 78]. In adult studies, use of dexamethasone has decreased the rate of CNS recurrence to 2% [79]. Two landmark pediatric studies, Children's Cancer Group CCG1922 and the UK Medical Research Council ALL97/99, demonstrated that transitioning prednisone to dexamethasone could decrease the risk of bone marrow and CNS relapse [77, 80]. While some follow-up studies in pediatrics suggest that dose matching of corticosteroids of prednisone and dexamethasone produces similar control of CNS disease with ratios of approximately 7 to 1 for prednisone to dexamethasone [81], additional studies demonstrate clear advantage of dexamethasone for minimizing risk of CNS relapse [62, 82]. Use of high-dose corticosteroids for prolonged periods during ALL therapy, however, is not without side effects. A meta-analysis evaluating efficacy and toxicity of corticosteroids during induction therapy demonstrated that in comparison to patients receiving prednisone, those receiving dexamethasone had higher risk of mortality during induction (RR 2.31, 95% CI 1.46–3.66), adverse neuropsychological events (RR 4.55, 95% CI 2.45–8.46), and myopathy (RR 7.05, 95% CI 3.00–16.58) [83]. This study did not find significant differences in osteonecrosis, sepsis rates, fungal infection, diabetes, or pancreatitis between the two groups [83]. Long-term follow-up studies of dexamethasone administration, not limited to induction therapy, found additional side effects including hyperlipidemia, hypertension, hyperglycemia, differences in bone health and body composition, and symptomatic osteonecrosis, which presents a major cause of morbidity, particularly in adolescent patients [77, 80, 84–87]. It is also known that there is increased neurocognitive and neuropsychological toxicities in both the short- and long-term follow-up of patients treated with dexamethasone compared to prednisone, but data are conflicting on the extent of this impact [71, 80, 88–92]. A study from St. Jude Children's Research Hospital (SJCRH) of long-term ALL survivors evaluated the etiology of these neuropsychological differences using functional MRI (fMRI) in adult survivors of childhood leukemia and found that patients treated with dexamethasone are at increased risk for memory deficits and there is correlating altered neural activity in regions associated with memory [91]. Nonetheless, for prophylaxis of CNS disease in acute leukemia, dexamethasone remains the corticosteroid of choice in most circumstances.

High-Dose Methotrexate and/or High-Dose Cytarabine

High-dose intravenous (IV) methotrexate (HDMTX) – generally defined as >1 g/m^2 [93] – was introduced as a treatment of ALL expected to prevent CNS relapse by crossing the BBB. Methotrexate is a classical folate antagonist that targets dihydrofolate reductase and when given in high doses can be associated with renal dysfunction, neurotoxicity including leukoencephalopathy and stroke-like symptoms, myelosuppression, and mucositis [94]. In a meta-analysis of eight studies that compared cranial radiation plus CSF-directed therapy with HDMTX plus intrathecal chemotherapy, HDMTX was shown to reduce hematologic relapse and improve EFS but only had a marginal effect on the control of CNS relapse [95]. High-dose methotrexate is given to children with ALL as 4–5 g/m^2 infusions over 24 h [96]. In adults, optimal dosing for HDMTX has not yet been determined, and doses will vary depending on treatment protocols [97].

Recent pediatric protocols have evaluated differing methods of methotrexate administration, comparing efficacy of HDMTX in various patient populations to Capizzi-based dose-escalating methotrexate plus PEG-asparaginase (C-MTX) with variable results. In patients with high-risk B-cell ALL evaluated in Children's Oncology Group (COG) trial AALL0232, there was a clear benefit of HDMTX and no increase in toxicity compared to C-MTX demonstrating 5-year EFS of 82%

versus 75.4% (p = 0.006) [96] and decrease in risk of bone marrow and CNS recurrences [98]. Despite a very clear advantage in high-risk B-cell ALL patients, these results were not corroborated in patients with T-cell ALL. The recent T-cell ALL trial, COG AALL0434, included a 2x2 randomization that compared regimens containing either C-MTX or HDMTX during an 8-week interim maintenance phase, with all patients except those with low-risk features receiving prophylactic (12 Gy) or therapeutic (18 Gy for CNS3) cranial radiation [99]. The 1031 patients with T-ALL without CNS3 disease or testicular leukemia were randomly assigned to receive C-MTX (n = 519) or HDMTX (n = 512). This study demonstrated increased 5-year disease-free survival and overall survival 91.5% (95% CI 88.1–94.8%) and 93.7% (95% CI 90.8–96.6%) for C-MTX compared to 85.3% (95% CI 88.1–94.8%) and 89.4% (95% CI 85.7–93.2%) for HDMTX [99]. Of these patients, C-MTX group had 32 relapses, 6 of which had CNS involvement (19%), and HDMTX had 59 relapses, 23 (39%) of which had CNS involvement, suggesting that T-cell ALL patients may benefit from C-MTX more than HDMTX [99]. This study, however, was not a direct comparison of C-MTX and HDMTX, with other differences between treatment groups. First, C-MTX includes two doses of PEG-asparaginase – known to be beneficial for CNS disease control (see next section) – not included in HDMTX blocks. Second, while both groups received the same dose and duration of CRT, those in the C-MTX group received it earlier in their course of therapy as concern regarding toxic interactions between HDMTX and CRT prompted investigators to delay radiation exposure in the HDMTX arm of the study. Future studies will hopefully better elucidate the exact mechanism of this C-MTX benefit observed in T-ALL patients [54].

Similar to HDMTX, high-dose cytarabine (HDAC) has also been successfully used for CNS prophylaxis and treatment. Cytarabine is an antimetabolite with an intracellular metabolite ara-CTP that is incorporated into DNA. After IV infusion, cytarabine rapidly distributes into total body water, and concentrations in the CSF reach 20–50% of simultaneous plasma concentration levels [100]. The half-life of cytarabine in the CSF is eight-fold greater than in plasma, and therefore cytotoxic concentrations can be achieved when administered at doses of 3 g/m^2 IV every 12 h [101]. Adult protocols often combine HDMTX and HDAC in addition to IT cytarabine to prevent CNS recurrence, but no consensus guidelines exist for optimal doses and number of cycles in adult patients. In pediatrics, HDAC is often reserved for relapsed or refractory patients. Toxicities of HDAC include myelosuppression, fever, rash, chemical conjunctivitis, and gastrointestinal disturbances, and given its distribution into the CNS, it also has rare but significant CNS toxicities including seizures, cerebral dysfunction, and cerebellar syndrome [100].

Intensive Asparaginase

Asparaginase is an enzyme which depletes extracellular asparagine, an amino acid ALL cells are unable to synthesize. This drug is a mainstay of ALL therapy and can contribute to effective CNS control. Asparaginase is omitted in some adult protocols secondary to particularly high rates of adverse effects such as hypersensitivity reactions, pancreatitis, and liver dysfunction [102]. Systemic asparaginase is known to lower CNS levels of asparagine, demonstrating ability to penetrate the BBB [103]. The efficacy of asparaginase in CNS prophylaxis is dependent on type and dose of asparaginase administered. Pegylated (PEG)-asparaginase is a modified version of the enzyme L-asparaginase, derived from *E. coli*, and is used in all pediatric ALL therapy due to its long half-life. PEG-asparaginase is administered at 2500 IU/m^2 IV early in induction therapy and then throughout pre-maintenance therapy in pediatric patients with ALL. Follow-up studies have demonstrated subsequent CSF asparagine concentrations decreased by 25–30% following this dose of PEG-asparaginase [104, 105]. Primary complications associated with PEG-asparaginase = include anaphylaxis, and patients with severe hypersensitivity reactions can be transitioned to *Erwinia*-derived products with a shorter half-life. In patients treated with *Erwinia* asparaginase =, the CNS relapse rate has been reported to be between two and six times the rate of patients treated with *E. coli*-derived preparations, further suggesting the impact of this medication in prevention of CNS relapse [106–108].

Thiopurines

Several studies have reported efficacy of both of the thiopurines mercaptopurine (6MP) and thioguanine (6TG) in the treatment of childhood ALL. One study comparing mercaptopurine (75 mg/m^2; n = 1017) and thioguanine (50–60 mg/m^2; n = 1010) demonstrated superior control of CNS relapse in patients treated with 6TG (p = 0.01) and improved 5-year EFS [109]. Another study reported a significantly lower risk of isolated CNS relapse with 6TG compared to 6MP at a lower dose of 6TG (40 mg) [110]. Follow-up studies have demonstrated risk of liver toxicity and veno-occlusive disease [109], limiting transition to 6TG entirely in ALL protocols, but most pediatric protocols still incorporate short blocks of 6TG.

Ifosfamide

Ifosfamide is an oxazaphosphorine alkylating agent and widely used in the treatment of solid tumors, with use now extending to some hematologic malignancies – specifically lymphoma [111]. Ifosfamide has been shown to have CNS penetration, although kinetics in CNS are not well understood [111]. Ifosfamide has been used in treatment of CNS malignancies due to its ability to cross the BBB and thus can be used in relapse or setting of refractory disease. One study evaluating relapsed, refractory CD20+ B-cell non-Hodgkin lymphoma and mature B-cell acute lymphoblastic leukemia showed the efficacy of combination therapy with one to three cycles of ifosfamide (300 mg/m^2) and etoposide (100 mg/m^2) given on days 3, 4, and 5 of each cycle and carboplatin (635 mg/m^2) on day 3, enhanced by rituximab [112].

Nelarabine

Nelarabine is a water-soluble prodrug of Ara-G, a deoxyguanosine analog that preferentially accumulates in T-cells where it is rapidly phosphorylated into ara-GTP which exerts cytotoxic effects [113]. In T-ALL and T-lymphoblastic lymphoma, it has been shown to be highly active [54]. In a phase I study of nelarabine administered as a 1-h infusion daily for 5 days in children and adults with refractory hematologic malignancies, a striking response rate was observed in patients with T-cell malignancies and limited response in those with B-cell malignancies [114]. A follow-up phase II trial sought to evaluate response rate to nelarabine in pediatric patients with first or subsequent T-cell ALL relapse [115]. In this study, a total of 121 patients were enrolled and evaluated, after two dose de-escalations to a dose of 650 mg/m^2 demonstrating tolerability. Interestingly in this study, 8 of 22 patients who had positive CSF cytology prior to study entry converted to negative CSF cytology by day 7 prior to their scheduled intrathecal chemotherapy, proving a role for nelarabine in treatment and possibly prophylaxis of CNS leukemia [115]. The subsequent COG study AALL0434 for de novo T-cell ALL patients included a nelarabine randomization wherein patients were randomized to receive 5-day blocks of nelarabine at 650 mg/m^2/day incorporated into two pre-maintenance cycles and four maintenance cycles of therapy. In this study of incorporating nelarabine up-front in T-cell ALL treatment, 4-year disease-free survival (DFS) and overall survival rates were 84.3% (+/−1.1%) and 90.2% (+/− 0.9%) for all patients. In the patients randomized to nelarabine ($n = 323$) versus no nelarabine ($n = 336$), 4-year DFS was 88.9% (+/− 2.2%) versus 83.3% (+/− 2.5%) ($p = 0.0332$), respectively, with a marked reduction in CNS relapses among patients receiving nelarabine (manuscript under review). These results have led to the incorporation of nelarabine into subsequent T-cell ALL treatment protocols. Nelarabine has been shown to have CNS penetration and associated side effects of neurotoxicity [116] including effects on both central and peripheral nervous system, most commonly seen in heavily pre-treated patients, but high-grade adverse effects are rare and the agent has been deemed tolerable in combination chemotherapy regimens [54].

Intrathecal Chemotherapy

Systemic chemotherapy alone is not adequate for CNS prophylaxis or treatment as, using this method of administration, it is difficult to produce and maintain prolonged therapeutic concentrations of drug in the CSF [117]. This can be overcome by direct injection of agents into the CSF compartment. This method has proven to be highly effective as high drug concentrations can be delivered into the CSF and meninges with low doses of medication and therefore minimal systemic toxicity [117]. All patients, regardless of CNS status, receive scheduled IT chemotherapy for the duration of treatment, but frequency is dependent on CNS disease at presentation and risk of relapse [15]. For patients with CNS1 disease or no evidence of CNS involvement at diagnosis, LPs with intrathecal chemotherapy occur at the beginning of each block of therapy and repeat with several weeks between treatments [16]. Patients who present with evidence of CNS disease require weekly to bi-weekly IT treatment until CSF is clear of lymphoblasts [16].

There are a limited number of agents that are routinely administered intrathecally. Most commonly used are antimetabolites methotrexate and cytarabine [15]. Less often used is the alkylating agent thiotepa [15, 117], which is reserved as a second-line agent for childhood meningeal disease [118–120] as it has a toxicity profile similar to IT methotrexate [118] but is rapidly cleared from the CNS. Intrathecal gemcitabine demonstrated significant cytotoxicity precluding direct CNS delivery [121], and intrathecal topotecan failed to demonstrate objective antitumor activity, despite being well tolerated in a phase II trial and demonstrating a favorable safety profile [122, 123].

The first IT treatment in patients with newly diagnosed ALL is often cytarabine [16]. Subsequent doses of IT chemotherapy consist of methotrexate or combinational therapy with methotrexate, cytarabine, and glucocorticoids (often hydrocortisone) in various combinations (termed “triple intrathecal therapy” or “TIT”) [15]. Intrathecal methotrexate has been in clinical use for over 50 years and is the most commonly used agent for intrathecal administration [117]. It is administered to patients with newly diagnosed ALL to prevent meningeal relapse and also can be used for the treatment of meningeal spread of disease. Bleyer and colleagues recommended an intrathecal dosage schedule for methotrexate based on age instead of body surface area, and as this regimen has proven to be less neurotoxic, it is now incorporated into frontline leukemia protocols [8]. There remain conflicting reports of antagonism and synergy of TIT [15, 124]. Results of the most recent high-risk pediatric ALL trial demonstrate no improvement in disease-free survival in patients who received triple intrathecal chemotherapy compared to those receiving intrathecal methotrexate [125]. An earlier randomized trial also demonstrated that despite reduction of isolated CNS relapse in patients receiving triple intrathecal chemotherapy compared to IT methotrexate alone, there was an increased frequency of bone marrow and testicular relapse resulting in inferior overall survival rates as medullary relapses are more difficult to salvage [126]. One explanation for this is isolated CNS relapse was a manifestation of systemic relapse and that improved CNS control secured with TIT favored overt leukemia relapse in other sites at later time points [15]. This suggests that more effective systemic chemotherapy will be needed for the full benefit of TIT to be demonstrated.

An alternative method of direct delivery of CNS therapy is through an Ommaya reservoir. This device is implanted subcutaneously and connected to a catheter in the lateral ventricle [127]. This reservoir allows for direct intraventricular administration of anticancer therapy which is a convenient and less painful method compared to lumbar puncture, does not require sedation, and requires lower doses of chemotherapy, usually 50% of the dose required via LP, with improved drug distribution [117, 128, 129]. The major limitation of Ommaya therapy is the inability to reliably screen for CSF clearance of lymphoblasts, as ventricular CSF may be negative for disease while lumbar CSF remains positive [117, 130, 131]. Therefore, these patients still require interval lumbar punctures for screening. While all patients receiving ALL therapy could have an Ommaya placed, these are often reserved for patients who have preclusions to lumbar punctures such as meningeal disease or challenging anatomy [130–132].

Repeated administration of IT chemotherapy is integral to treatment of the CNS compartment but can have significant side effects. The procedure alone, particularly in children, often requires sedation to be performed optimally, and over time, longer duration of anesthesia and higher cumulative doses of anesthetics (specifically propofol and fluranes) have resulted in slower processing speeds in a study of 212 long-term survivors of childhood ALL [133]. Intrathecal chemotherapy administration has additional effects on brain network efficiencies and processing, with highest risk in patients who receive more frequent intrathecal methotrexate administration [134] in a study done in patients who received chemotherapy only (no radiation). In a study of 571 adult survivors of ALL, neurocognitive tests and self reported neurocognitive symptoms were reviewed in multivariate analysis including exposure to intrathecal and high-dose methotrexate as covariates [67], but differences in neurocognitive and quality of life outcomes were only significant in groups receiving higher doses of cranial radiation therapy. A large study from 2003 to 2011 in the UK (UKALL2003) evaluated which patients are at highest risk for neurotoxicity secondary to chemotherapy administration with a multivariate analysis demonstrating that treatment allocation, female sex, CNS status, and age remained significant independent predictors of neurotoxicity [135].

It is clear that any method of treating the CNS may cause some real and significant untoward effects. However, it is also clear that any up-front ALL therapy with curative intent must contain intensive CNS-focused therapy. Using systemic therapy able to cross the BBB and IT therapy have greatly reduced effects seen in CRT, but additional improvements are needed.

Refractory CNS Disease and CNS Relapse

Despite increased intensity and efficacy of systemic chemotherapy and intrathecal chemotherapy, approximately 3–8% of patients will develop a CNS relapse [15]. At the time of CNS relapse, treatment options include a single or some combination of systemic re-induction chemotherapy, accentuated with therapies known to cross the BBB, intensified IT chemotherapy, with or without CRT, and hematopoietic stem cell transplant (HSCT). Relapse protocol choice is dependent on timing of relapse, location of relapse, host tolerability, and patient goals of care [14, 16].

As any relapsed therapy is going to be particularly toxic, accurately diagnosing a true CNS relapse is of critical importance. Despite its diagnostic limitations, as it is used in diagnosis at presentation, CSF cytology continues to be used in the initial diagnosis of relapsed and refractory CNS ALL [136]. In an attempt to improve on past diagnostic criteria, the COG recently put forth more stringent CNS relapse criteria for its most recent pre B-cell ALL studies AALL1731 and AALL1732 (clinicaltrials.gov identifiers NCT03914625 and NCT03959085, respectively). All relapses must occur after a complete remission (CR) is initially obtained. Definitive CNS relapse is diagnosed with a single CSF sample with CNS3 status; clinical signs of CNS leukemia such as facial nerve palsy, brain/eye involvement, or hypothalamic syndrome; or two consecutive CSF samples with CNS status confirmed by flow cytometry and/or fluorescence in situ hybridization (FISH). An equivocal CNS sample after obtaining a CR is defined as a single CSF sample with CNS2 status. In the case of equivocal CNS relapse, a CSF evaluation should be repeated as early as within 1 week but must be done within 4 weeks of the equivocal sample. On the repeat test, cytology, flow cytometric testing, and FISH (if applicable) should be sent. To convert to definitive relapse, the repeat CSF must either meet the criteria for definitive relapse or re-demonstrate CNS2 status but with lymphoblasts confirmed by flow cytometry and/or FISH. This system will hopefully improve both diagnostic accuracy and precision and lead to only those who truly require salvage CNS therapy to receive it.

If patients do get definitively defined as having a CNS relapse, while improvements are still required, refractory and first relapsed B-cell CNS disease is generally salvageable in children with current standard-of-care therapies, often without the need for HSCT. In these patients, better outcomes are seen in those with isolated CNS disease and/or late occurring relapse after achieving a first CR. Curative efforts, even in the setting of isolated CNS relapse, require the use of systemic chemotherapy in addition to CNS-directed therapy, as CNS disease in relapse of both B- and T-cell leukemias is known to occur largely in the presence of submicroscopic recurrence in the bone marrow, even when gold-standard clinical tests determine that the bone marrow is free of disease [137, 138]. On Pediatric Oncology Group (POG) trial 9061, 83 children ($n = 80$ (96%) with B-cell ALL) in first isolated CNS relapse who received CNS-directed systemic chemotherapy (intermediate-dose (1 g/m^2 over 24 h) methotrexate and high-dose cytarabine (3 g/m^2)), intensive IT therapy, and delayed CRT of 24 cGy achieved a 100% second CR rate and a 4-year EFS of 71.1% (±5.3%). Those who were ≥18 months from initial CR had a 4-year EFS of 83.3% (±5.3%), while those who remained in first remission <18 months had a 4-year EFS of 46.2% (±10.2%) [139]. St. Jude Children's Research Hospital achieved almost identical results on its R-11 protocol using a similar approach. They noted a 100% second CR and a 70% (±11%) 5-year disease-free survival (DFS) among all patients (15 of 17 (88%) of which had B-cell ALL). They also noted that 10 of 13 tested patients were found to retain normal intelligence quotient (IQ) scores after therapy [140]. B-cell patients on the POG 9061 successor study, POG 9412, achieved similar outcomes with reduced CRT (18 Gy) but included maximal intensity chemotherapy for 12 months prior to radiation [141]. Further attempts to intensify these relapsed backbones by increasing doses and frequency of chemotherapeutic agents have not improved outcomes dramatically but have increased toxicities [142, 143]. Therefore, current efforts aim to improve outcomes, particularly in early CNS relapse focus on offering novel systemic agents (e.g., blinatumomab), using intensified triple IT therapy and offering HSCT to early relapsed patients [144].

The excellent outcomes in childhood B-cell ALL are unfortunately not recapitulated in childhood T-ALL or in adult ALL of any lineage. In a recent large study, the 5-year OS for childhood T-ALL after first isolated CNS relapse ($n = 68$) was noted to be 51.7% (±6.2%) although if CNS relapse occurred in combination with overt relapse in the bone marrow ($n = 30$) the OS was 8.9% (±7.3%) – significantly worse than isolated bone marrow relapse ($n = 71$, 19.2% ±5%) [145]. Relapse in the CNS in adults has a dismal prognosis. Studies which have examined survival in adults with ALL after first CNS relapse note 4–5-year overall survival rates between 0% and 6% with median survivals after occurrence being <8 months [45, 146, 147] with no difference in survival based on phenotype [45]. In these patients, for whom outcome is particularly poor and for whom no current curative standard of care exists, there are more novel systemic and intrathecal medications that have proven to be efficacious for inducing remission.

Often first line treatment is intensive multiple-times-per-week administration of TIT [14, 16]. While a common approach, few well-controlled studies – particularly in the relapsed setting – have examined the benefit of TIT therapy over single-agent therapy. In children with de novo ALL, Children's Cancer Group (CCG) study 1952 randomized patients to standard IT methotrexate and TIT therapy. Although the use of TIT significantly improved CNS control with rates of isolated CNS relapse being 3.4% in the TIT group versus 5.9% in the IT methotrexate group ($p = 0.004$), there was no difference in 6-year EFS between the groups ($p = 0.2$) [126], and similar results were seen in the more recent high-risk pediatric ALL trial with no difference in disease-free survival of TIT compared to single-agent IT methotrexate [125]. On SJCRH Total Therapy XV, patients were non-randomly treated with TIT after which subjects had a historically low incidence of relapse either isolated to the CNS (2.7%) or combined CNS and systemic relapse (3.9%) despite using no CRT [68]. Based on this study, SJCRH studies now exclusively use TIT for CNS control [68].

Additional intrathecal options can be administered more centrally and intensively using an Ommaya reservoir. In adults, using an Ommaya reservoir, methotrexate (6–12 mg), cytarabine (30–50 mg), or both together can be injected twice weekly for six doses with good disease control [16]. In children, investigators at the Pediatric Oncology Branch of the National Cancer Institute pioneered using the Ommaya to provide increased exposure to therapeutic agents in a system called "concentration x time" ("CxT") [148]. They gave children, adolescents, and young adults (aged 3–24 years) with multiply relapsed or significantly refractory CNS leukemia methotrexate 2 mg daily for 3 days repeated every 10 days x 4, followed by cycles of cytarabine 15 mg daily for 3 days followed 15 days later by methotrexate 2 mg daily for 3 days for 46 days and finally cytarabine 15 mg daily for 3 days alternating with methotrexate 2 mg daily for 3 days every 29 days. With this system, they achieved at least a partial remission in 19 of 21 patients, and overall, patients were free of meningeal disease for a median of 15 months (range 2–89+ months) [149]. In addition, toxicities in this heavily pretreated cohort were minimal with few and minor incidences of chemical arachnoiditis, headache, and nausea noted [149]. There are some additional agents that can be used in the setting of relapse with increased intensity but do not require Ommaya placement, including liposomal cytarabine and thiotepa. Liposomal cytarabine (DepoCyt®) was created and tested in an effort to provide prolonged exposure and can be administered intrathecally without the need for a surgically implanted Ommaya reservoir. Compared with unencapsulated cytarabine, liposomal cytarabine has a longer half-life (141 h vs 3.4 h) and improved CSF distribution. Multiple studies in adults [150] (at a recommended dose of 50 mg) and children [151, 152] (at a recommended dose of 20 mg for children ≤1 year old, 25 mg for children >1 year and < 3 years old, 35 mg for children ≥3 and <14 years old, and 50 mg for children ≥14 years old) [153] have shown that its use is safe and effective in patients with relapsed or refractory CNS leukemia. Due to risk of chemical arachnoiditis, it must be administered with intrathecal dexamethasone and caution in concomitant use with systemic chemotherapy that can penetrate the BBB. In July, 2017 DepoCyt® was removed from the worldwide market due to the manufacturer's decision to stop its production [154]. Finally, both systemic and intrathecal thiotepas have been used to treat relapsed and refractory CNS lymphoblastic leukemia. Thiotepa is an alkylating agent and highly lipid-soluble, allowing for excellent CNS penetration [155]. However, after intraventricular administration thiotepa is removed from the CSF within approximately 3–4 h, and when administered by lumbar puncture, intraventricular delivery yields a lumbar area under the curve of 5% of that for ventricular CSF, likely due to rapid systemic absorption [120]. Despite these limitations, intrathecal thiotepa has been suggested as a possible therapeutic agent for leptomeningeal metastases in a number of diseases including solid tumors and hematologic malignancies [156–160], but data to support its use has been limited [161–163]. Systemic thiotepa, however, has been shown to be effective in treating CNS disease [141]. In a study of pediatric patients with isolated CNS relapse of ALL, a single-dose thiotepa up-front therapeutic window study was included to evaluate efficacy of blast clearance from CSF. In this study, 19 patients were evaluated and received a single IV dose of thiotepa administered over 5 min. Two dose levels were evaluated: ten patients received dose level 1 of thiotepa (50 mg/m^2), while an additional nine patients received dose level 2 (65 mg/m^2). Both groups demonstrated decrease in blast count in CSF within 1 week of single thiotepa dose (median blast count 85 decreased to 5 in the dose level 1 group; media blast count of 61 decreased to 4 in dose level 2 group), and dose level 2 resulted in 3 patients with CR, 4 patients with partial remission (clearing >50% of blasts), and minimal delay in proceeding to additional chemotherapy. This demonstrates the efficacy of single-agent thiotepa in CNS disease control, but a number of other studies have shown similar efficacy when combined with other chemotherapy (clofarabine or gemcitabine, topotecan, vinorelbine) in both pediatric and adult patients [164, 165].

New Therapeutic Approaches and Potential for CNS Treatment

New, targeted therapies are being developed for the treatment of primary and relapsed or refractory ALL, including small molecule inhibitors (such as tyrosine kinase inhibitors, CD4/CD6 inhibitors, and BCL-2 inhibitors) and immunotherapy (such as monoclonal antibodies, antibody-drug conjugates, and chimeric antigen receptor (CAR) T-cells). These therapies are often used in addition to systemic chemotherapy and intrathecal chemotherapy with or without radiation, depending on the patient and disease. In combination with additional therapy, extent of CNS penetration and effect in treating ALL in the CNS are still under investigation for most of these novel agents. However, preclinical studies, case series/reports, and even toxicity assessments have begun to suggest how these drugs may impact ALL in the CNS (Table 11.3).

Table 11.3 Novel ALL therapies and therapeutic potential for CNS leukemia

Class	Target	Drug	Preclinical/ Correlative[a]	ALL clinical[b]
Small molecule inhibitors	TKI (BCR-ABL)	Imatinib	No [167]	No [168]
		Dasatinib	Yes [169]	Yes [169]
		Nilotinib	Yes [170]	Yes [170]
		Ponatinib	No [173, 174]	No [173, 174]
	TKI (Jak)	Ruxolitinib	No [178]	*ND*
	CDK4/6 inhibitors	Ribociclib	No [179]	*ND*
		Palbociclib	No [179]	*ND*
	Proteasome inhibitors	Bortezomib	No [182]	No [182]
		Carfilzomib	No [182]	No [182]
		Ixazomib	No [182]	No [182]
		Marizomib	Yes [183]	*ND*
	mTOR inhibitors	Rapamycin	Yes [191–193]	*ND*
		Sirolimus	Yes [193]	*ND*
		Temsirolimus	Yes [193, 194]	*ND*
Antibodies	Monoclonal	Rituximab (CD20)	No [195]	No [195]
		Daratumumab (CD38)	No [196]	No [196]
		Epratuzumab (CD22)	No [197]	No [197]
	Monoclonal-drug conjugate	Inotuzumab (CD22-calichiamicin)	No [184]	No [188]
	BiTE	Blinatumomab (CD19-CD3)	No [184]	No [185, 198]
	CAR T-cells	CD19	Yes [189, 190, 199]	Yes [189, 190, 199]
		CD22	Yes [200]	*ND*
		CD19/22	Yes [199]	*ND*

[a]Preclinical or correlative – preclinical evidence or human subjects correlative biology evidence of agent's ability to cross the BBB
[b]ALL Clinical – evidence from human subjects clinical studies that systemic administration of the agent actively treats acute lymphoblastic leukemia in the CNS
ND no data

Imatinib revolutionized the treatment of t(9;11) Philadelphia chromosome-positive (Ph+) ALL. For example, historically <50% of pediatric patients with Ph + ALL would survive, even with HSCT. COG AALL0031, a landmark study, that showed backbone chemotherapy with the addition of continuous imatinib improved the 3-year EFS to 80% ± 11% compared to 35% ± 4% ($p < 0.0001$) in a historical cohort who received backbone chemotherapy alone [166]. However, the CNS remained a sanctuary site from imatinib [167], which preclinical studies showed did not cross the BBB well [168]. While data is sparse, the second-generation BCR-ABL tyrosine kinase inhibitors dasatinib and nilotinib appear to more effectively cross the BBB than their first-generation counterparts [169, 170]. There are clinical studies which have shown that both dasatinib and nilotinib have been effective in treating CNS-positive Ph+ ALL and even rescue patients who had residual or relapsed Ph+ CNS disease after failing imatinib [171, 172].

Unfortunately, most other small molecule inhibitors have efficacy similar to imatinib in penetrating the CNS. The third-generation TKI ponatinib does not appear to treat CNS Ph+ ALL [173], potentially secondary to its active rapid BBB efflux [174]. Ruxolitinib, a JAK1/2 inhibitor FDA approved for the treatment of myelofibrosis and polycythemia vera [175], is being investigated in the treatment of Philadelphia-like ALL [176], which, while preclinical studies suggest efficacy [177], does not clinically penetrate the CNS [178]. It has been shown that the BCL-2 inhibitor, venetoclax, does not cross the BBB [178] nor the CDK4/6 inhibitors such as ribociclib and palbociclib, which appear to either cross the BBB poorly or are actively and rapidly transported out of the CNS, making these drugs theoretically ineffective in CNS leukemia [179, 180]. Finally, the proteasome inhibitors advanced in clinical development such as bortezomib, carfilzomib, and ixazomib, which have shown great promise, particularly in relapsed ALL and T-ALL [181], have all failed to show BBB penetration [182]. However, a novel proteasome inhibitor, marizomib, not yet being tested in leukemias, does cross the BBB, making it an exciting agent to possibly treat proteasome inhibitor-sensitive CNS malignancies [183].

Generally, bispecific T-cell engagers (BiTEs), monocloncal antibodies, and antibody-drug conjugates are not able to penetrate into the CNS [184] limiting exciting new drugs such as blinatumomab, a CD19-CD3 bispecific antibody [185]; daratumumab, a CD38 monoclonal antibody [186, 187]; and inotuzumab, a CD22 antibody conjugated to calicheamicin [188] to the treatment of systemic disease only. However, CAR T-cells may be useful for treating CNS disease. CD19 CAR T-cells have been detected in the CSF in patients, and several reports support these agents being effective and safe in patients with CNS leukemia [189, 190]. Data on CAR T-cells targeting other antigens such as CD22 or dual-specific CD19/22 are lacking in data on penetration and/or efficacy into the CNS.

Conclusion

The provision of therapy specifically directed to the CNS, after its discovery as a sanctuary site for lymphoblasts, revolutionized the care of ALL. It is now considered a gold standard of care, in both children and adults, for ALL patients to receive early and intensive CNS-directed therapy either prophylactically or therapeutically. The meteoric rise of survival rates seen after the introduction of prophylaxis and treatment of the CNS, however, was not without cost of adverse effects. Advances and increased options in CNS-directed therapy have maintained and even improved CNS relapse rates and reduced toxicities. However, despite modern developments, CNS relapses continue to occur, and toxicities remain leading to significant morbidity and mortality in patients with ALL. Innovative therapies being developed for ALL should continue to focus on more effective and less toxic CNS-directed therapy to be a high priority.

References

1. Leonard J, Stock W. Progress in adult ALL: incorporation of new agents to frontline treatment. Hematology. 2017;2017(1):28–36. https://doi.org/10.1182/asheducation-2017.1.28.
2. Pui CH, Carroll WL, Meshinchi S, Arceci RJ. Biology, risk stratification, and therapy of pediatric acute leukemias: an update. J Clin Oncol Off J Am Soc Clin Oncol. 2011;29(5):551–65.
3. Pui CH, Evans WE. Treatment of acute lymphoblastic leukemia. N Engl J Med. 2006;354:166–78.
4. Thomas X, Boiron JM, Huguet F, Dombret H, Bradstock K, Vey N, et al. Outcome of treatment in adults with acute lymphoblastic leukemia: analysis of LALA-94 trial. J Clin Oncol Off J Am Soc Clin Oncol. 2004;22:4075–86. https://doi.org/10.1200/JCO.2004.10.050.
5. Thomas X, Le QH. Central nervous system involvement in adult acute lymphoblastic leukemia. Hematology. 2008;13:293–302. https://doi.org/10.1179/102453308X343374.
6. Izraeli S, Eckert C. Targeted therapy of CNS leukemia? Blood. 2017;130(5):562–3.
7. Price RA, Johnson WW. The central nervous system in childhood leukemia. I. The arachnoid. Cancer. 1973;31(3):520–33.
8. Bleyer WA. Biology and pathogenesis of CNS leukemia. Am J Pediatr Hematol Oncol. 1989;11(1):57–63.
9. Thomas LB. Pathology of leukemia in the brain and meninges: postmortem studies of patients with acute leukemia and of mice given inoculations of L1210 leukemia. Cancer Res. 1965;25(9):1555–71.
10. Frishman-Levy L, Izraeli S. Advances in understanding the pathogenesis of CNS acute lymphoblastic leukaemia and potential for therapy. Br J Haematol. 2017;176(2) https://doi.org/10.1111/bjh.1441.
11. Burger B, Zimmermann M, Mann G, Kühl J, Löning L, Riehm H, et al. Diagnostic cerebrospinal fluid examination in children with acute lymphoblastic leukemia: significance of low leukocyte counts with blasts or traumatic lumbar puncture. J Clin Oncol. 2003;21:184–8.
12. Simone JV. History of the treatment of childhood ALL: a paradigm for cancer cure. Best Pract Res Clin Haematol. 2006;19:353–9.
13. Henze G, v Stackelberg A, Eckert C. ALL-REZ BFM: the consecutive trials for children with relapsed acute lymphoblastic leukemia. Klin Padiatr. 2013;225:S73–8.
14. Pui CHaT, E. Central nervous system disease in hematological malignancies: historical perspective and practical applications. Semin Oncol. 2009;36:S2–S16.
15. Pui CH, Howard SC. Current management and challenges of malignant disease in the CNS in paediatric leukaemia. Lancet Oncol. 2008;9:257–68.
16. Larson RA. Managing CNS disease in adults with acute lymphoblastic leukemia. Leuk Lymphoma. 2018;59(1):3–13. https://doi.org/10.1080/10428194.2017.1326597.
17. Crespo-Solis E, López-Karpovitch X, Higuera J, Vega-Ramos B. Diagnosis of acute leukemia in cerebrospinal fluid (CSF-acute leukemia). Curr Oncol Rep. 2012;14(5):369–78. https://doi.org/10.1007/s11912-012-0248-6.

18. Stewart DJ, Keating MJ, McCredie KB, Smith TL, Youness E, Murphy SG, Bodey GP, Freireich EJ. Natural history of central nervous system acute leukemia in adults. Cancer. 1981;47(1):184–96.
19. Glass JP, Melamed M, Chernik NL, Posner JB. Malignant cells in cerebrospinal fluid (CSF): the meaning of a positive CSF cytology. Neurology. 1979;29(10):1369–75.
20. Zeiser R, Burger JA, Bley TA, Windfuhr-Blum M, Schulte-Monting J, Behringer DM. Clinical follow-up indicates differential accuracy of magnetic resonance imaging and immunocytology of the cerebral spinal fluid for the diagnosis of neoplastic meningitis - a single centre experience. Br J Haematol. 2004;124:762–8.
21. Hegde U, Filie A, Little RF, Janik JE, Grant N, Steinberg SM, et al. High incidence of occult leptomeningeal disease detected by flow cytometry in newly diagnosed aggressive B-cell lymphomas at risk for central nervous system involvement: the role of flow cytometry versus cytology. Blood. 2005;105:496–502.
22. Bromberg JEC, Breems DA, Kraan J, Bikker G, van der Holt B, Smitt PS, et al. CSF flow cytometry greatly improves diagnostic accuracy in CNS hematologic malignancies. Neurology. 2007;68:1674–9.
23. Bommer M, Nagy A, Schöpflin C, Pauls S, Ringhoffer M, Schmid M. Cerebrospinal fluid pleocytosis: pitfalls and benefits of combined analysis using cytomorphology and flow cytometry. Cancer Cytopathol. 2011;119(1):20–6. https://doi.org/10.1002/cncy.20127.
24. van der Velden VH, Hochhaus A, Cazzaniga G, Szczepanski T, Gabert J, van Dongen JJ. Detection of minimal residual disease in hematologic malignancies by real-time quantitative PCR: principles, approaches, and laboratory aspects. Leukemia. 2003;17(6):1013–34.
25. Rhodes CH, Glantz MJ, Glantz L, Lekos A, Sorenson GD, Honsinger C, et al. A comparison of polymerase chain reaction examination of cerebrospinal fluid and conventional cytology in the diagnosis of lymphomatous meningitis. Cancer. 1996;77:543–8.
26. Gleissner B, Siehl J, Korfel A, Reinhardt R, Thiel E. CSF evaluation in primary CNS lymphoma patients by PCR of the CDR III IgH genes. Neurology. 2002;58:390–6.
27. van Lochem EG, Wiegers YM, van den Beemd R, Hahlen K, van Dongen JJ, Hooijkaas H. Regeneration pattern of precursor-B-cells in bone marrow of acute lymphoblastic leukemia patients depends on the type of preceding chemotherapy. Leukemia. 2000;14(4):688–95. https://doi.org/10.1038/sj.leu.2401749.
28. van Wering ER, van der Linden-Schrever BE, Szczepanski T, Willemse MJ, Baars EA, van Wijngaarde-Schmitz HM, Kamps WA, van Dongen JJ. Regenerating normal B-cell precursors during and after treatment of acute lymphoblastic leukaemia: implications for monitoring of minimal residual disease. Br J Haematol. 2000;110(1):139–46. https://doi.org/10.1046/j.1365-2141.2000.02143.x.
29. Phillips ME, Ryals TJ, Kambhu SA, Yuh WT. Neoplastic vs inflammatory meningeal enhancement with Gd-DTPA. J Comput Assist Tomogr. 1990;14:536–41.
30. Levinsen M, Taskinen M, Abrahamsson J, et al. Clinical features and early treatment response of central nervous system involvement in childhood acute lymphoblastic leukemia. Pediatr Blood Cancer. 2014;61:1416–21. https://doi.org/10.1002/pbc.24981.
31. Howard SCGA, Cheng C, Kritchevsky SB, Somes GW, Harrison PL, et al. Risk factors for traumatic and bloody lumbar puncture in children with acute lymphoblastic leukemia. JAMA. 2002;288:2001–7.
32. Gajjar AHP, Sandlund JT, Rivera GK, Ribeiro RC, Rubnitz JE, et al. Traumatic lumbar puncture at diagnosis adversely affects outcome in childhood acute lymphoblastic leukemia. Blood. 2000;96:3381–4.
33. Gajjar A, Harrison PL, Sandlund JT, Rivera GK, Ribeiro RC, Rubnitz JE, et al. Traumatic lumbar puncture at diagnosis adversely affects outcome in childhood acute lymphoblastic leukemia. Blood. 2000;96:3381–4.
34. te Loo DM, Kamps WA, van der Does-van den Berg A, van Wering ER, de Graaf SS. Prognostic significance of blasts in the cerebrospinal fluid without pleiocytosis or a traumatic lumbar puncture in children with acute lymphoblastic leukemia: experience of the Dutch Childhood Oncology Group. J Clin Oncol. 2006;24:2332–6.

35. Nugent BD, Davis PJ, Noll RB, Tersak JM. Sedation practices in pediatric patients with acute lymphoblastic leukemia. Pediatr Blood Cancer. 2020;67(2):e28037. https://doi.org/10.1002/pbc.28037.
36. Flegal KM, Carroll MD, Kit BK, Ogden CL. Prevalence of obesity and trends in the distribution of body mass index among US adults, 1999-2010. JAMA. 2012;307(5):491–7. https://doi.org/10.1001/jama.2012.39.
37. Jaime-Perez JC, Sotomayor-Duque G, Aguilar-Calderon P, Salazar-Cavazos L, Gomez-Almaguer D. Impact of obesity on lumbar puncture outcomes in adults with acute lymphoblastic leukemia and lymphoma: experience at an academic reference center. Int J Hematol Oncol Stem Cell Res. 2019;13(3):146–52.
38. Gellhorn AC, Katz JN, Suri P. Osteoarthritis of the spine: the facet joints. Nat Rev Rheumatol. 2013;9(4):216–24. https://doi.org/10.1038/nrrheum.2012.199.
39. Pui CH, Mahmoud HH, Rivera GK, et al. Early intensification of intrathecal chemotherapy virtually eliminates central nervous system relapse in children with acute lymphoblastic leukemia. Blood. 1998;92:411.
40. Mastrangelo R, Poplack D, Bleyer A, et al. Report and recommendations of the Rome workshop concerning poor-prognosis acute lymphoblastic leukemia in children: biologic bases for staging, stratification, and treatment. Med Pediatr Oncol. 1986;14:191–4.
41. Mahmoud HH, Rivera GK, Jancock ML, et al. Low leukocyte counts with blast cells in cerebrospinal fluid of children with newly diagnosed acute lymphoblastic leukemia. N Engl J Med. 1993;329:314–9.
42. Winick N, Devidas M, Chen S, et al. Impact of initial CSF findings on outcome among patients with National Cancer Institute standard- and high-risk B-cell acute lymphoblastic leukemia: a report from the Children's Oncology Group. J Clin Oncol. 2017;35(22):2527–34.
43. Raetz EA, Loh ML, Devidas M, Maloney K, Mattano LA Jr, Larsen E, Carroll A, Heerema NA, Gastier-Foster JM, Wood B, Borowitz MJ, Winick N, Hunger SP, Carroll WL. Impact of corticosteroid pretreatment in pediatric patients with newly diagnosed B-lymphoblastic leukemia: a report from the Children's Oncology Group. Haematologica. 2019;104(11):e517–20. https://doi.org/10.3324/haematol.2018.215616.
44. Revesz T, Kardos G, Kajtar P, Schuler D. The adverse effect of prolonged prednisolone pretreatment in children with acute lymphoblastic leukemia. Cancer. 1985;55(8):1637–40. https://doi.org/10.1002/1097-0142(19850415)55:8<1637::aid-cncr2820550804>3.0.co;2-h.
45. JMR S, Oriol JM, Hernandez-Rivas A, Rivas JM, Bethencourt C, Parody C, Deben R, Bello G, Feliu JL, E. for the Programa para El Estudio y Tratamiento de Hemopatias Malignas Group. Central nervous system recurrence in adult patients with acute lymphoblastic leukemia. Cancer. 2006;106:2540–6. https://doi.org/10.1002/cncr.21948.
46. Del Principe MI, Maurillo L, Buccisano F, et al. Central nervous system involvement in adult acute lymphoblastic leukemia: diagnostic tools, prophylaxis, and therapy. Mediterr J Hematol Infect Dis. 2014;6(1):e2014075. https://doi.org/10.4084/MJHID.2014.075.
47. Lazarus HM, Richards SM, Chopra R, Litzow MR, et al. Central nervous system involvement in adult acute lymphoblastic leukemia at diagnosis: results from the international ALL trial MRC UKALL XII/ECOG E2993. Blood. 2006;108(2):465–72.
48. Asselin BL, Devidas M, Wang C, Pullen J, Borowitz MJ, Hutchison R, Lipshultz SE, Camitta BM. Effectiveness of high-dose methotrexate in T-cell lymphoblastic leukemia and advanced-stage lymphoblastic lymphoma: a randomized study by the Children's Oncology Group (POG 9404). Blood. 2011;118(4):874–83. https://doi.org/10.1182/blood-2010-06-292615.
49. Winter SS, Dunsmore KP, Devidas M, Wood BL, Esiashvili N, Chen Z, Eisenberg N, Briegel N, Hayashi RJ, Gastier-Foster JM, Carroll AJ, Heerema NA, Asselin BL, Gaynon PS, Borowitz MJ, Loh ML, Rabin KR, Raetz EA, Zweidler-Mckay PA, Winick NJ, Carroll WL, Hunger SP. Improved survival for children and young adults with T-lineage acute lymphoblastic leukemia: results from the Children's Oncology Group AALL0434 methotrexate randomization. J Clin Oncol Off J Am Soc Clin Oncol. 2018;36(29):2926–34. https://doi.org/10.1200/JCO.2018.77.7250.

50. Vora A, Andreano A, Pui CH, Hunger SP, et al. Influence of cranial radiotherpay on outcome in children with acute lymphoblastic leukemia treated with contemporary therapy. J Clin Oncol. 2016;34(9):919–26.
51. Vrooman LM, Blonquist TM, Harris MH, et al. Refining risk classification in childhood B acute lymphoblastic leukemia: results of DFCI ALL Consortium Protocol 05-001. Blood Adv. 2018;2(12):1449–58. https://doi.org/10.1182/bloodadvances.2018016584.
52. Jeha S, Pei D, Choi J, Cheng C, Sandlund JT, et al. Improved CNS control of childhood acute lymphoblastic leukemia without cranial irradiation: St Jude Total Therapy Study 16. J Clin Oncol Off J Am Soc Clin Oncol. 2019;37(35):3377–91. https://doi.org/10.1200/JCO.19.01692.
53. Hough R, Rowntree C, Goulden N, Mitchell C, Moorman A, Wade R, Vora A. Efficacy and toxicity of a paediatric protocol in teenagers and young adults with Philadelphia chromosome negative acute lymphoblastic leukaemia: results from UKALL 2003. Br J Haematol. 2016;172(3):439–51. https://doi.org/10.1111/bjh.13847.
54. Teachey DT, O'-Connor D. How I treat newly diagnosed T-cell acute lymphoblastic leukemia and T-cell lymphoblastic lymphoma in children. Blood. 2020;135(3):159–66. https://doi.org/10.1182/blood.2019001557.
55. Gossai N, Winter SS, Devidas M, Wood B, et al. SIOP19–1143 nelarabine abrogates relapse rates in CNS3 T-ALL: a report from Children's Oncology Group study AALL0434. Paper presented at the SIOP; 2019.
56. Gossai N, Winter SS, Devidas M, Wood B, et al. Nelarabine abrogrates relapse rates in CNS-3 T-ALL: a report from Children's Oncology Group ALL0434. Paper presented at the ASPHO 2019, New Orleans, LA.
57. Conter V, Schrappe M, Aricó M, Reiter A, Rizzari C, Dördelmann M, et al. Role of cranial radiotherapy for childhood T-cell acute lymphoblastic leukemia with high WBC and good response to prednisone. J Clin Oncol. 1997;15:2786–91.
58. Goldberg JM, Silverman LB, Levy DE, Dalton VK, Gelber RD, Lehmann L, et al. Childhood T-cell acute lymphoblastic leukemia: the Dana-Farber Cancer Institute acute lymphoblastic leukemia consortium experience. J Clin Oncol. 2003;21:3616–22.
59. Gossai NP, Gordon PM. The role of the central nervous system microenvironment in pediatric acute lymphoblastic leukemia. Front Pediatr. 2017;5:1–8.
60. Hoelzer D, Ludwig WD, Thiel E, Gassmann W, Löffler H, Fonatsch C, et al. Improved outcome in adult B-cell acute lymphoblastic leukemia. Blood. 1996;87:495–508.
61. Kantarjian HM, Walters RS, Smith TL, Keating MJ, Barlogie B, McCredie KB, et al. Identification of risk groups for development of central nervous system leukemia in adults with acute lymphocytic leukemia. Blood. 1998;72:1784–9.
62. Schrappe M, Reiter A, Ludwig WD, Harbott J, Zimmermann M, Hiddemann W, et al. Improved outcome in childhood acute lymphoblastic leukemia despite reduced use of anthracyclines and cranial radiotherapy: results of trial ALL-BFM 90. German-Austrian-Swiss ALL-BFM Study Group. Blood. 2000;95:3310–22.
63. Schafer ES, Hunger SP. Optimal therapy for acute lymphoblastic leukemia in adolescents and young adults. Nat Rev. 2011;8:417–24.
64. Stock W, La M, Sanford B, Bloomfield CD, et al. What determines the outcomes for adolescents and young adults with acute lymphoblastic leukemia treated on cooperative group protocols? A comparison of Children's Cancer Group and Cancer and Leukemia Group B studies. Blood. 2008;112(5):1646–54. https://doi.org/10.1182/blood-2008-01-130237.
65. Sison EAR, Silverman LB. CNS prophylaxis in pediatric acute lymphoblastic leukemia. Hematology. 2014;2014(1):198–201.
66. Geenen MM, Cardous-Ubbink MC, Kremer LC, et al. Medical assessment of adverse health outcomes in long-term survivors of childhood cancer. JAMA. 2007;297:2705–15.
67. Krull KR, Li C, Phillips NS, Cheung YT, Brinkman TM, Wilson CL, Armstrong GT, Khan RB, Merchant TE, Sabin ND, Srivastava D, Pui CH, Robison LL, Hudson MM, Sklar CA, Chemaitilly W. Growth hormone deficiency and neurocognitive function in adult survivors

of childhood acute lymphoblastic leukemia. Cancer. 2019;125(10):1748–55. https://doi.org/10.1002/cncr.31975.
68. Pui CH, Campana D, Pei D, et al. Treating childhood acute lymphoblastic leukemia without cranial irradiation. N Engl J Med. 2009;360(26):2730–41.
69. Wilejto M, Di Giuseppe G, Hitzler J, et al. Treatment of young children with CNS-positive acute lymphoblastic leukemia without cranial radiotherapy. Pediatr Blood Cancer. 2015;62:1881–5.
70. Waber DP, Turek J, Catania L, et al. Neuropsychological outcomes from a randomized trial of triple intrathecal chemotherapy compared with 18 Gy cranial radiation as CNS treatment in acute lymphoblastic leukemia: findings from Dana-Farber Cancer Institute ALL Consortium Protocol 95-01. J Clin Oncol Off J Am Soc Clin Oncol. 2007;25(31):4914–21.
71. Kadan-Lottick NS, Zeltzer LK, Liu Q, et al. Neurocognitive functioning in adult survivors of childhood non-central nervous system cancers. J Natl Cancer Inst. 2010;102(12):881–93.
72. Conklin HM, Krull KR, Reddick WE, Pei D, Cheng C, Pui CH. Cognitive outcomes following contemporary treatment without cranial irradiation for childhood acute lymphoblastic leukemia. J Natl Cancer Inst. 2012;104(18):1386–95.
73. Nachman J, Sather HN, Cherlow JM, et al. Response of children with high-risk acute lymphoblastic leukemia treated with and without cranial irradiation: a report from the Children's Cancer Group. J Clin Oncol. 1998;16(3):920–30.
74. Gaynon PS, Angiolillo AL, Carroll WL, et al. Long-term results of the children's cancer group studies for childhood acute lymphoblastic leukemia 1983-2002: a Children's Oncology Group report. Leukemia. 2010;24(2):285–97.
75. Schmiegelow K, Forestier E, Hellebostad M, et al. Long-term results of NOPHO ALL-92 and ALL-2000 studies of childhood acute lymphoblastic leukemia. Leukemia. 2010;24(2):345–54.
76. Sirvent N, Suciu S, Rialland X, et al. Prognostic significance of the initial cerebrospinal fluid (CSF) involvement of children with acute lymphoblastic leukaemia (ALL) treated without cranial irradiation: results of European Organization for Research and Treatment of Cancer (EORTC) Children Leukemia Group study 58881. Eur J Cancer. 2011;47(2):239–47.
77. Bostrom BC, Sensel MR, Sather HN, et al. Dexamethasone versus prednisone and daily oral versus weekly intravenous mercaptopurine for patients with standard-risk acute lymphoblastic leukemia: a report from the Children's Cancer Group. Blood. 2003;101(10):3809–17. https://doi.org/10.1182/blood-2002-08-2454
78. Jones B, Freeman AI, Shuster JJ, Jacquillat C, et al. Lower incidence of meningeal leukemia when prednisone is replaced by dexamethasone in the treatment of acute lymphocytic leukemia. Med Pediatr Oncol. 1991;19(4):269–75. https://doi.org/10.1002/mpo.2950190411
79. Annino L, Vegna ML, Camera A, Specchia G, Visani G, Fioritoni G, et al. GIMEMA group: treatment of adult acute lymphoblastic leukemia (ALL): long-term follow-up of the GIMEMA ALL 0288 randomized study. Blood. 2002;99:863–71. https://doi.org/10.1182/blood.V99.3.863
80. Mitchell CD, Richards SM, Kinsey SE, Lilleyman J, Vora A, Eden TO, et al. Benefit of dexamethasone compared with prednisolone for childhood acute lymphoblastic leukaemia: results of the UK Medical Research Council ALL97 randomized trial. Br J Haematol. 2005;129:734–45.
81. Igarashi S, Manabe A, Ohara A, Kumagai M, Saito T, Okimoto Y, et al. No advantage of dexamethasone over prednisolone for the outcome of standard- and intermediate-risk childhood acute lymphoblastic leukemia in the Tokyo Children's Cancer Study Group L95-14 protocol. J Clin Oncol. 2005;23:6489–98.
82. Balis FM, Lester CM, Chrousos GP, Heideman RL, Poplack DG. Differences in cerebrospinal fluid penetration of corticosteroids: possible relationship to the prevention of meningeal leukemia. J Clin Oncol. 1987;5:202–7.
83. Teuffel O, Kuster SP, Hunger SP, et al. Dexamethasone versus prednisone for induction therapy in childhood acute lymphoblastic leukemia: a systematic review and meta-analysis. Leukemia. 2011;25:1232–8.

84. Wallace AM, Tucker P, Williams DM, et al. Short-term effects of prednisolone and dexamethasone on circulating concentrations of leptin and sex hormone-binding globulin in children being treated for acute lymphoblastic leukaemia. Clin Endocrinol. 2003;58:770–6.
85. Ahmed SF, Tucker P, Mushtaq T, et al. Short-term effects on linear growth and bone turnover in children randomized to receive prednisolone or dexamethasone. Clin Endocrinol. 2002;57:185–91.
86. Mattano LAJ, Devidas M, Nachman JB, et al. Effect of alternate-week versus continuous dexamethasone scheduling on the risk of osteonecrosis in paediatric patients with acute lymphoblastic leukaemia: results from the CCG-1961 randomised cohort trial. Lancet Oncol. 2012;13:906–15.
87. te Winkel ML, Pieters R, Hop WC, et al. Prospective study on incidence, risk factors, and long-term outcome of osteonecrosis in pediatric acute lymphoblastic leukemia. J Clin Oncol. 2011;29:4143–50.
88. Waber DPMM, Sebree M, Forbes PW, et al. Neuropsychological outcomes of a randomized trial of prednisone versus dexamethasone in acute lymphoblastic leukemia: findings from Dana-farber cancer Institute ALL Consortium Protocol 00-01. Pediatr Blood Cancer. 2013;60:1785–91.
89. Mrakotsky CM, Silverman LB, Dahlberg SE, et al. Neurobehavioral side effects of corticosteroids during active treatment for acute lymphoblastic leukemia in children are age-dependent: Report from Dana-Farber Cancer Institute ALL Consortium Protocol 00-01. Pediatr Blood Cancer. 2011;57:492–8.
90. Kadan-Lottick NS, Brouwers P, Breiger D, et al. A comparison of neurocognitive functioning in children previously randomized to dexamethasone or prednisone in the treatment of childhood acute lymphoblastic leukemia. Blood. 2009;114:1746–52.
91. Edelmann MN, Ogg RJ, Scoggins MA, Tara M, et al. Dexamethasone exposure and memory function in adult survivors of childhood acute lymphoblastic leukemia: a report from the SJLIFE cohort. Pediatr Blood Cancer. 2013;60(11):1778–84. https://doi.org/10.1002/pbc.24644.
92. Warris LT, van den Heuvel-Eibrink MM, den Hoed MAH, et al. Does dexamethasone induce more neuropsychological side effects than prednisone in pediatric acute lymphoblastic leukemia? A systematic review. Pediatr Blood Cancer. 2014;61:1313–8. https://doi.org/10.1002/pbc.24988.
93. Widemann BC, Adamson PC. Understanding and managing methotrexate nephrotoxicity. Oncologist. 2006;11(6):694–703. https://doi.org/10.1634/theoncologist.11-6-694.
94. Bleyer WA. The clinical pharmacology of methotrexate: new applications of an old drug. Cancer. 1978;41(1):36–51.
95. Clarke M, Gaynon P, Hann I, Harrison G, Masera G, Peto R, et al. CNS-directed therapy for childhood acute lymphoblastic leukemia: childhood ALL Collaborative Group overview of 43 randomized trials. J Clin Oncol. 2003;21:1798–809.
96. Larsen EC, Devidas M, Chen S, et al. Dexamethasone and high-dose methotrexate improve outcome for children and young adults with high-risk B-acute lymphoblastic leukemia: a report from Children's Oncology Group study AALL0232. JCO. 2016;30:2380–8.
97. Jabbour E, Thomas D, Cortes J, et al. Central nervous system prophylaxis in adults with acute lymphoblastic leukemia: current and emerging therapies. Cancer. 2010;116:2290–300.
98. Larsen EC, Devidas M, Chen S, Salzer WL, et al. Dexamethasone and high-dose methotrexate improve outcome for children and young adults with high-risk B-acute lymphoblastic leukemia: a report from Children's Oncology Group Study AALL0232. J Clin Oncol Off J Am Soc Clin Oncol. 2016;34(10):2380–8. https://doi.org/10.1200/JCO.2015.62.4544.
99. Winter SS, Dunsmore KP, Devidas M, Wood BL, et al. Improved survival for children and young adults with T-lineage acute lymphoblastic leukemia: results from the Children's Oncology Group AALL0434 methotrexate randomization. J Clin Oncol Off J Am Soc Clin Oncol. 2018;36(29):2926–34. https://doi.org/10.1200/JCO.2018.77.7250.

100. Baker WJ, Royer GL Jr, Weiss RB. Cytarabine and neurologic toxicity. J Clin Oncol Off J Am Soc Clin Oncol. 1991;9(4):679–93. https://doi.org/10.1200/JCO.1991.9.4.679.
101. Cortes J, O'Brien SM, Pierce S, Keating MJ, Freireich EJ, Kantarjian HHM. The value of high-dose systemic chemotherapy and intrathecal therapy for central nervous system prophylaxis in different risk groups of adult acute lymphoblastic leukemia. Blood. 1995;86:2091–7.
102. Koprivnikar J, McCloskey J, Faderl S. Safety, efficacy, and clinical utility of asparaginase in the treatment of adult patients with acute lymphoblastic leukemia. Onco Targets Ther. 2017;10:1413–22. https://doi.org/10.2147/OTT.S106810.
103. Moghrabi A, Levy DE, Asselin B, Barr R, Clavell L, Hurwitz C, et al. Results of the Dana-Farber Cancer Institute ALL Consortium Protocol 95-01 for children with acute lymphoblastic leukemia. Blood. 2007;109:896–904.
104. Angiolillo AL, Schore RJ, Devidas M, et al. Pharmacokinetic and pharmacodynamic properties of calaspargase pegol Escherichia coli l-asparaginase in the treatment of patients with acute lymphoblastic leukemia: results from Children's Oncology Group study AALL07PA. JCO. 2014;32:3874–82.
105. Dinndorf PA, Gootenberg J, Cohen MH, et al. FDA drug approval summary: pegaspargase (Oncospar) for the first-line treatment of children with acute lymphoblastic leukemia (ALL). Oncologist. 2007;12:991–8.
106. Hofmans M, Suciu S, Ferster A, Van Vlierberghe P, Mazingue F, Sirvent N, Costa V, Yakouben K, Paillard C, Uyttebroeck A, Plantaz D, Plat G, Simon P, Millot F, Poiree M, van der Werff Ten Bosch J, Piette C, Minckes O, Rohrlich P, Girard S, Cave H, Bertrand Y, De Moerloose B. Results of successive EORTC-CLG 58 881 and 58 951 trials in paediatric T-cell acute lymphoblastic leukaemia (ALL). Br J Haematol. 2019;186(5):741–53. https://doi.org/10.1111/bjh.15983.
107. Pieters R, Hunger SP, Boos J, Rizzari C, Silverman L, Baruchel A, Goekbuget N, Schrappe M, Pui CH. L-asparaginase treatment in acute lymphoblastic leukemia: a focus on Erwinia asparaginase. Cancer. 2011;117(2):238–49. https://doi.org/10.1002/cncr.25489.
108. Sirvent NSS, Rialland X, et al. Prognostic significance of the initial cerebro-spinal fluid (CSF) involvement of children with acute lymphoblastic leukaemia (ALL) treated without cranial irradiation: results of European Organization for Research and Treatment of Cancer (EORTC) Children Leukemia Group study 58881. Eur J Cancer. 2011;47(2):239–47.
109. Stork LC, Sather H, Hutchinson R. Comparison of mercaptopurine (mp) with thioguanine (tg) and it methotrexate with it "triples" (ITT) in children with SR-ALL: results of CCG1952. Blood. 2002;100:156a.
110. Vora A, Mitchell CD, Lennard L, Eden TO, Kinsey SE, Lilleyman J, et al. Toxicity and efficacy of 6-thioguanine versus 6-mercaptopurine in childhood lymphoblastic leukaemia: a randomised trial. Lancet. 2006;368:1339–48.
111. Lewis LD. Ifosfamide pharmacokinetics. Investig New Drugs. 1991;9(4):305–11.
112. Griffin TC, Weitzman S, Weinstein H, Chang M, Cairo M, Hutchison R, Shiramizu B, Wiley J, Woods D, Barnich M, Gross TG, Children's Oncology Group. A study of rituximab and ifosfamide, carboplatin, and etoposide chemotherapy in children with recurrent/refractory B-cell (CD20+) non-Hodgkin lymphoma and mature B-cell acute lymphoblastic leukemia: a report from the Children's Oncology Group. Pediatr Blood Cancer. 2009;52(2):177–81. https://doi.org/10.1002/pbc.21753.
113. Buie LW, Epstein SS, Lindley CM. Nelarabine: a novel purine antimetabolite antineoplastic agent. Clin Ther. 2007;29(9):1887–99. https://doi.org/10.1016/j.clinthera.2007.09.002.
114. Kurtzberg J, Ernst TJ, Keating MJ, et al. Phase I study of 506U78 administered on a consecutive 5-day schedule in children and adults with refractory hematologic malignancies. J Clin Oncol Off J Am Soc Clin Oncol. 2005;23(15):3396–403.
115. Berg SL, Blaney SM, Devidas M, et al. Phase II study of nelarabine (compound 506U78) in children and young adults with refractory T-cell malignancies: a report from the Children's Oncology Group. J Clin Oncol Off J Am Soc Clin Oncol. 2005;23(15):3376–82.

116. Winter SS, Dunsmore KP, Devidas M, Eisenberg N, et al. Safe integration of nelarabine into intensive chemotherapy in newly diagnosed T-cell acute lymphoblastic leukemia: Children's Oncology Group study AALL0434. Pediatr Blood Cancer. 2015;62(7):1176–83. https://doi.org/10.1002/pbc.25470.
117. Adamson P, Blaney SM, Bagatell R, Skolnik JM, Balis FM. General principles of chemotherapy. In: Pizzo PA, Poplack DG, editors. Principles and practice of Pediatric oncology. 6th ed. Philadelphia: Wolters Kluwer; 2016. p. 294–7.
118. Grossman SA, Finkelstein JC, Ruckdeschel JC, et al. Randomized prospective comparison of intraventricular methotrexate and thiotepa in patients with previously untreated neoplastic meningitis. J Clin Oncol Off J Am Soc Clin Oncol. 1993;11:561–9.
119. Fisher PG, Kadan-Lottick NS, Korones DN. Intrathecal thiotepa: reappraisal of an established therapy. J Pediatr Hematol Oncol. 2002;24:274–8.
120. Strong JM, Collins JM, Lester C, et al. Pharmacokinetics of intraventricular and intravenous N, N[precedes], N″-triethylenethiophosphoramide (thiotepa) in rhesus monkeys and humans. Cancer Res. 1986;46:6101–4.
121. Bernardi RJ, Bomgaars L, Fox E, et al. Phase I clinical trial of intrathecal gemcitabine in patients with neoplastic meningitis. Cancer Chemother Pharmacol. 2008;62:355–61.
122. Potter SL, Berg S, Ingle AM, et al. Phase 2 clinical trial of intrathecal topotecan in children with refractory leptomeningeal leukemia: a Children's Oncology Group trial (P9962). Pediatr Blood Cancer. 2012;2012:362–5.
123. Blaney SM, Tagen M, Onar-Thomas A, et al. A phase-I pharmacokinetic optimal dosing study of intraventricular topotecan for children with neoplastic meningitis: a Pediatric Brain Tumor Consortium study. Pediatr Blood Cancer. 2013;60:627–32.
124. Akutsu M, Furukawa Y, Tsunoda S, et al. Schedule-dependent synergism and antagonism between methotrexate and cytarabine against human leukemia cell lines in vitro. Leukemia. 2002;16:1808–17.
125. Salzer WL, Burke MJ, Devidas M, et al. Triple intrathecal therapy (methotrexate/hydrocortisone/cytarabine) does not improve disease-free survival versus intrathecal methotrexate alone in children with high risk B-lymphoblastic leukemia: results of Children's Oncology Group study AALL1131. Blood. 2018;132(Supplement 1):35. https://doi.org/10.1182/blood-2018-99-116180.
126. Matloub Y, Lindemulder S, Gaynon PS, Sather H, La M, et al. Intrathecal triple therapy decreases central nervous system relapse but fails to improve event-free survival when compared with intrathecal methotrexate: results of the Children's Cancer Group (CCG) 1952 study for standard-risk acute lymphoblastic leukemia, reported by the Children's Oncology Group. Blood. 2006;108(4):1165–73. https://doi.org/10.1182/blood-2005-12-011809.
127. Ommaya AK. Subcutaneous reservoir and pump for sterile access to ventricular cerebrospinal fluid. Lancet. 1963;2(1735):983–4.
128. Peyrl A, Chocholous M, Azizi AA, et al. Safety of Ommaya reservoirs in children with brain tumors: a 20-year experience with 5472 intraventricular drug administrations in 98 patients. J Neuro-Oncol. 2014;120(1):139–45.
129. Wilson R, Osborne C, Halsey C. The use of Ommaya reservoirs to deliver central nervous system-directed chemotherapy in childhood acute lymphoblastic leukaemia. Paediatr Drugs. 2018;20(4):293–301. https://doi.org/10.1007/s40272-018-0298-9.
130. Bleyer WA, Pizzo PA, Spence AM, et al. The Ommaya reservoir: newly recognized complications and recommendations for insertion and use. Cancer. 1978;41(6):2431–7.
131. Lishner M, Perrin RG, Feld R, Messner HA, Tuffnell PG, Elhakim T, Matlow A, Curtis JE. Complications associated with Ommaya reservoirs in patients with cancer. The Princess Margaret Hospital experience and a review of the literature. Arch Intern Med. 1990;150(1):173–6.
132. Browne MJ, Dinndorf PA, Perek D, Commers J, Bleyer WA, Poplack DG, Pizzo PA. Infectious complications of intraventricular reservoirs in cancer patients. Pediatr Infect Dis J. 1987;6(2):182–9.

133. Banerjee P, Rossi MG, Anghelescu DL, Liu W, et al. Association between anesthesia exposure and neurocognitive and neuroimaging outcomes in long-term survivors of childhood acute lymphoblastic leukemia. JAMA Oncol. 2019; https://doi.org/10.1001/jamaoncol.2019.1094.
134. Kesler SR, Ogg R, Reddick WE, Phillips N, Scoggins M, Glass JO, Cheung YT, Pui CH, Robison LL, Hudson MM, Krull KR. Brain network connectivity and executive function in long-term survivors of childhood acute lymphoblastic leukemia. Brain Connect. 2018;8(6):333–42. https://doi.org/10.1089/brain.2017.0574.
135. Wahid QA, Hamadeh L, McGowan S, Hough R, et al. Acute neurotoxicity during ALL therapy is associated with treatment intensity, age and female sex – an analysis of SAE reports from the UKALL 2003 trial. Blood. 2018;132(Supplement 1):1379. https://doi.org/10.1182/blood-2018-99-113267.
136. Thastrup M, Marquart HV, Levinsen M, Grell K, Abrahamsson J, Albertsen BK, Frandsen TL, Harila-Saari A, Lahteenmaki PM, Niinimaki R, Pronk CJ, Ulvmoen A, Vaitkeviciene G, Taskinen M, Schmiegelow K, Nordic Society of Pediatric H, Oncology. Flow cytometric detection of leukemic blasts in cerebrospinal fluid predicts risk of relapse in childhood acute lymphoblastic leukemia: a Nordic Society of Pediatric Hematology and Oncology study. Leukemia. 2020;34(2):336–46. https://doi.org/10.1038/s41375-019-0570-1.
137. Goulden N, Langlands K, Steward C, Katz F, Potter M, Chessells J, Oakhill A. PCR assessment of bone marrow status in 'isolated' extramedullary relapse of childhood B-precursor acute lymphoblastic leukaemia. Br J Haematol. 1994;87(2):282–5. https://doi.org/10.1111/j.1365-2141.1994.tb04910.x.
138. Neale GA, Pui CH, Mahmoud HH, Mirro J Jr, Crist WM, Rivera GK, Goorha RM. Molecular evidence for minimal residual bone marrow disease in children with 'isolated' extra-medullary relapse of T-cell acute lymphoblastic leukemia. Leukemia. 1994;8(5):768–75.
139. Ritchey AK, Pollock BH, Lauer SJ, Andejeski Y, Barredo J, Buchanan GR. Improved survival of children with isolated CNS relapse of acute lymphoblastic leukemia: a pediatric oncology group study. J Clin Oncol Off J Am Soc Clin Oncol. 1999;17(12):3745–52.
140. Ribeiro RC, Rivera GK, Hudson M, Mulhern RK, Hancock ML, Kun L, Mahmoud H, Sandlund JT, Crist WM, Pui CH. An intensive re-treatment protocol for children with an isolated CNS relapse of acute lymphoblastic leukemia. J Clin Oncol Off J Am Soc Clin Oncol. 1995;13(2):333–8. https://doi.org/10.1200/JCO.1995.13.2.333.
141. Barredo JC, Devidas M, Lauer SJ, Billett A, Marymont M, Pullen J, et al. Isolated CNS relapse of acute lymphoblastic leukemia treated with intensive systemic chemotherapy and delayed CNS radiation: a pediatric oncology group study. J Clin Oncol. 2006;24:3142–9.
142. Lew G, Chen Y, Lu X, Rheingold SR, Whitlock JA, Devidas M, Hastings CA, Winick NJ, Carroll WL, Wood BL, Borowitz MJ, Pulsipher MA, Hunger SP. Outcomes after late bone marrow and very early central nervous system relapse of childhood B-acute lymphoblastic leukemia: a report from the Children's Oncology Group phase III study AALL0433. Haematologica. 2020; https://doi.org/10.3324/haematol.2019.237230.
143. Masurekar AN, Parker CA, Shanyinde M, Moorman AV, Hancock JP, Sutton R, Ancliff PJ, Morgan M, Goulden NJ, Fraser C, Hoogerbrugge PM, Revesz T, Darbyshire PJ, Krishnan S, Love SB, Saha V. Outcome of central nervous system relapses in childhood acute lymphoblastic leukaemia--prospective open cohort analyses of the ALLR3 trial. PLoS One. 2014;9(10):e108107. https://doi.org/10.1371/journal.pone.0108107.
144. Brown PA, Ji L, Xu X, Devidas M, et al. A randomized phase 3 trial of blinatumomab vs. chemotherapy as post-reinduction therapy in high and intermediate risk (HR/IR) first relapse of B-acute lymphoblastic leukemia (B-ALL) in children and adolescents/young adults (AYAs) demonstrates superior efficacy and tolerability of blinatumomab: a report from Children's Oncology Group study AALL1331. Blood. 2019;134(Supplement_2):LBA-1. https://doi.org/10.1182/blood-2019-132435.
145. Rheingold SR, Ji L, Xu X, Devidas M, et al (2019) Prognostic factors for survival after relapsed acute lymphoblastic leukemia (ALL): a Children's Oncology Group (COG) study. Paper presented at the ASCO Annual Meeting, 31 May 2019.

146. Surapaneni UR, Cortes JE, Thomas D, O'Brien S, Giles FJ, Koller C, Faderl S, Kantarjian H. Central nervous system relapse in adults with acute lymphoblastic leukemia. Cancer. 2002;94(3):773–9.
147. Fielding AK, Richards SM, Chopra R, Lazarus HM, Litzow MR, et al. Outcome of 609 adults after relapse of acute lymphoblastic leukemia (ALL); an MRC UKALL12/ECOG 2993 study. Blood. 2007;109(3):944–50. https://doi.org/10.1182/blood-2006-05-018192.
148. Bleyer WA, Poplack DG, Simon RM. "Concentration x time" methotrexate via a subcutaneous reservoir: a less toxic regimen for intraventricular chemotherapy of central nervous system neoplasms. Blood. 1978;51(5):835–42.
149. Moser AM, Adamson PC, Gillespie AJ, Poplack DG, Balis FM. Intraventricular concentration times time (C x T) methotrexate and cytarabine for patients with recurrent meningeal leukemia and lymphoma. Cancer. 1998;85(2):511–6.
150. Phuphanich S, Maria B, Braeckman R, Chamberlain M. A pharmacokinetic study of intra-CSF administered encapsulated cytarabine (DepoCyt) for the treatment of neoplastic meningitis in patients with leukemia, lymphoma, or solid tumors as part of a phase III study. J Neuro-Oncol. 2007;81(2):201–8. https://doi.org/10.1007/s11060-006-9218-x.
151. Bomgaars L, Geyer JR, Franklin J, Dahl G, Park J, Winick NJ, Klenke R, Berg SL, Blaney SM. Phase I trial of intrathecal liposomal cytarabine in children with neoplastic meningitis. J Clin Oncol Off J Am Soc Clin Oncol. 2004;22(19):3916–21. https://doi.org/10.1200/JCO.2004.01.046.
152. Seif AE, Reilly AF, Rheingold SR. Intrathecal liposomal cytarabine in relapsed or refractory infant and pediatric leukemias: the Children's Hospital of Philadelphia experience and review of the literature. J Pediatr Hematol Oncol. 2010;32(8):e349–52. https://doi.org/10.1097/MPH.0b013e3181ec0c25.
153. Parasole R, Petruzziello F, Messina C, Barisone E, et al. Toxicity and efficacy of intrathecal liposomal cytarabine in children with leukemia/lymphoma relapsing in the central nervous system: a retrospective multicenter study. Leuk Lymphoma. 2015;56(3):650–5. https://doi.org/10.3109/10428194.2014.927456.
154. Salehi B, Selamoglu Z, Mileski KS, Pezzani R, Redaelli M, Cho WC, Kobarfard F, Rajabi S, Martorell M, Kumar P, Martins N, Subhra Santra T, Sharifi-Rad J. Liposomal cytarabine as cancer therapy: from chemistry to medicine. Biomol Ther. 2019;9(12) https://doi.org/10.3390/biom9120773.
155. Heideman RL, Cole DE, Balis F, Sato J, Reaman GH, Packer RJ, et al. Phase I and pharmacokinetic evaluation of thiotepa in the cerebrospinal fluid and plasma of pediatric patients: evidence for dose- dependent plasma clearance of thiotepa. Cancer Res. 1989;49:736–41.
156. Chamberlain MC. A review of leptomeningeal metastases in pediatrics. J Child Neurol. 1995;10:191–9.
157. Balis FM, Holcenberg JS, Poplack DG. Intrathecal chemotherapy. In: Pizzo PA, Poplack DG, editors. Principles and practice of pediatric oncology. 3rd ed. Philadelphia: Lippincott-Raven; 1997. p. 256–7.
158. Blaney SM, Balis FM, Poplack DG. Pharmacologic approaches to the treatment of meningeal malignancy. Oncology. 1991;5:107–16.
159. DeAngelis LM. Current diagnosis and treatment of leptomeningeal metastasis. J Neuro-Oncol. 1998;38:245–52.
160. Grossman SA, Moynihan TJ. Neoplastic meningitis. Neurol Clin. 1991;4:843–56.
161. Chamberlain MC. Pediatric leptomeningeal metastases: outcome following combined therapy. J Child Neurol. 1997;12(1):53–9. https://doi.org/10.1177/088307389701200109.
162. Gutin PHWH, Wiernik PH, et al. Intrathecal N, N[precedes], N″-triethylenethiophosphoramide (thio-tepa [N6396]) in the treatment of malignant meningeal disease: phase I-II study. Cancer. 1976;38:1471–5.
163. Ochocka MBM, Ciepelewska D. Thiotepa in the treatment of central nervous system leukemia in children. Acta Haematol Pol. 1978;9:263–7.

164. Shukla N, Kobos R, Renaud T, Steinherz LJ, Steinherz PG. Phase II trial of clofarabine with topotecan, vinorelbine, and thiotepa in pediatric patients with relapsed or refractory acute leukemia. Pediatr Blood Cancer. 2014;61(3):431–5. https://doi.org/10.1002/pbc.24789.
165. Srour SA, Borders EB, Cherry MA, Holter J, et al. Role of topotecan, vinorelbine, thiotepa and gemcitabine chemotherapy in relapsed/refractory adult acute leukemia. Leuk Lymphoma. 2015;56(10):2962–4. https://doi.org/10.3109/10428194.2015.1018250.
166. Schultz KR, Bowman WP, Aledo A, Slayton WB, et al. Improved early event-free survival with imatinib in Philadelphia chromosome-positive acute lymphoblastic leukemia: a Children's Oncology Group study. J Clin Oncol Off J Am Soc Clin Oncol. 2009;27(31):5175–81. https://doi.org/10.1200/JCO.2008.21.2514.
167. Mele G, Pinna S, Melpignano A, Romano A, Brocca MC, Coppi MR, Quarta G. What is the best salvage therapy for treatment of isolated CNS relapse in elderly patients with imatinib-responsive Ph(+) ALL? Leuk Res. 2007;31(10):1445–7. https://doi.org/10.1016/j.leukres.2007.03.018.
168. Wolff NC, Richardson JA, Egorin M, Ilaria RL Jr. The CNS is a sanctuary for leukemic cells in mice receiving imatinib mesylate for Bcr/Abl-induced leukemia. Blood. 2003;101(12):5010–3. https://doi.org/10.1182/blood-2002-10-3059.
169. Porkka K, Koskenvesa P, Lundán T, et al. Dasatinib crosses the blood–brain barrier and is an efficient therapy for central nervous system Philadelphia chromosome-positive leukemia. Blood. 2008;112:1005–12.
170. Pagan FL, Hebron ML, Wilmarth B, Torres-Yaghi Y, et al. Pharmacokinetics and pharmacodynamics of a single dose Nilotinib in individuals with Parkinson's disease. Pharmacol Res Perspect. 2019;7(2):e00470. https://doi.org/10.1002/prp2.470.
171. Lai SW, Huang TC, Chen JH, Wu YY, Chang PY. Dasatinib as the salvage therapy for chronic myeloid leukemia with blast crisis and central nervous system involvement: a case report. Oncol Lett. 2015;9(4):1957–61. https://doi.org/10.3892/ol.2015.2928.
172. Reinwald M, Schleyer E, Kiewe P, Blau IW, et al. Efficacy and pharmacologic data of second-generation tyrosine kinase inhibitor nilotinib in BCR-ABL-positive leukemia patients with central nervous system relapse after allogeneic stem cell transplantation. Biomed Res Int. 2014:637059. https://doi.org/10.1155/2014/637059.
173. Abid MB, De Mel S. Does ponatinib cross the blood-brain barrier? Br J Haematol. 2017;179(3):497–8. https://doi.org/10.1111/bjh.14222.
174. Laramy JK, Kim M, Parrish KE, Sarkaria JN, Elmquist WF. Pharmacokinetic assessment of cooperative efflux of the multitargeted kinase inhibitor ponatinib across the blood-brain barrier. J Pharmacol Exp Ther. 2018;365(2):249–61. https://doi.org/10.1124/jpet.117.246116.
175. Ajayi S, Becker H, Reinhardt H, Engelhardt M, Zeiser R, von Bubnoff N, Wäsch R. Ruxolitinib. Recent Results Cancer Res. 2018;212:119–32. https://doi.org/10.1007/978-3-319-91439-8_6.
176. Maese L, Raetz EA. Can Ph-like ALL be effectively targeted? Best Pract Res Clin Haematol. 2019;32(4):101096. https://doi.org/10.1016/j.beha.2019.101096.
177. Tasian SK, Teachey DT, Li Y, Shen F, et al. Potent efficacy of combined PI3K/mTOR and JAK or ABL inhibition in murine xenograft models of Ph-like acute lymphoblastic leukemia. Blood. 2017;129(2):177–87. https://doi.org/10.1182/blood-2016-05-707653.
178. Walker KL, Kabakov SA, Zhu F, Bouchlaka MN, Olson SL, Cho MM, Quamine AE, Feils AS, Gavcovich TB, Rui L, Capitini CM. Efficacy of JAK1/2 and BCL2 inhibition on human T cell acute lymphoblastic leukemia in vitro and in vivo. bioRxiv. 2019:734913. https://doi.org/10.1101/734913.
179. Parrish KE, Pokorny J, Mittapalli RK, Bakken K, Sarkaria JN, Elmquist WF. Efflux transporters at the blood-brain barrier limit delivery and efficacy of cyclin-dependent kinase 4/6 inhibitor palbociclib (PD-0332991) in an orthotopic brain tumor model. J Pharmacol Exp Ther. 2015;355(2):264–71. https://doi.org/10.1124/jpet.115.228213.
180. Yin L, Li H, Liu W, Yao Z, Cheng Z, Zhang H, Zou H. A highly potent CDK4/6 inhibitor was rationally designed to overcome blood brain barrier in glioblastoma therapy. Eur J Med Chem. 2018;144:1–28. https://doi.org/10.1016/j.ejmech.2017.12.003.

181. Horton TM, Whitlock JA, Lu X, O'Brien MM, Borowitz MJ, Devidas M, Raetz EA, Brown PA, Carroll WL, Hunger SP. Bortezomib reinduction chemotherapy in high-risk ALL in first relapse: a report from the Children's Oncology Group. Br J Haematol. 2019;186(2):274–85. https://doi.org/10.1111/bjh.15919.
182. Gozzetti A, Papini G, Candi V, Brambilla CZ, Sirianni S, Bocchia M. Second generation proteasome inhibitors in multiple myeloma. Anti Cancer Agents Med Chem. 2017;17(7):920–6. https://doi.org/10.2174/1871520616666160902101622.
183. Harrison SJ, Mainwaring P, Price T, Millward MJ, Padrik P, Underhill CR, Cannell PK, Reich SD, Trikha M, Spencer A. Phase I clinical trial of marizomib (NPI-0052) in patients with advanced malignancies including multiple myeloma: study NPI-0052-102 final results. Clin Cancer Res. 2016;22(18):4559–66. https://doi.org/10.1158/1078-0432.CCR-15-2616.
184. Lampson LA. Monoclonal antibodies in neuro-oncology: getting past the blood-brain barrier. MAbs. 2011;3(2):153–60.
185. Kantarjian H, Stein A, Gökbuget N, Fielding AK, et al. Blinatumomab versus chemotherapy for advanced acute lymphoblastic leukemia. N Engl J Med. 2017;376(9):836–47. https://doi.org/10.1056/NEJMoa1609783.
186. Bride KL, Vincent TL, Im SY, Aplenc R, Barrett DM, et al. Preclinical efficacy of daratumumab in T-cell acute lymphoblastic leukemia. Blood. 2018;131(9):995–9. https://doi.org/10.1182/blood-2017-07-794214.
187. Ganzel C, Kharit M, Duksin C, Rowe JM. Daratumumab for relapsed/refractory Philadelphia-positive acute lymphoblastic leukemia. Haematologica. 2018;103(10):e489–90. https://doi.org/10.3324/haematol.2018.197640.
188. Kantarjian HM, DeAngelo DJ, Stelljes M, Martinelli G, et al. Inotuzumab ozogamicin versus standard therapy for acute lymphoblastic leukemia. N Engl J Med. 2016;375(8):740–53. https://doi.org/10.1056/NEJMoa1509277.
189. He X, Xiao X, Li Q, Jiang Y, et al. Anti-CD19 CAR-T as a feasible and safe treatment against central nervous system leukemia after intrathecal chemotherapy in adults with relapsed or refractory B-ALL. Leukemia. 2019;33(8):2102–4. https://doi.org/10.1038/s41375-019-0437-5.
190. Lee DW, Kochenderfer JN, Stetler-Stevenson M, Cui YK, et al. T cells expressing CD19 chimeric antigen receptors for acute lymphoblastic leukaemia in children and young adults: a phase 1 dose-escalation trial. Lancet. 2015;385(9967):517–28. https://doi.org/10.1016/S0140-6736(14)61403-3.
191. Supko JG, Malspeis L. Dose-dependent pharmacokinetics of rapamycin-28-N,N-dimethylglycinate in the mouse. Cancer Chemother Pharmacol. 1994;33(4):325–30. https://doi.org/10.1007/bf00685908.
192. Houchens DP, Ovejera AA, Riblet SM, Slagel DE. Human brain tumor xenografts in nude mice as a chemotherapy model. Eur J Cancer Clin Oncol. 1983;19(6):799–805. https://doi.org/10.1016/0277-5379(83)90012-3.
193. Gunosewoyo H, Yu L, Munoz L, Kassiou M. Kinase targets in CNS drug discovery. Future Med Chem. 2017;9(3):303–14. https://doi.org/10.4155/fmc-2016-0214.
194. Zhao H, Cui K, Nie F, et al. The effect of mTOR inhibition alone or combined with MEK inhibitors on brain metastasis: an in vivo analysis in triple-negative breast cancer models. Breast Cancer Res Treat. 2012;131(2):425–36. https://doi.org/10.1007/s10549-011-1420-7.
195. Rubenstein JL, Combs D, Rosenberg J, Levy A, et al. Rituximab therapy for CNS lymphomas: targeting the leptomeningeal compartment. Blood. 2003;101(2):466–8. https://doi.org/10.1182/blood-2002-06-1636.
196. Scheibe F, Ostendorf L, Reincke SM, Prüss H, von Brünneck AC, Köhnlein M, Alexander T, Meisel C, Meisel A. Daratumumab treatment for therapy-refractory anti-CASPR2 encephalitis. J Neurol. 2020;267(2):317–23. https://doi.org/10.1007/s00415-019-09585-6.
197. Wong ET. Monoclonal antibody therapy for central nervous system lymphomas: an emerging treatment paradigm. Expert Opin Pharmacother. 2005;6(7):1107–14. https://doi.org/10.1517/14656566.6.7.1107.

198. Aldoss I, Song J, Stiller T, Nguyen T, et al. Correlates of resistance and relapse during blinatumomab therapy for relapsed/refractory acute lymphoblastic leukemia. Am J Hematol. 2017;92(9):858–65. https://doi.org/10.1002/ajh.24783.
199. Schultz L, Gardner R. Mechanisms of and approaches to overcoming resistance to immunotherapy. Hematology Am Soc Hematol Educ Program. 2019;1:226–32. https://doi.org/10.1182/hematology.2019000018.
200. Fry TJ, Shah NN, Orentas RJ, et al. CD22-targeted CAR T cells induce remission in B-ALL that is naive or resistant to CD19-targeted CAR immunotherapy. Nat Med. 2018;24(1):20–8. https://doi.org/10.1038/nm.44412018.

Chapter 12
Late Effects of Therapy of Acute Lymphoblastic Leukemia

Liv Andrés-Jensen, Christoffer Johansen, and Kjeld Schmiegelow

Abbreviations

AAP	asparaginase-associated pancreatitis
ALL	acute lymphoblastic leukemia
BMD	bone mineral density
CCSS	Childhood Cancer Survivor Study
CIPN	chemotherapy induced peripheral neuropathy
CNS	central nervous system
CTCAE	United States National Cancer Institute Common Terminology Criteria for Adverse Events
HD	high dose
hSCT	hematopoietic stem cell transplantation
MetS	metabolic syndrome
MRI	magnetic resonance imaging
MTX	methotrexate

L. Andrés-Jensen
Department of Pediatrics and Adolescent Medicine, University Hospital Rigshospitalet, Copenhagen, Denmark

C. Johansen
Institute of Clinical Medicine, Faculty of Health and Medical Sciences, University of Copenhagen, Copenhagen, Denmark

Department of Oncology, University Hospital Rigshospitalet, Copenhagen, Denmark

K. Schmiegelow (✉)
Department of Pediatrics and Adolescent Medicine, University Hospital Rigshospitalet, Copenhagen, Denmark

Institute of Clinical Medicine, Faculty of Health and Medical Sciences, University of Copenhagen, Copenhagen, Denmark
e-mail: kschmiegelow@rh.dk

M. R. Litzow, E. A. Raetz (eds.), *Clinical Management of Acute Lymphoblastic Leukemia*, https://doi.org/10.1007/978-3-030-85147-7_12

NMDAR	N-methyl-D-aspartate receptor
ON	osteonecrosis
OS	overall survival
PEG	polyethylene glycol
PRES	posterior reversible encephalopathy syndrome
PTWG	Ponte di Legno Toxicity Working Group
QoL	quality of life
RCT	randomized controlled trial
SLS	stroke-like syndrome
SOS	sinusoidal obstruction syndrome
STFS	severe toxicity free survival
TBI	total body irradiation
TE	thromboembolism
UNL	upper normal limit

Introduction

The best contemporary chemotherapy for childhood acute lymphoblastic leukemia (ALL) yields 5-year overall survival (OS) rates above 90%, which reflects intensified chemotherapy with treatment stratification directed by the mutational landscape of the leukemic clone and the early response to chemotherapy, better use of conventional antileukemic agents, introduction of molecularly targeted drugs, refined strategies for hematopoietic stem cell transplantation (hSCT), and improved supportive care [1, 2]. However, the high cure rate has come at a price [3–5]. All patients encounter severe acute toxicities during therapy, mostly infections but frequently also severe organ dysfunctions [6], and a significant proportion of survivors are burdened by late effects [7]. Whereas high-throughput, cost-effective technologies have revolutionized our insight into the mutations driving ALL pathogenesis and drug resistance [8], our biological understanding of late effects remains limited, thus hindering further personalized therapy to reduce their incidence. This partly reflects their individual relative rarity (requiring multi-institutional and international research), complex pathogenesis, and uncertain associations with potential risk factors, including germline DNA variant profiles [9, 10].

The Toxicity Scenario

Toxicities have traditionally been defined and graded according to the United States National Cancer Institute Common Terminology Criteria for Adverse Events [11], although some research groups (e.g., St. Jude LIFE [12] and the PTWG [13]) have adapted these to better address toxicities relating to childhood cancer in general or to childhood ALL patients specifically. Several of the late effects are long-term consequences of acute toxicities that occurred during chemotherapy (e.g., insulin-dependent diabetes pancreatitis) [14], while others may emerge after discontinuation of therapy (e.g., osteonecrosis or second cancers) [15, 16].

Pattern of Late Effects

Parallel to changes in antileukemic therapy, the pattern of late effects has changed dramatically over the last decades [7]. Hematopoietic stem cell transplantation (hSCT) and prophylactic and therapeutic cranial irradiation are used less frequently with the latter being completely eliminated in many first-line protocols [17], while the use of glucocorticosteroids (including dexamethasone) and asparaginase has been intensified. Consequently, second cancers in the central nervous system (CNS), cognitive disturbances, reduced growth, and hypothalamic/pituitary dysfunction have become rarer, while osteonecrosis, musculoskeletal dysfunction, and endocrine disturbances have become more frequent (Fig. 12.1). The long-term impact on late effects of the more recently introduced immunotherapies, including chimeric antigen receptor modified T cells, is yet to be determined [18, 19].

Many late effect studies only address subsets of patients, one or a few specific late effects, are cross-sectional, or emerge from single institutions with limited study power. Since survival has become the most likely outcome for a child with

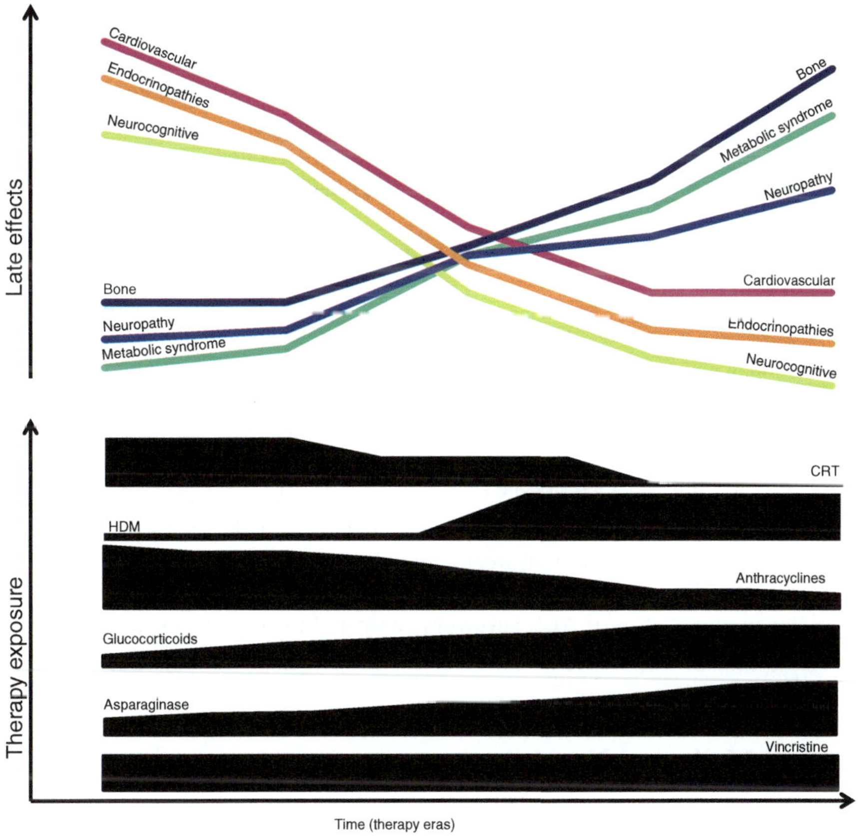

Fig. 12.1 Temporal changes in therapy exposure and late effects. *CRT* cranial radiation therapy, *HDM* high-dose methotrexate

ALL, systematic, longitudinal follow-up is of paramount importance. However, only a few very large (>10,000 patients), multi-institutional childhood cancer survivor cohort studies exist such as the US Childhood Cancer Survivor Study (www.ccss.stjude.org), the Nordic Adult Life after Childhood Cancer in Scandinavia (www.aliccs.org), and the British Childhood Cancer Survivor Study [20].

Severe Toxicity Free Survival

As survival rates are high for children with ALL, there is a need for supplementing traditional outcome measures (OS and EFS with events encompassing resistant disease, relapse and second malignancies) with severe and persisting late effects to reflect not only survival but also the cost of cure. Until recently, no international consensus have existed to guide a standardized capture of even the most severe late effects. Addressing this issue, the Ponte di Legno consortium, representing 17 major ALL childhood study groups and institutions across North America, Europe, Japan, Taiwan, and Australia, recently published a prioritized list and consensus definitions of 21 severe toxicities proposed to be captured and reported as an integrated part of the outcome evaluation of treatment protocols [21]. The measure of severe toxicity free survival (STFS) focuses on the most serious and objective late effects, while subsequent and more comprehensive (but also more complex) targets should include the lower-grade (equally burdensome), chronic, subjective late effects such as fatigue, pain, self-reported quality of life (QoL), and overall measures of the ability to comply with routine activities of daily living.

Late Deaths

Case-control and cohort studies of childhood cancer survivors have shown that even 15 years after cessation of therapy, the majority of deaths are caused by cancer or its treatment and only approximately 20% by non-neoplasia-related causes with an absolute excess risk of 6.2 per 1000 person-years [22, 23]. Importantly, for 5-year survivors of childhood ALL, the 15 years cumulative risk of recurrence has dropped from 10.2% in the 1970s to 2.2% for patients diagnosed in the 1990s parallel to the refinement and intensification of treatment, whereas the risk of death from health-related causes has stayed almost unchanged at 2–3% [24]. Accordingly, the life expectancy gap for 5-year ALL survivors compared to controls has dropped from 14.7 years in 1970–1979 to just 8 years in more recent years.

Second Malignant Neoplasm

In nationwide population- and register-based Nordic studies, the overall standardized incidence rate of second primary cancers is 3.3 times that of the background population, being increased in all age groups, even after the age of 70 years. Still, the reported frequency of second cancer (SMN) after ALL therapy is in the order of only 2% and dominated by second myeloid neoplasia. Importantly, the frequency of SMN is generally underestimated due to insufficient duration of follow-up. Thus, in a large international study of 642 childhood ALL survivors with SMN, 80% of hematological malignancies (3/4 being therapy-related acute myeloid leukemia (AML) and myelodysplasia (MDS)) occurred within 5 years from diagnosis of ALL, 80% of CNS tumors (except meningiomas) and sarcoma had occurred 12 years from diagnosis, while 16 years had to pass before 80% of carcinomas had been diagnosed (and even later for non-thyroid carcinomas) [16]. Patients with CNS tumors or therapy-related myeloid neoplasia had 5-year overall survival rates in the order of only 20%, but in contrast to CNS tumors, myeloid neoplasias demonstrated clear improvement in survival over time (34.1% ± 6.3% for AML and 48.2% ± 10.6% for MDS diagnosed after 2000) and were furthermore positively associated with the lag time from ALL diagnosis (10% drop in death hazard per year of interval). Importantly, 5-year survival rates were above 90% for patients with meningioma, Hodgkin lymphoma, thyroid carcinoma, basal cell carcinoma, and parotid gland tumor and were almost 70% for non Hodgkin lymphoma, i.e., very similar to their primary counterparts. Development of solid tumors is associated with cyclophosphamide exposure, whereas AML/MDS are associated with topoisomerase II inhibitor exposure and higher starting doses of methotrexate/mercaptopurine for maintenance therapy. The role of germline DNA variants is only beginning to emerge.

The Overall Burden of Antileukemic Therapy

According to the largest, prospective, clinical follow-up study among childhood ALL survivors, the 30-year-old survivor will have experienced an average of 5.7 recurring or chronic health events compared to only 2.0 in matched controls (at age 50 years, these figures have risen to 16.7 and 9.3, respectively) [7]. As the long-term morbidities we see today echo protocols used decades ago, further prospective, longitudinal research is needed to reveal the true burden of current childhood ALL regimens.

Endocrine Late Effects

Risk of hospital contact for endocrine disorders has been evaluated among >30.000 1-year Nordic childhood cancer survivors, revealing that survivors of leukemia and CNS tumors are the ones at highest risk [25]. The leukemia survivors were at significantly elevated risk for hospital contact relating to pituitary disorders, testicular dysfunction, and other disorders of puberty, reflecting therapy regimens using substantial amounts of cranial and testicular irradiation, which is becoming abandoned today.

Growth

Cranial and spinal irradiation causes the highest risk for reduced final height, as spinal irradiation inhibits vertebral growth directly resulting in reduced sitting height (larger impact with younger age), whereas cranial irradiation compromises growth via the hypothalamic-pituitary axis resulting in growth hormone deficiency, precocious puberty, and hypothyroidism [26]. Height reduction after cranial irradiation is dose-dependent and most consistently reported after doses ≥24 Gy, whereas no lower safe threshold has been determined [27]. Similarly, growth hormone deficiency has been reported more consistently after treatment with >24 Gy cranial irradiation than after doses of 18 Gy. The odds rate of clinical short stature below −2 SD is proportional to the extent of irradiation being 2.8 (95% confidence interval (CI) 1.9–4.0) for spinal irradiation, 2.9 (CI 2.0–4.2) for cranial irradiation, 8.0 (CI 3.7–17.4) for total body irradiation (TBI) in association with hSCT, and 10.6 (CI 4.25–25.3) for cranial irradiation and TBI [28].

Growth suppression from chemotherapy alone is frequently seen during treatment but is typically followed by subsequent catch-up growth and achievement of adult height within the normal range [26, 27, 29]. Risk factors associated with reduced final height in both irradiated and non-irradiated survivors include female gender and younger age at diagnosis [28, 29]. Importantly, most studies of final adult height reflect protocols used during the 1970s–1990s, and follow-up of more recently treated patients is needed.

Thyroid Dysfunction

TBI and craniospinal irradiation with scatter to the thyroid gland can cause hypo- and, more rarely, hyperthyroidism. Although the risk of hypothyroidism 15 years from ALL diagnosis is reported at only 1.6% (CI 1.1–2.1), the rate is significantly increased compared with siblings [30]. Importantly, survivors treated with cranial irradiation or chemotherapy only do not seem to be at increased risk of thyroid dysfunction [27, 30, 31].

Metabolic Syndrome

Although the applied definitions vary, several studies have reported increased rates of obesity, disproportional alterations in body composition (sarcopenic obesity), hypertension, dyslipidemia, and metabolic syndrome (MetS) among childhood ALL survivors [27, 29, 32–34]. One of the largest studies with 784 ALL survivors found MetS in 33% of adult survivors [35]. When compared to matched community controls ($N = 777$), survivors had a higher risk of MetS (relative risk [RR] 1.43, 95% [CI] 1.22–1.69), hypertension ([RR] 2.43, 95% [CI] 2.06–2.86), dyslipidemia ([RR]

1.40, 95% [CI] 1.23–1.59), obesity ([RR] 1.47, 95%[CI] 1.29–1.68), and insulin resistance (1.64, 95%[CI] 1.44–1.86). Risk factors include female gender, cranial irradiation, and older age at evaluation [33, 35]. The dysmetabolic effects of cranial irradiation is likely mediated by hypothalamic-pituitary dysregulation of leptin sensitivity and growth hormone deficiency [27, 32, 33]. Although radiotherapy is gradually being omitted from frontline childhood ALL protocols, it has been replaced by intensified glucocorticosteroid therapy and extended asparaginase exposure, thus replacing one risk factor for MetS by others [32, 36].

Corticosteroids can alter substrate oxidation and energy expenditure by suppressing growth hormone and inducing leptin resistance [27, 32, 37]. L-asparaginase reduces insulin secretion and plasma insulin levels while increasing insulin resistance, thereby acting synergistically with corticosteroids. In addition, asparaginase can cause acute pancreatitis (AAP) ultimately leading to insulin-dependent diabetes (type 3c). In a Nordic ALL cohort of 1285 patients exposed to 30 weeks of pegylated asparaginase, 6.8% developed AAP of whom 8% had persisting need of insulin therapy at a median follow-up of 4.6 years [38, 39]. In a study from the St. Jude Lifetime cohort including 1044 survivors with mean age at follow-up of 33.97 years, 7.5% were found to have type 2 diabetes mellitus (T2DM) compared to 3.8% in matched controls [40]. In that study, body mass index (BMI) $\geq$30 kg/m^2, older age, and drug-induced diabetes mellitus during ALL therapy were all associated with T2DM. Since dysmetabolic adverse effects generally emerge early during ALL therapy and furthermore are modifiable, they should be targeted throughout therapy and follow-up. There has been a lack of randomized clinical trials testing dietary and physical interventions to prevent or reduce MetS [41]; however such studies are now being performed.

Puberty and Fertility

In a large US-Canadian study of almost 11,000 5-year survivors of childhood cancer treated in 1970–1999 (median follow-up of 8 years (IQR 4–12)) and 4000 sibling controls, 38% of survivors reported a pregnancy, and 83% of these reported at least one live birth compared to 62% and 90% among siblings, respectively [42]. The most significant drugs associated with reduced likelihood of pregnancy were alkylating agents.

Male

Cranial irradiation disturbs the hypothalamic-pituitary-gonadal axis and can lead to pubertal disturbances, while antileukemic agents, especially alkylators, may cause testicular damage with the germinal epithelium being more sensitive than Leydig cells [43]. Thus, biopsy studies have found spermatogonia in only 50% of seminiferous tubuli and pathological sperm concentrations in patients with normal or only slightly reduced sex hormone levels [44, 45]. The most detrimental effects with azoospermia, Leydig cell insufficiency, and need for testosterone replacement are seen following direct testicular irradiation in cases of testicular relapse or as part of TBI [46]. Cranial irradiation does not seem to cause a higher frequency of oligo spermia or azoospermia when compared to chemotherapy only [47].

In survivors treated with chemotherapy only, Leydig cell function is rarely impaired, and survivors generally achieve normal puberty [44] with levels of gonadotropins and testosterone being similar to those of controls [46]. Cyclophosphamide is one of the most gonadotoxic antileukemic agents used; however risk of impaired sperm quality is considered to be low in survivors exposed to <8 mg/m^2 [46, 47]. Survivors treated with high doses of cyclophosphamide and/or testicular radiation have small chances of fathering a child unless using stored semen samples. However, for the remaining male ALL survivor population, risk of impaired fertility seems to be comparable to the background population [48]. According to the International Guideline Harmonization Group, survivors treated with one or more potentially gonadotoxic agents should be made aware of risk of testosterone deficiency and impaired spermatogenesis, those treated with irradiation exposing the testes to 12 Gy or more should be monitored for pubertal development, and those being exposed to cyclophosphamide and/or testicular radiation exposure should be offered semen analysis [49].

Females

In general, female ALL survivors who were premenarchal at diagnosis should expect to maintain ovarian function and achieve normal puberty (>90% achieve menarche within normal age range) [50, 51], unless exposed to high-dose alkylating agents and/or irradiation exposing the ovaries [52, 53].Thus, spinal irradiation with exposure of the ovaries and alkylating agents significantly increases the risk of premature ovarian failure and impaired fertility [54, 55]. One self-report study of fertility among 182 long-term ALL survivors indicated reduced fertility if treated with cranial radiation at any dose around the time of menarche [48]; however, ovarian dysfunction was not clinically validated. Two Danish studies examined ovarian function 10 years apart in 100 survivors of childhood cancer (47 with ALL) and found that survivors in spite of a reduced antral follicle count (AFC) in their mid-20s had a high chance of preserved ovarian function at least until their mid-30s, with more than 50% having achieved at least one live birth [56, 57]. However, as survivors generally had significantly lower AFC than age-matched controls, survivors may have a shortened reproductive span.

Risks relating to contemporary ALL therapy without spinal irradiation and with reduced doses of alkylating agents are more uncertain. Only a few clinical studies have investigated ovarian function in post-pubertal survivors treated with chemotherapy and no spinal irradiation at pre-pubertal age, finding subtle signs of ovarian insufficiency in some [58] and normal function in others [59]. International guidelines recommend systematic evaluations for signs indicating risk of premature menopause in post-pubertal survivors treated with potentially gonadotoxic chemotherapy and/or irradiation potentially exposing the ovaries [52].

Bone Morbidity

Osteoporosis

Although a few, small studies have reported little or no risk of osteoporosis among ALL survivors [60, 61], nearly all studies show that bone mineralization density (BMD) is frequently reduced. Risk factors include leukemia-related low BMD present at diagnosis [27], inadequate diet including lack of D-vitamin and calcium, low level of weight-bearing physical activity, intensive glucocorticosteroid and high-dose methotrexate exposure, and/or cranial irradiation. If patients fail to achieve expected normal peak bone mass during and following cessation of therapy, it is likely that reduced BMD and risk of osteoporotic fractures persist throughout life. Thus, a large St. Jude Lifetime Cohort study of 845 survivors found osteoporosis and osteopenia in 6% and 24%, respectively, at 31 years of age [62]. High-dose (≥24Gy) cranial or craniospinal irradiation was the strongest predictor of reduced BMD, while the cumulative dose of glucocorticoids was associated with significantly lower BMD in female survivors only. Importantly, 67% of those with osteoporosis improved by one or more BMD categories over a period of median 8.5 years, although the only provided advice consisted of physical activity and vitamin D and calcium supplementation. The clinical significance of low BMD has been emphasized in a prospective study of 186 ALL patients, finding that 16% had vertebral fractures at diagnosis and 26% had at least one low-trauma bone fracture within 4 years from diagnosis [63]. Significant risk factors predicting low-trauma fractures included corticosteroid exposure, low BMD z-score at diagnosis, and vertebral fracture at diagnosis. By 6 years follow-up, nearly 25% of patients had persistent vertebral deformity following vertebral fracture, more frequently affecting older children and cases with most severe vertebral collapse. Importantly, 23% had no or only partial vertebral body reshaping. Adults with vertebral deformity have been shown to be at high risk for chronic back pain and reduced mobility, but similar studies among childhood cancer survivors are lacking.

Osteonecrosis

Osteonecrosis (ON) is one of the most common and debilitating toxicities with potentially long-term impact on daily function and QoL. A marked rise in the incidence of ON coincided with the introduction of dexamethasone for delayed intensification. The overall incidence of clinical ON is reported as high as 17.6%, however with varying frequencies reflecting the proportion of adolescents (who are at highest risk), the antileukemic treatment regimens, and also the methodology for toxicity capture [64]. Prospective studies including only symptomatic cases report incidences of 10–16% among patients aged 10–15 years and 15–20% among patients aged >15 years [64]. Of note, the interval between diagnosis of ALL and of ON increases with older age [15]. The most common joints affected are knees (45–88% of cases) and hips (35–67%), followed by ankles (13–44%), shoulders (13–24%), and elbows (3–15%). Affection of multiple joints is seen in 29–90% of cases [64]. The underlying pathology of ON is poorly understood but is thought to reflect hypoperfusion caused by microvascular clotting (intraluminal obliteration), increased marrow pressure (extraluminal obliteration), and direct damage to the endothelial and smooth muscle cells in the nurturing arteries, caused by chemotherapy agents and systemic inflammation. In addition, chemotherapy, such as glucocorticoids, is thought to have a direct toxic effect on osteocytes and compromising normal osteogenesis. The strongest risk factors for ON is female sex and adolescent age, but also occurrence of hyperlipidemia [65], glucocorticoid exposure (cumulative dose and exposure time), cranial and gonadal irradiation, and race. The significance of obesity, BMI, and leukemic bone infiltration is so far insufficiently validated [64, 66]. Trials implementing shortening of continuous exposure to dexamethasone found a reduced occurrence of ON, however also significantly better EFS among the high-exposure patients with high incidence of ON [64]. Many ON cases occur after cessation of therapy, not least in the older patients [15], but few studies have addressed long-term incidence and impact of ON on QoL among childhood ALL survivors. One self-report study among 20-year survivors found a cumulative incidence of 0.2% in individuals aged <10 years at diagnosis and of 2.8% in patients ≥16 years at diagnosis, compared to 0.03% among siblings [66]. Studies among adults with ON indicate that lesions involving ≥30% of the articular surface are the most likely to cause joint collapse with need of arthroplasty surgery [67]; however long-term follow-up studies among children are lacking.

Teeth

Long-term dental abnormalities such as tooth agenesis, arrested root development, microdontia, and enamel dysplasia can occur in as many as 34–94%, not least among survivors treated with TBI and/or cranial irradiation and with age below 5 years being a significant risk factor [68, 69]. Even very low radiation doses (1–3 Gy) can permanently damage ameloblasts and halt tooth development, and cranial radiation may also cause craniofacial developmental disturbances due to deficient mandibular development. Still, few studies have addressed the long-term dental outcome among survivors treated with chemotherapy only. In one study of 111 survivors not receiving irradiation, 28–45% was found to have microdontia, disturbed root development, or enamel hypoplasia [70]. Diagnosis at or before 5 years of age and cumulative doses of anthracyclines >120 mg/m^2 (potentially reflecting the impact of severe mucositis and altered oral microbiome) were strongly associated with more severe dental aberrations, whereas survivors diagnosed with ALL above the age of 5 years experienced caries in their permanent dentition.

Neurotoxicity

Neurocognitive Effects

Significant proportions (16–50%) of childhood ALL survivors have impaired neurocognitive performance across a range of domains, which is associated with reduced chance of educational achievements and employment [71–73]. Neurocognitive impairment is predominantly found in non-verbal domains such as attention, visual perception, memory, and concept formation, while verbal skills are mostly spared [74]. Cranial irradiation has the most significant impact on brain morphology and neurocognitive outcome. Although there is a positive correlation between the dose of irradiation and degree of neurotoxicity, no lower safe limit has been defined. Furthermore, the neurotoxicity is enhanced, when irradiation is combined with neurotoxic chemotherapy, probably reflecting radiation-induced increased blood-brain barrier permeability. Even with decreasing use of irradiation, late neurotoxicity is reported in up to 10–30% of survivors [74, 75]. A meta-analysis of 10 studies, including a total of 509 survivors treated with chemotherapy only, concluded that compared to controls, at mean 8 years from diagnosis, survivors had moderate deficits in several neurocognitive domains including working memory, information procession speed, and fine motor functioning, with intelligence being most affected (IQ deficits of 6–8 points) [76]. Neurocognitive performance has rarely been evaluated longitudinally; however one study found that the pattern of affected neurocognitive domains changed over time and that degree and type of neurocognitive impairment at the end of therapy could not predict later impairment [77]. The three most neurotoxic chemotherapeutic agents responsible for late neurocognitive deficits are cytarabine, corticosteroids, and methotrexate given intrathecally or as high dose intravenously. The exact underlying pathophysiological pathways are not fully understood. Animal models have suggested that nucleoside analogs have a presynaptic depressant effect in neuronal tissues in addition to a direct toxic and apoptotic effect [74]. Antifolate disruption of normal folate physiology within the CNS causes direct neurotoxicity, including demyelination. Younger age at treatment is associated with Late effects of therapy neurotoxicity Neurotoxicity increased neurotoxicity of both CNS-directed chemotherapy and irradiation, potentially reflecting disturbed myelination in the maturing brain [73]. Intrathecal liposomal cytarabine could be less neurotoxic than methotrexate [78]. Corticosteroids are thought to exert deleterious effects on hippocampus, acting synergistically with the excitatory neurotransmitters which are seen elevated in cases of acute neurotoxicity.

Abnormalities are found in up to 78% of survivors, when systematic cerebral imaging is performed [74]; however no substantial longitudinal studies exist that describe persistence versus resolution over time. Findings include calcifications, atrophy, leukoencephalopathy, focal perfusion defects, and changes in glucose metabolism. Radiologic findings sometimes parallel histological abnormalities including demyelination, necrosis, and astrocytosis and can correlate with cerebral spinal fluid biomarkers of brain injury. However, correlations between imaging findings and neurocognitive outcome have in general not been found, although one study of 190 ALL survivors did find a significant association between screening-positive leukoencephalopathy during therapy and poorer neurocognitive performance at 5 years follow-up [79].

Peripheral Neuropathy

Chemotherapy-induced peripheral neuropathy (CIPN), experienced by most patients during treatment, is mainly caused by vincristine (VCR), and other antileukemic and supportive care drugs (such as antifungal azoles, increasingly used over the last decades) can modulate VCR pharmacokinetics and thus enhance both central and peripheral neurotoxicities. VCR exerts its antineoplastic effect by binding to mitotic β-tubulin, thereby disrupting mitotic microtubule aggregation in leukemic cells, leading to mitotic arrest and cell death. One β-tubulin subtype is found exclusively in neuronal axons, and the neurotoxic effect of VCR stems, in part, from the drug binding to these, causing demyelination [80], axonal degeneration, and compromised axonal transport [81]. Chemotherapy-induced peripheral neuropathy involves both small and large fibers resulting in sensory, motor, and autonomic nerve dysfunction. Sensory symptoms include hypo-, hyper-, and paresthesia, thermal hypoesthesia, and neuropathic pain with the affected area presenting with a "stocking and glove" type distribution, reflecting how longer axons are affected first. Motor dysfunction presents as distal muscle weakness and atrophy, while autonomic nerve dysfunction can result in orthostatic hypotension, constipation, and sexual dysfunction. At the time of therapy cessation, around 30% will have clinical findings, such as depressed tendon reflexes [82]. With time, symptoms resolve in most patients; however persisting neuropathy can be found among survivors even years off therapy, and some studies have suggested that CIPN can emerge several years after cessation of chemotherapy, known as the coasting effect [83, 84]. Two to 10 years post therapy, neuropathic symptoms are reported among 30–60% of survivors, while clinical signs of neuropathy are found in 10–41%, nerve conduction abnormalities (mixed motor and sensory) in 15–68% [82, 83, 85–89], and both clinical and electrophysiological findings in 16% [88]. There seems to be poor correlation between self-reported symptoms and objective findings. Except for the association between higher cumulative doses of VCR and risk of long-term CIPN

[88], other potential risk factors for CIPN, such as age, gender, and presence of CNS leukemia, are not reported consistently. Impact of CIPN on motor performance and QoL is present in some studies [85, 86], while absent in others [88, 89], emphasizing that larger prospective follow-up studies are warranted.

Cardiovascular Late Effects

Increased risk of long-term cardiac disease, characterized mainly by dilated or restrictive cardiomyopathy, increased afterload, and arrhythmia, has primarily been associated with anthracycline exposure with cumulative doses ≥300 mg/m^2 [90], although no lower safe dose has been established [91]. Cardiomyocytes have limited capacity to regenerate and are thus vulnerable to the cytotoxic effect of anthracyclines, which can lead to apoptosis and ventricular wall thinning. Heart failure is reported in 1–16% of survivors treated with high-dose anthracyclines, although even with the low doses currently used, evaluation of true risk will require long-term follow-up [92]. The Swiss Childhood Cancer Survivor Study (CCSS) assessed self-reported cardiovascular disease among 511 5-year survivors diagnosed between 1976 and 2005 and found an overall odds ratio for cardiovascular disease of 1.9 (CI 1.3–2.8) and for heart failure of 13.9 (CI 1.8–107.4), when compared to siblings [93]. In contrast, a recent St. Jude study of 911 30-year survivors found cardiomyopathy in only 3%, which was comparable to the rate among community controls [7], likely reflecting the lower dose of anthracycline exposure in that study (mean 105 mg/m^2). Importantly, cardiac abnormalities may progress with time, not least after higher cumulative doses of anthracycline but also after low dose exposure [94, 95]. Additional risk factors for cardiotoxicity include TBI (as low as 5 Gy cardiac irradiation), young age at diagnosis, female gender, and presence of hypertension, obesity, and endocrinopathies [90]. Potential cardioprotective strategies include continuous anthracycline infusion (versus bolus), but long-term validation of the benefit hereof is lacking. Co-administration of the iron-chelating agent dexrazoxane, which prevents formation of free radicals, has been associated with fewer and less severe cardiac abnormalities on echocardiography 5 years post therapy without compromising EFS and may represent a useful future strategy to reduce long-term cardiac morbidity in the subset of children with ALL for whom anthracyclines are needed to ensure cure [90]. The antileukemic effect of anthracyclines as a single drug is well-established; however it is unclear whether and to which extent use of anthracyclines in contemporary multi-drug ALL protocols improves outcome. A 2014 Cochrane review found no evidence from randomized controlled trials (RCTs) to favor the use of anthracyclines in ALL therapy; however, as pointed out by the authors, this could be due to low power and short follow-up in the review, and results from ongoing and unpublished RCTs are awaited [96].

Pulmonary Late Effects

Symptomatic pulmonary late effects, including obstructive and restrictive ventilatory defects and impaired diffusion capacity, are rare except following TBI and high-dose alkylating agents in the setting of hSCT [97–99]. Patients exposed to chemotherapy only have been shown to have slight, subclinical, restrictive ventilatory insufficiency, being associated with younger age at treatment and more intensive protocols that include higher cumulative doses of anthracyclines, cytarabine, and cyclophosphamide [100]. However, for these survivors, lung function is generally within normal range [98].

Immune Reconstitution

Chemotherapy-induced dysfunction of humoral and cellular immune function (including leuko-, neutro-, and lymphopenia, hypogammaglobinemia, and abnormal levels of lymphocyte subsets and natural killer cells) is generally thought to resolve within 6–12 months from therapy cessation. Some studies have found immune deficits several years later; however no larger studies with long follow-up exist. Normalization of cell counts occurs before serum immunoglobulin levels, reflecting a longer recovery phase for B-cell function [101]. Several studies have reported a correlation between younger age at diagnosis and degree of immune deficiency during follow-up. A significant proportion of survivors lose pre-existing immunity (e.g., against measles, mumps, rubella, VZV) [102]. Revaccination does not restore immunity in all; however even subtherapeutic levels of antibodies have been shown to offer some protection. There is consensus to revaccinate transplanted survivors; however, no international guidelines exist regarding revaccination of non-hSCT survivors. An association between chemotherapy-induced microbial dysbiosis and immune dysregulation has been reported in recent, smaller studies, indicating a role of the microbiome in both impaired immune function and increased inflammation [103]. The prevalence of long-term immune deficiencies, not least B-cell dysfunction, may increase second to the intensified chemotherapy and wider use of immunotherapy [104]. Research assessing long-term outcome will be key to the understanding of this field.

Cellular Aging

In addition to the well-characterized organ-specific late effects, survivors are at risk for less uniformly defined conditions including moderate cognitive dysfunction, reduced muscle strength, and poor exercise tolerance, resulting in frailty – a state of reduced physiological reserve and a predecessor of chronic disease and early death [105]. The overall pattern of morbidity in childhood ALL survivors mimics the aging phenotype, however appearing decades before expected among survivors [106]. The highly complex aging process at a cellular level is still poorly understood; however nine tentative hallmarks of aging include genomic instability, telomere attrition, epigenetic alterations, loss of proteostasis, deregulated nutrient-sensing, mitochondrial dysfunction, cellular senescence, stem cell exhaustion, and altered intercellular communication [107]. Chemotherapy has been found to accelerate aging, through epigenetic alterations, DNA damage, reduced telomere length, and cellular senescence [108–110]. Few studies have investigated these hallmarks in childhood cancer survivors; however, both shortened telomere length, senescence, and chronic inflammation (which can both induce and result from cellular senescence) have been reported among childhood leukemia survivors, who were found to have a cellular phenotype similar to that observed in controls who were two to three decades older [111–113]. There is no gold standard when estimating age at the cellular level, since this field is still exploratory. However, emerging research may uncover shared underlying cellular mechanisms leading to frailty and age-related disease across several organs and risk profiles. Such findings could facilitate development and testing of interventions (senolytics), aiming to reduce the overall treatment-related burden among survivors.

Leukemia Predisposition

Recent research has identified several germline mutations in genes that play a critical role in hematopoiesis and lymphoid development, many of which are also frequently somatically mutated in ALL, such as *RAS*, *TP53*, *PAX5* [114, 115], *ETV6* [116, 117], *RUNX11* [118], *IKZF1* [119] and *DDX41* [120], which align with the findings of high subtype concordance in familial cases of ALL [121]. Combined, these syndromes may account for 5% of ALL cases, and more are expected to emerge in parallel with the growing number of patients being germline DNA sequenced and with an increasing understanding of the continuum between germline and acquired mutations.

Several of these syndromes are dominated by their non-malignant phenotype, including Down syndrome, ataxia telangiectasia and Nijmegen breakage syndrome, Recklinghausen neurofibromatosis, Noonan syndrome, constitutional biallelic mismatch repair syndrome, and Fanconi anemia, although not all have been diagnosed at the time ALL emerges. The most common ALL prone syndrome is Down syndrome, accounting for 2–3% of all childhood ALL cases [122]. It has been associated with excessive risk of acute toxicity [123], including treatment-related mortality, but long-term follow-up studies to map their late effects are lacking.

In general, the impact of ALL predisposing germline DNA variants on acute and late effects is poorly explored, but a few (*TP53*, *ETV6*, and *RUNX1*) seem associated with an increased risk of SMN [124, 125]. Thus, any patient with unusual, severe acute toxicities and/or SMN should be explored for an underlying leukemia-prone syndrome [126].

Common Germline DNA Variants

Multiple variants in germline DNA have been associated with the pharmacology of antileukemic agents, including the risk of toxicities [9, 14, 127], but their individual hazard ratios are generally low (<2.0), the variants are rare, or they lack replication in independent patient cohorts. Thus, except for *TPMT* and *NUDT15* homozygous low-activity variants, treatment adaptation according to host DNA polymorphisms has so far not been implemented in childhood ALL therapy. As the *CEP72* TT genotype has been associated with an increased risk of peripheral neuropathy, the St. Jude Children's Research Hospital is currently exploring if reduced VCR dosing in patients with *CEP72* TT will reduce their risk of acute and long-term neuropathy without increasing their risk of relapse (www.clinicaltrials.gov ID: NCT03117751).

Furthermore, the international Ponte di Legno Toxicity Working Group is now collecting deep phenotypes of several acute toxicities (e.g. osteonecrosis, thromboembolism, and neurotoxicity with many hundreds of cases of each) to associate phenotypes with germline DNA variants [14] for which polygenic risk scores may identify DNA profiles that define patients for whom future antileukemic therapy should be individualized to avoid unacceptable short- and long-term toxicities.

Patient and Society

Danish population- and register-based studies have shown that compared with the background population, survivors of childhood leukemia leave their parental home at the same age range as their peers and have similar educational choices and partner at the same rate [128–130].

The work situation of parents during and immediately following cancer treatment of their child and the work situation of the childhood cancer survivors are significantly affected. Parental socioeconomic status is anticipated to influence education and labor market affiliation among childhood cancer survivors the same way as in their peers, but no study has thoroughly explored the issue. Bearing this in mind, a systematic review of 35 eligible papers revealed that hematological childhood cancers had a substantial impact on parent socioeconomic situation including disruptions in parental employment, particularly among mothers [131].

Whereas some countries provide full coverage of childhood cancer survivors through taxation-based health-care systems (e.g., most European countries and Canada), others primarily have a private insurance system (e.g., the USA), which may limit access to insurance and health care for adult survivors of childhood cancer [132, 133].

Although the social welfare and health insurance system of the surrounding society may affect the socioeconomic profiles of childhood ALL survivors, many studies across different countries have shown significant impact of childhood leukemia treatment on long-term socioeconomic outcomes.

A recent Canadian study, including more than 3900 childhood cancer survivors, showed significantly lower earnings compared to the background population [134]. In another cohort of 2844 adult survivors or childhood hSCT from the USA, South America, Europe, Asia, and Australia/New Zealand, unemployment rates persisted to be high at all attained ages [135]. Finally, a nationwide questionnaire study from the British Childhood Cancer Survivor Group (~10,000 childhood cancer survivors) showed that survivors were less likely to work than a control cohort with an odds ratio of 0.89 (95% CI, 0.81–0.98) [136].

Quality of Life (QoL)

Consensus measures of QoL for survivors of life-threatening disease are difficult to establish and furthermore prone to individual perceptions of the imagined future as well as the surrounding society's view on these individuals, which can influence both perceptions of and actual relationships, work, income, and daily life. Thus, QoL is a construct dwelling on other concepts that has no absolute beginning and no end in time or impact. Accordingly, one should observe the QoL critically and be cautious not to make too strong conclusions based on the available data. That being said, QoL survey studies generally indicate that ALL survivors have worse or equivalent health-related QoL compared with the background population [137]. The overall quality of life is typically influenced by treatment protocol and a number of phenotypic characteristics in parents and the patient [138].

However, risk factors for poor health-related QoL among childhood ALL survivors, including severity of late effects, disfigurement due to treatment, educational problems, and insecurity in establishing intimate relationships, are reported with wide variability.

Conclusion and Future Research

The currently obtained cure rates of 90% or more for childhood ALL are one of the most impressive successes of modern medicine, naturally leading to an increased focus on late effects. Exploration and prevention of significant treatment-related morbidity have become more relevant than ever before. Of equal importance is the implementation of a standardized reporting of consensus-defined severe toxicities that will allow an objective comparison of the burden of late effects across treatment protocols, thereby supplementing the traditional objective outcome measures.

Although EFS and OS are quite similar across the ALL study groups, there may be wide differences in the distribution of unacceptable acute, persisting, and late occurring morbidity. ALL trials generally register acute toxicities to assess the acute treatment burden, but with diverse focus on specific toxicities, which may influence the reported frequencies. The recent PTWG consensus definitions of relevant toxicities have simplified and even encouraged a unified capture strategy, allowing both powerful association studies, comparisons across treatment strategies, and long-term outcome of acute toxicities [13, 14, 139]. These efforts can ultimately result in novel treatment strategies with reduced toxicities. However, late effects are in general not captured in a consensus-based fashion, if captured at all. Thus, we are missing systematic and reliable registration of the long-term sequelae and the true chronic burden of treatment when assessing therapy outcome. The first steps toward solving this are to create and implement a consensus strategy for outcome analyses that integrate persistent, serious toxicities with the traditional cure rate measures. Subsequent international consensus on reporting these outcomes will allow reliable comparison of diverse treatment strategies, focusing not only on the traditional five events and OS but in addition the frequencies of unacceptable toxicities that are associated with significant costs for both the individual and society. As a starting point, the Ponte di Legno Toxicity Working Group has developed the measure of STFS which can facilitate reliable comparison of the frequency of unacceptable toxicities (e.g., osteonecrosis requiring joint replacement or renal failure requiring dialysis or kidney transplant) across treatment protocols [21]. The STFS measure is now beeing quantified in several large (>1000 patients) cohorts.

Although most long-term survivors can obtain an education, manage a job, and establish a family, including having children, many will be burdened by significant late effects requiring life-long medical attention. In addition, survivors could be at risk of premature aging (e.g., dementia or atherosclerosis), but little is known, since almost none was cured just a few decades ago. Thus, there is a need for systematic follow-up of the survivors, including identification of risk factors for adverse outcomes that can be integrated into future individualized therapy.

Disclosures

- *Liv Andres-Jensen:* No conflict of interest to declare.
- *Kjeld Schmiegelow:* Speaker and/or Advisory Board Honoraria from Jazz Pharmaceuticals, Servier, and Medscape. Educational grant from Servier.
- *Christoffer Johansen:* No conflict of interest to declare.

References

1. Starý J, Hrušák O. Recent advances in the management of pediatric acute lymphoblastic leukemia. F1000Research. 2016;5:2635.
2. Pui CH, Yang JJ, Hunger SP, et al. Childhood acute lymphoblastic leukemia: Progress through collaboration. J Clin Oncol. 2015;33(27):2938–48.
3. Lund B, Åsberg A, Heyman M, et al. Risk factors for treatment related mortality in childhood acute lymphoblastic leukaemia. Pediatr Blood Cancer. 2011;56(4):551–9.
4. Schmiegelow K, Müller K, Mogensen SS, et al. Non-infectious chemotherapy-associated acute toxicities during childhood acute lymphoblastic leukemia therapy. F1000Research. 2017;6:444.
5. Schmiegelow K, Frandsen TL. Comment: the cost of cure. Lancet Haematol. 2018;5(11):e504–5.
6. Toft N, Birgens H, Abrahamsson J, et al. Results of NOPHO ALL2008 treatment for patients 1-45 years with acute lymphoblastic leukemia. Leukemia. 2017;32(3(August)):606–15.

7. Mulrooney DA, Hyun G, Ness KK, et al. The changing burden of long-term health outcomes in survivors of childhood acute lymphoblastic leukaemia: a retrospective analysis of the St Jude Lifetime Cohort Study. Lancet Haematol. 2019;6(6):e306–16.
8. Mullighan CG. The molecular genetic makeup of acute lymphoblastic Leukemia. Hematol Am Soc Hematol Educ Progr. 2012;2012:389–96.
9. Moriyama T, Relling MV, Yang JJ. Inherited genetic variation in childhood acute lymphoblastic leukemia. Blood. 2015;125(26):3988–95.
10. Schmiegelow K, Attarbaschi A, Barzilai S, et al. Consensus definitions of 14 severe acute toxic effects for childhood lymphoblastic leukaemia treatment: a Delphi consensus. Lancet Oncol. 2016;17(17):231–9.
11. Common Terminology Criteria for Adverse Events (CTCAE) Version 4.0. US Department of Health and Human Services. National Institutes of Health National Cancer Institute. https://evs.nci.nih.gov/ftp1/CTCAE/CTCAE_4.03_2010.
12. Bhakta N, Liu Q, Ness KK, et al. The cumulative burden of surviving childhood cancer: an initial report from the St Jude Lifetime Cohort Study (SJLIFE). Lancet. 2017;390(10112):2569–82.
13. Schmiegelow K, Attarbaschi A, Barzilai S, et al. Consensus definitions of 14 severe acute toxic effects for childhood lymphoblastic leukaemia treatment: a Delphi consensus. Lancet Oncol. 2016;17(6):e231–9.
14. Wolthers BO, Frandsen TL, Baruchel A, et al. Asparaginase-associated pancreatitis in childhood acute lymphoblastic leukaemia: an observational Ponte di Legno Toxicity Working Group study. Lancet Oncol. 2017;2045(17):1–11.
15. Mogensen SS, Harila-Saari A, Mäkitie O, et al. Comparing osteonecrosis clinical phenotype, timing, and risk factors in children and young adults treated for acute lymphoblastic leukemia. Pediatr Blood Cancer. 2018;65(10):1–10.
16. Schmiegelow K, Levinsen MF, Attarbaschi A, et al. Second malignant neoplasms after treatment of childhood acute lymphoblastic leukemia. J Clin Oncol. 2013;31(19):2469–76.
17. Vora A, Andreano A, Pui CH, et al. Influence of cranial radiotherapy on outcome in children with acute lymphoblastic leukemia treated with contemporary therapy. J Clin Oncol. 2016;34(9):919–26.
18. Ruark J, Mullane E, Cleary N, et al. Patient-reported neuropsychiatric outcomes of long-term survivors after chimeric antigen receptor T cell therapy. Biol Blood Marrow Transplant. 2020;26(1):34–43.
19. Cordeiro A, Bezerra ED, Hirayama AV, et al. Late events after treatment with CD19-targeted chimeric antigen receptor modified T cells. Biol Blood Marrow Transplant. 2020;26(1):26–33.
20. Stevens M, Frobisher C, Hawkins M, et al. The British childhood cancer survivor study: objectives, methods, population structure, response rates and initial descriptive information. Pediatr Blood Cancer. 2008;50(February):1018–25.
21. Andrés-Jensen L, Attarbaschi A, Bardi E, et al. Severe toxicity free survival: physician-derived definitions of unacceptable long-term toxicities following acute lymphocytic leukaemia. Lancet Haematol. 2021 Jul;8(7):e513–e523. https://doi.org/10.1016/S2352-3026(21)00136-8. PMID: 34171282.
22. Mertens AC, Yasui Y, Neglia JP, et al. Late mortality experience in five-year survivors of childhood and adolescent cancer: the Childhood Cancer Survivor Study. J Clin Oncol. 2001;19(13):3163–72.
23. Garwicz S, Anderson H, Olsen JH, et al. Late and very late mortality in 5-year survivors of childhood cancer: changing pattern over four decades-experience from the Nordic countries. Int J Cancer. 2012;131(7):1659–66.
24. Armstrong GT, Chen Y, Yasui Y, et al. Reduction in late mortality among 5-year survivors of childhood cancer. N Engl J Med. 2016;374(9):833–42.
25. De Fine LS, Winther JF, Gudmundsdottir T, et al. Hospital contacts for endocrine disorders in Adult Life after Childhood Cancer in Scandinavia (ALiCCS): a population-based cohort study. Lancet. 2014;383(9933):1981–9.

26. Chow E, Friedman D, Yasui Y, et al. Decreased adult height in survivors of childhood acute lymphoblastic leukemia: a report from the Childhood Cancer Survivor Study. J Pediatr. 2007;150:370–5.
27. Howard SC, Pui CH. Endocrine complications in pediatric patients with acute lymphoblastic leukemia. Blood Rev. 2002;16(4):225–43.
28. Chow EJ, Liu W, Srivasta K, et al. Differential effects of radiotherapy on growth and endocrine function among acute leukemia survivors: a Childhood Cancer Survivor Study report. Pediatr Blood Cancer. 2013;60:110–5.
29. Bruzzi P, Predieri B, Corrias A, et al. Final height and body mass index in adult survivors of childhood acute lymphoblastic leukemia treated without cranial radiotherapy: a retrospective longitudinal multicenter Italian study. BMC Pediatr. 2014;14(1):236.
30. Chow EJ, Friedman DL, Stocall M, et al. Risk of thyroid dysfunction and subsequent thyroid cancer among survivors of acute lymphoblastic leukemia: a report from the Childhood Cancer Survivor Study. Pediatr Blood Cancer. 2009;53:432–7.
31. Delvecchio M, Cecinati V, Brescia LP, et al. Thyroid function and thyroid autoimmunity in childhood acute lymphoblastic leukemia off-therapy patients treated only with chemotherapy. J Endocrinol Investig. 2010;33(3):135–9.
32. Iughetti L, Bruzzi P, Predieri B, Paolucci P. Obesity in patients with acute lymphoblastic leukemia in childhood. Ital J Pediatr. 2012;38(1):1–11.
33. Gibson TM, Ehrhardt MJ, Ness KK. Obesity and metabolic syndrome among adult survivors of childhood leukemia. Curr Treat Options in Oncol. 2016;17(4):17.
34. Marriott CJC, Beaumont LF, Farncombe TH, et al. Body composition in long-term survivors of acute lymphoblastic leukemia diagnosed in childhood and adolescence: a focus on sarcopenic obesity. Cancer. 2018;124(6):1225–31.
35. Nottage KA, Ness KK, Li C, et al. Metabolic syndrome and cardiovascular risk among long-term survivors of acute lymphoblastic leukaemia - from the St. Jude Lifetime Cohort. Br J Haematol. 2014;165(3):364–74.
36. Ness KK, DeLany JP, Kaste SC, et al. Energy balance and fitness in adult survivors of childhood acute lymphoblastic leukemia. Blood. 2015;125(22):3411–9.
37. Skoczen S, Surmiak M, Strojny W. Survivors of acute lymphoblastic leukemia and body mass changes. Expert Opin Drug Saf. 2010;9(1):65–77.
38. Wolthers BO, Frandsen TL, Abrahamsson J, et al. Asparaginase-associated pancreatitis: a study on phenotype and genotype in the NOPHO ALL2008 protocol. Leukemia. 2017;31(2):325–32.
39. Wolthers BO, Mogensen PR, Frandsen TL, et al. Insulin-dependent diabetes: a chronic complication to acute pancreatitis in childhood acute lymphoblastic leukemia. Pediatr Blood Cancer. 2019;66(1):1–4.
40. Williams HE, Howell CR, Chemaitilly W, et al. Diabetes mellitus among adult survivors of childhood acute lymphoblastic leukemia: a report from the St. Jude Lifetime Cohort Study. Cancer. 2020;26(4):870–8.
41. Cohen JE, Wakefield CE, Cohn RJ. Nutritional interventions for survivors of childhood cancer. Cochrane Database Syst Rev. 2016;2016(8):CD009678.
42. Chow EJ, Stratton KL, Leisenring WM, et al. Pregnancy after chemotherapy in male and female survivors of childhood cancer treated between 1970 and 1999: a report from the Childhood Cancer Survivor Study cohort. Lancet Oncol. 2016;17(5):567–76.
43. Krawczuk-Rybak M, Solarz E, Wysocka J, et al. Testicular function after treatment for acute lymphoblastic leukemia (ALL) in prepubertal and pubertal boys. Pediatr Hematol Oncol. 2009;26(7):504–14.
44. Shalet SM, Lendon M, Jones PHM. Testicular function after chemotherapy for acute lymphoblastic leukemia. N Engl J Med. 1981;305(9):520.
45. Marquis A, Kuehni CE, Strippoli MPF, Kühne T, Brazzola P. Sperm analysis of patients after successful treatment of childhood acute lymphoblastic leukemia with chemotherapy. Pediatr Blood Cancer. 2010;55(1):208–10.

46. Jahnukainen K, Heikkinen R, Henriksson M, et al. Semen quality and fertility in adult long-term survivors of childhood acute lymphoblastic leukemia. Fertil Steril. 2011;96(4):837–42.
47. Green DM, Zhu L, Wang M, et al. Effect of cranial irradiation on sperm concentration of adult survivors of childhood acute lymphoblastic leukemia: a report from the St. Jude Lifetime Cohort Study. Hum Reprod. 2017;32(6):1192–201.
48. Byrne J, Fears TR, Mills JL, et al. Fertility of long-term male survivors of acute lymphoblastic leukemia diagnosed during childhood. Pediatr Blood Cancer. 2004;42(4):364–72.
49. Skinner R, Mulder RL, Kremer LC, et al. Recommendations for gonadotoxicity surveillance in male childhood, adolescent, and young adult cancer survivors: a report from the International Late Effects of Childhood Cancer Guideline Harmonization Group in collaboration with the PanCareSurFup Consort. Lancet Oncol. 2017;18(2):e75–90.
50. Mills JL, Fears TR, Robison LL, Ncholson SH, Sklar CA, Byrne J. Menarche in a cohort of 188 long-term survivors of acute lymphoblastic leukemia. J Pediatr. 1997;131(4):598–602.
51. Chow EJ, Friedman DL, Yasui Y, et al. Timing of menarche among survivors of childhood acute lymphoblastic leukemia: a report from the Childhood Cancer Survivor Study. Pediatr Blood Cancer. 2008;50:854–8.
52. Van Dorp W, Mulder RL, Kremer LCM, et al. Recommendations for premature ovarian insufficiency surveillance for female survivors of childhood, adolescent, and young adult cancer: a report from the International Late Effects of Childhood Cancer Guideline Harmonization Group in collaboration with the PanCareSurFup Consortium. J Clin Oncol. 2016;34(28):3440–50.
53. Wallace W, Shalet S, Tetlow L, Morris-Jones P. Ovarian function following the treatment of childhood acute lymphoblastic leukaemia. Med Pediatr Oncol. 1993;21(5):333–9.
54. Levine JM, Whitton JA, Ginsberg JP, et al. Nonsurgical premature menopause and reproductive implications in survivors of childhood cancer: a report from the Childhood Cancer Survivor Study. Cancer. 2018;124(5):1044–52.
55. Hamre MR, Robison LL, Nesbit ME, et al. Effects of radiation on ovarian function in long-term survivors of childhood acute lymphoblastic leukemia: a report from the Children's Cancer Study Group. J Clin Oncol. 1987;5(11):1759–65.
56. Larsen EC, Müller J, Schmiegelow K, Rechnitzer C, Andersen AN. Reduced ovarian function in long-term survivors of radiation- and chemotherapy-treated childhood cancer. J Clin Endocrinol Metab. 2003;88(11):5307–14.
57. Nielsen SN, Andersen AN, Schmidt KT, et al. A 10-year follow up of reproductive function in women treated for childhood cancer. Reprod Biomed Online. 2013;27(2):192–200.
58. Bath LE, Anderson RA, Critchley HOD, Kelnar CJH, Wallace WHB. Hypothalamic-pituitary-ovarian dysfunction after prepubertal chemotherapy and cranial irradiation for acute leukaemia. Hum Reprod. 2001;16(9):1838–44.
59. Krawczuk-Rybak M, Płonowski M, Leszczyńska E, et al. The influence of different intensity of treatment on hormonal markers of gonadal function in acute lymphoblastic leukemia survivors. Hematol Oncol. 2019;37(5):609–16.
60. Jain S, Jain S, Kapoor G, Virmani A, Bajpai R. No impact of disease and its treatment on bone mineral density in survivors of childhood acute lymphoblastic leukemia. Pediatr Blood Cancer. 2017;64(4):1–8.
61. Rohani F, Rafsanjani KA, Bahoush G, Sabzehparvar M, Ahmadi M. Bone mineral density in survivors of childhood acute lymphoblastic leukemia. Asian Pac J Cancer Prev. 2017;18(2):535–40.
62. Gurney JG, Kaste SC, Liu W, et al. Bone mineral density among long-term survivors of childhood acute lymphoblastic leukemia: results from the St. Jude Lifetime Cohort Study. J Pediatr Blood Cancer. 2014;61:1270–6.
63. Ward LM, Ma J, Lang B, et al. Bone morbidity and recovery in children with acute lymphoblastic leukemia: results of a six-year prospective cohort study. J Bone Miner Res. 2018;33(8):1435–43.
64. Kunstreich M, Kummer S, Laws HJ, Borkhardt A, Kuhlen M. Osteonecrosis in children with acute lymphoblastic leukemia. Haematologica. 2016;101(11):1295–305.

65. Mogensen SS, Schmiegelow K, Grell K, et al. Hyperlipidemia is a risk factor for osteonecrosis in children and young adults with acute lymphoblastic leukemia. Haematologica. 2017;102(5):e175–8.
66. Kadan-Lottick NS, Dinu I, Wasilewski-Masker K, et al. Osteonecrosis in adult survivors of childhood cancer: a report from the Childhood Cancer Survivor Study. J Clin Oncol. 2008;26(18):3038–45.
67. Kaste SC, Karmova EJ, Neel MD. Osteonecrosis in children after therapy for malignancy. AJR Am J Roentgenol. 2011;196(5):1011–8.
68. Sonis AL, Tarbell N, Valachovic RW, et al. Dentofacial development in long-term survivors of acute lymphoblastic leukemia: a comparison of three treatment modalities. Cancer. 1990;66(12):2645–52.
69. Kaste S, Hopkins K, Jones D, et al. Dental abnormalities in children treated for acute lymphoblastic leukemia. Leukemia. 1997;11(February):792–6.
70. Wilberg P, Kanellopoulos A, Ruud E, et al. Dental abnormalities after chemotherapy in long-term survivors of childhood acute lymphoblastic leukemia 7–40 years after diagnosis. Support Care Cancer. 2016;24(4):1497–506.
71. Kanellopoulos A, Andersson S, Zeller B, et al. Neurocognitive outcome in very long-term survivors of childhood acute lymphoblastic leukemia after treatment with chemotherapy only. Pediatr Blood Cancer. 2015;14(November 2014):1526–31.
72. Krull KR, Brinkman TM, Li C, et al. Neurocognitive outcomes decades after treatment for childhood acute lymphoblastic leukemia: a report from the St Jude Lifetime Cohort Study. J Clin Oncol. 2013;31(35):4407–15.
73. Jacola LM, Krull KR, Pui CH, et al. Longitudinal assessment of neurocognitive outcomes in survivors of childhood acute lymphoblastic leukemia treated on a contemporary chemotherapy protocol. J Clin Oncol. 2016;34(11):1239–47.
74. Cole PD, Kamen BA. Delayed neurotoxicity associated with therapy for children with acute lymphoblastic leukemia. Ment Retard Dev Disabil Res Rev. 2006;12(July):174–83.
75. Langer T, Martus P, Ottensmeier H, et al. CNS late-effects after ALL therapy in childhood. Part III: neuropsychological performance in long-term survivors of childhood ALL: impairments of concentration, attention, and memory. Med Pediatr Oncol. 2002;38(5):320–8.
76. Iyer NS, Balsamo LM, Bracken MB, Kadan-Lottick NS. Chemotherapy-only treatment effects on long-term neurocognitive functioning in childhood ALL survivors: a review and meta-analysis. Blood. 2015;126(3):346`–53.
77. Liu W, Cheung YT, Conklin HM, et al. Evolution of neurocognitive function in long-term survivors of childhood acute lymphoblastic leukemia treated with chemotherapy only. J Cancer Surviv. 2018;12(3):398–406.
78. Thomsen AM, Gulinello ME, Wen J, Schmiegelow K, Cole PD. Liposomal cytarabine induces less neurocognitive dysfunction than intrathecal methotrexate in an animal model. J Pediatr Hematol Oncol. 2018;40(2):e91–6.
79. Cheung YT, Sabin ND, Reddick WE, et al. Leukoencephalopathy and long-term neurobehavioural, neurocognitive, and brain imaging outcomes in survivors of childhood acute lymphoblastic leukaemia treated with chemotherapy: a longitudinal analysis. Lancet Haematol. 2016;3(10):e456–66.
80. Lehtinen SS, Huuskonen UE, Harila-Saari AH, et al. Motor nervous system impairment persists in long-term survivors of childhood acute lymphoblastic leukemia. Cancer. 2002;94(9):2466–73.
81. Kerckhove N, Collin A, Condé S, et al. Long-term effects, pathophysiological mechanisms, and risk factors of chemotherapy-induced peripheral neuropathies: a comprehensive literature review. Front Pharmacol. 2017;8(FEB):86.
82. Harila-Saari AH, Huuskonen UEJ, Tolonen U, Vainionpää LK, Lanning BM. Motor nervous pathway function is impaired after treatment of childhood acute lymphoblastic leukemia: a study with motor evoked potentials. Med Pediatr Oncol. 2001;36(3):345–51.
83. Lieber S, Blankenburg M, Apel K, et al. Small-fiber neuropathy and pain sensitization in survivors of pediatric acute lymphoblastic leukemia. Eur J Paediatr Neurol. 2018;3:457–69.

84. Verstappen C, Koeppen S, Heimans J, et al. Dose-related vincristine- induced peripheral neuropathy with unexpected off- therapy worsening. Neurology. 2005;64:1076–7.
85. Ramchandren S, Leonard M, Mody RJ, et al. Peripheral neuropathy in survivors of childhood acute lymphoblastic leukemia. J Peripher Nerv Syst. 2009;14(3):184–9.
86. Khan RB, Hudson MM, Ledet DS, et al. Neurologic morbidity and quality of life in survivors of childhood acute lymphoblastic leukemia: a prospective cross-sectional study. J Cancer Surviv. 2014;8(4):688–96.
87. Jain P, Gulati S, Seth R, et al. Vincristine-induced neuropathy in childhood all (acute lymphoblastic leukemia) survivors: prevalence and electrophysiological characteristics. J Child Neurol. 2014;29(7):932–7.
88. Tay CG, Lee VWM, Ong LC, et al. Vincristine-induced peripheral neuropathy in survivors of childhood acute lymphoblastic leukaemia. Pediatr Blood Cancer. 2017;64(8):1–7.
89. Varedi M, Lu L, Howell CR, et al. Peripheral neuropathy, sensory processing, and balance in survivors of acute lymphoblastic leukemia. J Clin Oncol. 2018;36(22):2315–22.
90. Hutchins KK, Siddeek H, Franco VI, Lipshultz SE. Prevention of cardiotoxicity among survivors of childhood cancer. Br J Clin Pharmacol. 2017;83(3):455–65.
91. Silverman LB. Balancing cure and long-term risks in acute lymphoblastic leukemia. Hematology. 2014;2014(1):191–7.
92. Bansal N, Amdani S, Lipshultz ER, Lipshultz SE. Chemotherapy-induced cardiotoxicity in children. Expert Opin Drug Metab Toxicol. 2017;13(8):817–32.
93. Hau EM, Caccia JN, Kasteler R, et al. Cardiovascular disease after childhood acute lymphoblastic leukaemia: a cohort study. Swiss Med Wkly. 2019;149(9–10):w20012.
94. Lipshultz SE, Lipsitz SR, Sallan SE, et al. Chronic progressive cardiac dysfunction years after doxorubicin therapy for childhood acute lymphoblastic leukemia. J Clin Oncol. 2005;23(12):2629–36.
95. Vandecruys E, Mondelaers V, de Wolf D, Benoit Y, Suys B. Late cardiotoxicity after low dose of anthracycline therapy for acute lymphoblastic leukemia in childhood. J Cancer Surviv. 2012;6(1):95–101.
96. van Dalen EC, Raphaël MF, Caron HN, Kremer LCM. Treatment including anthracyclines versus treatment not including anthracyclines for childhood cancer. Cochrane Database Syst Rev. 2014;2014(9):CD006647.
97. Dietz AC, Chen Y, Yasui Y, et al. Risk and impact of pulmonary complications in survivors of childhood cancer: a report from the Childhood Cancer Survivor Study. Cancer. 2016;122(23):3687–96.
98. Cerveri I, Fulgoni P, Giorgiani G, et al. Lung function abnormalities after bone marrow transplantation in children: has the trend recently changed? Chest. 2001;120(6):1900–6.
99. Gower WA, Collaco JM, Mogayzel PJ. Lung function and late pulmonary complications among survivors of hematopoietic stem cell transplantation during childhood. Paediatr Respir Rev. 2010;11(2):115–22.
100. Nysom K, Holm K, Olsen JH, Hertz H, Hesse B. Pulmonary function after treatment for acute lymphoblastic leukaemia in childhood. Br J Cancer. 1998;78(1):21–7.
101. Alanko S, Salmi TT, Pelliniemi TT. Recovery of blood t-cell subsets after chemotherapy for childhood acute lymphoblastic leukemia. Pediatr Hematol Oncol. 1994;11(3):281–92.
102. Bochennek K, Allwinn R, Langer R, et al. Differential loss of humoral immunity against measles, mumps, rubella and varicella-zoster virus in children treated for cancer. Vaccine. 2014;32(27):3357–61.
103. Chua LL, Rajasuriar R, Azanan MS, et al. Reduced microbial diversity in adult survivors of childhood acute lymphoblastic leukemia and microbial associations with increased immune activation. Microbiome. 2017;5(1):1–14.
104. McNeer JL, Rau RE, Gupta S, Maude SL, O'Brien MM. Cutting to the front of the line: immunotherapy for childhood acute lymphoblastic leukemia. Am Soc Clin Oncol Educ B. 2020;40:1–12.
105. Ness KK, Armstrong GT, Kundu M, et al. Frailty in childhood cancer survivors. Cancer. 2015;121(10):1540–7.

106. Armstrong GT, Kawashima T, Leisenring W, et al. Aging and risk of severe, disabling, life-threatening, and fatal events in the Childhood Cancer Survivor Study. J Clin Oncol. 2014;32(12):1218–27.
107. López-Otín C, Blasco MA, Partridge L, Serrano M, Kroemer G. The hallmarks of aging. Cell. 2013;153(6):1194–217.
108. Ness KK, Kirkland JL, Monica Gramatges M, et al. Premature physiologic aging as a paradigm for understanding increased risk of adverse health across the lifespan of survivors of childhood cancer. J Clin Oncol. 2018;36(21):2206–15.
109. Dong Y, Huang Y, Gutin B, et al. Associations between global DNA methylation and telomere length in healthy adolescents. Sci Rep. 2017;7(1):4210.
110. Mannava S, Moparthy KC, Wheeler LJ, et al. Depletion of deoxyribonucleotide pools is an endogenous source of DNA damage in cells undergoing oncogene-induced senescence. Am J Pathol. 2013;182(1):142–51.
111. Franceschi C, Campisi J. Chronic inflammation (inflammaging) and its potential contribution to age-associated diseases. J Gerontol Ser A Biol Sci Med Sci. 2014;69(Suppl 1):S4–9.
112. Marcoux S, Le ON, Langlois-Pelletier C, et al. Expression of the senescence marker p16 INK4a in skin biopsies of acute lymphoblastic leukemia survivors: a pilot study. Radiat Oncol. 2013;8:252.
113. Ariffin H, Azanan MS, Abd Ghafar SS, et al. Young adult survivors of childhood acute lymphoblastic leukemia show evidence of chronic inflammation and cellular aging. Cancer. 2017;123(21):4207–14.
114. Hyde RK, Liu PP. Germline PAX5 mutations and B cell leukemia. Nat Genet. 2013;45(10):1104–5.
115. Shah S, Schrader KA, Waanders E, et al. A recurrent germline PAX5 mutation confers susceptibility to pre-B cell acute lymphoblastic leukemia. Nat Genet. 2013;45(10):1226–31.
116. Moriyama T, Metzger ML, Wu G, et al. Germline genetic variation in ETV6 and risk of childhood acute lymphoblastic leukaemia: a systematic genetic study. Lancet Oncol. 2015;16(16):1659–66.
117. Topka S, Vijai J, Walsh MF, et al. Germline ETV6 mutations confer susceptibility to acute lymphoblastic leukemia and thrombocytopenia. PLoS Genet. 2015;11(6):e1005262.
118. Liew E, Owen C. Familial myelodysplastic syndromes: a review of the literature. Haematologica. 2011;96(10):1536–42.
119. Churchman ML, Qian M, te Kronnie G, et al. Germline genetic IKZF1 variation and predisposition to childhood acute lymphoblastic leukemia. Cancer Cell. 2018;33(5):937–948.e8.
120. Diness BR, Risom L, Frandsen TL, et al. Putative new childhood leukemia cancer predisposition syndrome caused by germline bi-allelic missense mutations in DDX41. Genes Chromosom Cancer. 2018;57(12):670–4.
121. Schmiegelow K, Lausten Thomsen U, Baruchel A, et al. High concordance of subtypes of childhood acute lymphoblastic leukemia within families: lessons from sibships with multiple cases of leukemia. Leukemia. 2012;26(4):675–81.
122. Zeller B, Gustafsson G, Forestier E, et al. Acute leukaemia in children with down syndrome: a population-based Nordic study. Br J Haematol. 2005;128(6):797–804.
123. Buitenkamp TD, Mathôt RAA, de Haas V, Pieters R, Michel ZC. Methotrexate-induced side effects are not due to differences in pharmacokinetics in children with down syndrome and acute lymphoblastic leukemia. Haematologica. 2010;95(7):1106–13.
124. Qian M, Cao X, Devidas M, et al. TP53 germline variations influence the predisposition and prognosis of b-cell acute lymphoblastic leukemia in children. J Clin Oncol. 2018;36(6):591–9.
125. Junk SV, Klein N, Schreek S, et al. TP53, ETV6 and RUNX1 germline variants in a case series of patients developing secondary neoplasms after treatment for childhood acute lymphoblastic leukemia. Haematologica. 2019;104(9):E402–5.
126. Ripperger T, Bielack SS, Borkhardt A, et al. Childhood cancer predisposition syndromes—a concise review and recommendations by the Cancer Predisposition Working

Group of the Society for Pediatric Oncology and Hematology. Am J Med Genet Part A. 2017;173(4):1017–37.
127. Davidsen ML, Dalhoff K, Schmiegelow K. Pharmacogenetics influence treatment efficacy in childhood acute lymphoblastic leukemia. J Pediatr Hematol Oncol. 2008;30(11):831–49.
128. Koch SV, Kejs AMT, Engholm G, Johansen C, Schmiegelow K. Educational attainment among survivors of childhood cancer: a population-based cohort study in Denmark. Br J Cancer. 2004;91(5):923–8.
129. Koch SV, Kejs AMT, Engholm G, et al. Leaving home after cancer in childhood: a measure of social independence in early adulthood. Pediatr Blood Cancer. 2006;47(1):61–70.
130. Koch SV, Kejs AMT, Engholm G, et al. Marriage and divorce among childhood cancer survivors. J Pediatr Hematol Oncol. 2011;33(7):500–5.
131. Roser K, Erdmann F, Michel G, Winther JF, Mader L. The impact of childhood cancer on parents' socio-economic situation—a systematic review. Psychooncology. 2019;28(6):1207–26.
132. Mueller EL, Park ER, Kirchhoff AC, et al. Insurance, chronic health conditions, and utilization of primary and specialty outpatient services: a Childhood Cancer Survivor Study report. J Cancer Surviv. 2018;12(5):639–46.
133. Nathan PC, Henderson TO, Kirchhoff AC, Park ER, Yabroff KR. Financial hardship and the economic effect of childhood cancer survivorship. J Clin Oncol. 2018;36(21):2198–205.
134. Tecklc P, Pcacock S, McBride ML, et al. Long-term effects of cancer on earnings of childhood, adolescent and young adult cancer survivors - a population-based study from British Columbia, Canada 11 Medical and Health Sciences 1117 Public Health and Health Services. BMC Health Serv Res. 2018;18(1):826.
135. Bhatt NS, Brazauskas R, Tecca HR, et al. Post-transplantation employment status of adult survivors of childhood allogeneic hematopoietic cell transplant: a report from the Center for International Blood and Marrow Transplant Research (CIBMTR). Cancer. 2019;125(1):144–52.
136. Frobisher C, Lancashire ER, Jenkinson H, et al. Employment status and occupational level of adult survivors of childhood cancer in Great Britain: the British Childhood Cancer Survivor Study. Int J Cancer. 2017;140(12):2678–92.
137. Vetsch J, Wakefield CE, Robertson EG, et al. Health-related quality of life of survivors of childhood acute lymphoblastic leukemia: a systematic review. Qual Life Res. 2018;27(6):1431–43.
138. Fardell JE, Vetsch J, Trahair T, et al. Health-related quality of life of children on treatment for acute lymphoblastic leukemia: a systematic review. Pediatr Blood Cancer. 2017;64(9)
139. Wolthers BO, Frandsen TL, Patel CJ, et al. Trypsin-encoding PRSS1-PRSS2 variations influence the risk of asparaginase-associated pancreatitis in children with acute lymphoblastic leukemia: a ponte di legno toxicity working group report. Haematologica. 2019;104(3):556–63.

Part III
New and Existing Modalities of Therapy

Chapter 13
Monoclonal Antibody-Based Treatment and Other New Agents for B-Lineage Acute Lymphoblastic Leukemia

John C. Molina and Nirali N. Shah

Introduction

Despite significant advances in the management of B-cell ALL (B-ALL) over the last several decades, particularly in pediatric patients where the 5-year overall survival (OS) reaches 90%, outcomes for the 10–15% with relapsed and refractory disease continue to be poor [1]. This is an even greater issue in adults where, with aggressive first-line treatment, adults aged 40–59 years or 60–69 years have very poor outcomes, with 5-year OS of 24% and 18%, respectively [2]. While the use of pediatric-inspired regimens has improved complete remission (CR) rates in younger adults, 20–30% will still relapse, following which, the 5-year OS rate is only 40–50% [3]. The median survival following relapse in adults ranges from 4.5 to 6 months with 5-year OS rates of 3–10%, and no uniformly accepted standard salvage treatment exists for relapsed ALL [2, 4].

The hallmark for frontline treatment of ALL remains the use of combination cytotoxic chemotherapies which improve anti-leukemia efficacy and reduce risk of relapse [5]. Nearly all medications used as the current standard of care for ALL were developed prior to the 1980s [3]. While advances in the 1990s and early 2000s for the sequence, dosing, and combination of cytotoxic therapies significantly improved outcomes, novel therapeutic approaches are required to improve outcomes for pediatric and adult B-ALL patients with relapsed and refractory or high-risk disease. Additionally, the toxicity associated with cytotoxic chemotherapy for

J. C. Molina
Pediatric Oncology Branch, Center for Cancer Research (CCR), National Cancer Institute (NCI), National Institutes of Health (NIH), Bethesda, MD, USA

Department of Pediatric Oncology, Johns Hopkins Hospital, Baltimore, MD, USA

N. N. Shah (✉)
Pediatric Oncology Branch, Center for Cancer Research (CCR), National Cancer Institute (NCI), National Institutes of Health (NIH), Bethesda, MD, USA
e-mail: Nirali.Shah@nih.gov

M. R. Litzow, E. A. Raetz (eds.), *Clinical Management of Acute Lymphoblastic Leukemia*, https://doi.org/10.1007/978-3-030-85147-7_13

relapsed B-ALL can be excessive due to prior chemotherapy exposure, particularly in older adults [6, 7].

This chapter will provide an overview of monoclonal antibody-based treatment for B-ALL with a focus on the new FDA-approved therapies and emerging strategies, including small molecule inhibitors and new cytotoxic drugs being used as single agents or in combination with chemotherapy.

Monoclonal Antibody-Based Treatment

Traditional cytotoxic chemotherapy functions primarily through inhibition of cell division and targets rapidly dividing cancer cells while also affecting normal tissue. In contrast, targeted therapies seek to optimize antitumor activity while minimizing systemic toxicities [6]. Monoclonal antibodies have emerged as one of the most promising class of novel, targeted therapeutic agents for the treatment of B-ALL [7].

Antibodies are produced by B lymphocytes to recognize the epitope region of an antigen with the fragment antigen binding (Fab) portion of monoclonal antibodies designed to recognize a single epitope. Once bound to a specific epitope, the Fc region of the monoclonal antibody engages different components of the host immune system leading to a targeted response [8]. Since the FDA approval in 1986 for the first monoclonal antibody, muromonab-CD3 (designed to prevent organ rejection after transplant by blocking T-cell function), monoclonal antibodies have become the most commonly approved and used cancer immunotherapy methodology [9].

Due to the high expression of cluster of differentiation (CD) surface markers on lymphoblasts with minimal or no expression on other cells, these antigens serve as the ideal monoclonal antibody target for B-ALL cells. As illustrated in Fig. 13.1, expression of various CD markers varies by the subtype of B-ALL. The percentage of cells expressing individual CD markers is also an important factor determining the efficacy of monoclonal antibody therapy [6]. The primary CD targets developed for B-ALL are the cell surface immunoglobulins CD19 and CD22 and the fixed

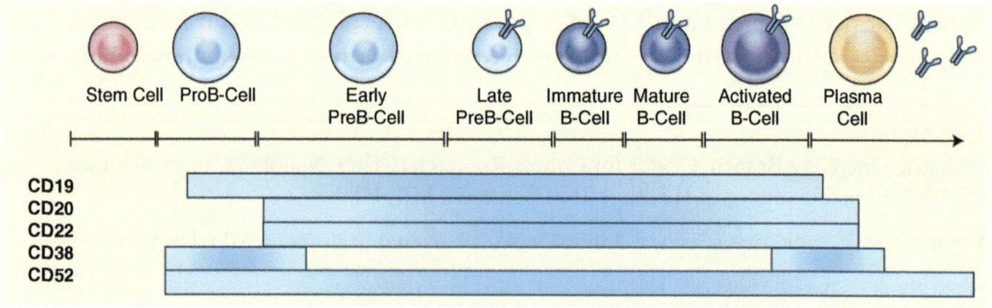

Fig. 13.1 Cluster of differentiation (CD) expression and B-cell maturation

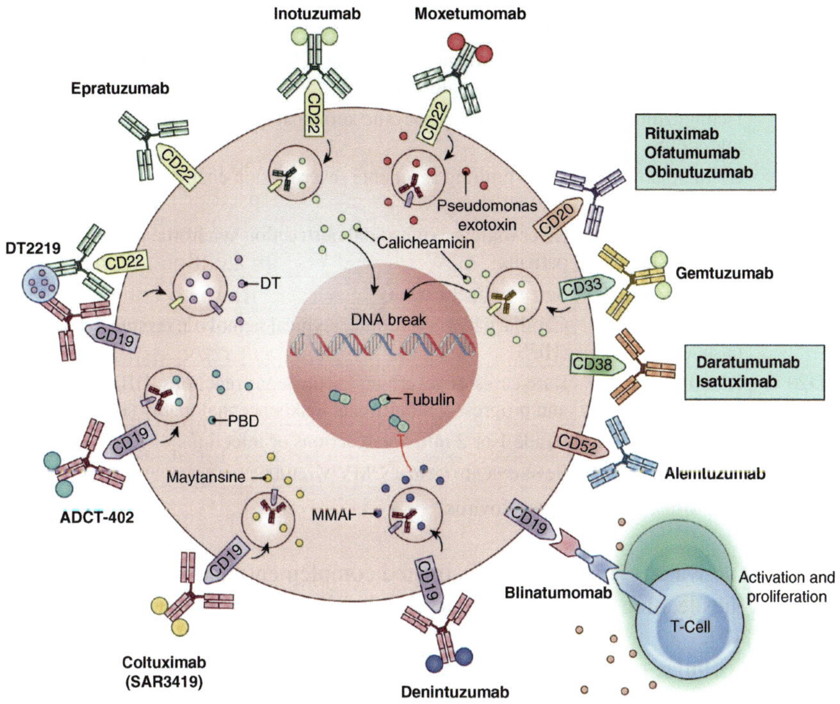

Fig. 13.2 Overview of monoclonal antibody-based therapy in B-ALL. Legend: *DT* diphtheria toxin, *PBD* pyrrolobenzodiazepine dimer toxin, *MMAF* monomethyl auristatin F

non-glycosylated transmembrane phosphoprotein CD20. The expression of CD19 and CD22 is fairly homogenously expressed on B lymphocytes with CD20 having a more heterogenous expression [10, 11].

Earlier generations of monoclonal antibodies targeting B-ALL CD markers have been non-conjugated antibodies that exerted an anticancer effect through three main mechanisms [12] (Fig. 13.2):

1. Antibody-dependent cellular cytotoxicity (ADCC)
2. Complement-dependent cytotoxicity (CDC)
3. Interruption of essential cancer cell processes by inhibiting receptors that activate the signaling pathways required for cell division

ADCC-induced apoptosis is mediated through the recognition of Fc receptors on cell-bound monoclonal antibodies by macrophages and natural killer (NK) cells. The cross-linking of macrophages and NK cells with monoclonal antibodies bound to antigens on the surface of target cells results in the release of cytotoxic agents like perforin and granzyme [13, 14]. Alternatively, in CDC, following monoclonal antibody binding to membrane surface antigens on the target cell, the complement

Table 13.1 Examples of unique side effects of monoclonal antibody-based therapies for B-ALL

Target	Medications	Side effects
CD19	Blinatumomab	Cytokine release syndrome (CRS), neurotoxicity, hypogammaglobulinemia
	Denintuzumab mafodotin	Superficial microcystic keratopathy
	Coltuximab ravtansine	Dose-limiting reversible severe vision changes associated with corneal changes
CD22	Inotuzumab ozogamicin	Liver toxicity, sinusoidal obstruction syndrome in transplant patients
	Epratuzumab	Seizure, liver toxicity
	Moxetumomab pasudotox	Capillary leak syndrome, atypical hemolytic uremic syndrome (HUS)
CD20	Rituximab	Rare cases of severe mucocutaneous reactions, HBV reactivation, and progressive multifocal leukoencephalopathy (PML)
	Ofatumumab	Grade 1 or 2 infusion reactions or infections
CD52	Alemtuzumab	Severe neutropenia, CMV viremia

HBV hepatitis B virus, *CMV* cytomegalovirus

cascade is activated. This results in activated complement binding to the monoclonal antibodies leading to lysis of the target cell following induction of a membrane complex [15].

Due to cellular targets like CD19 and CD22 being internalized upon binding, investigators began developing a second class of monoclonal antibodies with anticancer effects – antibody drug conjugates [16]. These monoclonal antibody and chemotherapeutic drug conjugates enhance the efficiency of antibody-based cancer cell killing by releasing a potent cytotoxin directly into the target cell [17]. Another recent class of medications are bispecific, or bifunctional, antibodies that are designed to engage two different target epitopes at the same time in order to function as T-cell engaging antibodies [18].

Although designed to produce less systemic toxicity, each monoclonal antibody with or without a drug conjugate has its own unique side effect depending on its target antigen and mechanism of action (see Table 13.1 [19]).

CD19-Directed Therapy

The human CD19 transmembrane protein is an essential component of the B-cell receptor multicomplex, and it is expressed on pre-B-cells through terminal differentiation to plasma cells [20]. It upregulates cell signaling primarily through the P13K and RAS pathways, and the expression of CD19 on B-cells is essential for their function and the maintenance of B-lineage cells [21]. CD19 is also the most reliable surface biomarker for B-cells, and it is present on 90% of pre-B and mature ALL lymphoblasts [22, 23]. As a result, CD19 is one of the most commonly targeted antigens for immunotherapy strategies for the treatment of hematological malignancies [24].

Blinatumomab

Blinatumomab is a novel, first-in-human bispecific T-cell engager (BiTE) antibody that binds both CD19 and CD3 [25]. It is designed to bring T-cells into proximity with B lymphoblasts leading to T-cell activation and a cytotoxic T-cell response against CD19-expressing cells [26, 27]. Blinatumomab was first studied in relapsed-refractory non-Hodgkin lymphoma (NHL) and chronic lymphocytic leukemia (CLL) with early study termination of early phase I NHL trials due to lack of efficacy and neurologic toxicity [28]. The success of subsequent trials in pre-B-cell ALL led to FDA approval for blinatumomab in three settings for both pediatric and adult patients with ALL: (1) positive minimal residual disease (MRD+) and (2) refractory and relapsed (r/r) Philadelphia-negative (Ph−) and (3) r/r Ph-positive (Ph+) B-ALL [29–35].

Mechanism of Action

Despite the critical role that T-cells play in the control of tumor growth, the lack of Fcγ receptors on T-cells results in the inability of conventional antibodies to recruit T-cells after binding target leukemia cells [36]. The bispecific T-cell engager blinatumomab is made up of two, unique recombinant monoclonal antibodies – an anti-CD19 fragment antigen-binding (Fab) region and an anti-CD3 Fab region – that are joined by a glycine-serine linker [27]. By binding CD19 on B-cells and CD3 primarily on cytotoxic $CD8^+$ T-cells (CTLs) [37], blinatumomab is able to engage the high cytotoxic potential of T-cells without the need for T-cell receptor (TCR) specificity, antigen processing and presentation, or major histocompatibility complex context [32]. The activation of T-cell by binding both CD19 and CD3 causes the release of granzymes and perforin leading to direct leukemia cell death via apoptosis, as well as the release of inflammatory cytokines resulting in serial T-cell activation, expansion, and enhanced B-cell-directed lysis [38].

Treatment-Specific Adverse Effects

Blinatumomab is generally well tolerated with its major therapy-associated toxicities being related to T-cell engagement, cytokine release syndrome (CRS), and immune activation [39, 40]. The most common side effects include CRS, neurotoxicity, and hypogammaglobulinemia:

Cytokine Release Syndrome (CRS) The CRS seen following blinatumomab is a similar phenomenon to that seen with chimeric antigen receptor T-cell therapy (CAR-T; see CAR T-cell chapter). Symptoms can be mild (fever, malaise, headache, or nausea) to severe (hypotension, hypoxia, renal dysfunction, transaminitis) and even life-threatening secondary to pulmonary edema, capillary leak syndrome, disseminated intravascular coagulation (DIC), or hemophagocytic lymphohistiocytosis (HLH) [41]. Like CAR-T, blinatumomab-associated CRS is mediated by IL-1 and IL-6 with anti-IL-6 targeted therapy (tocilizumab) being an effective strategy to decrease the severity and duration of symptoms [39]. In clinical trials, CRS occurred in 15% of the relapsed/refractory patients and 7% of MRD+ ALL with only a small percentage being grade 3 or higher [42]. The rate of CRS has been shown to be decreased following pretreatment cytoreduction [43].

Neurotoxicity Similar to CAR-T, the neurotoxicity following blinatumomab infusion is felt to be secondary to disruption of the blood-brain barrier by activated T-cells [44, 45]. Neurotoxicity was a common occurrence in clinical trial populations and was seen in 65% of patients with the median onset of 2 weeks following infusion. It can occur simultaneously with CRS or asynchronously. The most common symptoms were headache and tremors with grade 3 or greater (encephalopathy, confusion, seizures, speech disorders, coordination or balance abnormalities, and cranial nerve deficits) seen in 7–13% in adults and 4% of pediatric patients [41]. Unlike CAR-T, prophylaxis with anti-epileptics is not currently recommended given the low rate of seizures seen with blinatumomab [33].

Hypogammaglobulinemia As a result of blinatumomab-induced B-cell aplasia, hypogammaglobulinemia has been found to occur in 6% of patients, putting individuals at increased risk of infectious complications. Serial monitoring of IgG should be performed and treatment of hypogammaglobulinemia supported with IVIG as necessary [33, 46].

Administration

Due to its dose-dependent activity, linear time-dependent clearance, and short half-life of 2 h, prolonged exposure to blinatumomab is necessary for effective T-cell activation and resulting B-cell depletion [47]. As a result, blinatumomab is given through a continuous IV infusion pump for 28 days for enhanced efficacy and reduced toxicity followed by a treatment-free period of 2 weeks [33]. It is also recommended for the first cycle that blinatumomab is started in dose escalation manner in order to reduce neurotoxicity and minimize CRS [31–33]. Table 13.2 summarizes the dosing and schedules for blinatumomab's FDA-approved indications [48].

In order to monitor for possible adverse side effects, it is recommended that relapsed/refractory patients are observed inpatient for the initial 9 days of treatment (through the first 2 days of the dose escalation) before completing treatment as an outpatient. For patients who are MRD+, patients should be hospitalized for the first 3 days of cycle 1. For cycle 2, it is recommended that both relapsed/refractory and MRD+ patients are monitored for 2 days inpatient [30, 33]. Patients in the pediatric phase I/II trials with a high leukemic burden (i.e., bone marrow blasts >50%) were also given hydroxyurea or dexamethasone to decrease the risk of CRS [34].

Table 13.2 FDA-approved blinatumomab dosing for pre-B ALL

	Weight ≥ 45 kg (fixed dose)	Weight < 45 kg (BSA-based dose)
CR1 or CR2 with [a]MRD-positive patients (Gökbuget 2018)		
Cycles 1–4		
Days 1–28	28 mcg/day	15 mcg/m²/day (not to exceed 28 mcg/day)
Days 29–42	14-day treatment-free interval	14-day treatment-free interval
Relapsed or refractory Ph- and Ph+ patients (Kantarjian 2017)		
Induction cycle 1		
Days 1–7	9 mcg/day	5 mcg/m²/day (not to exceed 9 mcg/day)
Days 8–28	28 mcg/day	15 mcg/m²/day (not to exceed 28 mcg/day)
Days 29–42	14-day treatment-free interval	14-day treatment-free interval
Induction cycle 2		
Days 1–28	28 mcg/day	15 mcg/m²/day (not to exceed 28 mcg/day)
Days 29–42	14-day treatment-free interval	14-day treatment-free interval
Induction cycle 3–5		
Days 1–28	28 mcg/day	15 mcg/m²/day (not to exceed 28 mcg/day)
Days 29–42	14-day treatment-free interval	14-day treatment-free interval
Induction cycle 6–9		
Days 1–28	28 mcg/day	15 mcg/m²/day (not to exceed 28 mcg/day)
Days 29–84	56-day treatment-free interval	56-day treatment-free interval

CR complete remission, *MRD* minimal residual disease
[a]MRD is positive when blasts are ≥ 0.1% by flow cytometry in the bone marrow

Clinical Trial Results

Blinatumomab was approved for adults in the USA in 2014 under the FDA's Breakthrough Designation based on the results of Topp et al.'s single-arm, phase II clinical trial (NCT01466179) [32]. This was followed by regular approval in 2017 following the results of the randomized, phase III TOWER trial (NCT02013167) [33]. Pediatric labeling was also granted in 2017 based on the outcomes of a single phase I/II trial (NCT01471782) [34]. Compared to the adult trials, the CR rate (38.6%) and MRD-negative response rate (20%) were inferior to results seen in the adult trials [31]. See Table 13.3 for summary of the major blinatumomab trials' results.

Table 13.3 Blinatumomab trials leading to FDA approvals

Designation	Study	Phase	N	ORR	CR (CRh)	MRD RR	RFS	Median OS, mo	CRS (≥ grade 3)	Neurotoxicity (≥ grade 3)
FDA breakthrough	Topp et al (2014)	II	36	--	69%	88%	7.6 mo	9.8		
	Topp et al (2015)	II	189	43%	33% (10%)	82%	5.9 mo	6.1	2%	13%
R/R Ph-	TOWER (Kentarjian et al. 2017)	III	271	44%	34% (10%)	76%	6-month EFS = 31%	7.7	4.9%	9.4%
R/R Ph+	ALCANTARA (Martinelli et al. 2017)	II	45	36%	31% (4%)	88%	6.7 mo	7.1	0%	7%
MRD+	BLAST (Geokbuget et al. 2018)	II	113	--	--	78%	54% at 18 mo	36.5	2%	13%
Pediatric	von Stackelberg et al. (2016)	I/II	I: 49 II: 44	--	32%	--	4.4[a]	7.5	6%	4%

Abbreviations: N number, *ORR* overall response rate, *CR* complete response, *CRh* complete response with hematologic recovery, *MRD RR* minimal residual disease response rate, *RFS* relapse free survival, *OS* overall survival, *CRS* cytokine release syndrome

[a]Among responders

Recent results from the Children's Oncology Group's (COG) phase III study AALL 1331 found that blinatumomab was superior to standard chemotherapy for post-reinduction consolidation prior to hematopoietic stem cell transplantation (HSCT) in children and adolescent and young adult (AYA) patients with high and intermediate risk in first relapse. The use of blinatumomab resulted in higher rates of MRD response (32% vs. 75% after completing one cycle), increased likelihood of proceeding to HSCT (43% vs. 70%), improved 2-year disease-free (39% vs. 54.4%) and 2-year overall survival (58.4% vs. 71.3%) at 2 years, as well as fewer and less severe toxicities [49].

Mechanisms of Resistance

Despite its success in the treatment of relapsed/refractory and MRD+ ALL, a large proportion of patients treated with blinatumomab remain treatment-resistant; however, the mechanisms of resistance remain poorly understood. Although less common than rates seen with CD19 CAR-T, loss of CD19 antigen expression appears to be a major mechanism of blinatumomab resistance or cause of relapse following blinatumomab.

Multiple mechanisms of antigen loss secondary to CD19-directed therapy have been identified, including:

- Production of a truncated protein with either a nonfunctional or absent transmembrane domain seen in acquired mutations in CD19 exons 2–5 [50, 51]
- Intracellular accumulation of CD19 due to alteration in the chaperone protein CD81 [52]
- Lineage switch from sustained pressure against CD19, seen in patients with KMT2A, BCR-ABL1, or ZNF384 fusions [53–57]

Alternatively, CD19 escape may result from the selection of CD19-negative subclones that are able to maintain the ability to proliferate without CD19 expression [58].

Other proposed mechanisms of blinatumomab resistance include increased ALL cell expression of programmed death-ligand 1 (PD-L1) and activation of regulatory T-cells [59]. T-cell-mediated cell death may be inhibited by increased PD-L1 expression on lymphoblasts secondary to the cytokine release with blinatumomab exposure [60]. Additionally, by increasing IL-10 production, regulatory T-cells can suppress effector T-cell proliferation leading to decreased CD8 T-cell-mediated cytotoxic activity against leukemia cells. A lower rate of response to blinatumomab has been seen in patients with a higher percentage of regulatory T-cells in the peripheral blood [61].

Future Directions

Given the promising results of blinatumomab leading to its three FDA-approved indications, there are ongoing studies looking at combining blinatumomab with other therapies to increase its efficacy, as well as investigations looking to incorporate it as part of frontline therapy.

Several trials are evaluating the addition of the tyrosine kinase inhibitors (TKIs), dasatinib and ponatinib, to blinatumomab for the treatment of Ph+ ALL in hopes of developing chemo-sparing regimens. Based on retrospective analysis of blinatumomab and TKI combinations showing effectiveness and tolerability in relapsed Ph+ patients, prospective trials are underway to determine if these drug combinations can be a safe and effective consolidation regimen to bridge MRD+ Ph+ ALL patients to allogeneic HSCT [62]. In order to overcome inhibition of T-cell function due to upregulation and increased PD-L1 expression on lymphoblasts following blinatumomab-mediated cytokine release, several trials are looking to enhance blinatumomab with immune checkpoint inhibition (NCT02879695, NCT03160079). Initial phase I data has shown that the addition of nivolumab (anti-PD1) or ipilimumab (anti-CTLA-4) is safe and tolerable with an ongoing trial looking at combining one or both drugs with blinatumomab in poor-risk, relapsed, or refractory CD19+ B-ALL [63].

Additional trials are also underway to evaluate blinatumomab as part of frontline therapy for B-ALL. In a single-arm, phase II trial, blinatumomab was added as consolidation following four cycles of hyper-CVAD in an attempt to increase MRD negativity rates while reducing the amount of intensive chemotherapy and associated toxicities [43]. In the 14 evaluable patients on this study, the combination proved safe and effective with a CR rate of 100% and MRD-negative CR rate of 93%. Based on these results and a 1-year RFS rate of 77% and a 1-year OS rate of 90%, a current phase III trial is underway (NCT02003222). This randomized NCTN trial (E1910) will evaluate the effect on OS of adding blinatumomab for Ph-negative B-ALL patients who are MRD-negative following induction and intensification chemotherapy. Similarly, in pediatrics, the current phase III, COG study AALL1731 is investigating blinatumomab with chemotherapy as upfront therapy for subsets of children with standard-risk B-ALL and Down syndrome B-ALL (NCT03914625).

Additional CD19 Targeted Approaches

In addition to blinatumomab and CD19 CAR-T, other agents have been developed to utilize CD19 as a targeted approach for the treatment of relapsed/refractory ALL but have proved less successful.

Denintuzumab Mafodotin (SGN-CD19A) Denintuzumab is a humanized CD19 monoclonal antibody drug conjugate linked to monomethyl auristatin F (MMAF), a microtubule-disrupting agent. Following binding of CD19 and internalization of denintuzumab, MMAF is released and inhibits microtubule assembly leading to

G2/M growth arrest and apoptosis [64]. A phase I trial in children and adults with pre-B-ALL and aggressive lymphomas (NCT01786096) found a CR rate of 35% in B-ALL. Overall, the drug was well tolerated with the most frequently reported adverse events (AEs) being fever, nausea, fatigue, headaches, and superficial microcystic keratopathy requiring steroid eye drop prophylaxis [65]. There are currently no active clinical trials in adult or pediatric pre-B-ALL.

Coltuximab Ravtansine (SAR3419) Similar to denintuzumab, coltuximab is another antibody drug conjugate with a humanized anti-CD19 antibody this time conjugated to maytansin. Once internalized, the active maytansin metabolites function similar to vincristine with anti-tubulin activity leading to cell cycle arrest and apoptosis [66]. A phase I trial in CD19-positive NHL showed clinical activity, but a phase II trial (NCT01440179) in pre-B-ALL was terminated early due to limited activity compared to other new agents [67, 68].

DT2219 Designed as a bispecific monoclonal antibody targeting CD19 and CD22, DT2219 is made up of two sFv subunits that recognize CD19 and CD22 and are fused to the catalytic and translocation domains of diphtheria toxin (DT390) [69, 70]. A phase I/II trial in adults and children older than 12 years (NCT02370160) resulted in a complete response in only one of the six patients with pre-B-ALL [71].

CD22-Directed Therapy

Similar to CD19, CD22 is a transmembrane sialoglycoprotein found on 90% of B-ALL cells and mature B lymphocytes, but it is not expressed on non-B lymphoid cells, myeloid cells, hematopoietic stem cells, or non-hematopoietic lineage cells [11, 72, 73]. On B-cells, CD22 functions as an adhesion molecule for other leukocytes and increases the threshold for antigen/receptor stimulation by acting as a negative regulator of calcium channel signaling [10]. CD22 is rapidly internalized following antibody binding which allows anti-CD22 antibodies to function through several mechanisms including antibody drug conjugates (ADCs), modulation of B-cell signaling, and inhibition of proliferation [74]. It is an important target for relapsed/refractory ALL since it remains detected in most cases of CD19 antigen loss following CD19-directed BiTE (blinatumomab) and CAR-T-cell therapies [75, 76].

Inotuzumab Ozogamicin

Inotuzumab ozogamicin is an FDA-approved ADC for adults with relapsed/refractory ALL made up of a humanized IgG4 anti-CD22 monoclonal antibody covalently bound to a cytotoxic antitumor antibiotic, calicheamicin [77].

Mechanism of Action

Following binding of inotuzumab to the CD22 antigen on the surface of leukemia cells, the complex gets rapidly internalized by lysosomal vesicles whose acidic environment releases the potent antitumor antibiotic calicheamicin [78]. Calicheamicin is produced by *Micromonospora echinospora*, and it induces cell death in leukemia cells through its interactions with double-stranded DNA [78, 79]. Once liberated from the antibody drug conjugate, the calicheamicin binds the minor groove of DNA resulting in DNA cleavage and subsequent apoptosis [80].

Treatment-Specific Adverse Effects

Sinusoidal Obstruction Syndrome (SOS) Also known as veno-occlusive disease (VOD), SOS is the most concerning treatment-specific adverse effect seen with inotuzumab, particularly in patients who go on to receive an allogeneic HSCT [81]. SOS results from damage to the sinusoidal endothelium and hepatocytes typically seen with high-dose alkylating chemotherapy conditioning regimens in transplant. Severe VOD can have mortality rates as high as 84% [82]. The pathophysiology of SOS associated with inotuzumab is not fully understood but is felt to be secondary to direct effect of calicheamicin on sinusoidal endothelial cells similar to what has been reported with gemtuzumab, another ADC bound to calicheamicin [83, 84].

In the phase III INO-VATE trial, the incidence of SOS was 13% for any grade and 11% for grade 3 compared to <1% in the standard chemotherapy group. The median time to onset after the first dose of inotuzumab was 30 days. Risk for VOD with HSCT was increased with each cycle of inotuzumab received with a rate of 29% in patients receiving >2 cycles prior to transplant [85]. The only factor predicting VOD in HSCT transplant patients following inotuzumab was the use of a dual alkylator conditioning regimen [82].

Administration

The dosing schedule for inotuzumab is summarized in Table 13.4 [48]. Prior to the initial dose of inotuzumab, it is recommended that a combination of cytoreductive agents (hydroxyurea, steroids, and/or vincristine) is used for patients with

Table 13.4 FDA-approved inotuzumab dosing for pre-B ALL

	Day 1	Day 8	Day15
Induction			
Cycle 1 (21 days)	0.8 mg/m^2	0.5 mg/m^2	0.5 mg/m^2
Cycle 2[a] (28 days)			
Consolidation[b] (28 days)	0.5 mg/m^2	0.5 mg/m^2	0.5 mg/m^2

[a]Induction may be repeated if patients do not achieve CR/CRi with Cycle 1

[b]Patients going to allogenic transplant should be limited to 2 cycles, or the fewest number to achieve a CR/Cri

circulating lymphoblasts in order to decrease the peripheral blast count to ≤10,000/mm³ [82]. The recommended duration of therapy is two cycles for patients planning to proceed to HSCT with a potential third cycle if MRD negativity is not achieved [81]. Alternatively, for patients not proceeding to transplant, a maximum of six cycles is recommended. Patients should be premedicated with a corticosteroid, an antipyretic, and an antihistamine and observed for infusion reactions for at least an hour following the inotuzumab infusion [82].

Clinical Results

The initial phase I/II trial of inotuzumab had a goal dosing of 1.8 mg/m² administered once every 3 to 4 weeks based on prior data from studies in NHL [86]. Given the ORR of 57% but concerns for increased hepatic toxicity, future phase II trials utilized weekly doses of 0.8, 0.5, and 0.5 mg/m² with similar outcomes [87]. Inotuzumab was given FDA approval for adults with relapsed/refractory B-ALL in August 2017 based on the results from the randomized phase III study of inotuzumab ozogamicin versus investigator's choice of chemotherapy in patients with relapsed or refractory acute lymphoblastic leukemia (INO-VATE) which compared inotuzumab vs. chemotherapy in first or second salvage [88]. Table 13.5 outlines the results of the major inotuzumab trials in adults.

Table 13.5 Selected inotuzumab trials

Trial	Study	N	ORR (%)	CR (%)	MRD(-) ORR (%)	Median OS, mo	VOD
Phase I/II Kantarjian et al. (2013)	R/R B-ALL Ph+ included	90	58	36	72	6.2	6/90 6/36 (transplant)
Phase I/II DeAngelo et al. (2017)	R/R B-ALL Ph+ included	72	68	32	84	7.4	4
Phase II: InO + Chemo Jabbour et al. (2016)	R/R B-ALL Ph+ excluded	59	78	59	82	11.0	9/59
Phase II: InO + Chemo Kantarjian (2018)	New Diagnosis B-ALL Ph+ excluded	52	98	85	78	2-year OS 66%	4/52
Phase III: InO vs Chemo Kantarjian et al. (2016)	R/R B-ALL Ph+ included	326	81vs 29	36 vs 17	78 vs 28.1	7.7 mo vs 6.7 mo	11% vs 1%

Abbreviations: CR complete response, *InO* inotuzumab ozogamicin, *ORR* overall response rate, *OS* overall survival, *R/R* relapsed/refractory, *ALL* acute lymphoblastic leukemia, *VOD* veno-occlusive disease

ORR = CR + CR_p + CR_I CRi, complete response with incomplete recovery of peripheral blood counts; CRp, complete response with incomplete recovery of platelets

Inotuzumab is not currently FDA approved for children, but two trials are examining its efficacy in relapsed/refractory patients (phase II COG study AALL1621) and in newly diagnosed high-risk B-ALL patients (phase III COG AALL1732). A retrospective review of 51 pediatric patients receiving inotuzumab through the FDA's Expanded Access Program showed a CR rate of 67% with 71% of responders MRD-negative. However, over 50% of the patients who went on to allogeneic HSCT developed VOD which is much higher than the rates seen in adult studies [89]. In the ongoing phase II COG study, inotuzumab has been able to achieve a CR/CRi rate of 58% in heavily pretreated children and young adults with r/r CD22-positive B-ALL, of which 65.4% achieved MRD-negative remission [90].

Mechanisms of Resistance

Multiple steps are required for the inotuzumab to be clinically effective including the binding of the antibody drug conjugate to surface CD22 and receptor internalization, hydrolysis of the chemical linker, activation of calicheamicin, and the action of calicheamicin on DNA. Additionally, cellular efflux of inotuzumab can affect intracellular calicheamicin concentration and decrease efficacy [91]. Similar to the antigen loss seen with CD19 and blinatumomab, another mechanism of resistance for inotuzumab is downregulation of CD22 which has been reported in patients relapsing after treatment [92, 93]. The mechanism of CD22 antigen modulation remains poorly understood [94].

Future Directions

Given the success of inotuzumab in relapsed B-ALL, ongoing trials are combining the drug with additional therapies and evaluating its use in the frontline therapy in order to determine its best use. Active trials of inotuzumab include combination with TKIs for relapsed Ph+ ALL (NCT02311998), upfront use in adolescent and young adult patients to increase MRD-negative response rate and event-free survival (NCT03150693), efficacy of lower doses of weekly infusions in relapsed patients (NCT03094611), safety/efficacy to eliminate MRD in adult patients (NCT03441061), and tolerability/efficacy when combined with hyper-CVAD. There is also an ongoing trial combining inotuzumab with blinatumomab in older adults with previously untreated ALL in order to evaluate a "chemotherapy-free" regimen (NCT03739814).

Additional CD22 Targeted Approaches

Epratuzumab A humanized non-conjugated monoclonal anti-CD22 antibody that is internalized after binding to CD22, epratuzumab functions through CD22 phosphorylation, inhibition of proliferation, B-cell activation, and cytotoxicity [74]. It was the first CD22 targeted treatment for children, and an initial COG study (ADVL04P2) combining epratuzumab with standard four-drug reinduction chemotherapy following CD22+ relapse showed promising results with 7/15 patients achieving an MRD-negative remission [95]. A follow-up phase II COG trial, unfortunately, did not show improvement compared to historical controls and no statistically significant difference with MRD response [96]. Epratuzumab was evaluated in adult patients in combination with clofarabine and cytarabine in relapsed or refractory disease with an overall response rate of 40–52% compared to 17% with chemotherapy alone [97]. An international, randomized phase III trial in pediatric patients is currently underway studying the addition of epratuzumab to a standard chemotherapy backbone (NCT01802814).

Moxetumomab Pasudotox Developed at the National Cancer Institute (NCI) for the treatment of ALL, non-Hodgkin lymphoma, hairy cell leukemia, and CLL, moxetumomab pasudotox is a murine CD22 monoclonal antibody conjugated to a protein derivative of *Pseudomonas exotoxin A*. Similar to inotuzumab, it is designed to induce apoptosis following internalization by the leukemia cell and release of the exotoxin [98]. Despite evidence of clinical activity in B-ALL in a phase I trial [99], its phase II trial was terminated at interim analysis due to a failure of the CR rate to meet the stage 1 target. Additionally, serious adverse events occurred in a third of patients including capillary leak syndrome and hemolytic uremic syndrome (HUS) [100]. There are no clinical trials using moxetumomab for B-ALL currently underway. Given the very short half-life of this agent [101], future trials utilizing a continuous infusion model, akin to blinatumomab, may improve the therapeutic index of this agent, and preclinical efforts are underway [102].

CD20-Directed Therapy

CD20 also serves as a reliable biomarker for B-cell malignancies and is expressed in 30–50% of pre-B-ALL compared to 80–90% in mature B-cell or Burkitt type leukemia/lymphoma [103]. It functions as a calcium channel on B-cells that leads to upregulation of anti-apoptotic proteins and cell survival [104]. CD20 positivity, defined by the NCCN Guidelines as expression of CD20 on ≥20% of ALL blasts, is an independent predictor of higher relapse rate and is associated with lower overall survival [105, 106]. Three monoclonal antibodies developed to target CD20 expression and which have been tested in B-ALL include rituximab, ofatumumab, and obinutuzumab.

Rituximab First approved in 1997 for adults with NHL, rituximab is a chimeric anti-CD20 monoclonal antibody that functions through complement-mediated cytotoxicity, antibody-dependent cellular cytotoxicity, apoptosis induction, and increased chemotherapy sensitivity following its binding to CD20-positive cells [107]. Rituximab is one of the most studied immunotherapies, and its low toxicity profile makes it an ideal treatment for elderly patients or individuals unable to tolerate aggressive treatments [108]. Rituximab has limited activity when used as a monotherapy. Due to its inability to cross the blood-brain barrier, it is also not used to target CNS disease [109]. This has led investigators to incorporate it with standard chemotherapy regimens.

The addition of rituximab to standard or modified hyper-CVAD regimens in newly diagnosed, Ph-negative, CD20+ pre-B-ALL patients resulted in significantly improved 3-year CR rates (38% to 70%) and OS rates (47% to 75%) in patients <60 years old [110]. The German Multicenter Study Group for Adult ALL (GMALL) also showed increased rates of continuous CR at 3 years, OS, and MRD negativity in patients <55 years when added to a standard BFM-based regimen [111]. Following these trials, the Group for Research on Adult Acute Lymphoblastic Leukemia (GRAALL)-2005/R randomized study analyzed the benefit of adding rituximab to pediatric-inspired chemotherapy backbone of patients with CD20+ B-ALL. The addition of rituximab improved the 2-year EFS from 52% to 65% and the OS from 64% to 71% [112]. Based on the observation of CD20 upregulation during induction therapy, the more recent UKALL14 trial (NCT01085617) randomized 655 patients between 25 and 65 years of age to receive the addition of four doses of rituximab during standard induction therapy regardless of Ph status or CD20 expression [113]. In contrast to the GRAALL-2005/R study which gave rituximab during all phases of treatment for a total of 16–18 infusions, the addition of 4 infusions during induction did not lead to a statistically significant benefit. In addition to concluding that 16–18 doses may be required to achieve the full benefit of rituximab, the researchers found no difference in outcomes based on Ph status or CD20 expression level which suggests the GRAALL-2005/R results may be generalizable to all patients with B-ALL [113].

Data remains inconclusive for the benefits of adding rituximab to Ph-positive disease, and the observation of CD20 upregulation during induction therapy may prompt future trials looking at the benefit of adding rituximab for patients with a low CD20 expression at baseline [114].

Ofatumumab Ofatumumab is a second-generation anti-CD20 humanized, monoclonal antibody that was approved in 2009 for the treatment of CLL [115]. Its binding site is different from rituximab, instead targeting a membrane proximal small loop epitope on the CD20 molecule. Compared to rituximab, ofatumumab has more potent complement-dependent cytotoxicity and antibody-dependent cell-mediated toxicity but less direct cytotoxicity [116]. A phase II trial of 65 patients combining ofatumumab with hyper-CVAD for newly diagnosed pre-B CD20+ ALL patients was found to be highly effective, regardless of CD20 expression. The combination therapy resulted in a CR rate of 98% with MRD negativity in 93% and an estimated 2-year OS of 81% [117].

Obinutuzumab Like ofatumumab, obinutuzumab is another novel anti-CD20 humanized, monoclonal antibody that was engineered to have increased antibody-dependent cellular cytotoxicity cells compared to rituximab and ofatumumab through its enhanced binding affinity to the FcγRIII receptors on immune effector [116, 118]. Obinutuzumab is FDA approved for CLL and has been shown to be effective against B-ALL in preclinical studies with increased cell death [119]. No clinical trials in B-ALL have been carried out to date.

Other Pre-B-ALL Monoclonal Targets

Due to varying degrees of CD expression on B-ALL, additional antigen targeting has been or is actively being trialed in B-ALL including CD38 (daratumumab/isatuximab) (Clinicaltrials.gov NCT03384654/NCT03860844), CD52 (alemtuzumab [120, 121]), and CD33 (gemtuzumab ozogamicin) monoclonal antibodies for those cases with aberrant myeloid expression [122, 123]. A summary is provided in Table 13.6.

New Cytotoxic and Non-immunomodulatory Agents for B-Lineage ALL (Fig. 13.3)

Cytotoxic

While recent research and drug development has focused primarily on new antibody and small molecule chemotherapeutic agents, several novel cytotoxic agents have been studied as single agents or in combination with standard chemotherapy. There has also been the development of new formulations of established chemotherapy agents to improve efficacy and decrease toxicity.

Clofarabine Designed to overcome dose-limiting toxicities of cladribine and fludarabine, clofarabine is a second-generation purine nucleoside analog. Clofarabine inhibits DNA synthesis and repair through DNA polymerase and ribonucleotide reductase inhibition more effectively than cladribine and fludarabine. The drug also disrupts the mitochondrial membrane of leukemia cells that results in the release of cytochrome C and caspase leading to the apoptosis [124, 125]. Clofarabine was FDA approved in December 2004 through the Orphan Drug Program as a single agent for the treatment of relapsed/refractory pediatric B-ALL up to the age of 21 years who have received two prior lines of therapy [126, 127].

Additional clinical studies have evaluated clofarabine in combination with standard chemotherapies [128, 129]. Based on promising results from a phase II study utilizing clofarabine in patients with relapsed/refractory ALL [129], a prospective phase III study was initiated in newly diagnosed very high-risk B-ALL patients up through the age of 30 years (COG AALL1131). In this trial, following modified BFM induction, patients were randomized to one of the three arms for consolidation, one of which included cyclophosphamide, etoposide, and clofarabine.

Table 13.6 Summary table of other monoclonal antibody targets in relapsed/refractory B ALL

Antigen target	Drug	Clinicaltrials.gov identifier	Trial	Patients	Status	Results	Notes
CD38	*Daratumumab*	NCT03384654	Daratumumab + vincristine and prednisone	1–30 yo	Recruiting	NA	FDA approved for multiple myeloma
	Isatuximab	NCT03860844	Weekly isatuximab with induction chemotherapy, then biweekly with consolidation	<18 yo	Recruiting	NA	
CD52	*Alemtuzumab (Campath)*	Tibes et al. (2006)	Single-agent alemtuzumab	>18 yo	Completed	No observed effect in ALL patients	Significant AEs (CMV/HSV viremia, prolonged immunosuppression)
		NCT00089349	Single-agent alemtuzumab	<30 yo	Completed	1/13 with CR	
		NCT00061945	Alemtuzumab + intensified upfront chemotherapy	>15 yo	Completed	CRR ~80%	
CD33	*Gemtuzumab*	Case series only	Single agent and with combination chemotherapy	Adult and pediatric		Variable	Anti-CD33 antibody conjugated to calicheamicin, FDA approved for AML

Abbreviations: CR complete response, *CRR* complete response rate

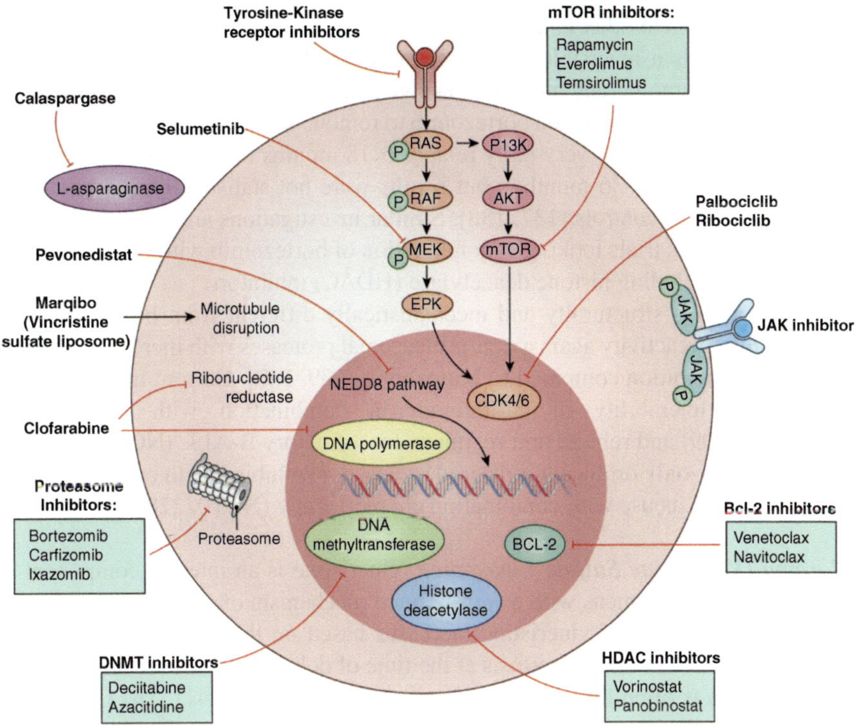

Fig. 13.3 Overview of new cytotoxic and non-immunomodulatory agents for B-ALL. Legend: *DNMT* DNA methyltransferase, *HDAC* histone deacetylase, *CDK* cyclin-dependent kinase, *mTOR* mammalian target of rapamycin, *MEK* mitogen-activated protein kinase kinase, *BCL-2* B-cell lymphoma 2

Ultimately, this regimen proved to be unacceptably toxic with higher rates of infection and more prolonged cytopenias over the two other consolidation arms (cyclophosphamide, cytarabine, mercaptopurine (standard arm) and cyclophosphamide, etoposide, vincristine, and pegaspargase (experimental arm 1)), and this arm was permanently closed to accrual following planned safety analysis and despite an amendment to incorporate a dose de-escalation [130]. In adults, the phase II GIMEMA LAL 1610 protocol studied the combination of clofarabine and cyclophosphamide as first salvage for Ph-negative patients that showed a median overall survival of 6.5 months and disease-free survival of 3.7 months [131].

Bortezomib/Carfilzomib/Ixazomib (Proteasome Inhibitors) The proteasome is responsible for the degradation of cellular proteins and plays an important role in cell survival and signaling. It was hypothesized that leukemia cells may be sensitive to proteasome inhibition due to increased protein turnover [132]. In particular, it has been shown that the deregulation of nuclear factor kappa-B (*NF-κB*) protects cells from apoptosis, and its inhibition by proteasome inhibitors (bortezomib, carfilzomib, and ixazomib) can both increase apoptosis of leukemia cells and increase sensitivity of malignant cells to other antitumor agents [133].

Bortezomib is a reversible 26S proteasome inhibitor shown to be effective in combination chemotherapy but not as a single agent [134–136]. The pediatric phase II trial COG AALL07P1 added bortezomib to reinduction therapy that showed overall CR2 rates of 63% for very early relapse (<18 months from diagnosis) and 72% for early relapse (18–36 months), but results were not statistically different compared to historical controls [137, 138]. Similar investigations are ongoing for adult patients as well as trials looking at combination of bortezomib with other classes of medications, including histone deacetylase (HDAC) inhibitors.

Carfilzomib is structurally and mechanistically different from bortezomib and has shown less reactivity against non-proteasomal proteases with increased levels of proteasome inhibition compared to bortezomib [139, 140]. Current trials are looking at the tolerability of carfilzomib in combination with hyper-CVAD (NCT02293109) and reinduction regimens for refractory B-ALL (NCT02228772). Ixazomib is the only orally administered proteasome inhibitor with ongoing phase I trials looking at its use with combination chemotherapy (NCT02228772).

Marqibo (Vincristine Sulfate Liposome) Vincristine is an integral component of standard B-ALL regimens with a well-defined mechanism of action and anticancer activity. The efficacy of vincristine increases based on the time of exposure and fraction of leukemia cells in mitosis at the time of delivery [2]. Unfortunately, dose intensification is often limited due to increased neuropathy [141]. The COG study AALL0433 looked to compare standard versus increased vincristine dosing in late bone marrow or very early isolated central nervous system relapse in pediatric B-ALL, but randomization was closed 3 years into the study due to excessive peripheral neuropathy in the experimental arm [142]. As a result, although the recommended dose of vincristine is 1.5–2 mg/m^2, dosing is typically capped at 2 mg to prevent severe vincristine-induced peripheral neuropathy resulting in the majority of adults and some pediatric patients receiving suboptimal dosing [2].

Marqibo, vincristine sulfate liposome injection (VSLI), is a sphingomyelin–/cholesterol-based liposome-encapsulated formulation designed to increase the therapeutic index of vincristine. By using liposome encapsulation, exposure to the drug can be prolonged at increased doses without increasing dose-limiting toxicities [141]. Based on phase II data from the RALLY study, Marqibo was given accelerated FDA approval in September 2012 for use in adult patients with Ph-negative B-ALL in second or greater relapse (2.25 mg/m2 weekly, without dose capping). The trial resulted in a CR (CR + CRi) rate with single-agent VSLI of 20% with a median duration of CR of 23 weeks [143]. A phase I trial in pediatric patients showed tolerability at the FDA-approved dose [141], and results from a pediatric trial looking at replacing standard vincristine in reinduction combination chemotherapy for children with relapsed/refractory ALL are forthcoming (Clinicaltrials.gov NCT02879643).

Calaspargase L-Asparaginase is a critical part of the upfront chemotherapy backbone for pediatric B-ALL, and it is often given in its pegylated form, pegaspargase

[4]. Pre-B-ALL cells are unable to synthesize adequate amounts of L-asparagine needed for DNA, RNA, and protein synthesis, and L-asparaginase depletes extracellular sources ultimately leading to cell death [144]. Calaspargase pegol is a newer formulation that uses a different linking molecule to increase hydrolytic stability and drug half-life compared to pegaspargase [145]. Based on the results of DFCI ALL Consortium Protocol 11-001, calaspargase was granted FDA approval in December 2018 as a component of multi-agent chemotherapy for pediatric patients up to the age of 21 years. Compared to pegaspargase given every 2 weeks, calaspargase administered every 3 weeks resulted in a similar EFS, OS, and safety profile [146]. No adult trials to date have examined the use of this formulation of L-asparaginase.

Epigenetic Modifiers

Epigenetic modification of gene expression can lead to transcriptional silencing of tumor suppressor genes and play a critical role in the malignant transformation of leukemia [147]. Epigenetic regulators, like histone deacetylase (HDAC) and DNA methyltransferase (DNMT) inhibitors, function to alter gene expression and the malignant phenotype and can help restore the chemosensitivity of relapsed B-ALL [148, 149].

HDAC Inhibitors (Vorinostat, Panobinostat) The deacetylation of histones results in a closed chromatin structure leading to the suppression of gene transcription and expression, including tumor suppressor genes. HDACs have been found to be both overexpressed and mutated in leukemia cells. By modifying gene expression, HDAC inhibitors can block proliferation, induce cell cycle arrest and apoptosis, and lead to cell differentiation [150]. The FDA-approved pan-HDAC inhibitors vorinostat and panobinostat are actively being studied in ALL in combination with DNA methyltransferase inhibitors and standard cytotoxic chemotherapeutic agents. Despite the role that HDACs play in numerous cell processes and the potential for a wide range of off-target effects, the side effect profile of HDAC inhibitors has been tolerable so far and includes gastrointestinal, neurological, and hematologic toxicities, as well as asymptomatic ECG changes [151].

DNMT Inhibitors (Azacitidine/Decitabine) DNA methylation is another major contributor to epigenetic modification, and DNA methyltransferases (DNMTs) have been found to be overexpressed in leukemia leading to tumorigenesis [152, 153]. 5-Azacytidine (azacitidine) and 5-aza-2′-deoxycytidine (decitabine) are cytosine analogs that once incorporated in the DNA lead to the depletion of DNMTs. This results in hypomethylation of DNA and induction of DNA damage [154]. Due to superior therapeutic outcomes, DNMT inhibitors are frequently combined with HDAC inhibitors that are known to increase DNMT1 acetylation and decrease the total DNMT1 protein [155]. Although most actively studied in AML, evaluations in B-ALL are warranted.

Other Targetable Pathways

Recently, the growing genomic landscape of B-ALL has led to the characterization of novel subtypes of ALL with various genetic alterations known to disrupt important cellular pathways including hematopoietic development, cell signaling or proliferation, and epigenetic regulation [156]. As a result, numerous targetable genes have been identified as potential therapeutic options for both established and emerging classes of medications with BCL-2 being the most studied to date.

BCL-2 Identified over 40 years ago in B-ALL, the oncogenic protein B-cell lymphoma 2 (BCL-2) blocks apoptosis and plays a key role in transformation of neoplastic cells to malignant cancers [157]. Unlike other oncogenic proteins that mediate cell growth and proliferation, BCL-2 dysregulation allows survival of cells by altering pro-apoptotic and anti-apoptotic intracellular signals [158]. With higher expression than normal B-cell, ALL cell lines with high BCL-2 expression are associated with slow response to treatment [159]. Navitoclax, a dual BCL-2/BCL-xL inhibitor, showed incredible preclinical efficacy in B-ALL, but thrombocytopenia and neutropenia proved to be dose-limiting toxicities [160, 161]. Due to the importance of BCL-xL as a pro-survival mechanism for megakaryocytes and platelets, the selective BCL-2 inhibitor venetoclax was developed with efficacy in both AML and ALL [162–164]. There are currently 13 active trials in adult and pediatric patients looking at the activity of venetoclax in pre-B-ALL in both relapsed and refractory patients and as potential frontline therapy in older patients. Preclinical data also supports a role for venetoclax in patients with hypodiploid ALL, warranting further study in this high-risk subgroup [165].

In addition to the ongoing trials looking into the use of BCL-2 inhibitors in pre-B-ALL, other targeted pathways have also been studied in relapsed and refractory disease including mTOR inhibitors (rapamycin, everolimus, temsirolimus), RAS pathway (selumetinib), NEDD8 inhibitor (pevonedistat), and CDK4/6 inhibitors (palbociclib, ribociclib). These trials are summarized in Table 13.7.

mTOR Pathway The activation of the pro-survival pathway PI3K/AKT/mTOR pathway provides relapsed ALL with a survival and proliferation advantage [5]. The PI3K/AKT/mTOR pathway is a major regulatory pathway of cell growth and survival and cellular metabolism and has been shown to be constitutively active in multiple malignancies, including B-ALL [166]. Despite the track record of mTOR inhibitors in solid tumors and promising preclinical data in B-ALL [167], the trials looking at the use of rapamycin, everolimus, and temsirolimus in relapsed ALL have demonstrated limited efficacy and raised concern for excessive toxicity [168–170].

RAS Pathway Similar to the PI3K/AKT/mTOR pathway, the RAS/Raf/MEK/ERK (MAPK) pathway provides relapsed ALL a survival and proliferation, as well as a migration, advantage [171]. Mutations in the MAPK pathway are highly prevalent

Table 13.7 Summary of other targeted therapies

Mechanism	Drug	Clinicaltrials.gov identifier	Trial	Disease	Patients	Status	Results
mTOR inhibitors							
	Rapamycin	NCT00874562	Rapamycin + corticosteroids	Relapsed ALL	>1 yo	Completed	NA
		NCT00776373	Rapamycin + High-dose etoposide and cytarabine	R/R ALL	Adult (>18 yo)	Terminated	NA
	Everolimus	NCT01523977	Everolimus + vincristine, prednisone, PEG-asparaginase and doxorubicin	Relapsed ALL	Pediatric: 18mo–21yo	Completed	NA
		NCT00968253	Everolimus + hyper-CVAD	R/R ALL	>10 yo	Completed	CR 39% Median OS 23 weeks
	Temsirolimus	NCT01614197	Temsirolimus + dexamethasone, cyclophosphamide and etoposide	Relapsed ALL	Pediatric: 1–21 yo	Recruiting	NA
		NCT01403415	Temsirolimus + dexamethasone, mitoxantrone, vincristine, and pegaspargase	Relapsed ALL	Pediatric: 1– 21yo	Completed	3/15 in MRD- remission (excessive toxicity, not deemed tolerable)
RAS pathway							
	Selumetinib (MEK inhibitor)	NCT03705507	Selumetinib + dexamethasone	R/R RAS- Mutated ALL	All ages	Recruiting	NA
CDK6 inhibitors							

(continued)

Table 13.7 (continued)

Mechanism	Drug	Clinicaltrials.gov identifier	Trial	Disease	Patients	Status	Results
	Palbociclib	NCT02310243	Single Agent Palbociclib	MLL-rearranged ALL	Adult (>18 yo)	Recruiting	NA
		NCT03515200	Palbociclib + dex, followed by bortezomib + doxorubicin	R/R ALL	Pediatric: < 21yo	Recruiting	NA
	Ribociclib	NCT03740334	Ribociclib + dex and everolimus	R/R ALL	1–30 yo	Active, not recruiting	NA
NEDD8 inhibitor							
	Pevonedistat	NCT03349281	Pevonedistat + VXLD	R/R ALL	16–39 yo	Recruiting	NA

VXLD vincristine, dexamethasone, PEG-asparaginase, doxorubicin, *CVAD* cyclophosphamide, vincristine, adriamycin (doxorubicin), and dexamethasone in relapsed ALL and have been shown to be associated with high-risk features and dismal prognosis [172, 173]. Currently, the MEK inhibitor selumetinib is being investigated in a phase I/II trial in combination with dexamethasone (SeluDex) in pediatric patients with relapsed/refractory RAS pathway mutated ALL (NCT03705507).

CDK-Rb Pathway Another therapeutic strategy is to inhibit the cyclin-dependent kinase-retinoblastoma (CDK-Rb) pathway which leads to loss of cell cycle control and unrestrained growth when in various malignancies [174]. Currently, trials are studying the effects of CDK4/CDK6 kinase inhibitors palbociclib and ribociclib as part of combination therapies. Of particular interest is *KMT2A*-rearranged infant ALL as the KMT2A fusion proteins activate CDK6 and drive its proliferation [175].

NEDD8 A form of posttranslational modification, the addition of the ubiquitin-like protein NEDD8 is required for two DNA repair pathways. The process of neddylation is regulated by various tumor suppressor genes and oncoproteins, namely, VHL, p53, and MDM2, and its inhibition can lead to deficient DNA repair, accumulation of DNA damage, and eventual cell death [176]. The addition of pevonedistat to a standard ALL induction regimen is currently being studied in relapsed/refractory B-ALL (NCT03349281).

Conclusion: The Future of B-ALL Therapy

The development of monoclonal antibodies for the treatment of B-ALL has led to improved outcomes in pediatric and adult patients, particularly in the relapsed/refractory setting. Similar to improvement in EFS and OS in the 1990s and early 2000s with modifications of the sequence, dosing, and combination of cytotoxic B-ALL therapies, attention must be turned to how emerging monoclonal, cytotoxic, and small drug therapies can be optimally combined with or without chemotherapy in both the relapsed/refractory and frontline treatment settings [17].

Ideally, integrating highly active agents like blinatumomab and inotuzumab in the frontline setting could lead to the reduction of intensive chemotherapy and decreased treatment-related mortality while maintaining or even improving treatment efficacy. Long-term studies will also need to evaluate the role HSCT plays in the management of different patient cohorts if similar OS can be achieved through the addition of novel therapeutic agents alone [17]. Given the emergence of CAR-T therapies for B-ALL, the proper sequence of these therapies must be further investigated as sequential targeting of single antigen can modulate antigen expressivity and effect of subsequent treatment with agents against the same antigen [177].

With monoclonal antibodies being approved at twice the rate of other new therapies, one can expect for the emergence of newer generations of targeted agents increasing the options available for B-ALL patients [178].

References

1. Locatelli F, Whitlock JA, Peters C, et al. Blinatumomab versus historical standard therapy in pediatric patients with relapsed/refractory Ph-negative B-cell precursor acute lymphoblastic leukemia. Leukemia. 2020;34(9):2473–8.
2. Douer D. Efficacy and safety of vincristine sulfate liposome injection in the treatment of adult acute lymphocytic Leukemia. Oncologist. 2016;21:840–7.
3. Man LM, Morris AL, Keng M. New therapeutic strategies in acute lymphocytic leukemia. Curr Hematol Malig Rep. 2017;12:197–206.
4. Brown P, Inaba H, Annesley C, et al. Pediatric acute lymphoblastic leukemia, version 2.2020, NCCN clinical practice guidelines in oncology. J Natl Compr Canc Netw. 2020;18:81.
5. Santiago R, Vairy S, Sinnett D, Krajinovic M, Bittencourt H. Novel therapy for childhood acute lymphoblastic leukemia. Expert Opin Pharmacother. 2017;18:1081–99.
6. Sikaria S, Aldoss I, Akhtari M. Monoclonal antibodies and immune therapies for adult precursor B-acute lymphoblastic leukemia. Immunol Lett. 2016;172:113–23.
7. Farhadfar N, Litzow MR. New monoclonal antibodies for the treatment of acute lymphoblastic leukemia. Leuk Res. 2016;49:13–21.
8. Harris TJ, Drake CG. Primer on tumor immunology and cancer immunotherapy. J Immunother Cancer. 2013;1:12.
9. Gerber DE. Targeted therapies: a new generation of cancer treatments. Am Fam Physician. 2008;77:311–9.
10. Raponi S, Stefania De Propris M, Intoppa S, et al. Flow cytometric study of potential target antigens (CD19, CD20, CD22, CD33) for antibody-based immunotherapy in acute lymphoblastic leukemia: analysis of 552 cases. Leuk Lymphoma. 2011;52:1098–107.
11. Shah NN, Stevenson MS, Yuan CM, et al. Characterization of CD22 expression in acute lymphoblastic leukemia. Pediatr Blood Cancer. 2015;62:964–9.
12. Kantarjian H, Thomas D, Wayne AS, O'Brien S. Monoclonal antibody-based therapies: a new dawn in the treatment of acute lymphoblastic leukemia. J Clin Oncol. 2012;30:3876–83.
13. Chung S, Lin YL, Reed C, et al. Characterization of in vitro antibody-dependent cell-mediated cytotoxicity activity of therapeutic antibodies - impact of effector cells. J Immunol Methods. 2014;407:63–75.
14. Wang W, Erbe AK, Hank JA, Morris ZS, Sondel PM. NK cell-mediated antibody-dependent cellular cytotoxicity in cancer immunotherapy. Front Immunol. 2015;6:368.
15. Zhou X, Hu W, Qin X. The role of complement in the mechanism of action of rituximab for B-cell lymphoma: implications for therapy. Oncologist. 2008;13:954–66.
16. Behrens CR, Liu B. Methods for site-specific drug conjugation to antibodies. MAbs. 2014;6:46–53.
17. Guerra VA, Jabbour EJ, Ravandi F, Kantarjian H, Short NJ. Novel monoclonal antibody-based treatment strategies in adults with acute lymphoblastic leukemia. Ther Adv Hematol. 2019;10:2040620719849496.
18. Zhang X, Yang Y, Fan D, Xiong D. The development of bispecific antibodies and their applications in tumor immune escape. Exp Hematol Oncol. 2017;6:12.
19. Wei G, Wang J, Huang H, Zhao Y. Novel immunotherapies for adult patients with B-lineage acute lymphoblastic leukemia. J Hematol Oncol. 2017;10:150.
20. Wang K, Wei G, Liu D. CD19: a biomarker for B cell development, lymphoma diagnosis and therapy. Exp Hematol Oncol. 2012;1:36.
21. Weiland J, Elder A, Forster V, Heidenreich O, Koschmieder S, Vormoor J. CD19: a multifunctional immunological target molecule and its implications for B lineage acute lymphoblastic leukemia. Pediatr Blood Cancer. 2015;62:1144–8.
22. Carter RH, Myers R. Germinal center structure and function: lessons from CD19. Semin Immunol. 2008;20:43–8.
23. Carter RH, Wang Y, Brooks S. Role of CD19 signal transduction in B cell biology. Immunol Res. 2002;26:45–54.

24. Im A, Pavletic SZ. Immunotherapy in hematologic malignancies: past, present, and future. J Hematol Oncol. 2017;10:94.
25. Nagorsen D, Kufer P, Baeuerle PA, Bargou R. Blinatumomab: a historical perspective. Pharmacol Ther. 2012;136:334–42.
26. Löffler A, Gruen M, Wuchter C, et al. Efficient elimination of chronic lymphocytic leukaemia B cells by autologous T cells with a bispecific anti-CD19/anti-CD3 single-chain antibody construct. Leukemia. 2003;17:900–9.
27. Loffler A, Kufer P, Lutterbuse R, et al. A recombinant bispecific single-chain antibody, CD19 x CD3, induces rapid and high lymphoma-directed cytotoxicity by unstimulated T lymphocytes. Blood. 2000;95:2098–103.
28. Goebeler ME, Knop S, Viardot A, et al. Bispecific T-Cell Engager (BiTE) antibody construct blinatumomab for the treatment of patients with relapsed/refractory non-Hodgkin lymphoma: final results from a phase I study. J Clin Oncol. 2016;34:1104–11.
29. Topp MS, Gokbuget N, Zugmaier G, et al. Long-term follow-up of hematologic relapse-free survival in a phase 2 study of blinatumomab in patients with MRD in B-lineage ALL. Blood. 2012;120:5185–7.
30. Gokbuget N, Dombret H, Bonifacio M, et al. Blinatumomab for minimal residual disease in adults with B-cell precursor acute lymphoblastic leukemia. Blood. 2018;131:1522–31.
31. Topp MS, Gökbuget N, Zugmaier G, et al. Phase II trial of the anti-CD19 bispecific T cell–engager blinatumomab shows hematologic and molecular remissions in patients with relapsed or refractory B-precursor acute lymphoblastic leukemia. J Clin Oncol. 2014;32:4134–40.
32. Topp MS, Gokbuget N, Stein AS, et al. Safety and activity of blinatumomab for adult patients with relapsed or refractory B-precursor acute lymphoblastic leukaemia: a multicentre, single-arm, phase 2 study. Lancet Oncol. 2015;16:57–66.
33. Kantarjian H, Stein A, Gökbuget N, et al. Blinatumomab versus chemotherapy for advanced acute lymphoblastic leukemia. N Engl J Med. 2017;376:836–47.
34. von Stackelberg A, Locatelli F, Zugmaier G, et al. Phase I/phase II study of blinatumomab in pediatric patients with relapsed/refractory acute lymphoblastic leukemia. J Clin Oncol. 2016;34:4381–9.
35. Martinelli G, Boissel N, Chevallier P, et al. Complete hematologic and molecular response in adult patients with relapsed/refractory Philadelphia chromosome-positive B-precursor acute lymphoblastic leukemia following treatment with blinatumomab: results from a phase II, single-arm, multicenter study. J Clin Oncol. 2017;35:1795–802.
36. Viardot A, Bargou R. Bispecific antibodies in haematological malignancies. Cancer Treat Rev. 2018;65:87–95.
37. Yin H, Huo Y, Sheng Z, et al. Blinatumomab-induced T cell activation at single cell transcriptome resolution. Blood. 2019;134:3886.
38. Nagorsen D, Bargou R, Ruttinger D, Kufer P, Baeuerle PA, Zugmaier G. Immunotherapy of lymphoma and leukemia with T-cell engaging BiTE antibody blinatumomab. Leuk Lymphoma. 2009;50:886–91.
39. Maude SL, Barrett D, Teachey DT, Grupp SA. Managing cytokine release syndrome associated with novel T cell-engaging therapies. Cancer J. 2014;20:119–22.
40. Teachey DT, Rheingold SR, Maude SL, et al. Cytokine release syndrome after blinatumomab treatment related to abnormal macrophage activation and ameliorated with cytokine-directed therapy. Blood. 2013;121:5154–7.
41. Jain T, Litzow MR. No free rides: management of toxicities of novel immunotherapies in ALL, including financial. Blood Adv. 2018;2:3393–403.
42. Rafei H, Kantarjian HM, Jabbour EJ. Recent advances in the treatment of acute lymphoblastic leukemia. Leuk Lymphoma. 2019;60:2606–21.
43. Richard-Carpentier G, Kantarjian HM, Short NJ, et al. A phase II study of the hyper-CVAD regimen in sequential combination with blinatumomab as frontline therapy for adults with B-Cell acute lymphoblastic leukemia (B-ALL). Blood. 2018;132:32.

44. Ribera JM, Ferrer A, Ribera J, Genesca E. Profile of blinatumomab and its potential in the treatment of relapsed/refractory acute lymphoblastic leukemia. Onco Targets Ther. 2015;8:1567–74.
45. Benjamin JE, Stein AS. The role of blinatumomab in patients with relapsed/refractory acute lymphoblastic leukemia. Ther Adv Hematol. 2016;7:142–56.
46. Zugmaier G, Topp MS, Alekar S, et al. Long-term follow-up of serum immunoglobulin levels in blinatumomab-treated patients with minimal residual disease-positive B-precursor acute lymphoblastic leukemia. Blood Cancer J. 2014;4:244.
47. Paul S, Rausch CR, Nasnas PE, Kantarjian H, Jabbour EJ. Treatment of relapsed/refractory acute lymphoblastic leukemia. Clin Adv Hematol Oncol. 2019;17:166–75.
48. Liu D, Zhao J, Song Y, Luo X, Yang T. Clinical trial update on bispecific antibodies, antibody-drug conjugates, and antibody-containing regimens for acute lymphoblastic leukemia. J Hematol Oncol. 2019;12:15.
49. Brown PA, Ji L, Xu X, et al. A randomized phase 3 trial of blinatumomab Vs. chemotherapy as post-reinduction therapy in high and intermediate risk (HR/IR) first relapse of B-acute lymphoblastic leukemia (B-ALL) in children and adolescents/young adults (AYAs) demonstrates superior efficacy and tolerability of blinatumomab: a report from Children's Oncology Group Study AALL1331. Blood. JAMA. 2021;134:LBA-1-LBA. https://doi.org/10.1001/jama.2021.0669. PMID: 33651090.
50. Sotillo E, Barrett DM, Black KL, et al. Convergence of acquired mutations and alternative splicing of CD19 enables resistance to CART-19 immunotherapy. Cancer Discov. 2015;5:1282–95.
51. Orlando EJ, Han X, Tribouley C, et al. Genetic mechanisms of target antigen loss in CAR19 therapy of acute lymphoblastic leukemia. Nat Med. 2018;24:1504–6.
52. Braig F, Brandt A, Goebeler M, et al. Resistance to anti-CD19/CD3 BiTE in acute lymphoblastic leukemia may be mediated by disrupted CD19 membrane trafficking. Blood. 2017;129:100–4.
53. Balducci E, Nivaggioni V, Boudjarane J, et al. Lineage switch from B acute lymphoblastic leukemia to acute monocytic leukemia with persistent t(4;11)(q21;q23) and cytogenetic evolution under CD19-targeted therapy. Ann Hematol. 2017;96:1579–81.
54. Nagel I, Bartels M, Duell J, et al. Hematopoietic stem cell involvement in BCR-ABL1-positive ALL as a potential mechanism of resistance to blinatumomab therapy. Blood. 2017;130:2027–31.
55. Gardner R, Wu D, Cherian S, et al. Acquisition of a CD19-negative myeloid phenotype allows immune escape of MLL-rearranged B-ALL from CD19 CAR-T-cell therapy. Blood. 2016;127:2406–10.
56. Oberley MJ, Gaynon PS, Bhojwani D, et al. Myeloid lineage switch following chimeric antigen receptor T-cell therapy in a patient with TCF3-ZNF384 fusion-positive B-lymphoblastic leukemia. Pediatr Blood Cancer. 2018;65:e27265.
57. Rayes A, McMasters RL, O'Brien MM. Lineage switch in MLL-rearranged infant leukemia following CD19-directed therapy. Pediatr Blood Cancer. 2016;63:1113–5.
58. Francis J, Dharmadhikari AV, Sait SN, et al. CD19 expression in acute leukemia is not restricted to the cytogenetically aberrant populations. Leuk Lymphoma. 2013;54:1517–20.
59. Kohnke T, Krupka C, Tischer J, Knosel T, Subklewe M. Increase of PD-L1 expressing B-precursor ALL cells in a patient resistant to the CD19/CD3-bispecific T cell engager antibody blinatumomab. J Hematol Oncol. 2015;8:111.
60. Feucht J, Kayser S, Gorodezki D, et al. T-cell responses against CD19+ pediatric acute lymphoblastic leukemia mediated by bispecific T-cell engager (BiTE) are regulated contrarily by PD-L1 and CD80/CD86 on leukemic blasts. Oncotarget. 2016;7:76902–19.
61. Duell J, Dittrich M, Bedke T, et al. Frequency of regulatory T cells determines the outcome of the T-cell-engaging antibody blinatumomab in patients with B-precursor ALL. Leukemia. 2017;31:2181–90.

62. King AC, Pappacena JJ, Tallman MS, Park JH, Geyer MB. Blinatumomab administered concurrently with oral tyrosine kinase inhibitor therapy is a well-tolerated consolidation strategy and eradicates measurable residual disease in adults with Philadelphia chromosome positive acute lymphoblastic leukemia. Leuk Res. 2019;79:27–33.
63. Webster J, Luskin MR, Prince GT, et al. Blinatumomab in combination with immune checkpoint inhibitors of PD-1 and CTLA-4 in adult patients with relapsed/refractory (R/R) CD19 positive B-cell acute lymphoblastic leukemia (ALL): preliminary results of a phase I study. Blood. 2018;132:557.
64. Van Epps HA, Heiser R, Cao A, et al. Denintuzumab mafodotin stimulates immune responses and synergizes with CD20 antibodies to heighten anti-tumor activity in preclinical models of non-Hodgkin lymphoma. Blood. 2016;128:4177.
65. Fathi AT, Borate U, DeAngelo DJ, et al. A phase 1 study of denintuzumab mafodotin (SGN-CD19A) in adults with relapsed or refractory B-lineage acute leukemia (B-ALL) and highly aggressive lymphoma. Blood. 2015;126:1328.
66. Blanc V, Bousseau A, Caron A, Carrez C, Lutz RJ, Lambert JM. SAR3419: an anti-CD19-Maytansinoid Immunoconjugate for the treatment of B-cell malignancies. Clin Cancer Res. 2011;17:6448–58.
67. Younes A, Kim S, Romaguera J, et al. Phase I multidose-escalation study of the anti-CD19 maytansinoid immunoconjugate SAR3419 administered by intravenous infusion every 3 weeks to patients with relapsed/refractory B-cell lymphoma. J Clin Oncol. 2012;30:2776–82.
68. Kantarjian HM, Lioure B, Kim SK, et al. A phase II study of coltuximab ravtansine (SAR3419) monotherapy in patients with relapsed or refractory acute lymphoblastic leukemia. Clin Lymphoma Myeloma Leuk. 2016;16:139–45.
69. Vallera DA, Todhunter DA, Kuroki DW, Shu Y, Sicheneder A, Chen H. A bispecific recombinant immunotoxin, DT2219, targeting human CD19 and CD22 receptors in a mouse xenograft model of B-cell leukemia/lymphoma. Clin Cancer Res. 2005;11:3879–88.
70. Vallera DA, Chen H, Sicheneder AR, Panoskaltsis-Mortari A, Taras EP. Genetic alteration of a bispecific ligand-directed toxin targeting human CD19 and CD22 receptors resulting in improved efficacy against systemic B cell malignancy. Leuk Res. 2009;33:1233–42.
71. Bachanova V, Cao Q, Weisdorf DJ, et al. Bispecific ligand-directed toxin targeting CD22 and CD19 (DT2219) for refractory B-cell malignancies: results of phase I-II trial. J Clin Oncol. 2019;37:e19066-e.
72. Piccaluga PP, Arpinati M, Candoni A, et al. Surface antigens analysis reveals significant expression of candidate targets for immunotherapy in adult acute lymphoid leukemia. Leuk Lymphoma. 2011;52:325–7.
73. Haso W, Lee DW, Shah NN, et al. Anti-CD22-chimeric antigen receptors targeting B-cell precursor acute lymphoblastic leukemia. Blood. 2013;121:1165–74.
74. Carnahan J, Wang P, Kendall R, et al. Epratuzumab, a humanized monoclonal antibody targeting CD22: characterization of in vitro properties. Clin Cancer Res. 2003;9:3982s–90s.
75. Ereno-Orbea J, Sicard T, Cui H, et al. Molecular basis of human CD22 function and therapeutic targeting. Nat Commun. 2017;8:764.
76. Libert D, Yuan CM, Masih KE, et al. Serial evaluation of CD19 surface expression in pediatric B-cell malignancies following CD19-targeted therapy. Leukemia. 2020;34(11):3064–9.
77. Lamb YN. Inotuzumab ozogamicin: first global approval. Drugs. 2017;77:1603–10.
78. DiJoseph JF, Armellino DC, Boghaert ER, et al. Antibody-targeted chemotherapy with CMC-544: a CD22-targeted immunoconjugate of calicheamicin for the treatment of B-lymphoid malignancies. Blood. 2004;103:1807–14.
79. de Vries JF, Zwaan CM, De Bie M, et al. The novel calicheamicin-conjugated CD22 antibody inotuzumab ozogamicin (CMC 544) effectively kills primary pediatric acute lymphoblastic leukemia cells. Leukemia. 2012;26:255–64.
80. Zein N, Sinha AM, McGahren WJ, Ellestad GA. Calicheamicin gamma 1I: an antitumor antibiotic that cleaves double-stranded DNA site specifically. Science. 1988;240:1198–201.

81. Marks DI, Kebriaei P, Stelljes M, et al. Outcomes of allogeneic stem cell transplantation after inotuzumab ozogamicin treatment for relapsed or refractory acute lymphoblastic leukemia. Biol Blood Marrow Transplant. 2019;25:1720–9.
82. Kebriaei P, Cutler C, de Lima M, et al. Management of important adverse events associated with inotuzumab ozogamicin: expert panel review. Bone Marrow Transplant. 2018;53:449–56.
83. Wadleigh M, Richardson PG, Zahrieh D, et al. Prior gemtuzumab ozogamicin exposure significantly increases the risk of veno-occlusive disease in patients who undergo myeloablative allogeneic stem cell transplantation. Blood. 2003;102:1578–82.
84. Rajvanshi P, Shulman HM, Sievers EL, McDonald GB. Hepatic sinusoidal obstruction after gemtuzumab ozogamicin (Mylotarg) therapy. Blood. 2002;99:2310–4.
85. Kantarjian HM, DeAngelo DJ, Advani AS, et al. Hepatic adverse event profile of inotuzumab ozogamicin in adult patients with relapsed or refractory acute lymphoblastic leukaemia: results from the open-label, randomised, phase 3 INO-VATE study. Lancet Haematol. 2017;4:e387–e98.
86. Kantarjian H, Thomas D, Jorgensen J, et al. Inotuzumab ozogamicin, an anti-CD22-calecheamicin conjugate, for refractory and relapsed acute lymphocytic leukaemia: a phase 2 study. Lancet Oncol. 2012;13:403–11.
87. Kantarjian H, Thomas D, Jorgensen J, et al. Results of inotuzumab ozogamicin, a CD22 monoclonal antibody, in refractory and relapsed acute lymphocytic leukemia. Cancer. 2013;119:2728–36.
88. Kantarjian HM, DeAngelo DJ, Stelljes M, et al. Inotuzumab ozogamicin versus standard therapy for acute lymphoblastic leukemia. N Engl J Med. 2016;375:740–53.
89. Bhojwani D, Sposto R, Shah NN, et al. Inotuzumab ozogamicin in pediatric patients with relapsed/refractory acute lymphoblastic leukemia. Leukemia. 2019;33:884–92.
90. O'Brien MM, Ji L, Shah NN, et al. A phase 2 trial of inotuzumab ozogamicin (InO) in children and young adults with relapsed or refractory (R/R) CD22+ B-acute lymphoblastic leukemia (B-ALL): results from Children's Oncology Group Protocol AALL1621. Blood. 2019;134:741.
91. Betts AM, Haddish-Berhane N, Tolsma J, et al. Preclinical to clinical translation of antibody-drug conjugates using PK/PD modeling: a retrospective analysis of inotuzumab ozogamicin. AAPS J. 2016;18:1101–16.
92. Kantarjian HM, Stock W, Cassaday RD, et al. Comparison of CD22 expression between baseline, end of treatment, and relapse among patients treated with inotuzumab ozogamicin who responded and subsequently relapsed in two clinical trials. Blood. 2018;132:2699.
93. Yates B, Shalabi H, Salem D, et al. Sequential CD22 targeting impacts CD22 CAR-T cell response. Blood. 2018;132:282.
94. Lanza F, Maffini E, Rondoni M, Massari E, Faini AC, Malavasi F. CD22 expression in B-cell acute lymphoblastic leukemia: biological significance and implications for inotuzumab therapy in adults. Cancers (Basel). 2020;12:303.
95. Raetz EA, Cairo MS, Borowitz MJ, et al. Chemoimmunotherapy reinduction with epratuzumab in children with acute lymphoblastic leukemia in marrow relapse: a Children's Oncology Group Pilot Study. J Clin Oncol. 2008;26:3756–62.
96. Raetz EA, Cairo MS, Borowitz MJ, et al. Re-induction chemoimmunotherapy with epratuzumab in relapsed acute lymphoblastic leukemia (ALL): phase II results from Children's Oncology Group (COG) study ADVL04P2. Pediatr Blood Cancer. 2015;62:1171–5.
97. Advani AS, McDonough S, Coutre S, et al. SWOG S0910: a phase 2 trial of clofarabine/cytarabine/epratuzumab for relapsed/refractory acute lymphocytic leukaemia. Br J Haematol. 2014;165:504–9.
98. Kreitman RJ, Pastan I. Antibody fusion proteins: anti-CD22 recombinant immunotoxin moxetumomab pasudotox. Clin Cancer Res. 2011;17:6398–405.
99. Wayne AS, Shah NN, Bhojwani D, et al. Phase 1 study of the anti-CD22 immunotoxin moxetumomab pasudotox for childhood acute lymphoblastic leukemia. Blood. 2017;130:1620–7.

100. Shah NN, Bhojwani D, August K, et al. Results from an international phase 2 study of the anti-CD22 immunotoxin moxetumomab pasudotox in relapsed or refractory childhood B-lineage acute lymphoblastic leukemia. Pediatr Blood Cancer. 2020:e28112.
101. Kreitman RJ, Tallman MS, Robak T, et al. Phase I trial of anti-CD22 recombinant immunotoxin moxetumomab pasudotox (CAT-8015 or HA22) in patients with hairy cell leukemia. J Clin Oncol. 2012;30:1822–8.
102. Muller F, Cunningham T, Beers R, Bera TK, Wayne AS, Pastan I. Domain II of pseudomonas exotoxin is critical for efficacy of bolus doses in a xenograft model of acute lymphoblastic leukemia. Toxins (Basel). 2018;10:210.
103. Zhou Y, You MJ, Young KH, et al. Advances in the molecular pathobiology of B-lymphoblastic leukemia. Hum Pathol. 2012;43:1347–62.
104. Jazirehi AR, Vega MI, Bonavida B. Development of rituximab-resistant lymphoma clones with altered cell signaling and cross-resistance to chemotherapy. Cancer Res. 2007;67:1270–81.
105. Maury S, Huguet F, Leguay T, et al. Adverse prognostic significance of CD20 expression in adults with Philadelphia chromosome-negative B-cell precursor acute lymphoblastic leukemia. Haematologica. 2010;95:324–8.
106. Thomas DA, O'Brien S, Jorgensen JL, et al. Prognostic significance of CD20 expression in adults with de novo precursor B-lineage acute lymphoblastic leukemia. Blood. 2009;113:6330–7.
107. McLaughlin P, Hagemeister FB, Grillo-Lopez AJ. Rituximab in indolent lymphoma: the single-agent pivotal trial. Semin Oncol. 1999;26:79–87.
108. Rai KR. Therapeutic potential of new B cell-targeted agents in the treatment of elderly and unfit patients with chronic lymphocytic leukemia. J Hematol Oncol. 2015;8:85.
109. Batchelor TT, Grossman SA, Mikkelsen T, Ye X, Desideri S, Lesser GJ. Rituximab monotherapy for patients with recurrent primary CNS lymphoma. Neurology. 2011;76:929–30.
110. Thomas DA, O'Brien S, Faderl S, et al. Chemoimmunotherapy with a modified hyper-CVAD and rituximab regimen improves outcome in de novo Philadelphia chromosome-negative precursor B-lineage acute lymphoblastic leukemia. J Clin Oncol. 2010;28:3880–9.
111. Hoelzer D, Huettmann A, Kaul F, et al. Immunochemotherapy with rituximab improves molecular CR rate and outcome in CD20+ B-lineage standard and high risk patients; results of 263 CD20+ patients studied prospectively in GMALL study 07/2003. Blood. 2010;116:170.
112. Maury S, Chevret S, Thomas X, et al. Rituximab in B-lineage adult acute lymphoblastic leukemia. N Engl J Med. 2016;375:1044–53.
113. Fielding AK, Alapi KZ, Wrench B, et al. First analysis of the UKALL14 phase 3 randomised trial to determine if the addition of rituximab to standard induction chemotherapy improves EFS in adults with precursor B-ALL (CRUK/09/006). Blood. 2019;134:739.
114. Dworzak MN, Schumich A, Printz D, et al. CD20 up-regulation in pediatric B-cell precursor acute lymphoblastic leukemia during induction treatment: setting the stage for anti-CD20 directed immunotherapy. Blood. 2008;112:3982–8.
115. Castillo J, Milani C, Mendez-Allwood D. Ofatumumab, a second-generation anti-CD20 monoclonal antibody, for the treatment of lymphoproliferative and autoimmune disorders. Expert Opin Investig Drugs. 2009;18:491–500.
116. Awasthi A, Ayello J, Van de Ven C, et al. Obinutuzumab (GA101) compared to rituximab significantly enhances cell death and antibody-dependent cytotoxicity and improves overall survival against CD20(+) rituximab-sensitive/-resistant Burkitt lymphoma (BL) and precursor B-acute lymphoblastic leukaemia (pre-B-ALL): potential targeted therapy in patients with poor risk CD20(+) BL and pre-B-ALL. Br J Haematol. 2015;171:763–75.
117. Bazarbachi AH, Yilmaz M, Ravandi F, et al. A phase 2 study of hyper-CVAD plus ofatumumab as frontline therapy in CD20+ acute lymphoblastic leukemia (ALL): updated results. J Clin Oncol. 2018;36:7041.

118. Herter S, Herting F, Mundigl O, et al. Preclinical activity of the type II CD20 antibody GA101 (obinutuzumab) compared with rituximab and ofatumumab in vitro and in xenograft models. Mol Cancer Ther. 2013;12:2031–42.
119. Goede V, Fischer K, Busch R, et al. Obinutuzumab plus chlorambucil in patients with CLL and coexisting conditions. N Engl J Med. 2014;370:1101–10.
120. Angiolillo AL, Yu AL, Reaman G, Ingle AM, Secola R, Adamson PC. A phase II study of Campath-1H in children with relapsed or refractory acute lymphoblastic leukemia: a Children's Oncology Group report. Pediatr Blood Cancer. 2009;53:978–83.
121. Tibes R, Keating MJ, Ferrajoli A, et al. Activity of alemtuzumab in patients with CD52-positive acute leukemia. Cancer. 2006;106:2645–51.
122. Chevallier P, Mahe B, Garand R, Talmant P, Harousseau JL, Delaunay J. Combination of chemotherapy and gemtuzumab ozogamicin in adult Philadelphia positive acute lymphoblastic leukemia patient harboring CD33 expression. Int J Hematol. 2008;88:209–11.
123. Papayannidis C, Derenzini E, Iacobucci I, et al. Successful combination treatment of clofarabine, cytarabine, and gemtuzumab-ozogamicin in adult refractory B-acute lymphoblastic leukemia. Am J Hematol. 2009;84:849–50.
124. Bonate PL, Arthaud L, Cantrell WR Jr, Stephenson K, Secrist JA 3rd, Weitman S. Discovery and development of clofarabine: a nucleoside analogue for treating cancer. Nat Rev Drug Discov. 2006;5:855–63.
125. Genini D, Adachi S, Chao Q, et al. Deoxyadenosine analogs induce programmed cell death in chronic lymphocytic leukemia cells by damaging the DNA and by directly affecting the mitochondria. Blood. 2000;96:3537–43.
126. Jeha S, Gaynon PS, Razzouk BI, et al. Phase II study of clofarabine in pediatric patients with refractory or relapsed acute lymphoblastic leukemia. J Clin Oncol. 2006;24:1917–23.
127. Jeha S, Razzouk B, Rytting M, et al. Phase II study of clofarabine in pediatric patients with refractory or relapsed acute myeloid leukemia. J Clin Oncol. 2009;27:4392–7.
128. Miano M, Pistorio A, Putti MC, et al. Clofarabine, cyclophosphamide and etoposide for the treatment of relapsed or resistant acute leukemia in pediatric patients. Leuk Lymphoma. 2012;53:1693–8.
129. Hijiya N, Thomson B, Isakoff MS, et al. Phase 2 trial of clofarabine in combination with etoposide and cyclophosphamide in pediatric patients with refractory or relapsed acute lymphoblastic leukemia. Blood. 2011;118:6043–9.
130. Salzer WL, Burke MJ, Devidas M, et al. Toxicity associated with intensive postinduction therapy incorporating clofarabine in the very high-risk stratum of patients with newly diagnosed high-risk B-lymphoblastic leukemia: a report from the Children's Oncology Group study AALL1131. Cancer. 2018;124:1150–9.
131. Bassan R, Fumagalli M, Chiaretti S, et al. Phase II trial with sequential clofarabine and cyclophosphamide for refractory and relapsed Philadelphia-negative adult acute lymphoblastic leukemia. Results of the GIMEMA LAL 1610 protocol. Leuk Lymphoma. 2019;60:3482–92.
132. Adams J, Palombella VJ, Sausville EA, et al. Proteasome inhibitors: a novel class of potent and effective antitumor agents. Cancer Res. 1999;59:2615–22.
133. Annesley CE, Brown P. Novel agents for the treatment of childhood acute leukemia. Ther Adv Hematol. 2015;6:61–79.
134. Cortes J, Thomas D, Koller C, et al. Phase I study of bortezomib in refractory or relapsed acute leukemias. Clin Cancer Res. 2004;10:3371–6.
135. Horton TM, Pati D, Plon SE, et al. A phase 1 study of the proteasome inhibitor bortezomib in pediatric patients with refractory leukemia: a Children's Oncology Group study. Clin Cancer Res. 2007;13:1516–22.
136. Messinger YH, Gaynon PS, Sposto R, et al. Bortezomib with chemotherapy is highly active in advanced B-precursor acute lymphoblastic leukemia: Therapeutic Advances in Childhood Leukemia & Lymphoma (TACL) Study. Blood. 2012;120:285–90.

137. Horton TM, Lu X, O'Brien MM, et al. Bortezomib reinduction therapy to improve response rates in pediatric ALL in first relapse: a Children's Oncology Group (COG) study (AALL07P1). J Clin Oncol. 2013;31:10003.
138. Horton TM, Whitlock JA, Lu X, et al. Bortezomib reinduction chemotherapy in high-risk ALL in first relapse: a report from the Children's Oncology Group. Br J Haematol. 2019;186:274–85.
139. Arastu-Kapur S, Anderl JL, Kraus M, et al. Nonproteasomal targets of the proteasome inhibitors bortezomib and carfilzomib: a link to clinical adverse events. Clin Cancer Res. 2011;17:2734–43.
140. Yang J, Wang Z, Fang Y, et al. Pharmacokinetics, pharmacodynamics, metabolism, distribution, and excretion of carfilzomib in rats. Drug Metab Dispos. 2011;39:1873–82.
141. Shah NN, Merchant MS, Cole DE, et al. Vincristine Sulfate liposomes injection (VSLI, Marqibo(R)): results from a phase I study in children, adolescents, and young adults with refractory solid tumors or leukemias. Pediatr Blood Cancer. 2016;63:997–1005.
142. Lew G, Chen Y, Lu X, et al. Outcomes after late bone marrow and very early central nervous system relapse of childhood B-acute lymphoblastic leukemia: a report from the Children's Oncology Group phase III study AALL0433. Haematologica. 2020;106(1):46–55.
143. O'Brien S, Schiller G, Lister J, et al. High-dose vincristine sulfate liposome injection for advanced, relapsed, and refractory adult Philadelphia chromosome-negative acute lymphoblastic leukemia. J Clin Oncol. 2013;31:676–83.
144. Egler RA, Ahuja SP, Matloub Y. L-asparaginase in the treatment of patients with acute lymphoblastic leukemia. J Pharmacol Pharmacother. 2016;7:62–71.
145. Angiolillo AL, Schore RJ, Devidas M, et al. Pharmacokinetic and pharmacodynamic properties of calaspargase pegol Escherichia coli L-asparaginase in the treatment of patients with acute lymphoblastic leukemia: results from Children's Oncology Group Study AALL07P4. J Clin Oncol. 2014;32:3874–82.
146. Vrooman LM, Blonquist TM, Supko JG, et al. Efficacy and toxicity of pegaspargase and calaspargase pegol in childhood acute lymphoblastic leukemia/lymphoma: results of DFCI 11-001. J Clin Oncol. 2019;37:10006.
147. Herman JG, Civin CI, Issa JP, Collector MI, Sharkis SJ, Baylin SB. Distinct patterns of inactivation of p15INK4B and p16INK4A characterize the major types of hematological malignancies. Cancer Res. 1997;57:837–41.
148. Gore SD. Combination therapy with DNA methyltransferase inhibitors in hematologic malignancies. Nat Clin Pract Oncol. 2005;2(Suppl 1):S30–5.
149. Burke MJ, Brown P, Sposto R, Gore L, Wayne AS. Pilot study of decitabine and vorinostat with chemotherapy for relapsed ALL: a report from the Therapeutic Advances in Childhood Leukemia & Lymphoma (TACL) Consortium. Blood. 2016;128:2781.
150. Bhatla T, Wang J, Morrison DJ, et al. Epigenetic reprogramming reverses the relapse-specific gene expression signature and restores chemosensitivity in childhood B-lymphoblastic leukemia. Blood. 2012;119:5201–10.
151. Subramanian S, Bates SE, Wright JJ, Espinoza-Delgado I, Piekarz RL. Clinical toxicities of histone deacetylase inhibitors. Pharmaceuticals (Basel). 2010;3:2751–67.
152. Dawson MA, Kouzarides T. Cancer epigenetics: from mechanism to therapy. Cell. 2012;150:12–27.
153. Irving JA. Towards an understanding of the biology and targeted treatment of paediatric relapsed acute lymphoblastic leukaemia. Br J Haematol. 2016;172:655–66.
154. Hollenbach PW, Nguyen AN, Brady H, et al. A comparison of azacitidine and decitabine activities in acute myeloid leukemia cell lines. PLoS One. 2010;5:e9001.
155. Cheng J, Yang H, Fang J, et al. Molecular mechanism for USP7-mediated DNMT1 stabilization by acetylation. Nat Commun. 2015;6:7023.
156. Grobner SN, Worst BC, Weischenfeldt J, et al. The landscape of genomic alterations across childhood cancers. Nature. 2018;555:321–7.

157. Cassier PA, Castets M, Belhabri A, Vey N. Targeting apoptosis in acute myeloid leukaemia. Br J Cancer. 2017;117:1089–98.
158. Ashkenazi A, Fairbrother WJ, Leverson JD, Souers AJ. From basic apoptosis discoveries to advanced selective BCL-2 family inhibitors. Nat Rev Drug Discov. 2017;16:273–84.
159. Stam RW, Den Boer ML, Schneider P, et al. Association of high-level MCL-1 expression with in vitro and in vivo prednisone resistance in MLL-rearranged infant acute lymphoblastic leukemia. Blood. 2010;115:1018–25.
160. Oltersdorf T, Elmore SW, Shoemaker AR, et al. An inhibitor of BCL-2 family proteins induces regression of solid tumours. Nature. 2005;435:677–81.
161. Tse C, Shoemaker AR, Adickes J, et al. ABT-263: a potent and orally bioavailable BCL-2 family inhibitor. Cancer Res. 2008;68:3421–8.
162. Schoenwaelder SM, Jarman KE, Gardiner EE, et al. Bcl-xL-inhibitory BH3 mimetics can induce a transient thrombocytopathy that undermines the hemostatic function of platelets. Blood. 2011;118:1663–74.
163. Kile BT. The role of apoptosis in megakaryocytes and platelets. Br J Haematol. 2014;165:217–26.
164. Souers AJ, Leverson JD, Boghaert ER, et al. ABT-199, a potent and selective BCL-2 inhibitor, achieves antitumor activity while sparing platelets. Nat Med. 2013;19:202–8.
165. Diaz-Flores E, Comeaux EQ, Kim KL, et al. BCL-2 is a therapeutic target for hypodiploid B-lineage acute lymphoblastic leukemia. Cancer Res. 2019;79:2339–51.
166. Fransecky L, Mochmann LH, Baldus CD. Outlook on PI3K/AKT/mTOR inhibition in acute leukemia. Mol Cell Ther. 2015;3:2.
167. Tasian SK, Teachey DT, Rheingold SR. Targeting the PI3K/mTOR pathway in pediatric hematologic malignancies. Front Oncol. 2014;4:108.
168. Place AE, Pikman Y, Stevenson KE, et al. Phase I trial of the mTOR inhibitor everolimus in combination with multi-agent chemotherapy in relapsed childhood acute lymphoblastic leukemia. Pediatr Blood Cancer. 2018;65:e27062.
169. Rheingold SR, Tasian SK, Whitlock JA, et al. A phase 1 trial of temsirolimus and intensive re-induction chemotherapy for 2nd or greater relapse of acute lymphoblastic leukaemia: a Children's Oncology Group study (ADVL1114). Br J Haematol. 2017;177:467–74.
170. Daver N, Boumber Y, Kantarjian H, et al. A phase I/II study of the mTOR inhibitor everolimus in combination with hyperCVAD chemotherapy in patients with relapsed/refractory acute lymphoblastic leukemia. Clin Cancer Res. 2015;21:2704–14.
171. Chang L, Karin M. Mammalian MAP kinase signalling cascades. Nature. 2001;410:37–40.
172. Irving J, Matheson E, Minto L, et al. Ras pathway mutations are prevalent in relapsed childhood acute lymphoblastic leukemia and confer sensitivity to MEK inhibition. Blood. 2014;124:3420–30.
173. Oshima K, Khiabanian H, da Silva-Almeida AC, et al. Mutational landscape, clonal evolution patterns, and role of RAS mutations in relapsed acute lymphoblastic leukemia. Proc Natl Acad Sci U S A. 2016;113:11306–11.
174. Bortolozzi R, Mattiuzzo E, Trentin L, Accordi B, Basso G, Viola G. Ribociclib, a Cdk4/Cdk6 kinase inhibitor, enhances glucocorticoid sensitivity in B-acute lymphoblastic leukemia (B-All). Biochem Pharmacol. 2018;153:230–41.
175. van der Linden MH, Willekes M, van Roon E, et al. MLL fusion-driven activation of CDK6 potentiates proliferation in MLL-rearranged infant ALL. Cell Cycle. 2014;13:834–44.
176. Watson IR, Irwin MS, Ohh M. NEDD8 pathways in cancer, Sine Quibus Non. Cancer Cell. 2011;19:168–76.
177. Pillai V, Muralidharan K, Meng W, et al. CAR T-cell therapy is effective for CD19-dim B-lymphoblastic leukemia but is impacted by prior blinatumomab therapy. Blood Adv. 2019;3:3539–49.
178. Hay M, Thomas DW, Craighead JL, Economides C, Rosenthal J. Clinical development success rates for investigational drugs. Nat Biotechnol. 2014;32:40–51.

Chapter 14
New Agents for the Treatment of T-Cell Acute Lymphoblastic Leukemia

Sunil S. Raikar, David T. Teachey, and Nathan P. Gossai

Introduction and Overview of the Treatment of T-Cell Acute Lymphoblastic Leukemia

The prognosis for children with acute lymphoblastic leukemia (ALL) has improved significantly over the past 50 years. ALL is often divided based upon immunophenotype into B-cell acute lymphoblastic leukemia (B-ALL) and T-cell acute lymphoblastic leukemia (T-ALL). Outcomes for children with B-ALL have historically been superior to T-ALL [1]. Yet, with modern chemotherapy backbones that include risk-stratified therapy, outcomes are similar. While comparable chemotherapy regimens have been used to treat T- and B-ALL, they are biologically distinct and have a different kinetic pattern of minimal residual disease (MRD) response [1]. Unlike in B-ALL, where treatment can be risk stratified based on several clinical variables as well as cytogenetic features, MRD response remains the driving prognostic determinant in T-ALL [1]. While outcomes for de novo T-ALL patients have improved, some patients relapse, and these patients often do not survive [2]. Systematic screening of T-ALL genomes by high-resolution copy number arrays and next-generation sequencing technologies has improved understanding of T-ALL

S. S. Raikar
Department of Pediatrics, Aflac Cancer and Blood Disorders Center, Emory University and Children's Healthcare of Atlanta, Atlanta, GA, USA
e-mail: sraikar@emory.edu

D. T. Teachey
Division of Oncology, Department of Pediatrics, Center for Childhood Cancer Research, Children's Hospital of Philadelphia and Perelman School of Medicine, University of Pennsylvania, Philadelphia, PA, USA
e-mail: teacheyd@email.chop.edu

N. P. Gossai (✉)
Department of Cancer and Blood Disorders, Children's Minnesota, Minneapolis, MN, USA
e-mail: nathan.gossai@childrensmn.org

M. R. Litzow, E. A. Raetz (eds.), *Clinical Management of Acute Lymphoblastic Leukemia*, https://doi.org/10.1007/978-3-030-85147-7_14

biology, providing novel attractive targets for therapy [3]. This review will outline our current understanding of T-ALL biology and describe the prospects for novel therapeutics.

Overview of the Biology of T-ALL

Over the past two decades, significant advances have been made in the understanding of biological mechanisms in T-ALL through genomic and transcriptomic analyses, identifying numerous signaling pathways that can potentially be targeted with novel agents [4–7]. T-ALL is a molecularly heterogeneous disease, and unique gene expression signatures are associated with T-ALL subgroups reflecting different stages of thymocyte developmental arrest [8]. Unfortunately, classifying T-ALL based on developmental stage has not had prognostic significance with modern chemotherapy regimens [1]. More recently, early T-cell precursor (ETP)-ALL was identified as a unique subgroup of T-ALL with a distinct molecular profile, with more similarities to myeloid disease compared to non-ETP T-ALL cases [9]. Several early studies showed that ETP-ALL had inferior outcomes compared to non-ETP T-ALL [10–12]. However, data from the Children's Oncology Group (COG) AALL0434 study demonstrated that while ETP-ALL had higher rates of induction failure, survival rates were excellent and comparable between ETP-ALL and non-ETP T-ALL groups [13].

The spectrum of genetic abnormalities seen in T-ALL is vast and diverse [3, 7, 8]. The various molecular pathways involved in T-ALL pathogenesis are reviewed in depth in this text by Dr. Adolfo Ferrando in the chapter entitled "Molecular Pathways and Targets in T Cell ALL." Here, we give a brief overview of the numerous genetic defects seen in T-ALL. One type of genetic abnormality seen includes chromosomal translocations of T-cell receptor genes, while another includes genetic mutations resulting in the aberrant expression of T-cell-specific transcription factors functioning as proto-oncogenes, thus leading to T-cell leukemogenesis [3, 8]. The proto-oncogenes most commonly overexpressed are *TAL1*, *TAL2*, *LYL1*, *BHLHB1*, *LMO1*, *LMO2*, *TLX1*, *TLX3*, *NKX2-1*, *NKX2-2*, *HOXA*, *MYC*, and *MYB* [3, 8]. Advanced sequencing techniques have now identified over a 100 genes that can be mutated in T-ALL [3, 7]. However, only two of these, *NOTCH1* and *CDKN2A/B*, are mutated in more than half of the cases [3, 8]. Notch1 signaling plays a critical role in the hematopoietic system and is crucial for normal T-cell development. Constitutive activation of the Notch1 signaling pathway represents the most common oncogenic event in the pathogenesis of T-ALL. This often occurs in combination with the loss of the *CDKN2A/B* locus, which encodes three tumor suppressor genes, $p14^{ARF}$, $p15^{INK4B}$, and $p16^{INK4A}$, and plays a critical role in cell cycle regulation. Further, common mutations seen in T-ALL may involve genes encoding cell cycle regulators *RB1* and *CDKN1B*, as well as alterations in signaling pathways such as Jak/Stat, MAPK, BRD4/MYC, PI3K/Akt/mTOR, and BCL-2 that are potentially targetable [8, 14]. One study showed the IL7R-JAK pathway was mutated in 27.7% of cases [15]. *JAK3* is frequently mutated (16.1%), and the majority of *JAK3* mutations identified in T-ALL have been confirmed as activating mutations [9, 16]. None of these alterations have been demonstrated to be prognostic independent of MRD response [15].

A recent large extensive genomic study of 264 children and young adults with T-ALL, as part of the Therapeutically Applicable Research to Generate Effective Treatments (TARGET) initiative, confirmed the genetic and molecular heterogeneity of this disease [7]. Using an integrated genomic analysis of whole exome sequencing (WES), copy number analysis, and RNA sequencing (RNAseq), they identified 106 potential oncogenic driver genes, half of which had not been previously described in childhood T-ALL [7]. They identified 83 different fusion events, 54 of which were from interchromosomal rearrangements, while the remaining 29 were from intrachromosomal events. The most common genes involved in translocations were *MLLT10*, *KMT2A*, *ABL1*, and *NUP98*. On average, 15.8 mutations per case were seen with a range from 2 to 50. Further analysis identified ten different functional pathways that were recurrently mutated in T-ALL (Fig. 14.1) [7, 17]. Mutations were seen in pathways involved in transcriptional regulation (91% of cases), cell cycle regulation and tumor suppression (84%), Notch1 signaling (79%), epigenetic regulation (68%), PI3K/Akt/mTOR signaling (29%), Jak/Stat signaling (25%), Ras signaling (14%), ribosomal function (13%), ubiquitination (9%), and RNA processing (9%) [7, 17]. This study was limited by analytic restrictions as only patients who had banked diagnostic and remission samples were analyzed. Thus, patients with refractory disease, which represents a high-risk subset, were excluded from analysis. Additionally, whole genome sequencing (WGS) was only performed on a small number of cases (n = 25) [7]. A number of recent studies, although small in sample size, have demonstrated the importance of genomic alterations in noncoding regions in T-ALL pathogenesis [18–21]. For example, three recent papers demonstrated multiple mechanisms of activation of the *TAL1* proto-oncogene in T-ALL by genomic alterations in noncoding regions [18–21]. These included mutations in the *TAL1* structural loop that can create super-enhancers, deletions of sequences in the CTCF-binding sites in the *TAL1* structural loop that allows an enhancer on an adjacent structural loop to activate *TAL1*, and an acquired interchromosomal interaction between cis-regulatory elements that can activate *TAL1* [19–21].

In the sections below, we will further discuss the various signaling pathways involved in T-ALL pathogenesis, describe potential newer approaches to targeting T-ALL, and review the current state of novel agents and ongoing clinical trials in this disease. A complete summary of these agents is presented in Table 14.1.

Review of Novel Agents by Type/Class

Notch

Notch proteins are highly conserved transmembrane receptors that regulate cell fate choices during the development of cell lineages, and the Notch1 pathway plays a critical role in multiple steps during T-cell development [22–24]. Furthermore,

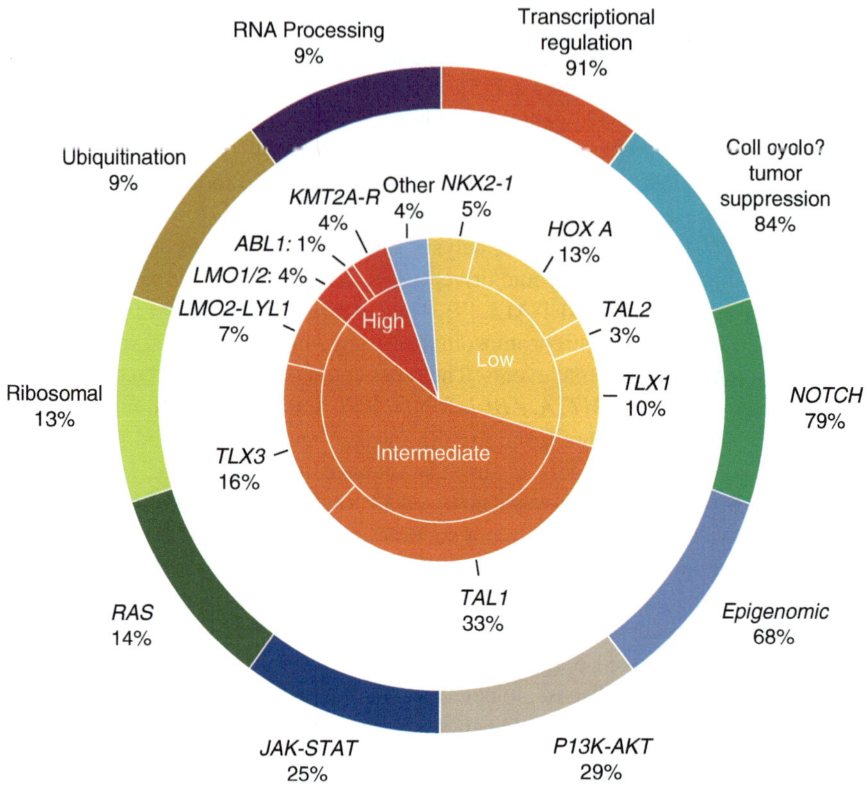

Fig. 14.1 *Estimated frequencies of specific genetic subtypes of childhood T-ALL.* The pie charts depict the estimated frequencies of each subtype among T-ALL patients who were studied as part of the TARGET initiative and treated in COG studies [7]. T-ALL cases were further divided based on the dysregulation of targetable functional pathways (outer ring). Subtypes are groups based on 5-year survival in low-risk, intermediate-risk, and high-risk categories: over 90%, 70% to 90%, and less than 70% event-free survival (EFS) in T-ALL, respectively. Of note, the EFS for T-ALL patients treated on the AALL0434 trial [128] that is used for risk grouping in this figure is superior to that found in most other published studies. Figure from *Teachey DT, Pui CH. Lancet Oncol. 2019;20(3):e142–e154* [17]

NOTCH1 was first identified in a gene involved in chromosomal translocations with the *TCRB* gene in a subset of cases of human T-ALL [22]. *NOTCH1*-induced T-ALLs require persistent Notch1 signaling for growth and survival [25]. More than 50% of human T-ALLs, including tumors from all major molecular oncogenic subtypes, have activating mutations that involve the extracellular heterodimerization domain and/or the C-terminal PEST domain of *NOTCH1* [4]. The high prevalence of *NOTCH1* mutations in T-ALL and the dependence of T-ALL cases on Notch1 pathway activation for unrestricted proliferation render this protein an excellent candidate for pharmacological intervention with gamma-secretase inhibitors (GSIs), which inhibit Notch activation [26]. T-ALL *NOTCH* mutations lead to upregulation

Table 14.1 Novel agents for the treatment of T-ALL

Target	Type of treatment	Available agents	Clinical trials in T-ALL
Notch	γ-Secretase inhibitors Soluble notch proteins Mastermind inhibiting peptides	MK-0752, LY3039478, BMS-906024 In development, preclinical only In development, preclinical only	NCT00100152, NCT02518113, NCT01363817
Jak/Stat	Jak inhibitors Stat inhibitors	Ruxolitinib, tofacitinib, peficitinib Pimozide	NCT03613428, NCT03117751
MAPK/Ras	MEK inhibitors Farnesyltransferase inhibitors Kv1.3 inhibitors	Selumetinib, trametinib, cobimetinib Tipifarnib PCARBTP	NCT03705507
PI3K/Akt/mTOR	PI3K inhibitors mTOR inhibitors Akt inhibitors mTORC1/2 inhibitors PI3K/mTOR dual inhibitors	Buparlisib, idelalisib Sirolimus, everolimus, temsirolimus MK-2206, ipatasertib, afuresertib Sapanisertib, vistusertib Dactolisib, gedatolisib	NCT01403415, NCT00981799, NCT03328104, NCT01523977, NCT01614197 NCT02484430 NCT01756118
Cell cycle regulation	CDK4/6 inhibitors Pan-CDK inhibitors	Ribociclib, palbociclib Roniciclib	NCT03515200, NCT03740334, NCT02310243, NCT03132454, NCT03792256
Proteasome	Proteasome inhibitors Neddylation inhibitors Deubiquitinating enzyme inhibitors E3 ubiquitin ligase inhibitors	Bortezomib, ixazomib, carfilzomib Pevonedistat In development, preclinical only In development, preclinical only	NCT00873093, NCT02112916, NCT02303821, NCT02228772, NCT03817320
BCL-2 apoptotic machinery	BCL-2 inhibitors BCL-XL and BCL-2 inhibitors MCL-1 inhibitors	Venetoclax Navitoclax S63845, AZD5991	NCT03808610, NCT00501826, NCT03504644, NCT03319901, NCT03236857 NCT03181126 NCT03218683

(continued)

Table 14.1 (continued)

Target	Type of treatment	Available agents	Clinical trials in T-ALL
Epigenetic	Demethylating agents HDAC inhibitors DOT1L inhibitors IDH1/2 inhibitors BRD4 inhibitors	Decitabine, 5-azacitidine Romidepsin, vorinostat Pinometostat AG-120 JQ1, OTX015, CPI203, BMS-986158	NCT00882206 NCT00882206, NCT02512497, NCT02083250 NCT01713582
Tyrosine kinase inhibitors	ABL class inhibitors	Dasatinib, imatinib, nilotinib	
Monoclonal antibodies	CD25 CD38 CD52 CD127	Basiliximab Daratumumab, isatuximab Alemtuzumab In development, preclinical only	NCT03384654, NCT02999633, NCT03860844 NCT00199030, NCT00061945
CAR T-cell therapy	CD5 CD7 TRBC1 CD1a	Preclinical and early phase trials Preclinical and early phase trials In development, preclinical only In development, preclinical only	NCT03081910 NCT03690011
Newer cytotoxics and other agents	Antimetabolites Vincas Alkylators CXCR4 antagonist	Nelarabine Liposomal vincristine OBI-3424 BL-8040	NCT00408005, NCT00684619, NCT00501826, NCT02881086, NCT02763384 NCT00495079, NCT01222780, NCT02518750, NCT03504644 NCT04315324 NCT02763384

of genes involved in anabolic pathways, and the *MYC* oncogene plays a major role in Notch-induced transformation. The oncogenic activity of Notch1 in T-ALL is strictly dependent on MYC upregulation, which further makes the Notch1-MYC regulatory circuit an attractive therapeutic target for the treatment of T-ALL [27]. GSIs can induce G0/G1 arrest, decrease cell viability, and cause apoptosis of T-ALL cell lines carrying *NOTCH1* activating mutations [28]. GSIs circumvent glucocorticoid resistance, but result in severe gastrointestinal (GI) toxicity due to accumulation of goblet cells in the gut. Yet, when GSIs were used in tandem with glucocorticoids (GCs), there was a dual benefit of avoiding glucocorticoid resistance and alleviating GI toxicity, as the GCs induced transcriptional upregulation of cyclin D2, thus preventing intestinal goblet cell metaplasia [29, 30]. These preclinical studies led to a trial of MK-0752, a potent gamma-secretase inhibitor, which was tolerated in a small number of patients on a phase I study and demonstrated temporary benefit in a T-ALL patient with Notch activation [28]. T-ALL maintenance is dependent on Notch activation, but not C-MYC expression, demonstrating that Notch is oncogenic dominant in T-ALL tumors [31]. A pediatric and adult phase I clinical trial (NCT02518113) was recently completed using the Notch inhibitor, LY3039478, in conjunction with dexamethasone; however, results are not yet published. Similarly, another phase I trial tested the pan-Notch inhibitor BMS-906024, either alone or in combination with dexamethasone, in adults with relapsed and refractory T-ALL (NCT01363817). This study is also now closed to recruitment, but results have not yet been reported. Interestingly, BMS-906024 was shown to induce a complete hematologic response in a patient with relapsed/refractory ETP-ALL [32]. Additional gamma-secretase inhibitors that have been identified but have not yet undergone clinical investigation include cowanin, DAPT, RO4929097, and PF0384014 [33–36]. As GSIs have not demonstrated activity in adult malignancies with aberrant Notch expression, including breast cancer, and considering the relative rarity of T-ALL, it remains unclear if translation of GSIs will be successful as pharmaceutical company investigations wane.

Jak/Stat

The Janus kinase (Jak)/signal transducer and activator of transcription (Stat) pathway is a mechanism by which extracellular signaling alters cell biology by inducing transcription activation [37]. The Jak/Stat pathway, when normal, is responsible for hematopoiesis and immune formulation but, when altered, has been implicated in hematological malignancies – including pediatric T-ALL [37]. Multiple mutations and upregulations of Jak/Stat activity have been identified, and somatic mutations of *JAK1* occur in 10–20% of T-ALL cases. In fact, some of the earliest descriptions of Jak/Stat lesions in cancer, such as a *TEL-JAK2* fusion, were first identified in pediatric T-ALL patients [38, 39]. *IL7R* mutational activation, including *IL7R-JAK* fusion, is involved in human T-cell leukemogenesis, and targeting of IL7R-mediated signaling may be a potential for therapeutic investigation. As *IL7R-JAK* lesions did not confer an adverse prognosis on the recent UKALL2003 pediatric clinical trial, studies focused on this population would be difficult based on a small sample size of relapsed and refractory patients [15, 40]. Alterations in Jak/Stat are more common in ETP-ALL. These alterations include mutations in *IL7R*. Based on the high frequency of alterations, preclinical studies evaluated the activity of the Jak1/2 inhibitor ruxolitinib [41]. Ruxolitinib was active in 6/6 patient-derived murine xenograft models of ETP-ALL [42]. Both Jak/Stat pathway activation and ruxolitinib efficacy were independent of the presence of Jak/Stat pathway mutations, raising the possibility that the therapeutic potential of ruxolitinib in ETP-ALL extends beyond those cases with JAK mutations [42]. Multiple studies have demonstrated that intrinsic or acquired resistance to steroids is correlated with worse outcomes in T-ALL. Recent preclinical work demonstrated that a combination of dexamethasone (glucocorticoid) and ruxolitinib may overcome IL7-induced resistance, which could in theory improve outcomes [43]. One group recently investigated the regulatory roles of the suppressor of cytokine signaling 5 (SOCS5) in T-ALL, showing that SOCS5 negatively regulates T-ALL cell growth and cell cycle progression [44]. Downregulation of SOCS5 expression enhanced activation of Jak/Stat signaling. Furthermore, when they inactivated SOCS5 leukemia engraftment, progression and burden all accelerated [44]. JAK1/2-mutated T-ALLs in patients aged 13–75 years are currently eligible for phase I study combining ruxolitinib and chemotherapy (NCT03613428). Other newer agents in this class that are yet to be tested in T-ALL include the Jak inhibitors tofacitinib and peficitinib and the Stat inhibitor pimozide.

MAPK/Ras

The Ras-mitogen-activated protein kinase (MAPK) signaling pathway is one of the most commonly mutated pathways in cancer. MAPK alterations are also common in T-ALL, affecting 13.6% of patients [7]. These alterations can be clonal or subclonal, are often not driver lesions, and are frequently enriched at relapse. A number of trials are investigating targeting MAPK in hematologic malignancies, including T-ALL [3]. The prospects of successful Ras inhibition in hematologic malignancies have been previously discussed, but recent indications demonstrate that Ras pathway mutations are more prevalent in relapsed disease and Ras targeting may be more useful at the time of T-cell ALL relapse [45, 46]. A current phase I/II trial of selumetinib, a MEK1/2 inhibitor that targets the MEK enzyme in the Ras pathway, with dexamethasone is open for patients of all ages with relapsed or refractory T-ALL with a *RAS* mutation (NCT03705507). The MAPK pathway has also been inhibited in lymphoid cells by alternative mechanisms including the farnesyltransferase inhibitor tipifarnib and the Kv1.3 inhibitor PCARBTP [47, 48].

PI3K/AKT/mTOR

The phosphatidylinositol 3-kinase (PI3K)/Akt/mammalian target of rapamycin (mTOR) signaling pathway plays a critical role in controlling cell metabolism, proliferation, and survival, and alterations leading to activation of this pathway are frequently seen in many cancers, including T-ALL [49–52]. Several novel drugs targeting this pathway are being investigated. The most common mechanism of activation of this pathway in T-ALL is through inactivation of phosphatase and tensin homolog (PTEN), which in turn results in Akt activation [51, 52]. PTEN inactivation in T-ALL can result from mutations and deletions in *PTEN* or through other signaling defects that affect PTEN expression; one study demonstrated abnormalities that inactivate PTEN may occur in as many as 36% of primary T-ALL cases [52]. There also has shown to be cross talk between activated NOTCH1 and PI3K/AKT activation [53–55]. HES1, a direct target of NOTCH1, binds to the *PTEN* promoter suppressing its expression, thereby promoting Akt activation [53]. Alternatively, mutations in *AKT1*, *PI3KCA*, *PI3KR1*, and *IL7R* have been shown to be associated with activation of this pathway [51]. Abnormalities in Jak/STAT and MAPK signaling also can indirectly lead to PI3K/AKT/mTOR activation [51].

Numerous preclinical studies in T-ALL have investigated targeting the PI3K/AKT/mTOR pathway. Initial studies primarily focused on the use of mTOR inhibitors. The first mTOR inhibitor to translate into the clinic, sirolimus (rapamycin), was shown to have efficacy as a single agent and when combined with conventional chemotherapy in T-ALL preclinical models [51, 56]. Importantly, sirolimus was shown to reverse corticosteroid resistance in multiple preclinical T-ALL studies [57, 58]. Newer mTOR inhibitors include everolimus, temsirolimus, and ridaforolimus. Treatment with mTOR inhibitors results in compensatory upregulation of feedback loops in the PI3K/Akt/mTOR pathway, thus reducing long-term efficacy. To overcome this, several new classes of drugs that target different parts of this signaling pathway are being investigated. These include PI3K/mTOR dual inhibitors, mTORC1/2 dual inhibitors, PI3K inhibitors, and Akt inhibitors [1, 51]. Numerous preclinical studies have shown these agents to have increased efficacy over targeting mTOR alone [51, 59–63]. Buparlisib (BKM120), a PI3K inhibitor, was shown to have acceptable tolerability and preliminary activity in a phase I trial of patients with advanced leukemias; however, no T-ALL patient was enrolled in this study [64]. Clinical trials are currently evaluating the use of mTOR inhibitors everolimus (NCT01523977, NCT03328104) and temsirolimus (NCT01614197) in combination with chemotherapy in children [65]. Newer agents being developed to target this pathway include the Akt inhibitors MK-2206, ipatasertib, and afuresertib, the mTORC1/2 inhibitors sapanisertib and vistusertib, and the PI3K/mTOR dual inhibitors dactolisib and gedatolisib. A phase II trial using sapanisertib was recently initiated for patients with relapsed/refractory ALL, in which T-ALL patients are eligible (NCT02484430).

D-Type Cyclins and Cyclin-Dependent Kinases

D-type cyclins (cyclins D1, D2, and D3) and their associated cyclin-dependent kinases CDK4 and CDK6 play an important role in both normal hematopoiesis and leukemogenesis [66, 67]. The cyclin D/CDK complex mediates phosphorylation of the retinoblastoma protein (Rb), thereby preventing it from binding to the transcription factor E2F1. This leads to the expression of E2F1-dependent genes and subsequent cell cycle progression from G1 to S phase. Loss of the *cyclin-dependent kinase inhibitor 2A (CDKN2A)* gene is among the most common genetic abnormalities seen in T-ALL [7, 8]. *CDKN2A* encodes two tumor suppressor proteins, p14^{ARF} and p16^{INK4A}, which selectively inhibit CDK4 and CDK6, thus preventing phosphorylation of Rb. [68, 69] Thus, deletions in *CDKN2A* disrupt the Rb tumor suppressor pathway through the D-type cyclin/CDK complex-mediated phosphorylation of Rb. Additionally, multiple preclinical studies have shown that cyclin D3 plays an important role in the initiation and progression of T-ALL in mouse models [70, 71].

Several groups have investigated the inhibition of the D-type cyclin/CDK complex as a potential therapeutic strategy in T-ALL. Two studies showed that treatment with a CDK4/6 inhibitor PD0332991 (palbociclib) resulted in reduction in tumor burden and improved survival in T-ALL xenograft models [71, 72]. Another study demonstrated the CDK4/6 inhibitor LEE001 (ribociclib) had a synergistic effect when combined with glucocorticoids and the mTOR inhibitor everolimus both in in vitro and in vivo T-ALL xenograft models [73]. However, the drug was found to be antagonistic when combined with methotrexate, mercaptopurine, doxorubicin, and L-asparaginase in vitro. It is unknown if the same antagonism would be seen in vivo. Based on these results, several early phase trials are investigating the use of CDK4/6 inhibitors in relapsed/refractory leukemias (NCT03515200, NCT03740334, NCT02310243, NCT03132454, NCT03792256) [14, 65]. For example, NCT03792256 is a phase I trial studying the use of palbociclib in combination with a standard re-induction chemotherapy backbone in children with relapsed ALL.

Ubiquitin-Proteasome Pathway

The ubiquitin-proteasome pathway (UPP) is the primary mechanism of protein degradation in cells and thus is a key driver in the regulation of cell cycle progression, apoptosis, and stress responses [74, 75]. One of the important regulatory proteins affected by the UPP is NF-κβ. In non-proliferating cells, the inhibitor protein Iκβ sequesters NF-Kβ in the cytoplasm [75]. However, in dividing cells, Iκβ is ubiquitinated and targeted for degradation, thus allowing NF-κβ to dimerize and move into the nucleus, where it acts as a transcription factor [75]. T-ALL blasts often have considerable activation of the NF-κβ pathway, frequently as a consequence of activated Notch1 [75, 76]. Thus, targeting the proteasome and disrupting the protein degradation pathway have been of considerable interest in T-ALL [1, 75].

Several preclinical studies have shown that the 26S proteasome inhibitor bortezomib has antitumor efficacy as a single agent in T-ALL [77–79]. It has shown to be synergistic with several conventional cytotoxic chemotherapy agents and also demonstrated the ability to reverse glucocorticoid resistance [77, 79]. Early phase clinical trials in relapsed B- and T-ALL had promising results [80, 81]. The COG phase II trial AALL07P1 tested bortezomib in combination with intensive re-induction chemotherapy for ALL or lymphoblastic lymphoma patients in the first relapse [81]. The study included 22 relapsed T-ALL and 10 T lymphoblastic lymphoma patients. Relapsed T-ALL patients had an encouraging remission rate of 68 ± 10% [81]. Based on these results, bortezomib was incorporated into a randomized phase III trial in de novo T-ALL through the COG (AALL1231). Results from this trial have not yet been published. Newer proteasome inhibitors include carfilzomib and ixazomib, both of which are currently being studied in early phase trials (NCT02303821, NCT02228772, NCT03817320). The ubiquitin-proteasome pathway can also be targeted by neddylation inhibitors, E3 ubiquitin ligase inhibitors, and deubiquitinating enzyme inhibitors; however, data are limited using these inhibitors in T-ALL.

BCL-2 Apoptotic Machinery

The B-cell lymphoma 2 (BCL-2) family of proteins consists of pro-survival and pro-apoptotic proteins that together play a critical role in maintaining tissue homeostasis [82, 83]. BCL-2, BCL-XL, and MCL-1 are the pro-survival members of the family, and its aberrant expression has been linked to a number of different cancers, including several hematological malignancies [82, 83]. Several studies have shown that BCL-2 expression in T-ALL is different based on its genetic and immunophenotypic subtype, with higher expression seen in more immature ETP-ALL or ETP-like T-ALL samples compared to other T-ALL samples in which BCL-XL expression was more prevalent [84, 85].

The BCL-2 inhibitors ABT-263 (navitoclax) and ABT-199 (venetoclax) have been tested against T-ALL in multiple preclinical studies. While navitoclax targets both BCL-2 and BCL-XL, venetoclax is more specific for BCL-2. Expectedly, a study showed that ETP-ALL samples showed greater sensitivity to ABT-199 both in in vitro and in vivo studies, while non-ETP-ALL samples were more sensitive to ABT-263 [84]. More recently, a new inhibitor selective for MCL-1, S63845, was shown to be active in a majority of T-ALL cell lines and interestingly was able to reverse venetoclax resistance [86]. There currently are several early phase trials testing the use of navitoclax and venetoclax in relapsed B- and T-ALL, including one trial that is testing the combination of both navitoclax and venetoclax [87]. Early results from a venetoclax trial for relapsed pediatric leukemia patients (NCT03236857) showed an overall response rate of 27% among ALL patients (3/11) [88]. These included five patients who received venetoclax monotherapy and six patients who received venetoclax in combination with chemotherapy. Seventy-three percent (8/11) had venetoclax-related adverse events, but no serious adverse event was attributed to venetoclax [88]. Thirty-six patients have been enrolled so far on the phase I navitoclax plus venetoclax combination trial (NCT03181126), including seven pediatric patients [87]. T-ALL has accounted for 44% (16/36) of enrolled study patients. The overall response rate was 56% in the total population, with a 38% (6/16) complete response rate in T-ALL patients. More encouragingly, however, there was an overall response rate of 86% (6/7) in pediatric patients, with five patients having a complete response [87].

Epigenetic Targeting

Recent genomic studies have demonstrated that epigenetic changes are frequently seen in T-ALL, thus making the targeting of epigenetic pathways an important consideration [7, 89]. The aforementioned TARGET analysis of T-ALL patients showed mutations associated with epigenetic regulation in 68% of patients [7]. Specific mutations were associated with certain genomic subtypes, such as *PHF6* mutations in cases with *TLX3* rearrangement and *USP7* alterations in *TAL1* cases, *CTCF* and *KDM6A* in *TLX3* cases, and *MLL1* in *HOXA* cases [7]. *HOXA* dysregulation when associated with *MLL-R* has been shown to confer a worse prognosis in T-ALL, with high rates of induction failure [90]. Other studies have previously identified mutations in numerous genes involved in DNA methylation (*DNMT3A*, *DNMT3B*, *TET1*, *IDH1*, *IDH2*), histone methylation (*EZH2*, *SUZ12*, *EED*, *JARID2*, *UTX*, *MLL1*, *MLL2*, *DOT1L*, *SETD2*), and histone acetylation (*CREBBP*, *EP300*, *NCOA2*, *HDACs*, *HDAC5*, *HDAC7*). Genome-wide promoter DNA methylation analysis in pediatric T-ALL has shown that low levels of global DNA methylation is associated with poor treatment outcomes [89, 91]. Given the high frequency of epigenetic changes in T-ALL, a number of epigenetic agents have been studied in preclinical models such as DNA methyltransferase inhibitors and histone deacetylase (HDAC) inhibitors. Two clinical trials studied the combination of the demethylating agent decitabine and the HDAC inhibitor vorinostat with re-induction chemotherapy in relapsed/refractory pediatric ALL patients (NCT00882206, NCT01483690) [92, 93]. While a clinical benefit was demonstrated in the first trial with tolerable toxicity [92], a high incidence of significant infectious toxicities were seen in the second trial resulting in early termination [93]. Only one patient with T-ALL was enrolled on study between the two trials. Interestingly, the HDAC inhibitor romidepsin is currently being studied to be given as maintenance therapy after allogeneic hematopoietic stem cell transplantation (HSCT) in adults with T-cell malignancies (NCT02512497). Other epigenetic drug classes of interest are IDH1 and IDH2 mutant inhibitors, DOT1L inhibitors, and BRD4 inhibitors [1, 89]. BRD4 inhibitors are discussed in detail below.

BRD4/MYC

Bromodomains (BRDs) are a diverse family of protein interaction modules, and proteins that use BRDs for their recruitment to specific regulatory complexes have been implicated in the development of cancer [94]. BRD4 is a member of the bromodomain and extraterminal (BET) subfamily of human bromodomain proteins [95]. Chromatin regulators, such as BRD4, are attractive as therapeutic targets for cancer because they are deregulated in numerous cancers and are amenable to small molecule inhibition [95]. One such cell-permeable small molecule (JQ1) was designed to bind competitively to acetyl-lysine recognition motifs of bromodomains [96]. JQ1 inhibited BRD4 and led to selective inhibition of the *MYC* oncogene in multiple myeloma [95]. *MYC* oncogene ongoing activity is necessary for T-ALL survival, and C-MYC inhibition results in efficient targeting of T-ALL-initiating cells [97]. C-MYC suppression by small hairpin RNA or pharmacologic approaches prevents leukemia initiation in mice by eliminating LIC activity [98]. Treatment with the BET bromodomain BRD4 inhibitor JQ1 reduced C-MYC expression and inhibited in vitro growth of relapsed and induction failure pediatric T-ALL samples [98]. It has been previously established that C-MYC is a developmentally regulated direct downstream target of Notch1 that contributes to the growth of T cells [4]. In functional assays, inhibitors of C-MYC interfere with the pro-growth effects of activated Notch1, and enforced expression of C-MYC rescues multiple Notch1-dependent T-ALL cell lines from Notch withdrawal [4]. Gamma-secretase inhibitors (GSIs) have been used to prevent Notch1 activation in T-ALL as described above, but response has not persisted [99]. It is thought that an epigenetic mechanism for the transient effect/response to GSI is present, so testing identified BRD4 as potential additional target to subvert an epigenetic resistance mechanism. GSI in combination with JQ1 was consistently effective in vivo [99]. JQ1 induced the downregulation of *MYC* transcription, the loss of BRD4 at the MYC promoter, and the reduced expression of C-MYC target genes [100]. JQ1 also downregulated *IL7R* transcription, depleted BRD4 from the IL7R promoter, and reduced JAK2 and STAT5 phosphorylation [100]. A novel oral inhibitor of BRD2/3/4, the thienotriazolodiazepine compound OTX015, is also under evaluation [101]. Treatment with OTX015 and JQ1 induced similar gene expression profiles in sensitive cell lines, including C-MYC downregulation [102]. OTX015 also induced a strong decrease of BRD2, BRD4, and C-MYC, supporting OTX015 evaluation in a phase I trial in relapsed/refractory leukemia patients (NCT01713582) [101, 102]. Unfortunately, no T-ALL patient was enrolled on this trial [103]. Study of a newer BRD/BET inhibitor (BMS-986158) in pediatric solid tumors, CNS tumors, and lymphoma is currently ongoing (NCT03936465).

Tyrosine Kinase Inhibitors

While tyrosine kinase inhibitors (TKIs) have not gained prominence in T-ALL as they have in other malignancies, they may have an important role in treating specific subsets of T-ALL patients, for example, those with *NUP214-ABL1* fusions, which account for 3.9–5.8% of all T-ALL cases [104, 105]. In these patients, the member of the nuclear pore complex NUP214 and the kinase ABL1 form a constitutively active fusion protein, thus making them sensitive to TKIs. The tyrosine kinase inhibitors imatinib, dasatinib, and nilotinib have all been shown to induce apoptosis in human *NUP214-ABL1*-positive T-ALL cell lines, and dasatinib was also shown to have activity in a xenograft model [106]. Rapid complete cytogenetic remission was seen after upfront dasatinib monotherapy in a patient with *NUP214-ABL1*-positive T-ALL [106]. In another similar case, a response was seen with imatinib, when used in combination with vincristine and prednisone [107]. A larger cohort of T-ALL patients with *NUP214-ABL1* fusions needs to be studied to better understand the efficacy of TKIs in this unique subset. Another rare subset of T-ALL cases that would potentially be responsive to TKIs are those with *PDGFRB* (platelet-derived growth factor receptor beta) fusions [108, 109].

Interestingly, a large ex vivo drug response profiling study identified a subset of T-ALL patient samples that were extremely sensitive to dasatinib, without the typical *ABL1* kinase translocation [110]. The drug response was seen in both diagnostic and relapsed samples, and surprisingly, the IC_{50} for dasatinib in these patient samples was at least tenfold lower than in any of the best B-ALL dasatinib responders tested [110]. No known genetic abnormality could be associated with this phenotype. Given that dasatinib is a dual ABL1/SRC inhibitor, the investigators hypothesized that the effect was due to SRC inhibition and demonstrated higher levels of activated, phosphorylated SRC in dasatinib-sensitive samples [110]. They validated these findings in an in vivo T-ALL xenograft model and then subsequently demonstrated that 40% (13/33) of adult and pediatric T-ALL samples responded to dasatinib with an IC50 of below 100 nM. Based on these findings, they initiated dasatinib therapy in combination with pegylated asparaginase in a refractory T-ALL patient. Asparaginase was discontinued after one dose due to intolerance, but continued dasatinib monotherapy was able to control the disease for 5 months [110]. Thus, further exploration of underlying molecular mechanisms is warranted in dasatinib-sensitive T-ALL.

Immunotherapy

While breakthroughs in immunotherapeutic approaches such as monoclonal antibodies, antibody-drug conjugates, bispecific T-cell engagers (BiTEs), and CAR T-cell therapy have changed the overall landscape of treating B-ALL, such advances in T-ALL have lagged behind [1, 65]. The principal problem in developing immunotherapies for T-ALL is the lack of a tumor-specific surface antigen on T lymphoblasts, as long-standing immunosuppression from T-cell aplasia would be life-threatening [1, 65, 111]. This is potentially less of a concern when using monoclonal antibodies compared to BiTEs or CAR T cells. However, single agent clinical trials targeting CD52 in T-ALL with the antibody alemtuzumab showed limited efficacy and were associated with significant infectious toxicity [112, 113]. Daratumumab, an anti-CD38 monoclonal antibody, has shown great efficacy in T-ALL xenograft models [114–116] and is currently being evaluated in an international multicenter phase II study for relapsed/refractory T-ALL in combination with chemotherapy (NCT03384654) [65]. Isatuximab is another monoclonal antibody targeting CD38 that is actively being studied in a phase II trial for children and young adults with relapsed/refractory T-ALL (NCT02999633). A potential antibody of interest in targeting T-ALL is the anti-CD25 monoclonal antibody basiliximab, given the known expression of CD25 in a majority of T-ALL blasts [1].

Additionally, two recent preclinical studies have shown that targeting the alpha chain of the interleukin 7 receptor (IL-7Rα, CD127) with monoclonal antibodies is efficacious in T-ALL [117, 118].

Apart from T-cell aplasia, there are two other significant challenges in the development of CAR T-cell therapy for T-ALL: the likelihood of fratricide, in which CAR T cells target each other, and the possibility of product contamination in which malignant T-ALL cells are inadvertently transduced with a CAR [111, 119]. One study showed that the accidental CAR transduction of a single B-ALL blast resulted in relapse, as the CD19 CAR bound to the CD19 epitope on the surface of leukemic cells, masking it from CAR T-cell recognition [120]. Thus, an "off-the-shelf" fratricide-resistant CAR T cell with a limited life span might be promising for T-ALL. Several preclinical studies have investigated the use of CAR T cells in T-cell malignancies with the most commonly targeted T-cell antigens being CD5 and CD7 [121–126]. Other T-cell antigens that have been targeted include CD30, TRBC1, CD37, and CD1a [111]. In order to overcome fratricide, several approaches have been used. These include targeting of downregulated antigens such as CD5, genome editing of target antigen, targeting antigens with limited expression on T cells (e.g., CD30, CD37, CD1a, TRBC1), Tet-OFF expression system, protein expression blockers (PEBLs), and using NK-92 cells [111]. A study showed that expression of a CD5 CAR with a CD28 costimulatory domain resulted in downregulation of CD5 from the T-cell surface, thereby causing only limited fratricide. Based on these findings, a phase I clinical trial is currently investigating the use of CD5 CAR T cells in relapsed T-cell malignancies (NCT03081910). Two studies have successfully shown that genome editing of CD7 using CRISPR/Cas9 resulted in fratricide-resistant CD7 CAR T cells [123, 126]. Another phase I clinical trial is investigating this approach (NCT03690011). In order to avoid long-term T-cell aplasia, investigators in both clinical trials recommend patients proceed to allogeneic HSCT after CAR T-cell therapy.

Nelarabine

Nelarabine, the prodrug for 9-β-D-arabinofuranosylguanine (araG), has shown great efficacy in T-ALL and was safely integrated into an intensive chemotherapy backbone in the phase III COG AALL0434 trial resulting in improved survival [127, 128]. It remains the only agent that has received US Food and Drug Administration (FDA) approval specifically for relapsed T-ALL [129].

The most recently completed Children's Oncology Group study for T-ALL patients, COG AALL0434, demonstrated outcomes not previously reached. AALL0434 was a phase III randomized clinical trial for children and young adults with T-ALL and T-cell acute lymphoblastic lymphoma (T-LL). It utilized a 2 x 2 pseudo-factorial randomization comparing Capizzi methotrexate (CMTX) vs. high-dose methotrexate (HDMTX), ± six 5-day courses of nelarabine. Post-induction, T-ALL patients were classified as low, intermediate, or high risk based on NCI risk group and early treatment response. All T-ALL patients were randomized to receive CMTX vs. HDMTX, and patients with intermediate- or high-risk T-ALL were also randomized to receive nelarabine or not. The 4-year disease-free survival (DFS) on the CMTX plus nelarabine arm for T-ALL patients was 92.2% ± 2.8%. In contrast, the 4-year DFS on the HDMTX/no nelarabine arm, which is the standard of care throughout much of the world, was 78.0% ± 3.7% [130]. In addition, AALL0434 demonstrated a nelarabine benefit in patients with central nervous system T-ALL [131].

Other Agents

Liposomal vincristine sulfate (Marqibo) was approved by the FDA in 2012 for the treatment of adults with Philadelphia chromosome-negative ALL in second or greater relapse [132]. The liposomal formulation increases the half-life and area under curve for vincristine sulfate, thus allowing for a higher concentration of drug in the blood compartment without increasing toxicity [132]. A phase II trial of liposomal vincristine monotherapy in adults included ten T-ALL patients, two (20%) of which achieved remission [133]. Subsequently, a phase I trial in children with relapsed and/or refractory acute leukemia and solid tumors demonstrated that children are able to safely tolerate the same dose of liposomal vincristine as adults [134]. A phase I/II trial testing the combination of venetoclax and liposomal vincristine in patients with relapsed/refractory T- or B-ALL is currently ongoing (NCT03504644).

A potential new target in this disease is the chemokine receptor CXCR4, which has been shown to be required for leukemia-initiating cell activity in T-ALL [135]. Preclinical data has demonstrated that inhibition of this receptor decreases the proliferation and survival of T-ALL cells and prevents homing to the bone marrow niche [135]. Based on these results, BL-8040, a short peptide CXCR4 antagonist, is currently being tested in a phase II trial in combination with nelarabine for patients with relapsed/refractory T-ALL (NCT02763384) [65]. Another novel agent that has gained recent interest in T-ALL is OBI-3424, a highly selective prodrug that is converted by aldo-keto reductase family 1 member C3 (AKR1C3) into a potent DNA-alkylating agent [136]. A recent study showed that AKR1C3 mRNA expression was significantly higher in primary T-ALL samples compared to B-ALL, and OBI-3424 showed potent cytotoxicity against both T-ALL cell lines and PDX models [136]. A phase I trial of this drug is currently ongoing in patients with solid tumors, hepatocellular carcinoma, and prostate cancer (NCT03592264).

Conclusion

Outcomes for pediatric T-ALL have steadily improved over the past 50 years; however, we have likely reached a plateau where further intensification of therapy is unlikely to increase survival. Recent studies using targeted agents provide hope of further improvement in outcomes while potentially mitigating toxicity. T-ALL has a well-established genetic heterogeneity, and the complexities of T-ALL biology provide many channels of investigation and much cause for optimism for those who treat pediatric patients with T-ALL. Additional genomic profiling in relapsed and refractory T-ALL may potentially identify novel targetable pathways.

References

1. Raetz EA, Teachey DT. T-cell acute lymphoblastic leukemia. Hematology Am Soc Hematol Educ Program. 2016;2016(1):580–8.
2. Rheingold SR, Ji L, Xu X, et al. Prognostic factors for survival after relapsed acute lymphoblastic leukemia (ALL): a Children's Oncology Group (COG) study. J Clin Oncol. 2019;37(15_suppl):10008.
3. Girardi T, Vicente C, Cools J, De Keersmaecker K. The genetics and molecular biology of T-ALL. Blood. 2017;129(9):1113–23.
4. Weng AP, Ferrando AA, Lee W, et al. Activating mutations of NOTCH1 in human T cell acute lymphoblastic leukemia. Science. 2004;306(5694):269–71.
5. Ferrando AA, Neuberg DS, Staunton J, et al. Gene expression signatures define novel oncogenic pathways in T cell acute lymphoblastic leukemia. Cancer Cell. 2002;1(1):75–87.
6. Homminga I, Pieters R, Langerak AW, et al. Integrated transcript and genome analyses reveal NKX2-1 and MEF2C as potential oncogenes in T cell acute lymphoblastic leukemia. Cancer Cell. 2011;19(4):484–97.
7. Liu Y, Easton J, Shao Y, et al. The genomic landscape of pediatric and young adult T-lineage acute lymphoblastic leukemia. Nat Genet. 2017;49(8):1211–8.
8. Belver L, Ferrando A. The genetics and mechanisms of T cell acute lymphoblastic leukaemia. Nat Rev Cancer. 2016;16(8):494–507.
9. Zhang J, Ding L, Holmfeldt L, et al. The genetic basis of early T-cell precursor acute lymphoblastic leukaemia. Nature. 2012;481(7380):157–63.
10. Coustan-Smith E, Mullighan CG, Onciu M, et al. Early T-cell precursor leukaemia: a subtype of very high-risk acute lymphoblastic leukaemia. Lancet Oncol. 2009;10(2):147–56.
11. Inukai T, Kiyokawa N, Campana D, et al. Clinical significance of early T-cell precursor acute lymphoblastic leukaemia: results of the Tokyo Children's Cancer Study Group study L99-15. Br J Haematol. 2012;156(3):358–65.
12. Patrick K, Wade R, Goulden N, et al. Outcome for children and young people with early T-cell precursor acute lymphoblastic leukaemia treated on a contemporary protocol, UKALL 2003. Br J Haematol. 2014;166(3):421–4.
13. Wood BL, Winter SS, Dunsmore KP, et al. T-Lymphoblastic Leukemia (T-ALL) shows excellent outcome, lack of significance of the Early Thymic Precursor (ETP) immunophenotype, and validation of the prognostic value of end-induction Minimal Residual Disease (MRD) in Children's Oncology Group (COG) study AALL0434. Blood. 2014;124(21):1–1.
14. Follini E, Marchesini M, Roti G. Strategies to overcome resistance mechanisms in T-cell acute lymphoblastic leukemia. Int J Mol Sci. 2019;20(12)
15. Vicente C, Schwab C, Broux M, et al. Targeted sequencing identifies associations between IL7R-JAK mutations and epigenetic modulators in T-cell acute lymphoblastic leukemia. Haematologica. 2015;100(10):1301–10.
16. Degryse S, de Bock CE, Cox L, et al. JAK3 mutants transform hematopoietic cells through JAK1 activation, causing T-cell acute lymphoblastic leukemia in a mouse model. Blood. 2014;124(20):3092–100.
17. Teachey DT, Pui CH. Comparative features and outcomes between paediatric T-cell and B-cell acute lymphoblastic leukaemia. Lancet Oncol. 2019;20(3):e142–e54.

18. Rivera-Reyes A, Hayer KE, Bassing CH. Genomic alterations of non-coding regions underlie human cancer: lessons from T-ALL. Trends Mol Med. 2016;22(12):1035–46.
19. Mansour MR, Abraham BJ, Anders L, et al. Oncogene regulation. An oncogenic super-enhancer formed through somatic mutation of a noncoding intergenic element. Science. 2014;346(6215):1373–7.
20. Hnisz D, Weintraub AS, Day DS, et al. Activation of proto-oncogenes by disruption of chromosome neighborhoods. Science. 2016;351(6280):1454–8.
21. Patel B, Kang Y, Cui K, et al. Aberrant TAL1 activation is mediated by an interchromosomal interaction in human T-cell acute lymphoblastic leukemia. Leukemia. 2014;28(2):349–61.
22. Deftos ML, Bevan MJ. Notch signaling in T cell development. Curr Opin Immunol. 2000;12(2):166–72.
23. Pear WS, Radtke F. Notch signaling in lymphopoiesis. Semin Immunol. 2003;15(2):69–79.
24. Adaki R, Raikar S, Shigli K, Gali S. Prosthetic rehabilitation of a geriatric patient with squamous cell carcinoma of the buccal mucosa: a report of clinical challenges. Int J Pharm Investig. 2017;7(2):107–10.
25. Weng AP, Nam Y, Wolfe MS, et al. Growth suppression of pre-T acute lymphoblastic leukemia cells by inhibition of notch signaling. Mol Cell Biol. 2003;23(2):655–64.
26. Sanchez-Martin M, Ferrando A. The NOTCH1-MYC highway toward T-cell acute lymphoblastic leukemia. Blood. 2017;129(9):1124–33.
27. Grabher C, von Boehmer H, Look AT. Notch 1 activation in the molecular pathogenesis of T-cell acute lymphoblastic leukaemia. Nat Rev Cancer. 2006;6(5):347–59.
28. Deangelo DJ, Stone RM, Silverman LB, et al. A phase I clinical trial of the notch inhibitor MK-0752 in patients with T-cell acute lymphoblastic leukemia/lymphoma (T-ALL) and other leukemias. J Clin Oncol. 2006;24(18_suppl):6585.
29. Real PJ, Ferrando AA. NOTCH inhibition and glucocorticoid therapy in T-cell acute lymphoblastic leukemia. Leukemia. 2009;23(8):1374–7.
30. Real PJ, Tosello V, Palomero T, et al. Gamma-secretase inhibitors reverse glucocorticoid resistance in T cell acute lymphoblastic leukemia. Nat Med. 2009;15(1):50–8.
31. Demarest RM, Dahmane N, Capobianco AJ. Notch is oncogenic dominant in T-cell acute lymphoblastic leukemia. Blood. 2011;117(10):2901–9.
32. Knoechel B, Bhatt A, Pan L, et al. Complete hematologic response of early T-cell progenitor acute lymphoblastic leukemia to the gamma-secretase inhibitor BMS-906024: genetic and epigenetic findings in an outlier case. Cold Spring Harb Mol Case Stud. 2015;1(1):a000539.
33. Arai MA, Akamine R, Tsuchiya A, et al. The Notch inhibitor cowanin accelerates nicastrin degradation. Sci Rep. 2018;8(1):5376.
34. Dovey HF, John V, Anderson JP, et al. Functional gamma-secretase inhibitors reduce beta-amyloid peptide levels in brain. J Neurochem. 2001;76(1):173–81.
35. Luistro L, He W, Smith M, et al. Preclinical profile of a potent gamma-secretase inhibitor targeting notch signaling with in vivo efficacy and pharmacodynamic properties. Cancer Res. 2009;69(19):7672–80.
36. Arcaroli JJ, Quackenbush KS, Purkey A, et al. Tumours with elevated levels of the Notch and Wnt pathways exhibit efficacy to PF-03084014, a gamma-secretase inhibitor, in a preclinical colorectal explant model. Br J Cancer. 2013;109(3):667–75.
37. Vainchenker W, Constantinescu SN. JAK/STAT signaling in hematological malignancies. Oncogene. 2013;32(21):2601–13.
38. Lacronique V, Boureux A, Valle VD, et al. A TEL-JAK2 fusion protein with constitutive kinase activity in human leukemia. Science. 1997;278(5341):1309–12.
39. Flex E, Petrangeli V, Stella L, et al. Somatically acquired JAK1 mutations in adult acute lymphoblastic leukemia. J Exp Med. 2008;205(4):751–8.
40. Zenatti PP, Ribeiro D, Li W, et al. Oncogenic IL7R gain-of-function mutations in childhood T-cell acute lymphoblastic leukemia. Nat Genet. 2011;43(10):932–9.

41. Treanor LM, Zhou S, Janke L, et al. Interleukin-7 receptor mutants initiate early T cell precursor leukemia in murine thymocyte progenitors with multipotent potential. J Exp Med. 2014;211(4):701–13.
42. Maude SL, Dolai S, Delgado-Martin C, et al. Efficacy of JAK/STAT pathway inhibition in murine xenograft models of early T-cell precursor (ETP) acute lymphoblastic leukemia. Blood. 2015;125(11):1759–67.
43. Delgado-Martin C, Meyer LK, Huang BJ, et al. JAK/STAT pathway inhibition overcomes IL7-induced glucocorticoid resistance in a subset of human T-cell acute lymphoblastic leukemias. Leukemia. 2017;31(12):2568–76.
44. Sharma ND, Nickl CK, Kang H, et al. Epigenetic silencing of SOCS5 potentiates JAK-STAT signaling and progression of T-cell acute lymphoblastic leukemia. Cancer Sci. 2019;110(6):1931–46.
45. Ward AF, Braun BS, Shannon KM. Targeting oncogenic Ras signaling in hematologic malignancies. Blood. 2012;120(17):3397–406.
46. Oshima K, Khiabanian H, da Silva-Almeida AC, et al. Mutational landscape, clonal evolution patterns, and role of RAS mutations in relapsed acute lymphoblastic leukemia. Proc Natl Acad Sci U S A. 2016;113(40):11306–11.
47. Ding H, Hackbarth J, Schneider PA, et al. Cytotoxicity of farnesyltransferase inhibitors in lymphoid cells mediated by MAPK pathway inhibition and Bim up-regulation. Blood. 2011;118(18):4872–81.
48. Bergermann T, Born L, Ferguson F, et al. Inhibition of PI-3-K and AKT amplifies Kv1.3 inhibitor-induced death of human T leukemia cells. Cell Physiol Biochem. 2019;53(S1):1–10.
49. Guertin DA, Sabatini DM. Defining the role of mTOR in cancer. Cancer Cell. 2007;12(1):9–22.
50. Yuan TL, Cantley LC. PI3K pathway alterations in cancer: variations on a theme. Oncogene. 2008;27(41):5497–510.
51. Tasian SK, Teachey DT, Rheingold SR. Targeting the PI3K/mTOR pathway in pediatric hematologic malignancies. Front Oncol. 2014;4:108.
52. Gutierrez A, Sanda T, Grebliunaite R, et al. High frequency of PTEN, PI3K, and AKT abnormalities in T-cell acute lymphoblastic leukemia. Blood. 2009;114(3):647–50.
53. Palomero T, Dominguez M, Ferrando AA. The role of the PTEN/AKT pathway in NOTCH1-induced leukemia. Cell Cycle. 2008;7(8):965–70.
54. Palomero T, Sulis ML, Cortina M, et al. Mutational loss of PTEN induces resistance to NOTCH1 inhibition in T-cell leukemia. Nat Med. 2007;13(10):1203–10.
55. Chan SM, Weng AP, Tibshirani R, Aster JC, Utz PJ. Notch signals positively regulate activity of the mTOR pathway in T-cell acute lymphoblastic leukemia. Blood. 2007;110(1):278–86.
56. Teachey DT, Grupp SA, Brown VI. Mammalian target of rapamycin inhibitors and their potential role in therapy in leukaemia and other haematological malignancies. Br J Haematol. 2009;145(5):569–80.
57. Gu L, Zhou C, Liu H, et al. Rapamycin sensitizes T-ALL cells to dexamethasone-induced apoptosis. J Exp Clin Cancer Res. 2010;29:150.
58. Zhang C, Ryu YK, Chen TZ, Hall CP, Webster DR, Kang MH. Synergistic activity of rapamycin and dexamethasone in vitro and in vivo in acute lymphoblastic leukemia via cell-cycle arrest and apoptosis. Leuk Res. 2012;36(3):342–9.
59. Chiarini F, Grimaldi C, Ricci F, et al. Activity of the novel dual phosphatidylinositol 3-kinase/mammalian target of rapamycin inhibitor NVP-BEZ235 against T-cell acute lymphoblastic leukemia. Cancer Res. 2010;70(20):8097–107.
60. Lonetti A, Antunes IL, Chiarini F, et al. Activity of the pan-class I phosphoinositide 3-kinase inhibitor NVP-BKM120 in T-cell acute lymphoblastic leukemia. Leukemia. 2014;28(6):1196–206.
61. Gutierrez A, Pan L, Groen RW, et al. Phenothiazines induce PP2A-mediated apoptosis in T cell acute lymphoblastic leukemia. J Clin Invest. 2014;124(2):644–55.

62. Hall CP, Reynolds CP, Kang MH. Modulation of glucocorticoid resistance in pediatric T-cell acute lymphoblastic Leukemia by increasing BIM expression with the PI3K/mTOR inhibitor BEZ235. Clin Cancer Res. 2016;22(3):621–32.
63. Janes MR, Limon JJ, So L, et al. Effective and selective targeting of leukemia cells using a TORC1/2 kinase inhibitor. Nat Med. 2010;16(2):205–13.
64. Ragon BK, Kantarjian H, Jabbour E, et al. Buparlisib, a PI3K inhibitor, demonstrates acceptable tolerability and preliminary activity in a phase I trial of patients with advanced leukemias. Am J Hematol. 2017;92(1):7–11.
65. McMahon CM, Luger SM. Relapsed T cell ALL: current approaches and new directions. Curr Hematol Malig Rep. 2019;14(2):83–93.
66. Kozar K, Ciemerych MA, Rebel VI, et al. Mouse development and cell proliferation in the absence of D-cyclins. Cell. 2004;118(4):477–91.
67. Sherr CJ, Beach D, Shapiro GI. Targeting CDK4 and CDK6: from discovery to therapy. Cancer Discov. 2016;6(4):353–67.
68. Carrasco Salas P, Fernandez L, Vela M, et al. The role of CDKN2A/B deletions in pediatric acute lymphoblastic leukemia. Pediatr Hematol Oncol. 2016;33(7-8):415–22.
69. Zhang W, Kuang P, Liu T. Prognostic significance of CDKN2A/B deletions in acute lymphoblastic leukaemia: a meta-analysis. Ann Med. 2019;51(1):28–40.
70. Sicinska E, Lee YM, Gits J, et al. Essential role for cyclin D3 in granulocyte colony-stimulating factor-driven expansion of neutrophil granulocytes. Mol Cell Biol. 2006;26(21):8052–60.
71. Choi YJ, Li X, Hydbring P, et al. The requirement for cyclin D function in tumor maintenance. Cancer Cell. 2012;22(4):438–51.
72. Sawai CM, Freund J, Oh P, et al. Therapeutic targeting of the cyclin D3:CDK4/6 complex in T cell leukemia. Cancer Cell. 2012;22(4):452–65.
73. Pikman Y, Alexe G, Roti G, et al. Synergistic drug combinations with a CDK4/6 inhibitor in T-cell acute lymphoblastic Leukemia. Clin Cancer Res. 2017;23(4):1012–24.
74. Motegi A, Murakawa Y, Takeda S. The vital link between the ubiquitin-proteasome pathway and DNA repair: impact on cancer therapy. Cancer Lett. 2009;283(1):1–9.
75. Niewerth D, Dingjan I, Cloos J, Jansen G, Kaspers G. Proteasome inhibitors in acute leukemia. Expert Rev Anticancer Ther. 2013;13(3):327–37.
76. Vilimas T, Mascarenhas J, Palomero T, et al. Targeting the NF-kappaB signaling pathway in Notch1-induced T-cell leukemia. Nat Med. 2007;13(1):70–7.
77. Horton TM, Gannavarapu A, Blaney SM, D'Argenio DZ, Plon SE, Berg SL. Bortezomib interactions with chemotherapy agents in acute leukemia in vitro. Cancer Chemother Pharmacol. 2006;58(1):13–23.
78. Houghton PJ, Morton CL, Kolb EA, et al. Initial testing (stage 1) of the proteasome inhibitor bortezomib by the pediatric preclinical testing program. Pediatr Blood Cancer. 2008;50(1):37–45.
79. Koyama D, Kikuchi J, Hiraoka N, et al. Proteasome inhibitors exert cytotoxicity and increase chemosensitivity via transcriptional repression of Notch1 in T-cell acute lymphoblastic leukemia. Leukemia. 2014;28(6):1216–26.
80. Messinger YH, Gaynon PS, Sposto R, et al. Bortezomib with chemotherapy is highly active in advanced B-precursor acute lymphoblastic leukemia: therapeutic advances in childhood leukemia & lymphoma (TACL) study. Blood. 2012;120(2):285–90.
81. Horton TM, Whitlock JA, Lu X, et al. Bortezomib reinduction chemotherapy in high-risk ALL in first relapse: a report from the Children's oncology group. Br J Haematol. 2019;
82. Cory S, Huang DC, Adams JM. The Bcl-2 family: roles in cell survival and oncogenesis. Oncogene. 2003;22(53):8590–607.
83. Adams JM, Cory S. The Bcl-2 apoptotic switch in cancer development and therapy. Oncogene. 2007;26(9):1324–37.
84. Chonghaile TN, Roderick JE, Glenfield C, et al. Maturation stage of T-cell acute lymphoblastic leukemia determines BCL-2 versus BCL-XL dependence and sensitivity to ABT-199. Cancer Discov. 2014;4(9):1074–87.

85. Peirs S, Matthijssens F, Goossens S, et al. ABT-199 mediated inhibition of BCL-2 as a novel therapeutic strategy in T-cell acute lymphoblastic leukemia. Blood. 2014;124(25):3738–47.
86. Li H, Pauza CD. Rapamycin increases the yield and effector function of human gammadelta T cells stimulated in vitro. Cancer Immunol Immunother. 2011;60(3):361–70.
87. Lacayo NJ, Pullarkat VA, Stock W, et al. Safety and efficacy of venetoclax in combination with navitoclax in adult and pediatric relapsed/refractory acute lymphoblastic leukemia and lymphoblastic lymphoma. Blood. 2019;134(Supplement_1):285.
88. Karol SE, Cooper TM, Bittencourt H, et al. Safety, efficacy, and PK of the BCL2 inhibitor venetoclax in combination with chemotherapy in pediatric and young adult patients with relapsed/refractory acute myeloid leukemia and acute lymphoblastic leukemia: phase 1 study. Blood. 2019;134(Supplement_1):2649.
89. Peirs S, Van der Meulen J, Van de Walle I, et al. Epigenetics in T-cell acute lymphoblastic leukemia. Immunol Rev. 2015;263(1):50–67.
90. Matlawska-Wasowska K, Kang H, Devidas M, et al. MLL rearrangements impact outcome in HOXA-deregulated T-lineage acute lymphoblastic leukemia: a children's oncology group study. Leukemia. 2016;30(9):1909–12.
91. Borssen M, Palmqvist L, Karrman K, et al. Promoter DNA methylation pattern identifies prognostic subgroups in childhood T-cell acute lymphoblastic leukemia. PLoS One. 2013;8(6):e65373.
92. Burke MJ, Lamba JK, Pounds S, et al. A therapeutic trial of decitabine and vorinostat in combination with chemotherapy for relapsed/refractory acute lymphoblastic leukemia. Am J Hematol. 2014;89(9):889–95.
93. Burke MJ, Kostadinov R, Sposto R, et al. Decitabine and vorinostat with chemotherapy in relapsed pediatric acute lymphoblastic leukemia: a TACL pilot study. Clin Cancer Res. 2020;
94. Muller S, Filippakopoulos P, Knapp S. Bromodomains as therapeutic targets. Expert Rev Mol Med. 2011;13:e29.
95. Loven J, Hoke HA, Lin CY, et al. Selective inhibition of tumor oncogenes by disruption of super-enhancers. Cell. 2013;153(2):320–34.
96. Filippakopoulos P, Qi J, Picaud S, et al. Selective inhibition of BET bromodomains. Nature. 2010;468(7327):1067–73.
97. Reynolds C, Roderick JE, LaBelle JL, et al. Repression of BIM mediates survival signaling by MYC and AKT in high-risk T-cell acute lymphoblastic leukemia. Leukemia. 2014;28(9):1819–27.
98. Roderick JE, Tesell J, Shultz LD, et al. c-Myc inhibition prevents leukemia initiation in mice and impairs the growth of relapsed and induction failure pediatric T-ALL cells. Blood. 2014;123(7):1040–50.
99. Knoechel B, Roderick JE, Williamson KE, et al. An epigenetic mechanism of resistance to targeted therapy in T cell acute lymphoblastic leukemia. Nat Genet. 2014;46(4):364–70.
100. Ott CJ, Kopp N, Bird L, et al. BET bromodomain inhibition targets both c-Myc and IL7R in high-risk acute lymphoblastic leukemia. Blood. 2012;120(14):2843–52.
101. Braun T, Coude MM, Berrou J, et al. Preclinical study of the bromodomain inhibitor OTX015 In acute myeloid (AML) and lymphoid (ALL) leukemias. Blood. 2013;122(21):4218.
102. Coude MM, Braun T, Berrou J, et al. BET inhibitor OTX015 targets BRD2 and BRD4 and decreases c-MYC in acute leukemia cells. Oncotarget. 2015;6(19):17698–712.
103. Berthon C, Raffoux E, Thomas X, et al. Bromodomain inhibitor OTX015 in patients with acute leukaemia: a dose-escalation, phase 1 study. Lancet Haematol. 2016;3(4):e186–95.
104. Graux C, Cools J, Melotte C, et al. Fusion of NUP214 to ABL1 on amplified episomes in T-cell acute lymphoblastic leukemia. Nat Genet. 2004;36(10):1084–9.
105. Burmeister T, Gokbuget N, Reinhardt R, Rieder H, Hoelzer D, Schwartz S. NUP214-ABL1 in adult T-ALL: the GMALL study group experience. Blood. 2006;108(10):3556–9.
106. Quintas-Cardama A, Tong W, Manshouri T, et al. Activity of tyrosine kinase inhibitors against human NUP214-ABL1-positive T cell malignancies. Leukemia. 2008;22(6):1117–24.

107. Clarke S, O'Reilly J, Romeo G, Cooney J. NUP214-ABL1 positive T-cell acute lymphoblastic leukemia patient shows an initial favorable response to imatinib therapy post relapse. Leuk Res. 2011;35(7):e131–3.
108. Zabriskie MS, Antelope O, Verma AR, et al. A novel AGGF1-PDGFRb fusion in pediatric T-cell acute lymphoblastic leukemia. Haematologica. 2018;103(2):e87–91.
109. Heilmann AM, Schrock AB, He J, et al. Novel PDGFRB fusions in childhood B- and T-acute lymphoblastic leukemia. Leukemia. 2017;31(9):1989–92.
110. Frismantas V, Dobay MP, Rinaldi A, et al. Ex vivo drug response profiling detects recurrent sensitivity patterns in drug-resistant acute lymphoblastic leukemia. Blood. 2017;129(11):e26–37.
111. Fleischer LC, Spencer HT, Raikar SS. Targeting T cell malignancies using CAR-based immunotherapy: challenges and potential solutions. J Hematol Oncol. 2019;12(1):141.
112. Angiolillo AL, Yu AL, Reaman G, Ingle AM, Secola R, Adamson PC. A phase II study of Campath-1H in children with relapsed or refractory acute lymphoblastic leukemia: a children's oncology group report. Pediatr Blood Cancer. 2009;53(6):978–83.
113. Portell CA, Advani AS. Novel targeted therapies in acute lymphoblastic leukemia. Leuk Lymphoma. 2014;55(4):737–48.
114. Bride KL, Vincent TL, Im SY, et al. Preclinical efficacy of daratumumab in T-cell acute lymphoblastic leukemia. Blood 2018; 131(9): 995-9.
115. Naik J, Themeli M, de Jong-Korlaar R, et al. CD38 as a therapeutic target for adult acute myeloid leukemia and T-cell acute lymphoblastic leukemia. Haematologica. 2019;104(3):e100–e3.
116. Vogiatzi F, Winterberg D, Lenk L, et al. Daratumumab eradicates minimal residual disease in a preclinical model of pediatric T-cell acute lymphoblastic leukemia. Blood. 2019;134(8):713–6.
117. Hixon JA, Andrews C, Kashi L, et al. New anti-IL-7Ralpha monoclonal antibodies show efficacy against T cell acute lymphoblastic leukemia in pre-clinical models. Leukemia. 2020;34(1):35–49.
118. Akkapeddi P, Fragoso R, Hixon JA, et al. A fully human anti-IL-7Ralpha antibody promotes antitumor activity against T-cell acute lymphoblastic leukemia. Leukemia. 2019;33(9):2155–68.
119. Alcantara M, Tesio M, June CH, Houot R. CAR T-cells for T-cell malignancies: challenges in distinguishing between therapeutic, normal, and neoplastic T-cells. Leukemia. 2018;32(11):2307–15.
120. Ruella M, Xu J, Barrett DM, et al. Induction of resistance to chimeric antigen receptor T cell therapy by transduction of a single leukemic B cell. Nat Med. 2018;24(10):1499–503.
121. Mamonkin M, Rouce RH, Tashiro H, Brenner MK. A T-cell-directed chimeric antigen receptor for the selective treatment of T-cell malignancies. Blood. 2015;126(8):983–92.
122. Raikar SS, Fleischer LC, Moot R, et al. Development of chimeric antigen receptors targeting T-cell malignancies using two structurally different anti-CD5 antigen binding domains in NK and CRISPR-edited T cell lines. Onco Targets Ther. 2018;7(3):e1407898.
123. Gomes-Silva D, Srinivasan M, Sharma S, et al. CD7-edited T cells expressing a CD7-specific CAR for the therapy of T-cell malignancies. Blood. 2017;130(3):285–96.
124. Png YT, Vinanica N, Kamiya T, Shimasaki N, Coustan-Smith E, Campana D. Blockade of CD7 expression in T cells for effective chimeric antigen receptor targeting of T-cell malignancies. Blood Adv. 2017;1(25):2348–60.
125. Mamonkin M, Mukherjee M, Srinivasan M, et al. Reversible transgene expression reduces fratricide and permits 4-1BB costimulation of CAR T cells directed to T-cell malignancies. Cancer Immunol Res. 2017;
126. Cooper ML, Choi J, Staser K, et al. An "off-the-shelf" fratricide-resistant CAR-T for the treatment of T cell hematologic malignancies. Leukemia. 2018;32(9):1970–83.
127. Winter SS, Dunsmore KP, Devidas M, et al. Safe integration of nelarabine into intensive chemotherapy in newly diagnosed T-cell acute lymphoblastic leukemia: children's oncology group study AALL0434. Pediatr Blood Cancer. 2015;62(7):1176–83.

128. Dunsmore KP, Winter S, Devidas M, et al. COG AALL0434: a randomized trial testing nelarabine in newly diagnosed t-cell malignancy. J Clin Oncol. 2018;36(15_suppl):10500.
129. Cohen MH, Johnson JR, Justice R, Pazdur R. FDA drug approval summary: nelarabine (Arranon) for the treatment of T-cell lymphoblastic leukemia/lymphoma. Oncologist. 2008;13(6):709–14.
130. Winter SS, Dunsmore KP, Devidas M, et al. Improved survival for children and young adults with T-lineage acute lymphoblastic Leukemia: results from the children's oncology group AALL0434 methotrexate randomization. J Clin Oncol. 2018;36(29):2926–34.
131. Gossai NWS, Devidas M, Wood B, Zweidler-McKay P, Rabin KR, Loh M, Raetz E, Winick N, Burke MJ, Carroll WL, Esiashvili N, Heerema NA, Carroll A, Hunger SP, Dunsmore KP, Teachey D. AW05 SIOP19-1143 nelarabine abrogates relapse rates in CNS3 T-ALL: a report from children's oncology group study AALL0434. Pediatr Blood Cancer. 2019;66(S4):e27989.
132. Silverman JA, Deitcher SR. Marqibo(R) (vincristine sulfate liposome injection) improves the pharmacokinetics and pharmacodynamics of vincristine. Cancer Chemother Pharmacol. 2013;71(3):555–64.
133. O'Brien S, Schiller G, Lister J, et al. High-dose vincristine sulfate liposome injection for advanced, relapsed, and refractory adult Philadelphia chromosome-negative acute lymphoblastic leukemia. J Clin Oncol. 2013;31(6):676–83.
134. Shah NN, Merchant MS, Cole DE, et al. Vincristine sulfate liposomes injection (VSLI, Marqibo(R)): results from a phase I study in children, adolescents, and young adults with refractory solid tumors or leukemias. Pediatr Blood Cancer. 2016;63(6):997–1005.
135. Passaro D, Irigoyen M, Catherinet C, et al. CXCR4 is required for leukemia-initiating cell activity in T cell acute lymphoblastic Leukemia. Cancer Cell. 2015;27(6):769–79.
136. Evans K, Duan J, Pritchard T, et al. OBI-3424, a novel AKR1C3-activated prodrug, exhibits potent efficacy against preclinical models of T-ALL. Clin Cancer Res. 2019;25(14):4493–503.

Chapter 15
The Development and Management of Treatment with Chimeric Antigen Receptor T Cell (CAR T)

Colleen Annesley and Rebecca Gardner

Introduction to CAR T Cell Therapy

Chimeric antigen receptor (CAR) T cell therapy consists of genetically modified T cells that are re-engineered to recognize surface-expressed proteins. CARs are composed of an antigen-binding domain that is derived from a single-chain variable fragment (scFv) from an immunoglobulin against the protein of interest, a transmembrane domain, and an intracellular signaling domain. This technology has allowed for flexibility in targeting tumor cells with cytotoxic T cells in a non-HLA-dependent manner. Initial first-generation CARs consisted of an intracellular CD3ζ signal which was insufficient for in vivo activity [1]. Second-generation CARs encoded for a second signal, most frequently CD28 or 4-1BB, in addition to the CD3ζ signal. Second-generation CARs entered clinical trials in the late 2000s, and clinical responses began to occur in B cell acute lymphoblastic leukemia (B-ALL), chronic lymphocytic leukemia (CLL), and B cell non-Hodgkin lymphoma (B NHL) [2–5]. The most remarkable responses with the use of CAR T cell therapy have been seen in pediatric B-ALL, leading to the first Food and Drug Administration (FDA) approval of a gene-modified cell therapy for cancer [6].

Commonalities of CAR T cell manufacturing to date include apheresis for autologous T cell collection, gene modification through viral transduction, and cell growth for approximately 1–2 weeks [7, 8]. Non-viral methods of gene modification are starting to come to clinic, which may enable faster and cheaper manufacturing [9]. Recent technology advances have also enhanced production ability. With

C. Annesley · R. Gardner (✉)
Department of Pediatrics, University of Washington, Seattle, WA, USA

Cancer and Blood Disorders Center, Seattle Children's Hospital, Seattle, WA, USA
e-mail: colleen.annesley@seattlechildrens.org; rebecca.gardner@SeattleChildrens.org

M. R. Litzow, E. A. Raetz (eds.), *Clinical Management of Acute Lymphoblastic Leukemia*, https://doi.org/10.1007/978-3-030-85147-7_15

the CliniMACS Prodigy, point-of-care CAR T cell manufacturing is becoming possible without the expense of a dedicated good manufacturing practice (GMP) facility, and currently several clinical trials are making use of the CliniMACS Prodigy for cell manufacturing [10]. Following the initial trials in the late 2000s, CAR T cell products under clinical investigation have expanded to greater than 1000 studies on clinicaltrials.gov targeting solid, brain, and liquid tumors.

Validated Targets in B-ALL

A key component of CAR T cell therapy is choosing a target protein which is expressed on the cell surface of the tumor cell and has minimal or no expression on normal tissue, in order to minimize the risks of on-target off-tumor toxicity. The two main targets meeting this criterion that have been exploited for therapeutic efficacy in B-ALL are CD19 and CD22.

CD19 is expressed on human B lymphocytes at all stages of maturation. It is an attractive target, as it is expressed on the majority of B-ALL and is not expressed on normal tissues other than B cells [11]. Engraftment assays in NOD/SCID mice have indicated that leukemia repopulating cells are uniformly CD34+ and CD19+ in the common forms of B-ALL [12]. In certain subtypes of B-ALL, such as BCR/ABL1-positive ALL, there are some reports that the leukemia-initiating cells are CD19 negative, although this is not definitive [13].

CD19 became a validated target in B-ALL initially through the development of blinatumomab, a CD19/CD3 bispecific T cell-engaging antibody that binds to CD3+ T cells and co-localizes them with CD19+ B cells, thereby activating the T cells and inducing perforin-mediated death of the targeted B cells [14]. Blinatumomab has been shown to have efficacy in both the minimal residual disease (MRD) and bulk disease settings. In a phase 2 study of blinatumomab in adults with B-ALL, 43% achieved a complete remission (CR) or CRh [15].

Similar to CD19, CD22 is expressed on all human B cells from the early pre-B phase [16] and is expressed in 96% of B-ALL cases [17]. However, CD22 expression is differentially expressed on certain subgroups of B-ALL. BCR/ABL1- and *KMT2A*-rearranged B-ALL have lower CD22 site density, which may impact the ability to respond to CD22 targeting. Inotuzumab ozogamicin (InO) is an anti-CD22 antibody conjugated to calicheamicin, a cytotoxic agent. Reports of InO in relapsed and refractory B-ALL have demonstrated CR rates of 80.7% in adults and 67% in a pediatric retrospective review. [18, 19] Although those with less than 100% expression of CD22 responded similarly to those with 100% expression, those with *KMT2A* or BCR/ABL1 mutations were less responsive to InO in the adult study [20].

Clinical Trial Insights

The ELIANA trial was the pivotal phase 2 registration trial for tisagenlecleucel in pediatric relapsed/refractory B-ALL and led to the first FDA approval of a CAR T cell product [21]. Tisagenlecleucel is a second-generation CAR T cell product, initially developed at the University of Pennsylvania (UPENN) and investigated academically in pediatrics at the Children's Hospital of Philadelphia (CHOP) as CTL019 [22]. Tisagenlecleucel is generated from patient-obtained leukapheresis material; expanded and transduced to express a second-generation CAR with the scFv domain derived from the murine anti-CD19 antibody, FMC63; and has 4-1BB co-stimulation. Eligibility criteria for the ELIANA trial included patients who were refractory or in second or greater relapse, with at least 5% lymphoblasts in the bone marrow at screening. Age requirements included at least 3 years of age at the time of enrollment and no greater than 21 years of age at diagnosis. Patients were treated with doses of 0.2–5.4 × 10^6 CAR+ T cells/kg. Of the 75 infused patients, 81% achieved a CR, and an intention-to-treat analysis of all enrolled patients showed a 66% CR rate. Of those who achieved a CR, the estimated relapse-free survival at 1 year was 59%. Most relapses were caused by loss of target antigen expression. The loss of CD19 was encountered early in the development of CAR T cell therapy, and the mechanism of antigen loss appears to be multifactorial [23–25]. Interrogation of the CD19-negative relapses from this group of patients showed that most had loss of surface CD19 expression due to truncating mutations, resulting in a protein that lacked the transmembrane domain [23].

Major learnings from the ELIANA trial included that CAR T cell therapy could be given across multiple hospitals and countries with central manufacturing and maintain high rates of remission. However, a significant portion of patients (18%) were unable to receive a CAR T cell product, either due to issues with manufacturing a CAR T cell product or encountering medical complications during the time of cell manufacturing that precluded infusion of the product. The manufacturing failure rate was 7.6%, and the median time from enrollment to infusion was 45 days (range, 30–105). Following commercialization, details regarding manufacturing failure rates are unavailable, but initial commercial tisagenlecleucel products generated for B-ALL had a median turnaround time of 23 days (range, 21–37 days) from the time the apheresis material was received at the manufacturing facility until it was returned to the patients [7].

Prior to commercialization of CAR T cell therapy, several academic centers conducted trials of varying CAR constructs in both pediatric and adult B-ALL that have led to varying insights on the use of CAR T cell therapy in this population [22, 26–29]. Collectively, these trials demonstrated high rates of remission across varying CAR products. Although the rates of remission have been high in adults, the rates of toxicity have also been high, which has slowed down the development of CD19 CAR T cell therapy for adult B-ALL.

Maintenance of remission is crucial to the ability to provide a long-term cure. It has been well established that the ongoing persistence of CAR T cells can be protective against CD19-positive recurrence [22, 28, 30]. Constructs that utilize CD28 co-stimulation, such as those developed at the National Cancer Institute (NCI) [26] and Memorial Sloan Kettering Cancer Center (MSKCC) [29], have shortened duration of in vivo persistence compared to those that use 4-1BB co-stimulation, such as UPENN [31], CHOP [22], the Fred Hutchinson Cancer Research Center (FHCRC) [27], and Seattle Children's Hospital (SCH) [28]. The 4-1BB co-stimulation appears to be protective against exhaustion with enhanced in vivo persistence. In addition to prolonged persistence, 4-1BB co-stimulation has demonstrated higher rates of CR in B-ALL of 82–94% [22, 27, 28] compared to 60–83% [26, 29]. This may reflect that 4-1BB co-stimulation leads to less exhaustion, allowing for repeated lytic activity in high disease burden patients, whereas the CD28 co-stimulation leads to exhausted T cells prior to obtaining a CR.

Aside from a small single-institution study comparing 4-1BB versus CD28 co-stimulation in NHL [32], there has not been a direct comparison of which product provides a superior overall outcome. Products that have longer in vivo persistence have higher rates of CD19-negative relapse, whereas those with short persistence have higher rates of CD19-positive relapse. In addition to higher rates of initial remission, the durability of the responses seems enhanced in products with 4-1BB co-stimulation. For adults, the 6-month event-free survival (EFS) with CD28 co-stimulation was 50% [29], compared with a 1-year disease-free survival (DFS) of 65% with 4-1BB co-stimulation [27]. Similarly in pediatrics, the median overall survival (OS) following CD28 co-stimulation was 13.3 months [26, 33] compared to 1-year EFS of 50% in two studies of 4-1BB co-stimulation [21, 28].

With loss of CD19 antigen emerging as a major barrier to durable remissions, the NCI embarked on a trial of CD22-directed CAR T cells with 4-1BB co-stimulation. The initial experience demonstrated remission rates of 73% at doses of $\geq 1 \times 10^6$ CD22 CAR T cells/kg [34]. The median duration of remission of 6 months following CD22-directed CAR T cell therapy is inferior to that following CD19-directed therapy. The mechanism of escape is predominately down-modulation of CD22, rather than loss of the target. This leads to diminished likelihood that CD22-directed therapy can be administered as definitive therapy. It remains to be determined whether specific subgroups of ALL with lower site density of CD22 expression, such as BCR/ABL1- and *KMT2A*-rearranged ALL, will have differential responses to CD22 CAR T cell therapy, as has been seen with InO.

Approaches to Overcoming Barriers to Therapeutic Efficacy

Several parameters should be considered when gauging the likelihood for CAR T cell therapy to be successful. One is to determine the expression of target antigen on the patient's leukemia cells. If there is a pre-existing antigen-negative population, CAR T cell therapy will not effectively eradicate the disease, and alternative therapies should be sought. Additionally, a patient must have adequate T cells to collect. In certain subgroups of patients, manufacture of an autologous CAR T cell product remains a challenge. Infants with refractory leukemia may not be able to feasibly undergo apheresis or other cell collection protocol given their smaller size. Patients may have poor bone marrow function related to prior disease-directed therapy or ongoing active disease, which precludes recovery of peripheral lymphocytes. Certain chemotherapy agents are strongly lymphodepleting, such as clofarabine and fludarabine. Proximal use of these agents prior to apheresis may inhibit successful manufacturing and should be avoided when CAR T cell therapy is being considered. Some groups have started recommending apheresis, cryopreservation, and storage of mononuclear cells for high-risk patients, with the possibility of later pursuing CAR T cell therapy.

Universal Products

For patients in whom lymphocytes are not able to be collected or waiting the required time for cell manufacturing is not feasible, alternative therapies are needed. One possible solution is the manufacture and delivery of an "off-the-shelf" allogeneic CAR T cell product. Allogeneic T cells must first be modified to reduce the risk of graft-versus-host disease (GVHD) in the recipient, as well as to mitigate the risk of the T cells being rejected. UCART19 is an allogeneic T cell product with TALEN-mediated knockout of the constant region of the T cell receptor α chain and disruption of CD52, rendering these T cells resistant to alemtuzumab while also lacking expression of a native TCR. Loss of the TCR minimizes the risk of developing GVHD, and knockout of CD52 allows for significant lymphodepletion with alemtuzumab to prevent rejection of the allogeneic T cells by the host. Preliminary results in two infants with refractory B-ALL treated with UCART19 demonstrated remission and subsequent ability to proceed with transplant [35]. Pooled clinical trial data of 20 patients on adult and pediatric clinical trials of UCART19 were presented at ASH in 2018 (NCT02746952 and NCT02808442) [36]. No expansion of UCART19 was observed in three patients who did not receive alemtuzumab, due to presumed rejection of the product by the patient. Fourteen of sixteen patients who received alemtuzumab achieved a CR or CRi, of which 86% (12 of 14) were MRD negative. Two grade 1 skin GVHD events were reported, of unclear attribution to the UCART19 cells. Because UCART19 has a relatively short engraftment with a median duration of persistence of 28 days, patients must be quickly bridged to transplant. Although these findings are encouraging, UCART19 does not seem as efficacious as autologous CAR T cells for B-ALL with the currently available data and requires significant lymphodepletion which carries the risk of severe viral infections.

CAR-expressing natural killer (NK) cells from the group at MD Anderson have been recently described. NK cells can exhibit lytic function through CAR expression, similar to cytotoxic T cells. Additionally, NK cells do not require HLA matching, allowing for a universal cell product without the requirements for additional gene modification. Eleven adult patients with relapsed or refractory CD19+ cancers (B-NHL or CLL) were treated with HLA-mismatched anti-CD19 CAR-NK cells derived from cord blood on a phase 1/2 trial [37]. In addition to CAR expression, the CAR NK cells were manufactured to secrete IL-15 to enhance in vivo expansion and persistence and contained an inducible caspase-9 to trigger apoptosis in the case of toxicity. Following infusion, no associated CRS, neurotoxicity, or GVHD was observed among three dose levels. Eight of 11 patients (73%) had a response, and 7 (4 with B-NHL and 3 with CLL) had a CR. Importantly, CAR-NK cells demonstrated expansion and persistence at low levels for at least 12 months. CAR-NK products could have future applicability for B-ALL with multiple advantages over off-the-shelf CAR T cells, including the ability to generate many products from a single cord unit, off-the-shelf timely availability, and a low toxicity profile. It is unclear how CAR-NK cells would compare overall with autologous CAR T cells.

Advances in Manufacturing Platforms

Manufacturing failure rates of up to 25% have been reported, thought to be related to the quality of the lymphocytes collected. In order to overcome manufacturing failure, a variety of groups have focused on manufacturing platforms that can rescue poor starting material and potentially provide a more homogenous final product. Non-T cells, such as monocytes, that are obtained at the time of apheresis and present at the initiation of cell culture, can be inhibitory toward cell expansion. One potential benefit to the upfront selection of T cells is the depletion of monocytes and other potentially inhibitory cells from culture. The addition of homeostatic cytokines such as IL-7 and IL-15 has been shown to rescue a poorly expanding product [38]. In a pediatric trial of CD19 CAR T cells, the manufacturing success rate was 100% in a group of heavily pretreated patients with the combination of upfront T cell selection and use of IL-7 and IL-15 in culture [28].

The CD22 CAR T cell trial at the NCI made a manufacturing change midway through their phase 1 trial. After a manufacturing failure, the manufacturing platform was amended to include upfront T cell selection prior to initiation of expansion [39]. This change led to not only higher rates of manufacturing success but also a more potent product. The trial then underwent dose de-escalation to accommodate the higher potency of the product.

Because persistence of the CAR T cell product is of the utmost importance in providing a durable remission, defining CAR T cell product attributes that are capable or predictive of long-term engraftment is desirable. Aside from the already defined addition of 4-1BB co-stimulation to the CAR construct to prevent exhaustion, there may be specifics of manufacturing that enable long-term persistence of a product. One example is the manufacture of CAR T cells from central memory CD8+ T cells (T_{CM}) via lineage marker selection [40], based on prior data demonstrating that T_{CM} have enhanced in vivo persistence [41]. Similar work has shown that there may be advantages to using naïve T cells as the starting T cell population [42]. At this time, it remains unclear if selecting specific T cell populations leads to enhanced persistence of CAR T cell products.

Another emerging advantage of upfront selection is that it can effectively remove leukemia blasts from the cell culture. A case report described the unintentional transduction of a leukemia cell that resulted in a CAR-expressing leukemic clone. Nine months following infusion, a patient experienced relapse, and the leukemic cells were noted to express both the CAR and CD19; however, the expression of the CAR on the leukemic cell surface bound to the CD19, preventing its recognition by CAR+ T cells [43].

Identification of Risk Factors for Lack of Response

In addition to manufacturing challenges, new insights have indicated product and leukemia intrinsic factors as barriers to response to CAR T cell therapy. One report found that higher LAG-3 expression and lower TNFα production in the starting T cell product were associated with lack of a response [30]. If further validated, this could potentially prospectively identify patients who are less likely to respond to autologous CAR T cell therapy. The same study showed that there were product characteristics that predicted more durable engraftment of the CAR T cells in patients. The products with long persistence had decreased TIM-3 expression and high TNFα production when compared to those with shortened persistence.

Early investigations are underway to identify leukemic intrinsic properties, other than antigen loss, that prohibit a response. Singh et al. utilized a CRISPR-based genome-wide loss-of-function screen to determine that impaired death receptor signaling in leukemia cells causes resistance to T cell cytotoxicity, as well as impairment of CAR T cell function, resulting in rapidly progressive leukemia [44]. Another recent report used exomic, single-cell genomic and epigenomic analyses to compare four pediatric cases of dysfunctional responders versus five responders to CD19 CAR T cell therapy and found that CREBBP fusions, methylation-based upregulation of JUND/JUN regulation, and a significant increase in open chromatin regions correlated with dysfunctional responders [45].

Overcoming Antigen Loss

Antigen loss is a well-reported barrier to the success of targeted therapy. CD19 epitope and trafficking modification following blinatumomab and CD19 CAR T cell therapy converts CD19 to an unrecognizable antigen target, and CD22 downregulation has been observed following CD22-targeted therapy. At present, there is not a predictive algorithm for who will develop antigen escape. The first report of

CD19-"negative" relapse occurred in a patient who had received blinatumomab prior to CD19 CAR T cell therapy, leading to questions about the relationship of successive CD19 antigen targeting and development of CD19-negative disease [46]. A retrospective analysis of 166 patients receiving CD19 CAR T cells showed that the brightness of CD19 antigen expression did not impact response to CAR T cell therapy as long as the entire population was CD19 positive, but prior blinatumomab therapy was associated with a higher rate of failure to achieve MRD-negative remission and CD19-negative relapse [47]. Weaknesses of this study included the retrospective nature as well as the small number of patients who were treated with blinatumomab prior to CAR T cell therapy. Conversely, a retrospective review of 24 adult patients treated with CD19 CAR T therapy showed no impact of prior blinatumomab on response [48]. As the immunotherapy field evolves, it will be important to prospectively identify factors that are predictive of CD19 antigen escape.

To address the issue of CD22 site density downregulation after CD22 targeting therapy, certain compounds such as bryostatin 1 are reported to upregulate CD22 and may provide increased efficacy of CD22 targeting therapy [49, 50]. Although CD19 and CD22 are the most commonly used targets for B-ALL, additional targets are also being developed. These include TSLPR, which is often overexpressed in a subset of Philadelphia-like ALL [51], CD123 [52], and BAFF-R [53]. Using multiple targets and pharmacologic upregulation of a target may both be strategies to overcome antigen escape or potentially limit the impact of antigen loss on durable remissions.

Multiple groups are investigating dual-targeting CAR therapy, and the most experience has been targeting both CD19 and CD22. Some have used a tandem CAR approach, with a bivalent construct containing both CD19 and CD22 scFvs in the extracellular domain and a single intracellular signaling domain. Clinical trials for both adults and pediatrics are underway (NCT03241940 and NCT03233854), and results were presented at ASH 2019 [54]. Eleven of twelve evaluable patients achieved a CR, and 3 patients subsequently relapsed with CD19+ disease; however, CD19-negative relapses were also reported. Another option is to incorporate two CARs in a single T cell. One approach uses dual transduction of two separate vectors, each encoding for a single CAR construct. This technique results in a heterogeneous population of T cells with both single and dual CAR expression, and preliminary results show an 83% CR rate in a phase 1 trial (NCT03330691) [55]. AUTO3 is a product manufactured with a bicistronic construct, resulting in one population of dual expressing CD19 x CD22 CAR T cells. Preliminary results from the phase 1 study of AUTO3 reported that seven of seven CAR-naïve patients treated at the highest dose levels achieved an MRD-negative CR (NCT03289455) [56]. However, after a median follow-up of 8 months, four subjects had emergence of MRD, three of which demonstrated loss of CAR T cell persistence and one with CD19-negative, CD22 low expressing relapsed disease. Each of these dual-targeting products has demonstrated manufacturing feasibility and good tolerability; however, it has yet to be demonstrated that dual-targeting CAR T cell products provide a more durable remission. Whether dual targeting can maintain the same level of specificity for each of the targets remains to be seen.

Promoting Long-Term Persistence

Early loss of persistence is a barrier to CD19 CAR T cell success and increases the risk for CD19+ relapse. Aside from the abovementioned product-related phenotypes and CAR constructs that may help predict long-term CAR T cell engraftment, one report demonstrated that low CD19 antigen burden (<15% CD19+ cells prior to CAR T cell infusion, inclusive of malignant and normal B cells) increases the risk of early loss of persistence [28]. An ongoing pilot clinical trial provides episodic antigen stimulation to CD19 CAR T cells in vivo through the use of patient-derived, CD19-expressing T cell antigen-presenting cells (T-APCs) (NCT03186118). Secondary expansions of CD19-specific CAR T cells have been observed following sequential doses of CD19 T-APCs [57]. The first 12 treated subjects, all with a predictive factor to experience early loss of CAR T cell engraftment by 2 months, showed prolonged engraftment with a median duration of CAR T cell persistence of 8.1 months. Importantly, T-APC doses have been well tolerated without recrudescence of CRS. As CAR T cell therapy moves toward upfront treatment, more patients may receive treatment in the low antigen burden setting, necessitating alternative therapies, such as T-APCs, to enhance long-term persistence.

Another explanation for short persistence of CAR T cells is the development of an immune-mediated rejection of the CAR construct, typically directed at the murine-based scFv domain [27]. To attempt to prevent this rejection, groups have developed humanized and fully human CD19 scFv-containing CARs. CHOP presented their results of a phase 1 trial of a humanized CD19 CAR (NCT2374333) in 30 children and young adults, which showed an excellent 100% MRD-negative CR rate in CAR-naïve subjects and a 45% MRD-negative CR rate in those with prior CAR exposure [58]. Although encouraging responses were seen in the CAR-naïve group, the lack of responses to those with prior CAR exposure suggests that there is some overlap in epitope recognition with shared rejection responses. Several early phase clinical trials are underway using a fully human CD19 scFvs that do not share sequences with the murine-based FMC63 scFv (NCT03684889, NCT02659943, NCT03103971), which may further mitigate the phenomenon of rejection, allow for repeat infusions if necessary, and potentially prolong durable responses.

Finally, blinatumomab has been given in combination with checkpoint inhibitors to attempt to enhance efficacy (NCT02879695, NCT03605589), with promising tolerability reports [59]. Similarly, ongoing early phase clinical trials are investigating the use of checkpoint blockade with pembrolizumab or nivolumab following CAR T cell therapy (NCT02879695, NCT04205409). In one report, three of six patients with early B cell recovery had return of B cell aplasia following checkpoint blockade, suggesting return of functional persistence of CAR T cells, and two of four subjects with bulky extramedullary disease and ongoing systemic functional persistence had complete responses following checkpoint blockade [60].

CAR T Cell Therapy Indications and Role of Consolidation Therapy

With initial FDA approval of tisagenlecleucel for refractory and second or greater relapse, many groups are now interested in how to further develop this therapy and expand the indications. In partnership with Novartis, the Children's Oncology Group is now conducting a study (NCT03876769) to administer tisagenlecleucel to those pediatric and young adult patients who are MRD positive at the end of consolidation. This group of patients has inferior outcomes with standard chemotherapy with 5-year disease-free survival of <40% [61].

A controversial question is whether additional therapy is warranted following CAR T cell-induced remission. In part, this is determined by the target antigen of the CAR T cells and the patient. With CD19 targeting, it is now clear that a subset of patients can be cured with CAR T cell therapy. However, the ability to prospectively determine who will be cured has been elusive. Patients with functional CAR T cell persistence are protected against CD19-positive relapse but remain at risk for CD19-negative disease. For these reasons, various groups have sought to define the role for consolidative transplant following CD19-directed CAR T cell therapy.

In a landmark analysis of the UPENN trial, adult subjects who underwent consolidative hematopoietic cell transplant (HCT) had superior leukemia-free and overall survival [31]. In the FHCRC trial, adult subjects who underwent HCT after CAR T cell therapy saw a protective impact on EFS with a hazard ratio of 0.39 ($P = 0.088$) [62]. Both of these trials utilized constructs with 4-1BB co-stimulation. In contrast, there was no benefit of HCT shown in adults in long-term follow-up of the MSKCC trial [29]. The SCH trial showed that there was an advantage to consolidation with HCT after CAR T cell therapy ($P = 0.01$) in pediatric patients. This effect was concentrated among those who had not received a prior HCT, with 2-year leukemia-free survival (LFS) of 91% versus 33% ($P = 0.005$). Among those with early loss of CAR T cell persistence (prior to 2 months), those who underwent consolidative HCT showed an improved LFS, regardless of prior history of HCT ($P = 0.003$) [63]. However, these reports should be interpreted with caution, due to the non-randomized assignment of consolidative HCT.

In an analysis of patients on the ELIANA trial, those who were MRD negative by next-generation sequencing (NGS) at 1-month post-CAR T cell infusion had a PFS of 80% compared to 30% [64]. This may represent one tool to distinguish those who may benefit from additional therapy post-CAR T cells; those who obtain early NGS negativity have a higher chance of long-term remission without further therapy. Similarly, in the adult FHCRC study, those who were NGS MRD negative by 3 weeks after CAR T cell infusion had improved EFS with median of 8.4 vs. 3.6 months ($P = 0.036$) [65].

The role of transplant is likely to vary based on the population and the target. Because down-modulation of CD22 following CD22 CAR T cell therapy is nearly universal, the ability to stay in remission without additional therapy is negligible [34]. For this reason, it is generally recommended to proceed with HCT following

CD22-directed CAR T cell therapy, regardless of CAR T cell persistence or history of prior transplantation.

Toxicity and Management of Toxicity

Cytokine release syndrome (CRS) and neurotoxicity, now termed immune effector cell-associated neurotoxicity syndrome (ICANS), are the two most common and severe toxicities associated with CAR T cell therapy in hematologic malignancies.

Cytokine Release Syndrome

CRS is characterized by a hallmark finding of fever and is frequently accompanied by hypotension and respiratory compromise in the setting of elevated serum cytokines, predominantly IL-6 [66]. Other lab abnormalities during CRS include elevation of acute-phase proteins such as CRP and ferritin. A consumptive coagulopathy is also described, though with a relatively low incidence of clinical bleeding. The onset of CRS generally occurs within the first 2 weeks following infusion.

Grading of CAR T cell-related toxicities has proven challenging, as the toxicity grading for CRS in the Common Terminology Criteria for Adverse Events (CTCAE) was more applicable to characterizing infusion-related reactions with monoclonal antibody therapy. As a result, separate groups developed independent grading scales for cytokine release syndrome in early CAR T cell clinical trials, making comparisons among groups more difficult. In 2014, Lee et al. published a suggested CRS grading scale, which became the most frequently adopted scale by multiple groups [67]. More recently, consensus guidelines on the grading of CRS were published in 2019 by the American Society for Transplantation and Cellular Therapy (ASTCT) [68]. The recent publication of the consensus grading system from the ASTCT group will hopefully further align the grading systems across various protocols and products.

The severity of CRS has correlated with the dose of CAR T cells and the amount of disease burden prior to CAR T cell infusion across multiple studies [6, 26–28]. Initially, adults seemed to have more complicated CRS than pediatric patients. Over time, the ability to safely administer CD19 CAR T cell therapy to adults has improved. The group at the FHCRC has trialed disease burden-based dosing, with a lower dose administered to patients with high disease burden [27]. Alternatively, UPENN has focused on split dosing [31]. With these strategies, both groups have been able to retain high rates of remission while allowing for manageable toxicity.

Several algorithms have been developed to predict the development of severe CRS, inclusive of both clinical features and serum cytokine levels at early time points following infusion. One model for pediatric patients showed that disease burden $\geq$51% and early IL-10 levels >11.7457 pg/mL was 91% sensitive and 96%

specific for the development of severe CRS [58]. Another group demonstrated that fever ≥38.9 °C within 36 h after infusion and MCP-1 ≥ 1343.5 pg/mL was 100% sensitive and 95% predictive of ≥ grade 4 CRS in adults with CD19+ malignancies [69]. Further validation will be needed to determine if these algorithms are predictive across varying CAR T cell products. For example, one group has already shown that a pediatric algorithm, while predictive for CRS after CTL019, is not predictive for CRS following a different CAR T cell product, SCRI-CAR19, in a similar patient population [70].

The first reports of treatment success for severe CRS described the administration of tocilizumab, an IL-6 receptor (IL-6R) antagonist [46]. This recombinant monoclonal antibody blocks the binding of IL-6 to the IL-6R, preventing IL-6 activity, but subsequently increases the serum concentration of IL-6, as clearance of IL-6 requires binding to the IL-6R. Tocilizumab is now widely used to treat severe CRS associated with CAR T cell therapy [71]. In addition to IL-6 blockade, glucocorticoids are the most common intervention given for CRS.

The optimal timing and use of tocilizumab and steroids during CRS have yet to be determined. Several groups are working on the mitigation of CAR T cell toxicity, both during and prior to its development. Initially, there was concern that intervening too early following CAR T cell infusion could negatively impact CAR T cell engraftment and efficacy. In Seattle, an early intervention strategy was implemented in which tocilizumab and dexamethasone were given for mild but persistent CRS, to prevent severe CRS. This small study showed that the early use of tocilizumab and dexamethasone led to an increase in the use of tocilizumab (22% vs. 60% of patients after implementation of early use) and steroids (17% vs. 25%) but resulted in an approximately 50% decrease in the rate of severe CRS [70]. Importantly, there did not appear to be any untoward effect from using tocilizumab and dexamethasone earlier in the course of CRS, including no increased incidence of ICANS or diminished T cell function. The rates of CAR T cell engraftment and persistence were maintained in patients who received intervention with tocilizumab and steroids, as were the rates of responses. CHOP is investigating the use of early tocilizumab given to children with ≥40% disease burden (NCT02906371). In the ZUMA studies, a subset of B-NHL patients who received axicabtagene ciloleucel (CD19-specific CAR T cells with CD28 co-stimulation) were given prophylactic tocilizumab. Results showed a reduction in ≥ grade 3 CRS (28% to 3%) but raised concern for increased neurotoxicity [72]. Several groups are working on publishing consensus treatment guidelines, similar to the grading guidelines, to unify the approach to mitigate toxicity.

Neurotoxicity

Neurological symptoms related to CAR T cell infusion tend to occur simultaneously with CRS, or days to weeks following resolution of CRS, and encompass a wide range of symptoms and severity, including headache, tremor, confusion, delirium, language disturbances, seizures, and rarely cerebral edema [73]. Neurological symptoms were initially thought to be a manifestation of CRS, but these symptoms have been described in the absence of CRS, and neurotoxicity is now known as a distinct toxicity. The severity of neurological toxicities has also been graded differently in different trials. Along with CRS consensus grading, the ASTCT also provided a consensus grading scale for neurotoxicity under the comprehensive terminology of ICANS [68].

The incidence of reported neurotoxicity has varied widely between trials and may be affected by differences in disease, CAR T cell product, age, interventions used to mitigate toxicity, and other factors. In pediatric trials, the incidence of neurotoxicity has been 40–44% (13–21% ≥ grade 3) using a 4-1BB CAR construct and 30% (5% ≥ grade 3) with a CD28 construct [21, 26, 28]. Adult trials using a 4-1BB construct have reported neurotoxicity in 50% (50% ≥ grade 3) in ALL [27], 28–39% (11–28% ≥ grade 3) in B-NHL [74, 75], and 6–33% (0–25% ≥ grade 3) in CLL [76, 77]. Adult trials using a CD28 construct have reported neurotoxicity in 44% (42% ≥ grade 3) in ALL [29] and up to 64% (28–45% ≥ grade 3) in B-NHL [78, 79]. Neurotoxicity is also described after treatment with blinatumomab for ALL [15], leading some to suggest that neurotoxicity may be linked to targeting CD19. Although the incidence of neurotoxicity has been reported in up to 25% of patients treated with non-CD19 targeting CAR therapy in varying hematologic malignancies, only 0–8% has been ≥ grade 3 [34, 80–83].

Some groups have attempted to develop a predictive algorithm for the development of severe neurotoxicity. Gust et al. found that adult patients with fever ≥38.9 °C, serum IL-6 ≥ 16 pg/mL, and MCP-1 ≥ 1343.5 pg/mL in the first 36 h after CAR T cell infusion were at high risk of subsequent ≥ grade 4 neurotoxicity following CD19 CAR T cell therapy for B-ALL, although these factors were also predictive of severe CRS in this patient group [84]. Santomasso et al. found that serum cytokine levels on day 3 following CAR T cell infusion were predictive of severe neurotoxicity, specifically IL-15 > 50 pg/mL, EGF (produced by platelets) < 120 pg/mL, and IL-10 > 200 pg/mL [85]. Clinical predictors of ICANS include the occurrence of severe CRS.

Due to the lack of definitive cause of ICANS, treatment and management of ICANS are unclear. Unlike CRS, neurotoxicity does not appear to be responsive to tocilizumab. Additionally, since tocilizumab is not thought to cross the blood-brain barrier (BBB), and administration of tocilizumab is predicted to increase serum IL-6 levels following its administration, some groups have avoided use of tocilizumab in neurotoxicity. However, the role of elevated levels of IL-6 in neurotoxicity has not been established. For now, glucocorticoids, either dexamethasone or high-dose methylprednisolone, remain the standard for treatment of ICANS.

The role of CAR T cells present in the CSF in neurotoxicity also remains unclear. There does not appear to be a correlation with neurotoxicity and central nervous system (CNS) disease involvement. Although it has been shown that CAR T cells egress into the CSF, CAR T cells are detected in the CSF of both patients with and without neurotoxicity [86]. In a non-human primate model of neurotoxicity following CD20 targeting CAR T cells, both CAR and non-CAR T cells were seen in the

CSF as well as the brain parenchyma at necropsy, and pan-encephalitis with pro-inflammatory cytokines was postulated as the driver of neurotoxicty [87]. Other proposed mechanisms include endothelial injury and disruption of the BBB. Patients with severe neurotoxicity have demonstrated elevated biomarkers of endothelial cell activation (Ang-2 and von Willebrand factor), systemic capillary leak, and disruption of the BBB [84].

It remains unclear if the pathophysiology of cerebral edema development is different from that of the other neurological symptoms associated with CAR T cell therapy. Acute cerebral edema represents a rare but life-threatening subset of cases of neurotoxicity and has only been reported following CD19 CAR T cells. Five fatal cases of cerebral edema resulted in the early termination of one clinical trial investigating CD19-specific CAR T cells (JCAR015) in adult ALL [88], though cerebral edema has been reported in other trials as well [75, 84]. The investigation of JCAR015 reported that cerebral edema was associated with rapid early expansion of CAR T cells and a rise in serum IL-15 levels. In two cases at autopsy, breakdown of the BBB was evident, with endothelial damage, astrocyte damage, and microglial activation, although CAR T cell infiltration was not seen. Autopsy of another case without neurotoxicity did not show breakdown of the BBB. Prior CNS radiation, CNS disease, intrathecal chemotherapy, transplant, and blinatumomab were not associated with development of cerebral edema [88].

As clinical trials have begun to empirically treat CRS and ICANS, more work has focused on the development of animal models to gain further insights into mechanisms and uncover new treatment strategies. In a mouse model of CRS following human CAR T cell infusion, researchers found that CAR T cells appear to recruit and activate murine myeloid cells [89]. Further, although GM-CSF and IFN-γ were produced from the human CAR T cells, other cytokines such as IL-6 were of murine origin, and IL-6 was specifically produced by tumor-associated macrophages. RNA-seq data also demonstrated upregulation of IL-1R1 in tumor-associated myeloid cells during CRS, which is required for functional IL-1 signaling. Both IL-6 blockage and IL-1 blockade abrogated CRS-related mortality in this model. In a humanized mouse model engrafted with human hematopoietic stem and progenitor cells (HSPCs), CAR T cells were engineered from engrafted T cells and produced a reliable model of CRS and ICANS when challenged with human leukemia cells [90]. CAR T cells released GM-CSF and TNF-α upon tumor recognition, whereas monocytes were found to be the main source of IL-1 and IL-6 during CRS. Monocyte depletion abrogated CRS, but also impeded CAR T cell expansion and anti-leukemia effect. In this model, both tocilizumab and anakinra, administered either prophylactically prior to CAR T cell infusion or after onset of fever following infusion, were effective at preventing CRS without impeding leukemia clearance. Interestingly, only anakinra was effective at abrogating delayed neurotoxicity in this model, both in the prophylactic and treatment settings.

Several clinical trials are now investigating the use of anakinra, a synthetic IL-1 receptor antagonist, to mitigate or prevent the development of CRS and/or neurotoxicity in patients with B-ALL or B-NHL (NCT04148430, NCT04205838, NCT04150913). Hopefully, continued experience and gained knowledge will lead to predictive models and effective interventions that will ultimately diminish the rates of severe CRS and neurotoxicity.

Infectious Complications

Patients receiving CAR T cell therapy are at risk for infectious complications. This is in part due to an immunocompromised state prior to treatment, compounded by the use of lymphodepleting chemotherapy, and followed by ongoing B cell aplasia related to functional CAR T cell persistence. There is also a subset of patients who experience prolonged bone marrow aplasia following CAR T cell infusion that is not related to their underlying disease and may render these patients at higher risk of infection. Recommendations for immunoglobulin replacement for ongoing hypogammaglobulinemia related to B cell aplasia have varied based on patient populations, with pediatric providers more frequently providing replacement. Further investigations are needed to optimize the screening and prevention of CAR T cell-related infections.

Conclusions

The landscape of treatment for relapsed and refractory B-ALL has forever been changed with the advent of CAR T cell therapy. With improved toxicity profiles and greater understanding of the biology of CRS and ICANS, higher-risk patients, including adults, will be able to safely receive CAR T cell therapy. As the field advances, additional targets may be validated and multi-targeted approaches taken. With more experience, "off-the-shelf" products are likely to become more refined, expanding access of CAR therapy to greater numbers of patients. Ultimately, it seems increasingly likely that CAR T cell and other immunotherapy treatments will replace at least parts of conventional treatment in the near future.

References

1. Jensen MC, Popplewell L, Cooper LJ, et al. Antitransgene rejection responses contribute to attenuated persistence of adoptively transferred CD20/CD19-specific chimeric antigen receptor redirected T cells in humans. Biol Blood Marrow Transplant. 2010;16(9):1245–56.
2. Kochenderfer JN, Wilson WH, Janik JE, et al. Eradication of B lineage cells and regression of lymphoma in a patient treated with autologous T cells genetically engineered to recognize CD19. Blood. 2010;116(20):4099–102.
3. Grupp SA, Kalos M, Barrett D, et al. Chimeric antigen receptor-modified T cells for acute lymphoid leukemia. N Engl J Med. 2013;368(16):1509–18.

4. Porter DL, Levine BL, Kalos M, Bagg A, June CH. Chimeric antigen receptor-modified T cells in chronic lymphoid Leukemia. N Engl J Med. 2011;
5. Savoldo B, Ramos CA, Liu E, et al. CD28 costimulation improves expansion and persistence of chimeric antigen receptor-modified T cells in lymphoma patients. J Clin Invest. 2011;121(5):1822–6.
6. Maude SL. Tisagenlecleucel in pediatric patients with acute lymphoblastic leukemia. Clin Adv Hematol Oncol. 2018;16(10):664–6.
7. Tyagarajan S, Spencer T, Smith J. Optimizing CAR-T cell manufacturing processes during pivotal clinical trials. Mol Ther Methods Clin Dev. 2020;16:136–44.
8. Stock S, Schmitt M, Sellner L. Optimizing manufacturing protocols of chimeric antigen receptor T cells for improved anticancer immunotherapy. Int J Mol Sci. 2019;20(24)
9. Kebriaei P, Singh H, Huls MH, et al. Phase I trials using sleeping beauty to generate CD19-specific CAR T cells. J Clin Invest. 2016;126(9):3363–76.
10. Zhu F, Shar NN, Schneider D, Xu H, Chaney K, Luib L, Keever-Taylor CA, Dropulic B, Orentas R, Hari P, Johnson B. Point-of-care manufacturing of CD20.19 bi-specific chimeric antigen receptor T (CAR-T) cells in a standard academic cell processing facility for a phase I clinical trial in relapsed, refractory NHL. Blood. 2018;132(Supplement 1)
11. Katz BZ, Herishanu Y. Therapeutic targeting of CD19 in hematological malignancies: past, present, future and beyond. Leuk Lymphoma. 2014;55(5):999–1006.
12. Kong Y, Yoshida S, Saito Y, et al. CD34+CD38+CD19+ as well as CD34+CD38-CD19+ cells are leukemia-initiating cells with self-renewal capacity in human B-precursor ALL. Leukemia. 2008;22(6):1207–13.
13. Hotfilder M, Rottgers S, Rosemann A, et al. Leukemic stem cells in childhood high-risk ALL/t(9;22) and t(4;11) are present in primitive lymphoid-restricted CD34+CD19- cells. Cancer Res. 2005;65(4):1442–9.
14. Loffler A, Kufer P, Lutterbuse R, et al. A recombinant bispecific single-chain antibody, CD19 x CD3, induces rapid and high lymphoma-directed cytotoxicity by unstimulated T lymphocytes. Blood. 2000;95(6):2098–103.
15. Topp MS, Gokbuget N, Stein AS, et al. Safety and activity of blinatumomab for adult patients with relapsed or refractory B-precursor acute lymphoblastic leukaemia: a multicentre, single-arm, phase 2 study. Lancet Oncol. 2015;16(1):57–66.
16. Shah NN, Stevenson MS, Yuan CM, et al. Characterization of CD22 expression in acute lymphoblastic leukemia. Pediatr Blood Cancer. 2015;62(6):964–9.
17. Gudowius S, Recker K, Laws HJ, et al. Identification of candidate target antigens for antibody-based immunotherapy in childhood B-cell precursor ALL. Klin Padiatr. 2006;218(6):327–33.
18. Kantarjian HM, DeAngelo DJ, Stelljes M, et al. Inotuzumab ozogamicin versus standard therapy for acute lymphoblastic Leukemia. N Engl J Med. 2016;375(8):740–53.
19. Bhojwani D, Sposto R, Shah NN, et al. Inotuzumab ozogamicin in pediatric patients with relapsed/refractory acute lymphoblastic leukemia. Leukemia. 2019;33(4):884–92.
20. Kantarjian H, Thomas D, Jorgensen J, et al. Results of inotuzumab ozogamicin, a CD22 monoclonal antibody, in refractory and relapsed acute lymphocytic leukemia. Cancer. 2013;119(15):2728–36.
21. Maude SL, Laetsch TW, Buechner J, et al. Tisagenlecleucel in children and young adults with B-cell lymphoblastic Leukemia. N Engl J Med. 2018;378(5):439–48.
22. Maude SL, Frey N, Shaw PA, et al. Chimeric antigen receptor T cells for sustained remissions in leukemia. N Engl J Med. 2014;371(16):1507–17.
23. Orlando EJ, Han X, Tribouley C, et al. Genetic mechanisms of target antigen loss in CAR19 therapy of acute lymphoblastic leukemia. Nat Med. 2018;24(10):1504–6.
24. Bagashev A, Sotillo E, Tang CH, et al. CD19 alterations emerging after CD19-directed immunotherapy cause retention of the misfolded protein in the endoplasmic reticulum. Mol Cell Biol. 2018;38(21)

25. Sotillo E, Barrett DM, Black KL, et al. Convergence of acquired mutations and alternative splicing of CD19 enables resistance to CART-19 immunotherapy. Cancer Discov. 2015;5(12):1282–95.
26. Lee DW, Kochenderfer JN, Stetler-Stevenson M, et al. T cells expressing CD19 chimeric antigen receptors for acute lymphoblastic leukaemia in children and young adults: a phase 1 dose-escalation trial. Lancet. 2015;385(9967):517–28.
27. Turtle CJ, Hanafi LA, Berger C, et al. CD19 CAR-T cells of defined CD4+:CD8+ composition in adult B cell ALL patients. J Clin Invest. 2016;126(6):2123–38.
28. Gardner RA, Finney O, Annesley C, et al. Intent-to-treat leukemia remission by CD19 CAR T cells of defined formulation and dose in children and young adults. Blood. 2017;129(25):3322–31.
29. Park JH, Riviere I, Gonen M, et al. Long-term follow-up of CD19 CAR therapy in acute lymphoblastic leukemia. N Engl J Med. 2018;378(5):449–59.
30. Finney OC, Brakke HM, Rawlings-Rhea S, et al. CD19 CAR T cell product and disease attributes predict leukemia remission durability. J Clin Invest. 2019;130
31. Frey NV, Shaw PA, Hexner EO, et al. Optimizing chimeric antigen receptor T-cell therapy for adults with acute lymphoblastic leukemia. J Clin Oncol. 2019:JCO1901892.
32. Ramos CA, Rouce R, Robertson CS, et al. In vivo fate and activity of second- versus third-generation CD19-specific CAR-T cells in B cell non-Hodgkin's lymphomas. Mol Ther. 2018;26(12):2727–37.
33. Lee DW, Stetler-Stevenson M, Yuan CM et al. Long-term outcomes following CD19 CAR T cell therapy for B-ALL are superior in patients receiving a fludarabine/cyclophosphamide preparative regimen and post-CAR hematopoietic stem cell transplantation. Blood 2016;128(22):218–218
34. Fry TJ, Shah NN, Orentas RJ, et al. CD22-targeted CAR T cells induce remission in B-ALL that is naive or resistant to CD19-targeted CAR immunotherapy. Nat Med. 2018;24(1):20–8.
35. Qasim W, Zhan H, Samarasinghe S, et al. Molecular remission of infant B-ALL after infusion of universal TALEN gene-edited CAR T cells. Sci Transl Med. 2017;9(374)
36. Benjamin R, Graham C, Yallop D, et al. Preliminary data on safety, cellular kinetics and anti-leukemic activity of UCART19, an allogeneic anti-CD19 CAR T-cell product, in a pool of adult and pediatric patients with high-risk CD19+ relapsed/refractory B-cell acute lymphoblastic leukemia. Blood 2018;132(Suppl 1):896–896
37. Liu E, Marin D, Banerjee P, et al. Use of CAR-transduced natural killer cells in CD19-positive lymphoid tumors. N Engl J Med. 2020;382(6):545–53.
38. Singh N, Perazzelli J, Grupp SA, Barrett DM. Early memory phenotypes drive T cell proliferation in patients with pediatric malignancies. Sci Transl Med. 2016;8(320):320ra323.
39. Shah NH, SL.; Shalabi, H; Yates, B; Kane, E; Fellowes V; Delbrook C; Ren J; Jin J; Stroncek D; Fry TJ. CD4/CD8 T-cell selection enhances CD22 CAR-T cell transduction and in vivo CAR-T expansion: updated results on phase I anti-CD22 CAR dose expansion cohort. Blood. 2017;130:809.
40. Sommermeyer D, Hudecek M, Kosasih PL, et al. Chimeric antigen receptor-modified T cells derived from defined CD8+ and CD4+ subsets confer superior antitumor reactivity in vivo. Leukemia. 2016;30(2):492–500.
41. Berger C, Jensen MC, Lansdorp PM, Gough M, Elliott C, Riddell SR. Adoptive transfer of effector CD8+ T cells derived from central memory cells establishes persistent T cell memory in primates. J Clin Invest. 2008;118(1):294–305.
42. Hinrichs CS, Borman ZA, Cassard L, et al. Adoptively transferred effector cells derived from naive rather than central memory CD8+ T cells mediate superior antitumor immunity. Proc Natl Acad Sci U S A. 2009;106(41):17469–74.
43. Ruella M, Xu J, Barrett DM, et al. Induction of resistance to chimeric antigen receptor T cell therapy by transduction of a single leukemic B cell. Nat Med. 2018;24(10):1499–503.
44. Singh N, Lee YG, Shestova O, et al. Impaired death receptor signaling in leukemia causes antigen-independent resistance by inducing CAR T cell dysfunction. Cancer Discov. 2020;

45. Masih KE, Gardner R, Gryder B, Lack J, Stanton B, Wilson A, Sindiri S, Song Y, Rae Z, Kelly M, Chaoyu W, Wen X, Cheuk A, Wei J, Jensen MC, Khan J, Orentas R. Detailed multi-method analysis of bone marrow from pediatric pre-B-ALL patients prior to CD19-CAR-T therapy subsequently evidencing OVert CAR-T resistance. Blood. 2019;134(Suppl 1)
46. Grupp SA, Kalos M, Barrett D, et al. Chimeric antigen receptor-modified T cells for acute lymphoid Leukemia. N Engl J Med. 2013;
47. Pillai V, Rosenthal J, Muralidharan K, Wertheim GB, Paessler M, Maude SL, Rheingold SR, Grupp SA. Correlation of pre-CAR CD19 expression with responses and relapses after CAR T cell therapy. J Clin Oncol. 2018;36(Suppl):3051.
48. Shah BD, Oluwole OO, Baer MR, Bishop MR, Holmes HE, Schiller GJ. Outcomes of patients (pts) treated with prior blinatumomab (Blin) in ZUMA-3: a study of KTE-C19, an anti-CD19 chimeric antigen receptor (CAR) t cell therapy, in adult pts with relapsed/refractory acute lymphoblastic leukemia (R/R ALL). J Clin Oncol 2018;36(15):7006–7006
49. Ramakrishna S, Highfill SL, Walsh Z, et al. Modulation of target antigen density improves CAR T cell functionality and persistence. Clin Cancer Res. 2019.
50. Biberacher V, Decker T, Oelsner M, et al. The cytotoxicity of anti-CD22 immunotoxin is enhanced by bryostatin 1 in B-cell lymphomas through CD22 upregulation and PKC-betaII depletion. Haematologica. 2012;97(5):771–9.
51. Qin H, Cho M, Haso W, et al. Eradication of B-ALL using chimeric antigen receptor-expressing T cells targeting the TSLPR oncoprotein. Blood. 2015;126(5):629–39.
52. Ruella M, Barrett DM, Kenderian SS, et al. Dual CD19 and CD123 targeting prevents antigen-loss relapses after CD19-directed immunotherapies. J Clin Invest. 2016;126(10):3814–26.
53. Qin H, Dong Z, Wang X, et al. CAR T cells targeting BAFF-R can overcome CD19 antigen loss in B cell malignancies. Sci Transl Med. 2019;11(511)
54. Schultz LM, Muffly LS, Spiegel JY, Ramakrishna S, Hossain N, Baggott C, Sahaf B, Patel S, Craig J, Yoon J, Kadapakkam M, Majzner RG, Frank MJ, Erickson C, Marcy AC, Fujimoto M, Bhatia N, Meyer EH, Kong KA, Egeler E, Marvroukakis S, Zin H, Fry TJ, Feldman SA, Miklos DB, Mackall CL, Davis KL. Phase I trial using CD19/CD22 bispecific CAR T cells in pediatric and adult acute lymphoblastic leukemia (ALL). Blood. 2019;134(Suppl 1):744.
55. Gardner R, Annesley C, Finney O, et al. Early clinical experience of CD19 x CD22 dual specific CAR T cells for enhanced anti-leukemic targeting of acute lymphoblastic leukemia. Blood 2018;132(Suppl 1):278–278
56. Amrolia PJ, Wynn R, Hough RE, Vora A, Bonney D, Veys P, Chiesa R, Rao K, Clark L, Al-Hajj M, Cordoba SP, Onuoha S, Kotsopoulou E, Khokhar NZ, Pule M, VGR P. Phase 1 study of AUO3, a bicistronic chimeric antigen receptor (CAR) T-cell therapy targeting CD19 and CD22, in pediatric patients with relapsed/refractory B-cell acute lymphoblastic leukemia (r/r/B-ALL): amelia study. Blood. 2019;134(Suppl 1):2620.
57. Annesley C, Gardner R, Wilson A, Summers C, Lamble AJ, Rivers J, Wu QV, Brand A, Johnson A, Spratt K, Mgebroff S, Brown C, Lindgren C, Park JR, Jensen MC. Novel CD19t T-antigen presenting cells expand CD19 CAR T cells in vivo. Blood. 2019;134(Suppl 1):223.
58. Teachey DT, Lacey SF, Shaw PA, et al. Identification of predictive biomarkers for cytokine release syndrome after chimeric antigen receptor T-cell therapy for acute lymphoblastic leukemia. Cancer Discov. 2016;6(6):664–79.
59. Webster J, Luskin MR, Prince TG, DeZern AE, DeAngelo DJ, Sharon E, Streicher H, Luznik L, Gojo I. Blinatumomab in combination with immune checkpoint inhibitors. Blood. 2018;132
60. Li AM, Hucks GE, Dinofia AM, et al. Checkpoint inhibitors augment CD19-directed chimeric antigen receptor (CAR) T cell therapy in relapsed B-cell acute lymphoblastic leukemia. Blood 2018;132(Suppl 1):556–556
61. Borowitz MJ, Wood BL, Devidas M, et al. Prognostic significance of minimal residual disease in high risk B-ALL: a report from children's oncology group study AALL0232. Blood. 2015;126(8):964–71.
62. Ahmad S, Zhao W, Renstrom F, et al. Physical activity, smoking, and genetic predisposition to obesity in people from Pakistan: the PROMIS study. BMC Med Genet. 2015;16:114.

63. Summers C, Annesley C, Bleakley M, Dahlberg A, Jensen MC, Gardner R. Long term follow-up after SCRI-CAR19v1 reveals late recurrences as well as a survival advantage to consolidation with HCT after CAR T cell induced remission. Blood 2018;132(Suppl 1):967–967
64. Pulsipher MS, Han X, Quigley M, Kari G, Rives S, Laetsch TW, Myers GD, Hiramatsu J, Yanik GA, Qayed M, Driscoll R, Boyer MW, Stefanski H, Buchner J, Baruchel A, Bader P, Yi L, Kalfoglou C, Robins H, Yusko E, Gorgun G, Bleikardt E, Wong S, Grupp SA. Molecular detection of minimal residual disease precedes morphological relapse and could be used to identify relapse in pediatric and young adult B-cell acute lymphoblastic leukemia patients treated with tisagenlecleucel. Blood. 2018;132(Suppl 1):1551.
65. Hay KA, Gauthier J, Hirayama AV, et al. Factors associated with durable EFS in adult B-cell ALL patients achieving MRD-negative CR after CD19 CAR T-cell therapy. Blood. 2019;133(15):1652–63.
66. Brudno JN, Kochenderfer JN. Toxicities of chimeric antigen receptor T cells: recognition and management. Blood. 2016;127(26):3321–30.
67. Lee DW, Gardner R, Porter DL, et al. Current concepts in the diagnosis and management of cytokine release syndrome. Blood. 2014;124(2):188–95.
68. Lee DW, Santomasso BD, Locke FL, et al. ASTCT consensus grading for cytokine release syndrome and neurologic toxicity associated with immune effector cells. Biol Blood Marrow Transplant. 2019;25(4):625–38.
69. Hay KA, Hanafi LA, Li D, et al. Kinetics and biomarkers of severe cytokine release syndrome after CD19 chimeric antigen receptor-modified T cell therapy. Blood. 2017;
70. Gardner RA, Ceppi F, Rivers J, et al. Preemptive mitigation of CD19 CAR T-cell cytokine release syndrome without attenuation of antileukemic efficacy. Blood. 2019;134(24):2149–58.
71. Le RQ, Li L, Yuan W, et al. FDA approval summary: tocilizumab for treatment of chimeric antigen receptor T cell-induced severe or life-threatening cytokine release syndrome. Oncologist. 2018;23(8):943–7.
72. Locke FLNS, Bartlett NL, Lekakis LJ, Jacobson CA, Braunschweig I, Oluwole OO, Siddiqi T, Lin Y, Timmerman JM, Reagan PM, Bot A, Rossi JM, Sherman M, Navale L, Jian Y, Aycock JS, Elias M, Wiezorek JS, Go WY, Miklos DB. Preliminary results of prophylactic tocilizumab after axicabtagencilolecel (axi-cel; KTE-C19) treatment for patients with refractory, aggressive non-hodgkin lymphoma (NHL). Blood. 2017;130(Suppl 1):1547.
73. Gofshteyn JS, Shaw PA, Teachey DT, et al. Neurotoxicity after CTL019 in a pediatric and young adult cohort. Ann Neurol. 2018;84(4):537–46.
74. Turtle CJ, Hanafi LA, Berger C, et al. Immunotherapy of non-Hodgkin's lymphoma with a defined ratio of CD8+ and CD4+ CD19-specific chimeric antigen receptor-modified T cells. Sci Transl Med. 2016;8(355):355ra116.
75. Schuster SJ, Svoboda J, Chong EA, et al. Chimeric antigen receptor T cells in refractory B-cell lymphomas. N Engl J Med. 2017;377(26):2545–54.
76. Turtle CJ, Hay KA, Hanafi LA, et al. Durable molecular remissions in chronic lymphocytic leukemia treated with CD19-specific chimeric antigen receptor-modified T cells after failure of Ibrutinib. J Clin Oncol. 2017;35(26):3010–20.
77. Fraietta JA, Lacey SF, Orlando EJ, et al. Determinants of response and resistance to CD19 chimeric antigen receptor (CAR) T cell therapy of chronic lymphocytic leukemia. Nat Med. 2018;24(5):563–71.
78. Kochenderfer JN, Dudley ME, Kassim SH, et al. Chemotherapy-refractory diffuse large B-cell lymphoma and indolent B-cell malignancies can be effectively treated with autologous T cells expressing an anti-CD19 chimeric antigen receptor. J Clin Oncol. 2015;33(6):540–9.
79. Neelapu SS, Locke FL, Bartlett NL, et al. Axicabtagene Ciloleucel CAR T-cell therapy in refractory large B cell lymphoma. N Engl J Med. 2017;377(26):2531–44.
80. Ramos CA, Ballard B, Zhang H, et al. Clinical and immunological responses after CD30-specific chimeric antigen receptor-redirected lymphocytes. J Clin Invest. 2017;127(9):3462–71.
81. Ritchie DS, Neeson PJ, Khot A, et al. Persistence and efficacy of second generation CAR T cell against the LeY antigen in acute myeloid leukemia. Mol Ther. 2013;21(11):2122–9.

82. Ali SA, Shi V, Maric I, et al. T cells expressing an anti-B-cell maturation antigen chimeric antigen receptor cause remissions of multiple myeloma. Blood. 2016;128(13):1688–700.
83. Wang CM, Wu ZQ, Wang Y, et al. Autologous T cells expressing CD30 chimeric antigen receptors for relapsed or refractory Hodgkin lymphoma: an open-label phase I trial. Clin Cancer Res. 2017;23(5):1156–66.
84. Gust J, Hay KA, Hanafi LA, et al. Endothelial activation and blood-brain barrier disruption in neurotoxicity after adoptive immunotherapy with CD19 CAR-T cells. Cancer Discov. 2017;7(12):1404–19.
85. Santomasso BD, Park JH, Salloum D, et al. Clinical and biological correlates of neurotoxicity associated with CAR T-cell therapy in patients with B-cell acute lymphoblastic Leukemia. Cancer Discov. 2018;8(8):958–71.
86. Gust J, Finney OC, Li D, et al. Glial injury in neurotoxicity after pediatric CD19-directed chimeric antigen receptor T cell therapy. Ann Neurol. 2019;86(1):42–54.
87. Taraseviciute A, Tkachev V, Ponce R, et al. Chimeric antigen receptor T cell-mediated neurotoxicity in nonhuman primates. Cancer Discov. 2018;8(6):750–63.
88. DeAngelo DJ, Ghobadi A, Park JH, Dinner SN, Mannis GN, Lunning MA, Khaled SK, Fathi AT, Gojo I, Wang ES, Bishop MR, Hughes H, Blackman S, Whitmore J, Trede NS, Gilber M, Wierda WG. Clinical outcomes for the phase 2, single-arm, multicenter trial of JCAR015 in adult B-ALL (ROCKET study). SITC Ann Meet. 2017;
89. Giavridis T, van der Stegen SJC, Eyquem J, Hamieh M, Piersigilli A, Sadelain M. CAR T cell-induced cytokine release syndrome is mediated by macrophages and abated by IL-1 blockade. Nat Med. 2018;24(6):731–8.
90. Norelli M, Camisa B, Barbiera G, et al. Monocyte-derived IL-1 and IL-6 are differentially required for cytokine-release syndrome and neurotoxicity due to CAR T cells. Nat Med. 2018;24(6):739–48.

Chapter 16
Hematopoietic Stem Cell Transplantation in Adults with Acute Lymphoblastic Leukemia

Erik L. Kimble and Ryan D. Cassaday

Introduction

Despite significant advances in the frontline management of acute lymphoblastic leukemia (ALL) in adults, relapse rates remain high, and long-term survival rates are inferior compared to children. Allogeneic hematopoietic stem cell transplantation (HSCT) has established an important role in the treatment of patients with ALL and offers the potential to improve rates of long-term remission or cure. However, the decision to proceed to HSCT in first remission has become increasingly complex, as the optimal candidates and timing of HSCT are controversial. Furthermore, while HSCT has historically been considered the only therapy associated with a realistic chance of long-term survival in relapsed/refractory disease, the development of more potent novel agents may be changing this viewpoint. This chapter will review the evolving role of HSCT in adult patients with ALL.

Current Indications for HSCT in ALL

HSCT certainly offers a survival benefit in a selected group of adult patients with ALL. In general, HSCT is considered the standard of care for the treatment of ALL in CR2. In CR1, HSCT has traditionally been reserved for patients with high-risk

Research reported in this publication was supported by the NHLBI under award number T32HL007093.

E. L. Kimble · R. D. Cassaday (✉)
Department of Medicine, University of Washington School of Medicine, Seattle, WA, USA

Clinical Research Division, Fred Hutchinson Cancer Research Center, Seattle, WA, USA
e-mail: ekimbl@uw.edu; cassaday@uw.edu

M. R. Litzow, E. A. Raetz (eds.), *Clinical Management of Acute Lymphoblastic Leukemia*, https://doi.org/10.1007/978-3-030-85147-7_16

Table 16.1 High-risk factors in adult ALL

Category	Adverse risk factor
Age	Varies, but minimally >35 years
High WBC	>30,000 (B-ALL)/>100,000 (T-ALL)
Immunophenotype	Pro-B-ALL (i.e., CD10 negative) Early and mature T-ALL
Cytogenetics/ molecular genetics	Complex karyotype Low hypodiploid/near tetraploid t(4;11)/*KMT2A-AF4* t(9;22)/*BCR-ABL* t(1;19)/*E2A-PBX1* Other *KMT2A* rearrangements *BCR-ABL1*-like or Ph-like *IKZF1* deletion Unmutated *NOTCH1*
Miscellaneous	CNS involvement
Treatment response	Late CR (>1 cycle) MRD-positive remission (>10^{-3})

Modified from Hoelzer et al. [146]

features, although the definition of "high-risk" has evolved over time, and different criteria have been used in clinical trials and across transplant centers (Table 16.1).

Recently, there has been an increasing emphasis on the evaluation of post-induction MRD, as it has proven to be the most important prognostic factor for relapse in ALL and is independent of the presence of some conventional risk factors at diagnosis. As experience with the use of pediatric-inspired regimens in young adults has increased, there is now increasing equipoise around the decision-making for ALL in CR1. In this subgroup of patients, the evaluation of MRD is critical and is heavily weighted in the decision for HSCT.

Evidence-based reviews and consensus recommendations have been published and recently updated [1–4]. Current recommendations highlight the finding that HSCT is believed to offer a survival advantage compared to chemotherapy in high-risk patients and in those in CR2. Disease-related outcomes for patients with MRD-positive CR are often inferior to patients without MRD, and HSCT may improve outcomes for these patients. It has become increasingly clear that for adult patients with MRD-negative CR after pediatric-inspired chemotherapy protocols, the use of HSCT in CR1 may not be required despite the presence of other high-risk factors. The latest consensus recommendations of the American Society for Transplantation and Cellular Therapy (ASTCT) for the indication for HSCT in adults with ALL are summarized in Table 16.2.

HSCT Outcomes in Adults with ALL

Overall, treatment outcomes for adults with ALL have improved over the last 30 years. This is likely attributable to improved rates of CR with optimized chemotherapy regimens incorporating frontline targeted agents and the adoption of

Table 16.2 Evidence-based indications for transplant in patients with ALL

Clinical scenario	HSCT recommended
Ph-negative ALL	
Standard-risk CR1	Unclear
High-risk CR1[a]	Yes
CR2 or later	Yes
Refractory	Unclear
MRD-negative CR1 after pediatric-inspired regimens	No
Ph-positive ALL	
CR1 if received TKI	Yes
MRD-negative CR1 and received TKI	Unclear

Adapted from DeFilipp et al. [3]
[a]Includes MRD-positive CR1

pediatric-inspired regimens in young adults, improved risk stratification with the use of MRD, the development of novel therapies for relapsed or refractory disease, progress in HSCT, and improvements in supportive care [5]. OS after HSCT, which incorporates transplant-related mortality (TRM) and the impact of relapsed disease, has nearly doubled, according to data from the Center for International Blood and Marrow Transplant Research (CIBMTR). The 3-year OS after a matched sibling donor (MSD) HSCT is now 61%, 40%, and 29% for adult patients with early, intermediate, and advanced disease, respectively. Matched unrelated donor (MUD) HSCTs showed similar outcomes [6].

Despite these advances, whereas the long-term OS in children with ALL is currently approaching 90%, adults with ALL have a higher risk of relapse and long-term survival rates of 30–60% [5, 7–9]. This discrepancy is likely multifactorial. As adults are poorly tolerant of intensive chemotherapy regimens, less intensive regimens are often utilized in older populations. In addition, there are biological differences in the disease, with adults presenting more often with high-risk features that are associated with an increased risk for relapse.

Transplantation Versus Chemotherapy

There is conflicting evidence in the literature defining the role of allogeneic HSCT in management of ALL. Generally, trials have attempted to stratify patients into dichotomous risk-defined groups (i.e., high-risk vs low-risk); however, there is significant variability in the definition of high-risk, which contributes to inconsistencies in reported outcomes due to various confounders. Thus, the applicability of trial data for clinical decision-making is hindered.

Another issue inherent to historical HSCT trials for ALL is that there is no true randomization; rather, patients were often allocated to treatment based on the availability of a suitable donor, a process known as genetic randomization. The assumption is made that the availability or non-availability of a donor is sufficiently random that the results of the trial would mimic a purely randomized trial. Of course, this type of randomization is subject to confounding as well.

Transplantation in CR1

A summary of the major trials evaluating allogeneic HSCT vs chemotherapy or autologous HSCT can be found in Table 16.3. The LALA-87 trial compared post-remission therapy strategies for unselected adult ALL patients. They investigated the use of allogeneic HSCT, autologous HSCT, or consolidation chemotherapy for adult patients with ALL in CR1. Patients underwent genetic randomization, and thus, those who were <40 years old and had a MSD were allocated to allogeneic HSCT. Other patients received either an autologous HSCT or further consolidation. There was no demonstrable benefit for autologous HSCT vs maintenance chemotherapy as a post-remission strategy [10]. In a donor versus no-donor comparison of the allogeneic HSCT-eligible group, there was no significant difference in disease-free survival (DFS) or OS at 5 years. However, a subgroup analysis demonstrated that high-risk patients (defined as Ph positive, $CD10^{-}/CD20^{-}$ phenotype, age > 35 years, WBC > 30 × 10^9/L, or time to CR >4 weeks) had superior OS and DFS after allogeneic HSCT compared with the control group [11, 12].

The LALA-94 trial then utilized a risk-adapted approach where allogeneic HSCT was considered only in high-risk patients with an available donor. In the donor vs no-donor analysis, allogeneic HSCT was associated with an improvement in DFS [13]. Subsequent studies comparing allogeneic HSCT, autologous HSCT, and chemotherapy in CR1 for high-risk ALL were conducted by the PETHEMA and EORTC groups; however, neither study was able to identify a differential survival benefit to HSCT [14, 15].

The benefit of allogeneic HSCT in standard-risk ALL was demonstrated in the UKALLXII/ECOG 2993 trial. In an intent-to-treat, donor vs no-donor analysis, Ph-negative ALL patients with a donor had an improved 5-year OS and lower relapse risk. However, subgroup analysis demonstrated that the survival benefit was limited to the standard-risk patients, and this benefit was not extended to the high-risk population (defined as Ph positive, age > 35 years, and WBC ≥30 × 10^9/L for B-ALL or ≥ 100 × 10^9/L for T-ALL). The lack of survival benefit in the high-risk population was attributed to an increased non-relapse mortality (NRM) [16].

A Cochrane systematic review and meta-analysis of 14 controlled trials using a donor vs no-donor comparison for adult ALL in CR1 showed improved DFS and OS in the patients with an available donor [17]. In 2013, Gupta et al. published a meta-analysis with the incorporation of individual patient data. It suggested that there is a 10% absolute overall survival benefit favoring HSCT in CR1 for patients with Ph-negative ALL who are <35 years old (OR 0.79, $p = 0.0003$). Otherwise, there were no differences in survival associated with other patient- and disease-related variables (Fig. 16.1) [18].

Table 16.3 Major trials assessing the benefit of allogeneic HSCT compared to chemotherapy or autologous HSCT in CR1 in a donor vs no-donor analysis

Trial	Treatment arms	Sample size (n)	Age (years)	Analysis includes Ph + t(9;22)	Risk category	NRM/ TRM	Relapse	Significance	EFS/ DFS/ LFS	Significance	OS	Significance
LALA-87 [11]	Donor (MSD allo-HSCT) vs no donor (chemo or auto-HSCT)	257	15–40	Yes	Overall	16% vs 3%	NR	NR	5-YR DFS 45% vs 31%	NS	5-YR OS 48% vs 35%	NS
					High risk	NR	NR	NR	5-YR DFS 39% vs 14%	$P = 0.01$	5-YR OS 44 vs 20%	$P = 0.03$
LALA-94 [13]	Donor (MSD allo-HSCT) vs no donor (chemo or auto-HSCT)	259	15–55	No	High risk	18% vs 7%	5-YR CIR 36% vs 62%	$P = 0.001$	5-YR DFS 45% vs 23%	$P = 0.007$	NR	NR
EORTC ALL-3 [14]	Donor (MSD allo-HSCT) vs no donor (chemo or auto-HSCT)	184	14–50	Yes	Overall	24% vs 7%	6-YR CIR 38% vs 56%	$P = 0.001$	6-YR DFS 38% vs 36%	NS	6-YR OS 41% vs 39%	NS
					High	NR	NR	NR	DFS HR 1.04	NS	NR	NR
					Standard	NR	NR	NR	DFS HR 0.82	NS	NR	NR

(continued)

Table 16.3 (continued)

Trial	Treatment arms	Sample size (n)	Age (years)	Analysis includes Ph + t(9;22)	Risk category	NRM/TRM	Relapse	Significance	EFS/DFS/LFS	Significance	OS	Significance
PETHEMA ALL-93 ([15])	Donor (MSD allo-HSCT) vs no donor (chemo or auto-HSCT)	222	15–50	Yes	High	10% vs 2%	5-YR CIR 62% vs 51%%	NS	5-year DFS 33% vs 39%	NS	5-YR OS 35% vs 44%	NS
EORTC ALL-4 [147]	Donor (MSD allo-HSCT) vs no donor (chemo or auto-HSCT)	325	15–50	Yes	Overall	22 vs 3%; $p < 0.05$	5-YR CIR 38% vs 58%	$P < 0.05$	5-YR DFS 41% vs 36%	$P = 0.38$	5-YR OS 42% vs 38%	NS
	Donor (MSD allo-HSCT) vs no donor (chemo or auto-HSCT)	1031	15–64	No	Overall	NR	NR	$P < 0.001$	NR	NR	5-YR OS 53% vs 45%	$P = 0.01$
UKALLXII/ECOG 2993 [16]					High risk	36% vs 14%	10-YR CIR 37% vs 63%	$P < 0.00005$	NR	NR	5-YR OS 41% vs 35%	NS
					Standard risk	20% vs 7%	10-YR CIR 24% vs 49%	$P < 0.00005$	NR	NR	5-YR OS 62 vs 52%	$P = 0.02$

CIR cumulative incidence of relapse
NS non-significant
NR not reported
YR year

Stratum	Deaths/Patients Donor	Deaths/Patients No donor	Statistics (O–E)	Statistics Var.	O.R. & 99% CI[2] (Donor : No donor)
Age <35	337/731	717/1303	-55.9	241.8	0.79 (0.67, 0.94)
Age 35+	229/366	359/562	0.8	135.8	1.01 (0.81, 1.26)
Female	225/418	384/690	-5.7	139.2	0.96 (0.77, 1.19)
Male	341/679	692/1175	-49.1	239.2	0.81 (0.69, 0.96)
B-Lineage	386/739	748/1266	-37.1	260.1	0.87 (0.74, 1.02)
T-Lineage	137/286	263/472	-23.1	92.9	0.78 (0.60, 1.02)
WBC <10	219/458	445/804	-25.2	151.7	0.85 (0.69, 1.04)
WBC 10-29	97/207	214/373	-19.2	70.0	0.76 (0.56, 1.03)
WBC 30-99	118/215	212/368	-6.4	75.1	0.92 (0.68, 1.24)
WBC 100+	121/196	186/284	-6.4	71.0	0.91 (0.67, 1.24)
Standard risk	369/770	755/1358	-45.1	257.7	0.84 (0.72, 0.99)
High risk	192/319	315/496	-12.8	118.3	0.90 (0.71, 1.14)
T411	37/60	42/66	1.2	16.2	1.08 (0.57, 2.05)
T814	5/6	10/15	0.8	1.6	1.64 (0.21, 12.70)
T119	9/24	25/41	-4.7	7.1	0.51 (0.20, 1.35)
High hyperdiploid	19/57	35/72	-5.5	12.1	0.63 (0.30, 1.33)
Low hyperdiploid	11/15	22/34	1.6	5.4	1.34 (0.44, 4.04)
Complex karyotype	15/28	39/65	-4.9	10.5	0.62 (0.28, 1.38)
Overall	**566/1097 (51.6%)**	**1076/1865 (57.7%)**	**-53.4**	**380.1**	**0.87 (0.79, 0.96) 2P = 0.006**

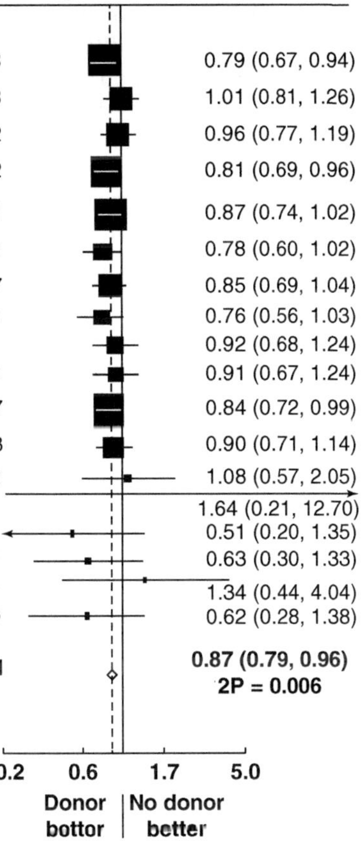

99% or 95% limits

Test for heterogeneity (18 groups): $\chi^2_{17} = 16.8$; P = 0.5

Fig. 16.1 Meta-analysis supporting the benefit of allogeneic HSCT in a donor vs no-donor comparison of Ph-negative ALL. Reprinted from "Allogeneic, but not autologous, hematopoietic cell transplantation improves survival only among younger adults with acute lymphoblastic leukemia in first remission: an individual patient data meta-analysis," by Gupta et al. (2013), Blood, Vol. 121, No. 2, Copyright 2013. The American Society of Hematology. Reprinted with permission [18]

Transplantation After Pediatric-Inspired Chemotherapy

In addition to disease biology, the improved outcomes seen in pediatric patients with ALL are due to their ability to tolerate the intensity of pediatric regimens. Pediatric regimens adapted for adults often contain asparaginase and more dose-intensive agents which are thought to contribute to higher CR rates and improved survival. In the GRAALL-2003 and GRAALL-2005 trials, adults <55 years old with high-risk ALL in CR1 after pediatric-inspired therapy were eligible for HSCT (high risk was defined as CNS involvement, low hypodiploidy/near triploidy, >5%

BM blasts after 1 week of induction, WBC > 1.0×10^9/L after pre-phase steroids, refractory disease requiring salvage to reach CR, MRD-positive CR by Ig/TCR PCR $\geq 10^{-2}$, WBC $\geq 30 \times 10^9$/L, *KMT2A* rearrangement, t(4;11) [*KMT2A-AF4* fusion], t(1;19) [*E2A-PBX1* fusion], complex karyotype, or CD10$^-$ phenotype). Though there was an observed decrease in relapse risk associated with allogeneic HSCT, its effect on OS was offset by an increased NRM (HR 1.46, $p = 0.001$). In a subset analysis, allogeneic HSCT demonstrated an improvement in both OS and relapse-free survival (RFS) in patients with MRD-positive CR prior to transplant (HR 0.40, $p = 0.001$). This benefit was not seen in the patients who were MRD negative, indicating that early MRD response may better predict who may benefit from allogeneic HSCT in the context of pediatric-inspired therapy [19].

In a retrospective study from the Dana-Farber Cancer Institute, adults with Ph-negative ALL treated with a pediatric-inspired non-HSCT regimen were compared with patients from the CIBMTR database who underwent contemporaneous allogeneic HSCT in CR1. Long-term incidence of relapse was similar between the groups; however, the allogeneic HSCT cohort had a higher TRM (37% vs 6%, $p < 0.0001$) and worse OS (45% vs 73%, $p < 0.0001$) [20].

Subsequently, the CALGB 10403 trial assessed the feasibility and efficacy of a pediatric treatment regimen for adolescent and young adult (AYA) patients with newly diagnosed ALL administered by adult treatment teams. The regimen was well tolerated and showed promising outcomes, with a 3-year EFS of 59% and estimated 3-year OS of 73% (95% CI, 68–78%) [21]. In a secondary analysis, the outcomes of those who received post-remission chemotherapy were compared with a contemporary matched AYA cohort from the CIBMTR database who underwent myeloablative allogeneic HSCT. HSCT was associated with inferior OS (HR 1.99, $p < 0.001$), inferior DFS (HR 1.51, $p = 0.002$), and increased NRM (HR 3.93, $p < 0.001$) [22].

Thus, while randomized data are lacking, these results suggest that the outcomes for allogeneic HSCT after pediatric-inspired therapy may be inferior compared to continued chemotherapy, particularly if MRD-negative CR is achieved.

Transplantation in CR2

The outcomes of patients with relapsed ALL have been historically poor, even in those able to achieve a subsequent CR [23]. Retrospective data suggest that HSCT in unselected patients in CR2 or beyond is associated with improved survival. For instance, for participants in the ECOG 2993 trial who sustained their first relapse and had not undergone transplant in CR1, allogeneic HSCT was associated with improved 5-year OS compared to chemotherapy alone (23% vs <5%, respectively, $p < 0.001$) [24]. Therefore, in most patients who can achieve a CR2 or beyond, allogeneic HSCT has been generally considered the standard of care.

Emerging novel therapies are associated with increased CR rates in the salvage setting, allowing more patients to successfully proceed to transplant in CR. Whether HSCT is still needed in these patients is an area of active investigation [5]. MRD retains its prognostic significance in CR2, and perhaps the use of MRD to allocate patients to transplant after salvage therapy may improve outcomes [25].

HSCT for Refractory Disease

Patients with refractory disease have an exceedingly poor prognosis. When transplanted in this context, historical OS is between 16 and 25% [26, 27]. Therefore, HSCT in patients with active disease is rarely recommended, and clinical trial participation should be encouraged when possible. Innovative strategies to improve the efficacy of HSCT in refractory disease, such as radioimmunotherapy with ^{131}I-anti-CD45 prior to HSCT conditioning, are in development and hold promise for improved long-term outcomes [28].

Philadelphia Chromosome-Positive ALL

The t(9;22), also known as the Philadelphia chromosome, is the most common recurrent cytogenetic abnormality in adults with ALL, and it has historically been associated with poor long-term outcomes [29, 30]. Thus, early HSCT trials stratified patients with this cytogenetic abnormality into the high-risk cohorts.

The treatment and outcomes of Ph-positive ALL have changed dramatically since the introduction of tyrosine kinase inhibitors (TKIs). In the pre-TKI era, several studies demonstrated the superiority of allogeneic HSCT over autologous HSCT or chemotherapy alone [13, 31, 32]. In the LALA-94 trial, the 3-year OS of patients with Ph-positive ALL with a donor was double that of the no-donor groups (36% vs 17%, respectively, $p = 0.009$) [13, 32]. Similar improvements in survival were seen in the UKALLXII/ECOG 2993 study, although the donor vs no-donor analysis did not achieve statistical significance. Since then, allogeneic transplant has remained the standard consolidation strategy for Ph-positive ALL.

After several publications demonstrated the safety and potential benefit of imatinib in ALL, the UKALLXII/ECOG 2993 study was amended to incorporate imatinib in combination with chemotherapy upfront in patients with Ph-positive ALL [33–37]. Patients then proceeded to allogeneic HSCT if they had a suitable donor. Imatinib was restarted post-HSCT and continued for 2 years. Compared to the pre-imatinib cohort, patients in this study had improved CR rates, and there was a marked improvement in 4-year OS in patients who received an allogeneic HSCT compared to those who did not (50% vs 19%, respectively). RFS was also significantly improved (69% vs 18%, respectively) [38]. In the GRAAPH-2005 study, allogeneic HSCT after imatinib plus either hyper-CVAD or reduced-intensity induction was also associated with significant benefits in RFS and OS [39].

A recent US intergroup study evaluated the safety and efficacy of dasatinib in adult patients <50 years old with Ph-positive ALL. Patients who achieved a CR1 after hyper-CVAD and dasatinib induction underwent TBI-based allogeneic HSCT

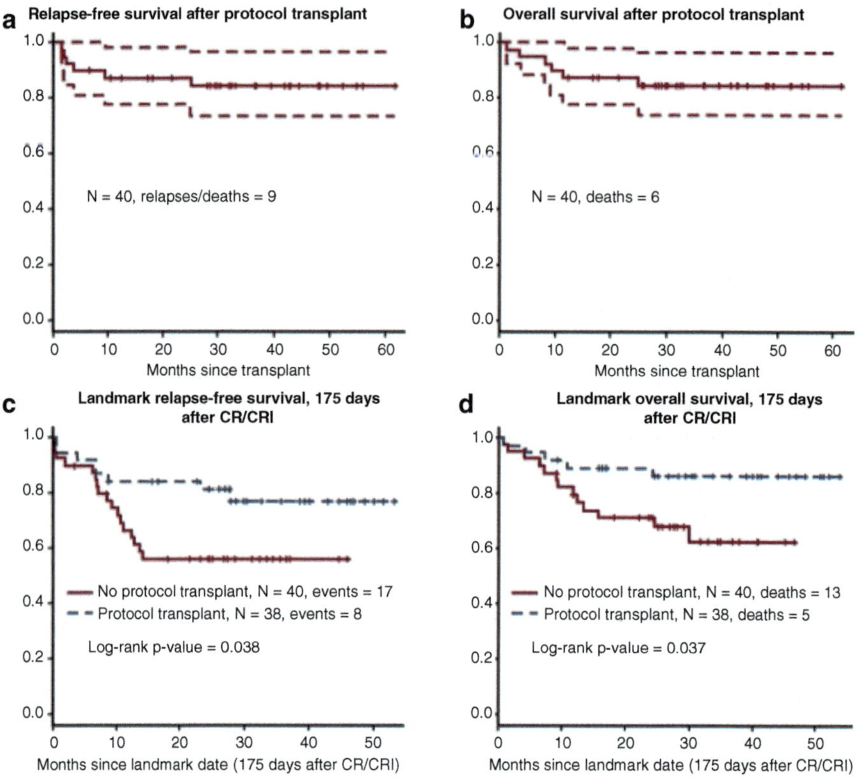

Fig. 16.2 Landmark analysis of adults with Ph-positive ALL treated with hyper-CVAD and dasatinib followed by protocol HSCT. (**a**) RFS after protocol-specified HSCT. (**b**) OS after protocol-specified HSCT. (**c**) RFS; landmark analysis of HSCT versus no HSCT; hazard ratio (HR) 0.42, 95% CI (0.18–0.97). (**d**) OS; landmark analysis HSCT versus no HSCT; HR 0.35, 95% CI (0.12–0.97). Reprinted from "US intergroup study of chemotherapy plus dasatinib and allogeneic stem cell transplant in Philadelphia chromosome positive ALL," by Ravandi et al. (2016), Blood Advances, Vol. 1, No. 3, Copyright 2016. The American Society of Hematology. Reprinted with permission [40]

if a donor was available. Others received standard maintenance chemotherapy. A landmark analysis, performed 175 days after CR1, showed a sustained benefit in favor of allogeneic HSCT vs no HSCT, with improved OS (HR 0.35, 95% CI 0.12–0.97) and RFS (HR 0.42, 95% CI 0.18–0.97) (Fig. 16.2) [40].

Perhaps one of the major limitations of these trials was the absence of data regarding MRD prior to HSCT. This precludes our ability to draw conclusions about the benefit of HSCT in patients who are MRD negative. There are accumulating data that suggest that patients who receive a TKI with adult-inspired chemotherapy and achieve a CR with no detectable BCR/ABL1 transcript (complete molecular response or CMR) have superior OS compared to those who did not [41, 42]. Recent studies assessing the efficacy of newer-generation TKIs, such as ponatinib, combined with chemotherapy upfront, show encouraging outcomes even in the absence of HSCT [43]. However, prospective randomized data are lacking.

Overall, the results and pitfalls of these trials illustrate the current controversy of allogeneic HSCT in the era of modern TKIs. Whereas allogeneic HSCT in CR1 remains the standard approach to patients with Ph-positive ALL, its benefits merit careful consideration. This is particularly true for those patients who achieve a CMR.

T-Cell ALL

T-ALL is a rare entity representing 25% of all new cases of adult ALL. The outcomes with chemotherapy alone are generally considered superior to the B-cell ALL counterpart [44]. Allogeneic HSCT is typically recommended in CR2, although it can be considered in CR1 if there are high-risk features [45].

Data on the outcomes of allogeneic HSCT in T-ALL are limited. In a subgroup analysis of the UKALLXII/ECOG 2993 trial, MSD HSCT for patients in CR1 with T-ALL was associated with improved 5-year OS (61% vs 46%, $p = 0.02$) and decreased relapse risk. Overall, having a donor had a similar effect on protection from relapse in patients with T-ALL (25 vs 51%, $p < 0.001$) vs B-ALL (30 vs 55%, $p < 0.001$) [46]. A more recent multicenter retrospective study suggested that the 5-year OS of adults with T-ALL who underwent allogeneic HSCT in CR1 was 44% and the corresponding cumulative incidence of NRM and relapse was 25% and 38%, respectively. Those in CR2 and beyond had similar outcomes [47].

There has been much interest in the early T-cell precursor (ETP) subtype T-ALL which is associated with chemotherapy resistance and inferior outcomes [48]. In adults treated in the GRAALL-2003 and GRAALL-2005 studies, there was no difference in outcomes in ETP T-ALL vs non-ETP subtypes. This was due in large part to the high rate of allogeneic HSCT in CR1, suggesting that early HSCT may abrogate the poor prognosis of ETP T-ALL [49].

Factors Impacting Outcomes of HSCT for ALL

Preparative Regimen

The optimal preparative regimen for allogeneic HSCT in the treatment of ALL remains unknown. The ideal regimen for an individual patient will maximize disease-related outcomes while minimizing TRM and long-term toxicity. Total body irradiation (TBI)-based regimens are considered the standard by many, as TBI has several advantages including its effectiveness against resistant leukemic cells, the ability to treat sanctuary sites, and the reported increased immunosuppressive properties compared to chemotherapy alone [50]. Historically, the most commonly used ablative regimen has been cyclophosphamide (Cy) and full-intensity TBI (12 Gy) [51, 52]. Over the years, there have been several attempts to optimize conditioning regimens for the treatment of ALL.

In an effort to improve the efficacy of conditioning and potentially impact disease-related outcomes, investigators from the City of Hope developed the etoposide (VP16)/TBI regimen [53]. A retrospective study in 2006 suggested an advantage in substituting VP16 for Cy for the treatment of ALL in CR2, particularly if the TBI dose was <13 Gy. There was no difference between Cy/TBI and VP16/TBI in CR1 [54]. A recent comparison of VP16 vs Cy in combination with TBI was performed using data from the European Society for Blood and Marrow Transplantation (EBMT) registry. It included only adults with Ph-negative ALL in CR1 or CR2. The use of VP16/TBI was associated with a reduced incidence of relapse at 5 years (17% vs 30%, $p = 0.007$), increased LFS (60% vs 50%, $p = 0.04$), and improved *graft-*versus-*host disease- and relapse-free survival* (GRFS) (43% vs 33%, $p = 0.04$). In the multivariate model, however, only the reduced risk of relapse maintained significance [55]. In all, VP16/TBI appears to be an active regimen with some suggestion that it may be more effective in patients in CR2.

TBI-containing regimens are associated with acute and long-term toxicities, as well as an increased risk for GVHD and TRM [55–60]. With the objective to reduce the TRM, the Johns Hopkins group developed busulfan (Bu)/Cy as a TBI-free conditioning regimen [61, 62]. A SWOG study comparing VP16/TBI vs Bu/Cy in patients with leukemia in CR2 or beyond showed no difference in TRM, DFS, nor OS [63]. In a subsequent retrospective analysis, IV Bu vs TBI-containing conditioning regimens in CR1 or CR2 were compared. The adjusted 3-year outcomes showed that IV Bu was associated with less TRM (19 vs 25%, $p = 0.04$), but higher risk of relapse (37% vs 28%, p = 0.007). Despite these differences, overall survival was comparable (57% vs 53%, $p = 0.35$) [64].

In young patients with T-cell ALL, the benefit of TBI-based conditioning is more pronounced. In an EBMT registry study of adults with T-ALL, patients <35 years old had improved 5-year OS and LFS with TBI-based regimens compared to Bu/Cy (OS 53% vs 21%, $p < 10^{-5}$; LFS 50% vs 18%, $p < 10^{-5}$). There was no difference in NRM. In patients >35 years old, there was no benefit to TBI-based regimens despite improved relapse risk given the higher risk for NRM (38% vs 9%, $p = 0.01$) [65].

Thus, while chemotherapy-only regimens are active in ALL, there appears to be no benefit in OS compared to TBI-based conditioning. Importantly, young patients with T-ALL likely derive a differential benefit from TBI compared to chemotherapy alone.

Conditioning Intensity

For younger adult patients, the randomized data supporting the use of allogeneic HSCT in ALL used myeloablative conditioning (MAC) regimens [11, 13, 16]. In contrast, the long-term benefit of allogeneic HSCT for the treatment of ALL in older adults is offset by a higher incidence of NRM [16]. Reduced-intensity conditioning (RIC) regimens have been developed to decrease treatment toxicities and harness the graft-vs-leukemia (GVL) effect of allogeneic HSCT [66]. To date, there are no randomized data comparing the outcomes of older adults undergoing allogeneic

HSCT with MAC vs RIC. Therefore, the use of RIC in ALL has been justified by the results of several retrospective studies.

Using data from the CIBMTR, Marks et al. compared the outcomes of MAC and RIC regimens for the treatment of Ph-negative ALL in CR1–2. Neither TRM nor relapse rates differed, and the 3-year OS and DFS between the two regimen groups were comparable despite the older age of the patients who received RIC (median age of 28 vs 45 years, respectively) [67].

In a subsequent EBMT report, RIC was associated with lower NRM compared to MAC for ALL in CR1–2 (HR 0.59, $p = 0.03$). Accordingly, despite an increase in relapse rates in the RIC group (HR 1.98, $p = 0.0001$), the 2-year OS was similar between the regimens (OS 45% vs 48%, $p = 0.56$) [68]. A report from the Japan Society for Hematopoietic Stem Cell Transplantation (JSHCT) also demonstrated similar findings [69].

There is a single significant study establishing the role of RIC in patients with Ph-positive ALL. Bachanova et al. compared the outcomes of adults in the CIBMTR registry who underwent allogeneic HSCT in CR1 with either MAC or RIC. The groups were matched for age, donor type, and year of HSCT. Similar to the reports from the EBMT and the JSHCT, RIC was associated with a lower TRM, higher incidence of relapse (HR 1.84, $p = 0.011$), and similar 3-year OS (39% vs 35%, $p = 0.062$). Pre-HSCT TKI therapy was associated with a decreased risk of relapse in the RIC group, while this was not apparent in the patients who received MAC. In patients who were MRD positive pre-HSCT, RIC was associated with a higher risk of relapse compared to MAC (HR 1.97, $p = 0.026$). However, those patients with an MRD-negative CR had a similar relapse risk independent of their conditioning intensity (HR 1.0, $p = 0.13$) (Fig. 16.3). Thus, the study encourages the use of RIC as an alternative strategy for adult patients with Ph-positive ALL who are ineligible for MAC and achieve MRD-negative CR1 [70].

While a randomized trial comparing MAC to RIC is unlikely to occur, these key registry studies have established a role for RIC in the management of adults with ALL who are not candidates for MAC, such as older (e.g., >55 years old), less fit patients. Together, they suggest a lower TRM with RIC, at the expense of a higher incidence of relapse. Yet, OS is similar with either strategy. In Ph-positive disease, the presence of MRD prior to transplant may negate the summative benefit of RIC; perhaps alternative strategies should be considered in these patients. The role of MRD status prior to RIC in Ph-negative patients is not well established.

Donor Source

Matched Sibling Donor vs Unrelated Donor

The initial studies demonstrating the benefit of allogeneic HSCT in the treatment of adult patients with ALL utilized genetic randomization, whereby patients with an available MSD proceeded to HSCT [11, 13, 16]. However, only approximately 25–30% of HSCT candidates will have a MSD. Meanwhile, depending on the race

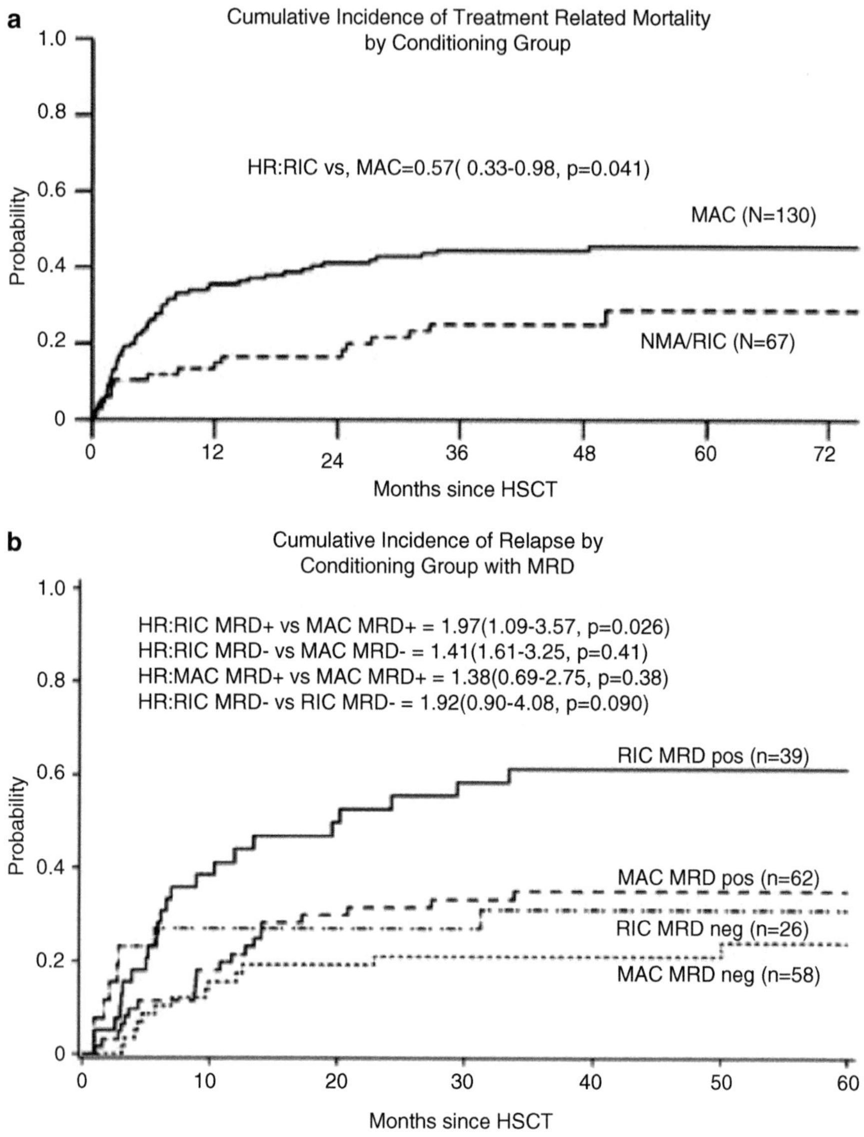

Fig. 16.3 Outcomes of Ph-positive ALL according to conditioning intensity and MRD. (**a**) Cumulative incidence of TRM by conditioning intensity. (**b**) Cumulative incidence of relapse by pre-HSCT MRD and conditioning intensity. (**c**) Kaplan-Meier estimate of OS according to conditioning intensity and MRD status. Reprinted from "Ph+ ALL patients in first complete remission have similar survival after reduced intensity and myeloablative allogeneic transplantation: impact of tyrosine kinase inhibitor and minimal residual disease," by Bachanova et al. (2014), Leukemia, Vol. 28, Copyright 2013. Springer Nature. Reprinted with permission [70]

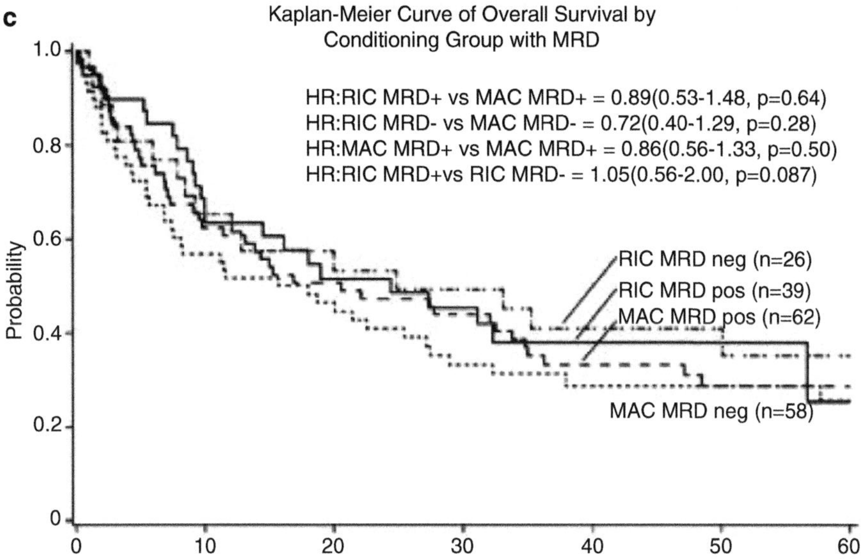

Fig. 16.3 (continued)

and ethnicity of the recipient, the probability of finding a fully HLA-matched unrelated donor ranges from 16% to 75% [71]. Nonetheless, with the development of allele-level HLA typing of unrelated donors, as well as modern post-transplant immunosuppression regimens and supportive care, there have been improved outcomes with MUDs [72–74]. MUDs now represent the most common donor source for allogeneic HSCTs worldwide [6].

While there are no randomized studies comparing MSD vs MUD HSCTs in adults with ALL, several retrospective studies exist [75–79]. In the largest study to date, the outcomes of 1458 adults with B-ALL who underwent MSD or MUD HSCT were compared. MUD recipients had similar TRM (HR 1.16, $p = 0.23$) and OS (HR 1.01, $p = 0.93$) compared with MSD recipients. This was not true for mismatched unrelated donor (MMUD) recipients, who had a greater risk of TRM (HR 1.92, $p < 0.0001$) and worse OS (HR 1.29, $p = 0.01$). Compared to MSD recipients, both MUD and MMUD recipients appeared to have a lower risk of relapse (33% and 31% vs 43%, respectively, $p = 0.002$) with a corresponding higher risk of acute GVHD (HR 2.18, $p < 0.0001$, and HR 2.65, $p < 0.0001$, respectively) and chronic GVHD (HR 1.28, $p = 0.01$, and HR 1.46, $p = 0.003$, respectively) [77].

Alternative Donor Sources

There has been increasing interest in alternative donor sources for patients without a MSD or MUD. This is often seen in the case of racial and ethnic minorities, who are unlikely to have unrelated donors available [71, 80]. In this setting, umbilical cord blood (UCB) and haplo-identical related donor (HID) transplants have emerged as viable graft sources.

Umbilical Cord Blood

UCB is a promising donor source for allogeneic HSCT with several putative advantages. First, matching requirements for UCB are less stringent, allowing for mismatched UCB units which can be well tolerated without negatively impacting long-term outcomes [81]. Second, UCB HSCT may be associated with a lower risk of GVHD and at least similar LFS compared to matched donors [79, 82–89].

Notably, there is evidence supporting the use of UCB for patients who do not have a matched donor and are MRD positive prior to transplant. The Seattle group compared the outcomes of 582 adult patients with acute leukemia or myelodysplastic syndrome who underwent HSCT with an UCB donor, MUD, or MMUD. Among patients with MRD pre-HSCT, the risk of relapse was higher in the two unrelated donor groups compared to UCB (MMUD vs UCB, HR 3.01, $p = 0.02$; MUD vs UCB, HR 2.92, $p = 0.007$). The risk of death was also higher with MMUD (HR 2.92, $p = 0.001$), while there was no difference in the OS of UCB vs MUD recipients [90]. In a subsequent study, the use of UCB in 67 ALL patients with a median age of 22 years was assessed. Prior to transplant, 32% were MRD positive. The overall DFS at 5 years was 74% (CI 95%, 60–83%) with no difference in relapse risk or DFS between MRD-negative and MRD-positive patients [91]. This suggests that the prognostic significance of MRD pre-HSCT may be abrogated by the use of UCB allografts.

Haplo-Identical Related Donor

Resurrected by the pioneering work on CD34+ selection with ex vivo T-cell depletion by the group from Perugia University and then further advanced by the development of the post-transplant Cy regimens at Johns Hopkins, HID allogeneic HSCTs are now routinely performed [92–95]. While there are no prospective randomized trials addressing the net benefit of HID allografts in adult ALL, several retrospective studies have been published.

Srour et al. reported the outcome of 109 adult patients with high-risk ALL in CR1 and beyond, undergoing HID HSCT. OS and LFS at 3 years were 37% and 31%, respectively. Those patients in CR1 had 52% DFS at 3 years [96]. Santoro et al. analyzed 208 adult ALL patients transplanted with HID allografts. The post-transplant GVHD prophylaxis in this study included PT-Cy in only 57% of the patients, while the rest were given ATG. In the overall cohort, OS, LFS, and GRFS at 3 years were 33%, 31%, and 26%, respectively. When restricted to patients in CR1, results were superior with reported OS, LFS, and GRFS of 52%, 47%, and 40%, respectively [97]. Finally, in a large EBMT registry analysis, HID recipients appeared to have similar LFS, OS, incidence of relapse, NRM, and acute and chronic GVHD when compared to MUD and MMUD [98].

There are limited comparisons of HID vs UCB HSCT for ALL. One retrospective study showed no differences in relapse incidence (HR 0.82, $p = 0.31$), NRM (HR 1.23, $p = 0.23$), and LFS (HR 1.00, $p = 0.84$) between HID and UCB allograft recipients [99]. The Bone Marrow Transplant Clinical Trials Network prospective randomized trial of HID vs UCB grafts in adults with hematologic malignancies (NCT01597778) may further address this knowledge gap.

KIR Typing

Killer cell immunoglobulin-like receptors (KIRs) allow natural killer (NK) cells to interact with HLA class I alleles which modulate NK cell-mediated donor-versus-recipient alloreactivity and cytotoxicity. KIR mismatching is proposed to increase the GVL effect without increasing GVHD ([100, 101, 102]). However, ALL blasts appear to be resistant to NK cell-mediated cytotoxicity, unlike AML ([100], [101], [103]). The exact role of KIR-ligand interactions and haplotypes requires further evaluation and cannot currently be incorporated into the decision-making process for donor selection in ALL.

Minimal Residual Disease

MRD is prognostic in the pre- and post-HSCT setting and thus represents an attractive tool to risk-stratify patients who may benefit from HSCT. A retrospective analysis from the Seattle group suggested that the presence of MRD pre-HSCT is associated with increased relapse risk (HR 3.64, $p = 0.0001$) and mortality (HR 2.39, $p = 0.0005$). MRD retains its prognostic significance even when adjusting for CR status (CR1 vs CR2) [104]. Similar results were described in a retrospective study from the MD Anderson Cancer Center [105].

As noted in the previous section, young adults with Ph-negative ALL who achieve MRD-negative remissions with pediatric-inspired regimens are not recommended to undergo HSCT. One potential exception is patients with *KMT2A*-rearranged disease: these patients are often directed to HSCT regardless of depth of response, so relatively little is known about their outcomes in the absence of HSCT [21].

Less is known about how to use MRD to risk-stratify those who receive adult-inspired therapy. The group in Seattle published their experience in adults undergoing myeloablative, reduced-intensity, or deferred HSCT in CR1 following adult-inspired therapy for ALL. Relapse was reduced significantly by undergoing HSCT with MAC in MRD-negative CR1 (HR 0.19, $p = 0.001$). Yet, those who underwent HSCT in MRD-negative remission after salvage therapy had similar outcomes for both relapse and survival compared to patients who underwent HSCT in MRD-negative CR1. This may be attributable to the higher risk of TRM with HSCT and the potential to salvage relapses with HSCT beyond CR1 [25].

Most studies have utilized multiparameter flow cytometry (MFC) to define MRD. However, newer technologies are now available to detect disease at lower thresholds. A retrospective analysis from Stanford showed detectable disease $>10^{-4}$ pre-HSCT or $>10^{-6}$ post-HSCT using high-throughput sequencing (HTS) had a significantly greater risk of relapse ([106]). While HTS has a higher level of sensitivity for residual disease than MFC, the dominant clone-specific sequence must be known in order to detect it. Patients who are in morphologic remission, and do not already have this sequence identified, may not have this testing performed unless archived material of sufficient quality is available.

In patients with Ph-positive ALL, MRD detection by RT-PCR for *BCR-ABL1* transcripts is the standard and can be used for risk stratification. In the CIBMTR analysis by Bachanova et al., which is described in previous sections of this chapter, MRD positivity was independently associated with an increased risk of relapse post-HSCT (HR 1.60, $p = 0.070$) [70].

In light of the fairly consistent results emphasizing the importance of MRD pre-HSCT, one important question is whether or not an attempt to eliminate MRD prior to HSCT will improve outcomes. Unfortunately, there has not been a study in adult ALL to date that shows this with confidence. It may be that persistent MRD implies particularly high-risk disease, and its elimination will not actually modify a patient's risk of relapse post-HSCT. Further, if the therapy administered to eliminate MRD is ineffective, the patient's disease burden may increase beyond the point where HSCT is indicated. Although novel agents for relapsed/refractory B-ALL appear to be a more appealing strategy for MRD-positive disease as opposed to proceeding directly to HSCT, it is important to recognize the high risk of relapse in this situation. Therefore, until quality data exist to guide this decision, treatment to eliminate MRD prior to HSCT must be done with caution.

Pre-Transplant Consolidation Strategy

Time from CR to the first post-remission therapy is an independent predictor of relapse and OS [107]. Although many ALL treatment regimens for adults outline consolidation regimens, the post-remission strategy prior to allogeneic HSCT varies among protocols. The UKALLXII/ECOG 2993 and LALA-94 trials, for instance, mandated consolidation chemotherapy prior to HSCT, even if CR1 was achieved after the initial induction cycle [13, 16]. In contrast, trials such as the CALGB 19802 and those utilizing the hyper-CVAD regimen allowed for patients to proceed to HSCT soon after a CR was achieved ([40, 43, 108, 109]). Thus, the need for consolidation of patients in CR prior to HSCT is not well established.

A recent CIBMTR registry study determined there was no difference in the incidence of relapse, LFS, nor OS regardless of whether adults with ALL in CR1 received 0, 1, or ≥ 2 cycles of consolidation. Furthermore, the number of consolidation cycles was not associated with TRM, suggesting that in patients who do not have a donor readily available, consolidation can be administered without increasing the risk of TRM [110].

Post-Transplant Prophylaxis

Ph-Positive ALL

As previously discussed, outcomes in Ph-positive ALL have improved dramatically since the introduction of TKIs into frontline therapy. However, relapse remains a significant cause of treatment failure, and the risk is significantly higher with detectable *BCR-ABL1* transcripts post-HSCT [32, 38, 111, 112]. While the use of TKIs to prevent relapse after HSCT appears to be a logical intervention, their use is variable, and the benefit remains poorly defined. Two distinct post-HSCT treatment strategies have been described: preemptive and prophylactic therapy [36, 40, 113–117]. In the former, TKI therapy is prompted by the detection of measurable *BCR-ABL1* transcripts in the absence of relapsed disease, while the latter is started post-HSCT regardless of the results of MRD testing.

There are no prospective randomized data to establish the benefit of TKI prophylaxis. In what remains the largest analysis to date, the EBMT published their review of 473 adult patients with Ph-positive ALL who received an allogeneic HSCT in CR1. Post-HSCT TKI use was associated with improved OS (HR 0.42, $p = 0.004$) and LFS (HR 0.44, $p = 0.002$) as well as a reduced risk of relapse (HR 0.40, $p = 0.01$) [118].

The GMALL study group performed the only randomized multicenter study comparing the use of prophylactic vs MRD-triggered use of imatinib post-HSCT for Ph-positive ALL. Prophylactic imatinib was associated with a lower incidence of molecular recurrence (40 vs 69%, respectively, $p = 0.046$). Yet, the relapse rates were not different between treatment strategies, and the 5-year OS was comparable (80% vs 75%, respectively, $p = 0.84$). Notably, imatinib was eventually discontinued in over 65% of patients due to toxicity. Thus, while imatinib appears to be poorly tolerated in the post-HSCT setting, even limited administration seemed to be associated with favorable long-term outcomes [119].

The cumulative results of these studies and others have led the EBMT and ASTCT to recommend the use of TKIs post-HSCT in all patients with Ph-positive ALL, acknowledging the limited prospective evidence [3, 120]. Currently, there are no commonly accepted standards with respect to the choice of TKI, dosage, time of initiation, nor treatment duration. Both prophylactic and preemptive strategies are equally endorsed, and it is not unreasonable to choose the TKI based on the presence or history of ABL kinase domain mutations, if known [3, 120].

Ph-Negative ALL

There is currently no standard prophylaxis regimen for Ph-negative ALL. Clinical trials evaluating the role of blinatumomab maintenance post-HSCT are currently enrolling, and preliminary results suggest that it is a feasible approach. More patients and follow-up are needed to establish efficacy [121].

CNS Prophylaxis

The CNS represents the most common site of extramedullary relapse after HSCT for ALL [122]. Although routine CNS prophylaxis is now part of modern ALL induction therapies, in the post-HSCT setting, prophylaxis is not standard.

In a large multicenter retrospective study addressing the role of CNS prophylaxis post-HSCT, 457 adult patients with ALL who received their first allogeneic HSCT in CR1 or CR2 were reviewed. Overall, 47% of patients received post-HSCT intrathecal CNS prophylaxis. There was no benefit to post-HSCT CNS prophylaxis as the 4-year cumulative incidence of CNS relapse was 6% vs 1.5% for patients with and without CNS prophylaxis, respectively ($p = 0.08$) [123.] A major limitation of this analysis was the lack of any description of the degree of CNS prophylaxis administered pre-HSCT, which likely impacts the risk of CNS relapse post-HSCT. A subsequent study from the City of Hope reviewed 87 patients with a history of CNS involvement who then went on to HSCT. Neither pre-HSCT cranial irradiation, use of TBI-based conditioning, nor post-HSCT prophylactic intrathecal chemotherapy was associated with a reduction of CNS relapse risk [124]. Thus, in their most recent position statement, the ASTCT does not support the use of CNS prophylaxis post-HSCT for adult patients with ALL [125].

A distinct intervention not addressed in the described studies is the administration of low-dose cranial boost during TBI-based HSCT conditioning to reduce the risk of CNS relapse. The published data have yielded conflicting results, although it appears to be a well-tolerated procedure [126–129].

HSCT and the Use of Novel Therapies for ALL

Blinatumomab

Blinatumomab, a bispecific T-cell engager (BiTE) targeted to CD19 and CD3, is approved for the treatment of relapsed/refractory B-ALL. In 2018, it became the first FDA-approved therapy for MRD-positive B-ALL [130–132].

The role of HSCT in the era of blinatumomab is not well-defined. In the phase 2 study published by Gökbuget et al., 67% of the patients in a continuous remission after receiving blinatumomab for MRD underwent allogeneic HSCT. After 2 years of median follow-up, 25% of the MRD responders who did not proceed to HSCT had durable remissions compared to 49% of those who received a HSCT [133]. Similarly, a post hoc analysis of the TOWER study showed that responders to blinatumomab given for relapsed/refractory B-ALL did not derive a significant survival benefit from consolidation with HSCT [134]. Considering the toxicity of allogeneic HSCT, these provocative results have led to questions about the need for HSCT in patients who clear MRD after treatment with blinatumomab.

Recent data from the AALL1331 trial provided some evidence in favor of HSCT post-blinatumomab. In this phase 3 trial, pediatric and AYA Ph-negative B-ALL patients in first relapse received standard induction chemotherapy. Those with early or late relapse with high levels of MRD were randomized to chemotherapy or blinatumomab and then underwent HSCT. The trial was stopped early after patients in the blinatumomab arm had improved rates of MRD clearance, OS, and DFS with significantly less toxicity. Further analysis demonstrated that perhaps the benefit of blinatumomab was its ability to successfully bridge patients to HSCT compared to the control arm (73 vs 45%, respectively, $p = 0.0001$) [135].

CAR T-Cell Therapy

Autologous T cells engineered to express a chimeric antigen receptor (CAR) specific for CD19 have produced high rates of CR in patients with relapsed/refractory B-ALL. Unfortunately, many patients eventually relapse. The durability of the treatment response is associated with the kinetics and persistence of CAR T cells, which may be influenced by many factors, including the lymphodepleting regimen, cell dose, tumor burden, T-cell composition, and specific costimulatory domain [136, 137]. In addition, leukemia-dependent factors may lead to relapse, including antigen-negative escape and lineage switching [138]. This has led to the consideration of consolidation with allogeneic HSCT post-CAR T-cell therapy for many patients. However, this practice varies by institution, with reported transplant rates between 10% and 78% [139].

Recently, investigators from the Seattle group published data on the safety of allogeneic HSCT after CD19-directed CAR T-cell therapy for B-cell malignancies. Of the patients with B-ALL (n = 19), 74% received MAC, with the majority receiving MUD allografts. The toxicity profile observed in this cohort was not higher than expected, with the 1-year cumulative incidences of NRM reported to be 21% [140]. Multivariate analysis demonstrated a non-significant reduction in the risk for treatment failure in patients who underwent allogeneic HSCT after CAR T-cell therapy compared with those who did not (HR 0.39, $p = 0.088$) [141]. Together, these data suggest that HSCT is feasible, may improve long-term outcomes, and is not necessarily associated with an increased risk for toxicity after CAR T-cell therapy.

In contrast, reports from the Memorial Sloan Kettering Cancer Center experience found no significant benefit in EFS nor OS in favor of consolidative post-CAR T-cell HSCT [137]. It is possible that this finding may be explained by the differences in CAR constructs which incorporate different costimulatory domains.

Overall, given the small size of these studies and several potential confounding variables, the role of consolidative HSCT after CAR T-cell therapy remains to be defined. At the Fred Hutchinson Cancer Research Center in Seattle, patients are referred to HSCT if they achieve an MRD-negative CR and they do not have a history of a prior allogeneic HSCT. Patients with a previous allogeneic HSCT are considered on a case-by-case basis. This practice may not apply to other centers utilizing a different cellular product.

Inotuzumab Ozogamicin

Inotuzumab ozogamicin (InO), a humanized anti-CD22 monoclonal antibody conjugated to calicheamicin, is approved for the treatment of relapsed/refractory B-ALL. It is associated with a higher rate of reaching allogeneic HSCT compared to salvage chemotherapy (41% vs 11%, $P < 0.001$) [142]. Marks et al. analyzed pooled data from patients who underwent HSCT after InO. The 2-year OS after HSCT was 41%, and those who went directly to HSCT upon remission without additional salvage therapy fared better [143].

There is, however, a well-established risk of hepatic sinusoidal obstruction syndrome (SOS, formerly veno-occlusive disease) associated with HSCT after treatment with InO that appears to increase with each cycle of therapy. In the above pooled analysis, 19 patients (18.8%) developed SOS, 5 of which were fatal. Conditioning with dual alkylating therapy (HR 8.6, $p = 0.015$), elevated bilirubin (HR 15.3, $p = 0.009$), and pre-HSCT transaminase elevation (HR 0.027, $p = 0.039$) were all associated with a risk of SOS [144]. Thus, although HSCT contributes to the improved outcomes with InO for relapsed/refractory B-ALL, its use should be well planned, and close monitoring for SOS is indicated. If feasible, the number of cycles of InO should be limited to two or less, and careful consideration should be taken when selecting the conditioning regimen [145].

Future of HSCT for ALL

As long as there remains a high risk of relapse, HSCT will continue to have a role in the management of adults with ALL. Efforts will need to focus on identifying those patients most likely to benefit from this approach, balancing the potential for relapse risk reduction and the risk of TRM. This is being investigated in a variety of ways, including new approaches to graft manipulation, GVHD prophylaxis, and post-HSCT supportive care. More sensitive assays for MRD detection may also better identify those patients likely to do well or not with continued chemotherapy. These principles will remain true even if novel agents become part of the standard-of-care frontline therapy. A similar argument could be viable even in the setting of relapsed/refractory disease, as antithetical as it may have been to make such a claim as recently as 2015. This is particularly true among those with B-ALL who may respond favorably to agents like blinatumomab and CAR T cells. Ultimately, HSCT is likely to remain part of the routine armamentarium in the treatment of adults with ALL, though the timing and manner in which it is performed will continue to evolve.

References

1. Hahn T, Wall D, Camitta B, Davies S, Dillon H, Gaynon P, et al. The role of cytotoxic therapy with hematopoietic stem cell transplantation in the therapy of acute lymphoblastic leukemia in adults: an evidence-based review. Biol Blood Marrow Transplant. 2006;12(1):1–30.
2. Oliansky DM, Larson RA, Weisdorf D, Dillon H, Ratko TA, Wall D, et al. The role of cytotoxic therapy with hematopoietic stem cell transplantation in the treatment of adult acute lymphoblastic leukemia: update of the 2006 evidence-based review. Biol Blood Marrow Transplant. 2012;18(1):18–36. e6
3. DeFilipp Z, Advani AS, Bachanova V, Cassaday RD, Deangelo DJ, Kebriaei P, et al. Hematopoietic cell transplantation in the treatment of adult acute lymphoblastic Leukemia: updated 2019 evidence-based review from the American Society for Transplantation and Cellular Therapy. Biol Blood Marrow Transplant. 2019;25(11):2113–23.
4. Giebel S, Marks DI, Boissel N, Baron F, Chiaretti S, Ciceri F, et al. Hematopoietic stem cell transplantation for adults with Philadelphia chromosome-negative acute lymphoblastic leukemia in first remission: a position statement of the European Working Group for Adult Acute Lymphoblastic Leukemia (EWALL) and the acute leukemia working party of the European Society for Blood and Marrow Transplantation (EBMT). Bone Marrow Transplant. 2019;54(6):798–809.
5. Jabbour E, Pui CH, Kantarjian H. Progress and innovations in the Management of Adult Acute Lymphoblastic Leukemia. JAMA Oncol. 2018;4(10):1413–20.
6. D'Souza AFC. Current uses and outcomes of hematopoietic cell transplantation (HCT): CIBMTR summary slides, 2019. 2019
7. Pui CH, Yang JJ, Hunger SP, Pieters R, Schrappe M, Biondi A, et al. Childhood acute lymphoblastic Leukemia: progress through collaboration. J Clin Oncol. 2015;33(27):2938–48.
8. Lennmyr E, Karlsson K, Ahlberg L, Garelius H, Hulegardh E, Izarra AS, et al. Survival in adult acute lymphoblastic leukaemia (ALL): a report from the Swedish ALL registry. Eur J Haematol. 2019;103(2):88–98.
9. Pulte D, Jansen L, Gondos A, Katalinic A, Barnes B, Ressing M, et al. Survival of adults with acute lymphoblastic leukemia in Germany and the United States. PLoS One. 2014;9(1):e85554.
10. Fiere D, Lepage E, Sebban C, Boucheix C, Gisselbrecht C, Vernant JP, et al. Adult acute lymphoblastic leukemia: a multicentric randomized trial testing bone marrow transplantation as postremission therapy. The French Group on Therapy for Adult Acute Lymphoblastic Leukemia. J Clin Oncol. 1993;11(10):1990–2001.
11. Sebban C, Lepage E, Vernant JP, Gluckman E, Attal M, Reiffers J, et al. Allogeneic bone marrow transplantation in adult acute lymphoblastic leukemia in first complete remission: a comparative study. French Group of Therapy of Adult Acute Lymphoblastic Leukemia. J Clin Oncol. 1994;12(12):2580–7.

12. Thiebaut A, Vernant JP, Degos L, Huguet FR, Reiffers J, Sebban C, et al. Adult acute lymphocytic leukemia study testing chemotherapy and autologous and allogeneic transplantation. A follow-up report of the French protocol LALA 87. Hematol Oncol Clin North Am. 2000;14(6):1353–66. x
13. Thomas X, Boiron JM, Huguet F, Dombret H, Bradstock K, Vey N, et al. Outcome of treatment in adults with acute lymphoblastic leukemia: analysis of the LALA-94 trial. J Clin Oncol. 2004;22(20):4075–86.
14. Labar B, Suciu S, Zittoun R, Muus P, Marie JP, Fillet G, et al. Allogeneic stem cell transplantation in acute lymphoblastic leukemia and non-Hodgkin's lymphoma for patients <or=50 years old in first complete remission: results of the EORTC ALL-3 trial. Haematologica. 2004;89(7):809–17.
15. Ribera JM, Oriol A, Bethencourt C, Parody R, Hernandez-Rivas JM, Moreno MJ, et al. Comparison of intensive chemotherapy, allogeneic or autologous stem cell transplantation as post-remission treatment for adult patients with high-risk acute lymphoblastic leukemia. Results of the PETHEMA ALL-93 trial. Haematologica. 2005;90(10):1346–56.
16. Goldstone AH, Richards SM, Lazarus HM, Tallman MS, Buck G, Fielding AK, et al. In adults with standard-risk acute lymphoblastic leukemia, the greatest benefit is achieved from a matched sibling allogeneic transplantation in first complete remission, and an autologous transplantation is less effective than conventional consolidation/maintenance chemotherapy in all patients: final results of the International ALL Trial (MRC UKALL XII/ECOG E2993). Blood. 2008;111(4):1827–33.
17. Pidala J, Djulbegovic B, Anasetti C, Kharfan-Dabaja M, Kumar A. Allogeneic hematopoietic cell transplantation for adult acute lymphoblastic leukemia (ALL) in first complete remission. Cochrane Database Syst Rev. 2011;10:CD008818.
18. Gupta V, Richards S, Rowe J. Acute Leukemia stem cell transplantation Trialists' collaborative G. allogeneic, but not autologous, hematopoietic cell transplantation improves survival only among younger adults with acute lymphoblastic leukemia in first remission: an individual patient data meta-analysis. Blood. 2013;121(2):339–50.
19. Dhedin N, Huynh A, Maury S, Tabrizi R, Beldjord K, Asnafi V, et al. Role of allogeneic stem cell transplantation in adult patients with Ph-negative acute lymphoblastic leukemia. Blood. 2015;125(16):2486–96. quiz 586
20. Seftel MD, Neuberg D, Zhang MJ, Wang HL, Ballen KK, Bergeron J, et al. Pediatric-inspired therapy compared to allografting for Philadelphia chromosome-negative adult ALL in first complete remission. Am J Hematol. 2016;91(3):322–9.
21. Stock W, Luger SM, Advani AS, Yin J, Harvey RC, Mullighan CG, et al. A pediatric regimen for older adolescents and young adults with acute lymphoblastic leukemia: results of CALGB 10403. Blood. 2019;133(14):1548–59.
22. Wieduwilt MJ, Stock W, Advani AS, Luger SM, Larson RA, Tallman MS, et al. Superior survival with post-remission pediatric-inspired chemotherapy compared to myeloablative allogeneic hematopoietic cell transplantation in adolescents and young adults with Ph-negative acute lymphoblastic leukemia in first complete remission: comparison of CALGB 10403 to patients reported to the CIBMTR. Blood. 2019;134(Supplement_1):261.
23. Kantarjian HM, Thomas D, Ravandi F, Faderl S, Jabbour E, Garcia-Manero G, et al. Defining the course and prognosis of adults with acute lymphocytic leukemia in first salvage after induction failure or short first remission duration. Cancer. 2010;116(24):5568–74.
24. Fielding AK, Richards SM, Chopra R, Lazarus HM, Litzow MR, Buck G, et al. Outcome of 609 adults after relapse of acute lymphoblastic leukemia (ALL); an MRC UKALL12/ECOG 2993 study. Blood. 2007;109(3):944–50.
25. Cassaday RD, Alan Potts D Jr, Stevenson PA, Bar M, Georges GE, Shustov AR, et al. Evaluation of allogeneic transplantation in first or later minimal residual disease – negative remission following adult-inspired therapy for acute lymphoblastic leukemia. Leuk Lymphoma. 2016;57(9):2109–18.
26. Duval M, Klein JP, He W, Cahn JY, Cairo M, Camitta BM, et al. Hematopoietic stem-cell transplantation for acute leukemia in relapse or primary induction failure. J Clin Oncol. 2010;28(23):3730–8.

27. Pavlu J, Labopin M, Zoellner AK, Sakellari I, Stelljes M, Finke J, et al. Allogeneic hematopoietic cell transplantation for primary refractory acute lymphoblastic leukemia: a report from the acute leukemia working party of the EBMT. Cancer. 2017;123(11):1965–70.
28. Orozco JJ, Gooley T, Rajendran JG, Fisher DR, Deeg HJ, Storb RF, et al. Anti-CD45 radioimmunotherapy followed by haploidentical allogeneic hematopoietic cell transplantation for advanced acute leukemia or high-risk MDS. Blood. 2017;130(Supplement 1):2048.
29. Moorman AV, Harrison CJ, Buck GA, Richards SM, Secker-Walker LM, Martineau M, et al. Karyotype is an independent prognostic factor in adult acute lymphoblastic leukemia (ALL): analysis of cytogenetic data from patients treated on the Medical Research Council (MRC) UKALLXII/Eastern Cooperative Oncology Group (ECOG) 2993 trial. Blood. 2007;109(8):3189–97.
30. Westbrook CA, Hooberman AL, Spino C, Dodge RK, Larson RA, Davey F, et al. Clinical significance of the BCR-ABL fusion gene in adult acute lymphoblastic leukemia: a Cancer and Leukemia Group B Study (8762). Blood. 1992;80(12):2983–90.
31. Laport GG, Alvarnas JC, Palmer JM, Snyder DS, Slovak ML, Cherry AM, et al. Long-term remission of Philadelphia chromosome-positive acute lymphoblastic leukemia after allogeneic hematopoietic cell transplantation from matched sibling donors: a 20-year experience with the fractionated total body irradiation-etoposide regimen. Blood. 2008;112(3): 903–9.
32. Dombret H, Gabert J, Boiron JM, Rigal-Huguet F, Blaise D, Thomas X, et al. Outcome of treatment in adults with Philadelphia chromosome-positive acute lymphoblastic leukemia--results of the prospective multicenter LALA-94 trial. Blood. 2002;100(7):2357–66.
33. de Labarthe A, Rousselot P, Huguet-Rigal F, Delabesse E, Witz F, Maury S, et al. Imatinib combined with induction or consolidation chemotherapy in patients with de novo Philadelphia chromosome-positive acute lymphoblastic leukemia: results of the GRAAPH-2003 study. Blood. 2007;109(4):1408–13.
34. Thomas DA, Faderl S, Cortes J, O'Brien S, Giles FJ, Kornblau SM, et al. Treatment of Philadelphia chromosome-positive acute lymphocytic leukemia with hyper-CVAD and imatinib mesylate. Blood. 2004;103(12):4396–407.
35. Towatari M, Yanada M, Usui N, Takeuchi J, Sugiura I, Takeuchi M, et al. Combination of intensive chemotherapy and imatinib can rapidly induce high-quality complete remission for a majority of patients with newly diagnosed BCR-ABL-positive acute lymphoblastic leukemia. Blood. 2004;104(12):3507–12.
36. Ribera JM, Oriol A, González M, Vidriales B, Brunet S, Esteve J, et al. Concurrent intensive chemotherapy and imatinib before and after stem cell transplantation in newly diagnosed Philadelphia chromosome-positive acute lymphoblastic leukemia. Final results of the CSTIBES02 trial. Haematologica. 2010;95(1):87–95.
37. Wassmann B, Pfeifer H, Goekbuget N, Beelen DW, Beck J, Stelljes M, et al. Alternating versus concurrent schedules of imatinib and chemotherapy as front-line therapy for Philadelphia-positive acute lymphoblastic leukemia (Ph+ ALL). Blood. 2006;108(5):1469–77.
38. Fielding AK, Rowe JM, Buck G, Foroni L, Gerrard G, Litzow MR, et al. UKALLXII/ECOG2993: addition of imatinib to a standard treatment regimen enhances long-term outcomes in Philadelphia positive acute lymphoblastic leukemia. Blood. 2014;123(6):843–50.
39. Chalandon Y, Thomas X, Hayette S, Cayuela JM, Abbal C, Huguet F, et al. Randomized study of reduced-intensity chemotherapy combined with imatinib in adults with Ph-positive acute lymphoblastic leukemia. Blood. 2015;125(24):3711–9.
40. Ravandi F, Othus M, O'Brien SM, Forman SJ, Ha CS, Wong JYC, et al. US intergroup study of chemotherapy plus dasatinib and allogeneic stem cell transplant in Philadelphia chromosome positive ALL. Blood Adv. 2016;1(3):250–9.
41. Short NJ, Jabbour E, Sasaki K, Patel K, O'Brien SM, Cortes JE, et al. Impact of complete molecular response on survival in patients with Philadelphia chromosome-positive acute lymphoblastic leukemia. Blood. 2016;128(4):504–7.
42. Kim DY, Joo YD, Lim SN, Kim SD, Lee JH, Lee JH, et al. Nilotinib combined with multiagent chemotherapy for newly diagnosed Philadelphia-positive acute lymphoblastic leukemia. Blood. 2015;126(6):746–56.

43. Jabbour E, Short NJ, Ravandi F, Huang X, Daver N, DiNardo CD, et al. Combination of hyper-CVAD with ponatinib as first-line therapy for patients with Philadelphia chromosome-positive acute lymphoblastic leukaemia: long-term follow-up of a single-centre, phase 2 study. Lancet Haematol. 2018;5(12):e618–e27.
44. Boucheix C, David B, Sebban C, Racadot E, Bene MC, Bernard A, et al. Immunophenotype of adult acute lymphoblastic leukemia, clinical parameters, and outcome: an analysis of a prospective trial including 562 tested patients (LALA87). French Group on Therapy for Adult Acute Lymphoblastic Leukemia. Blood. 1994;84(5):1603–12.
45. Marks DI, Rowntree C. Management of adults with T-cell lymphoblastic leukemia. Blood. 2017;129(9):1134–42.
46. Marks DI, Paietta EM, Moorman AV, Richards SM, Buck G, DeWald G, et al. T-cell acute lymphoblastic leukemia in adults: clinical features, immunophenotype, cytogenetics, and outcome from the large randomized prospective trial (UKALL XII/ECOG 2993). Blood. 2009;114(25):5136–45.
47. Hamilton BK, Rybicki L, Abounader D, Adekola K, Advani A, Aldoss I, et al. Allogeneic hematopoietic cell transplantation for adult T cell acute lymphoblastic leukemia. Biol Blood Marrow Transplant. 2017;23(7):1117–21.
48. Jain N, Lamb AV, O'Brien S, Ravandi F, Konopleva M, Jabbour E, et al. Early T-cell precursor acute lymphoblastic leukemia/lymphoma (ETP-ALL/LBL) in adolescents and adults: a high-risk subtype. Blood. 2016;127(15):1863–9.
49. Bond J, Graux C, Lhermitte L, Lara D, Cluzeau T, Leguay T, et al. Early response-based therapy stratification improves survival in adult early thymic precursor acute lymphoblastic Leukemia: a group for research on adult acute lymphoblastic leukemia study. J Clin Oncol. 2017;35(23):2683–91.
50. Storb R, Georges GE, Gooley TA. Total body irradiation-based versus chemotherapy-based myeloablative conditioning for allogeneic hematopoietic cell transplant. Biol Blood Marrow Transplant. 2019;25(12):e356–e62.
51. Thomas ED, Sanders JE, Flournoy N, Johnson FL, Buckner CD, Clift RA, et al. Marrow transplantation for patients with acute lymphoblastic leukemia in remission. Blood. 1979;54(2):468–76.
52. Giebel S, Miszczyk L, Slosarek K, Moukhtari L, Ciceri F, Esteve J, et al. Extreme heterogeneity of myeloablative total body irradiation techniques in clinical practice: a survey of the acute leukemia working party of the European Group for Blood and Marrow Transplantation. Cancer. 2014;120(17):2760–5.
53. Blume KG, Forman SJ, O'Donnell MR, Doroshow JH, Krance RA, Nademanee AP, et al. Total body irradiation and high-dose etoposide: a new preparatory regimen for bone marrow transplantation in patients with advanced hematologic malignancies. Blood. 1987;69(4):1015–20.
54. Marks DI, Forman SJ, Blume KG, Perez WS, Weisdorf DJ, Keating A, et al. A comparison of cyclophosphamide and total body irradiation with etoposide and total body irradiation as conditioning regimens for patients undergoing sibling allografting for acute lymphoblastic leukemia in first or second complete remission. Biol Blood Marrow Transplant. 2006;12(4):438–53.
55. Czyz A, Labopin M, Giebel S, Socie G, Apperley J, Volin L, et al. Cyclophosphamide versus etoposide in combination with total body irradiation as conditioning regimen for adult patients with Ph-negative acute lymphoblastic leukemia undergoing allogeneic stem cell transplant: on behalf of the ALWP of the European Society for Blood and Marrow Transplantation. Am J Hematol. 2018;93(6):778–85.
56. Flowers ME, Inamoto Y, Carpenter PA, Lee SJ, Kiem HP, Petersdorf EW, et al. Comparative analysis of risk factors for acute graft-versus-host disease and for chronic graft-versus-host disease according to National Institutes of Health consensus criteria. Blood. 2011;117(11):3214–9.
57. Sutton L, Kuentz M, Cordonnier C, Blaise D, Devergie A, Guyotat D, et al. Allogeneic bone marrow transplantation for adult acute lymphoblastic leukemia in first complete remission: factors predictive of transplant-related mortality and influence of total body irradiation modalities. Bone Marrow Transplant. 1993;12(6):583–9.

58. Baker KS, Leisenring WM, Goodman PJ, Ermoian RP, Flowers ME, Schoch G, et al. Total body irradiation dose and risk of subsequent neoplasms following allogeneic hematopoietic cell transplantation. Blood. 2019;133(26):2790–9.
59. Majhail NS, Ness KK, Burns LJ, Sun CL, Carter A, Francisco L, et al. Late effects in survivors of Hodgkin and non-Hodgkin lymphoma treated with autologous hematopoietic cell transplantation: a report from the bone marrow transplant survivor study. Biol Blood Marrow Transplant. 2007;13(10):1153–9.
60. Armenian SH, Sun CL, Mills G, Teh JB, Francisco L, Durand JB, et al. Predictors of late cardiovascular complications in survivors of hematopoietic cell transplantation. Biol Blood Marrow Transplant. 2010;16(8):1138–44.
61. Santos GW, Tutschka PJ, Brookmeyer R, Saral R, Beschorner WE, Bias WB, et al. Marrow transplantation for acute nonlymphocytic leukemia after treatment with busulfan and cyclophosphamide. N Engl J Med. 1983;309(22):1347–53.
62. Tutschka PJ, Copelan EA, Klein JP. Bone marrow transplantation for leukemia following a new busulfan and cyclophosphamide regimen. Blood. 1987;70(5):1382–8.
63. Blume KG, Kopecky KJ, Henslee-Downey JP, Forman SJ, Stiff PJ, LeMaistre CF, et al. A prospective randomized comparison of total body irradiation-etoposide versus busulfan-cyclophosphamide as preparatory regimens for bone marrow transplantation in patients with leukemia who were not in first remission: a Southwest Oncology Group study. Blood. 1993;81(8):2187–93.
64. Kebriaei P, Anasetti C, Zhang MJ, Wang HL, Aldoss I, de Lima M, et al. Intravenous busulfan compared with total body irradiation pretransplant conditioning for adults with acute lymphoblastic leukemia. Biol Blood Marrow Transplant. 2018;24(4):726–33.
65. Cahu X, Labopin M, Giebel S, Aljurf M, Kyrcz-Krzemien S, Socie G, et al. Impact of conditioning with TBI in adult patients with T-cell ALL who receive a myeloablative allogeneic stem cell transplantation: a report from the acute leukemia working party of EBMT. Bone Marrow Transplant. 2016;51(3):351–7.
66. Storb R, Sandmaier BM. Nonmyeloablative allogeneic hematopoietic cell transplantation. Haematologica. 2016;101(5):521–30.
67. Marks DI, Wang T, Perez WS, Antin JH, Copelan E, Gale RP, et al. The outcome of full-intensity and reduced-intensity conditioning matched sibling or unrelated donor transplantation in adults with Philadelphia chromosome-negative acute lymphoblastic leukemia in first and second complete remission. Blood. 2010;116(3):366–74.
68. Mohty M, Labopin M, Volin L, Gratwohl A, Socie G, Esteve J, et al. Reduced-intensity versus conventional myeloablative conditioning allogeneic stem cell transplantation for patients with acute lymphoblastic leukemia: a retrospective study from the European Group for Blood and Marrow Transplantation. Blood. 2010;116(22):4439–43.
69. Tanaka J, Kanamori H, Nishiwaki S, Ohashi K, Taniguchi S, Eto T, et al. Reduced-intensity vs myeloablative conditioning allogeneic hematopoietic SCT for patients aged over 45 years with ALL in remission: a study from the Adult ALL Working Group of the Japan Society for Hematopoietic Cell Transplantation (JSHCT). Bone Marrow Transplant. 2013;48(11):1389–94.
70. Bachanova V, Marks DI, Zhang MJ, Wang H, de Lima M, Aljurf MD, et al. Ph+ ALL patients in first complete remission have similar survival after reduced intensity and myeloablative allogeneic transplantation: impact of tyrosine kinase inhibitor and minimal residual disease. Leukemia. 2014;28(3):658–65.
71. Gragert L, Eapen M, Williams E, Freeman J, Spellman S, Baitty R, et al. HLA match likelihoods for hematopoietic stem-cell grafts in the U.S. registry. N Engl J Med. 2014;371(4):339–48.
72. Nademanee A, Schmidt GM, Parker P, Dagis AC, Stein A, Snyder DS, et al. The outcome of matched unrelated donor bone marrow transplantation in patients with hematologic malignancies using molecular typing for donor selection and graft-versus-host disease prophylaxis regimen of cyclosporine, methotrexate, and prednisone. Blood. 1995;86(3):1228–34.
73. Speiser DE, Tiercy JM, Rufer N, Grundschober C, Gratwohl A, Chapuis B, et al. High resolution HLA matching associated with decreased mortality after unrelated bone marrow transplantation. Blood. 1996;87(10):4455–62.

74. Gooley TA, Chien JW, Pergam SA, Hingorani S, Sorror ML, Boeckh M, et al. Reduced mortality after allogeneic hematopoietic-cell transplantation. N Engl J Med. 2010;363(22):2091–101.
75. Dahlke J, Kroger N, Zabelina T, Ayuk F, Fehse N, Wolschke C, et al. Comparable results in patients with acute lymphoblastic leukemia after related and unrelated stem cell transplantation. Bone Marrow Transplant. 2006;37(2):155–63.
76. Kiehl MG, Kraut L, Schwerdtfeger R, Hertenstein B, Remberger M, Kroeger N, et al. Outcome of allogeneic hematopoietic stem-cell transplantation in adult patients with acute lymphoblastic leukemia: no difference in related compared with unrelated transplant in first complete remission. J Clin Oncol. 2004;22(14):2816–25.
77. Segal E, Martens M, Wang HL, Brazauskas R, Weisdorf D, Sandmaier BM, et al. Comparing outcomes of matched related donor and matched unrelated donor hematopoietic cell transplants in adults with B-cell acute lymphoblastic leukemia. Cancer. 2017;123(17):3346–55.
78. Nishiwaki S, Inamoto Y, Sakamaki H, Kurokawa M, Iida H, Ogawa H, et al. Allogeneic stem cell transplantation for adult Philadelphia chromosome-negative acute lymphocytic leukemia: comparable survival rates but different risk factors between related and unrelated transplantation in first complete remission. Blood. 2010;116(20):4368–75.
79. Tomblyn MB, Arora M, Baker KS, Blazar BR, Brunstein CG, Burns LJ, et al. Myeloablative hematopoietic cell transplantation for acute lymphoblastic leukemia: analysis of graft sources and long-term outcome. J Clin Oncol. 2009;27(22):3634–41.
80. Pidala J, Kim J, Schell M, Lee SJ, Hillgruber R, Nye V, et al. Race/ethnicity affects the probability of finding an HLA-A, -B, -C and -DRB1 allele-matched unrelated donor and likelihood of subsequent transplant utilization. Bone Marrow Transplant. 2013;48(3):346–50.
81. Brunstein CG, Petersdorf EW, DeFor TE, Noreen H, Maurer D, MacMillan ML, et al. Impact of allele-level HLA mismatch on outcomes in recipients of double umbilical cord blood transplantation. Biol Blood Marrow Transplant. 2016;22(3):487–92.
82. Marks DI, Woo KA, Zhong X, Appelbaum FR, Bachanova V, Barker JN, et al. Unrelated umbilical cord blood transplant for adult acute lymphoblastic leukemia in first and second complete remission: a comparison with allografts from adult unrelated donors. Haematologica. 2014;99(2):322–8.
83. Laughlin MJ, Eapen M, Rubinstein P, Wagner JE, Zhang MJ, Champlin RE, et al. Outcomes after transplantation of cord blood or bone marrow from unrelated donors in adults with leukemia. N Engl J Med. 2004;351(22):2265–75.
84. Rocha V, Labopin M, Sanz G, Arcese W, Schwerdtfeger R, Bosi A, et al. Transplants of umbilical-cord blood or bone marrow from unrelated donors in adults with acute leukemia. N Engl J Med. 2004;351(22):2276–85.
85. Brunstein CG, Gutman JA, Weisdorf DJ, Woolfrey AE, Defor TE, Gooley TA, et al. Allogeneic hematopoietic cell transplantation for hematologic malignancy: relative risks and benefits of double umbilical cord blood. Blood. 2010;116(22):4693–9.
86. Takahashi S, Ooi J, Tomonari A, Konuma T, Tsukada N, Oiwa-Monna M, et al. Comparative single-institute analysis of cord blood transplantation from unrelated donors with bone marrow or peripheral blood stem-cell transplants from related donors in adult patients with hematologic malignancies after myeloablative conditioning regimen. Blood. 2007;109(3):1322–30.
87. Takahashi S, Iseki T, Ooi J, Tomonari A, Takasugi K, Shimohakamada Y, et al. Single-institute comparative analysis of unrelated bone marrow transplantation and cord blood transplantation for adult patients with hematologic malignancies. Blood. 2004;104(12):3813–20.
88. Gutman JA, Leisenring W, Appelbaum FR, Woolfrey AE, Delaney C. Low relapse without excessive transplant-related mortality following myeloablative cord blood transplantation for acute leukemia in complete remission: a matched cohort analysis. Biol Blood Marrow Transplant. 2009;15(9):1122–9.
89. Eapen M, Rocha V, Sanz G, Scaradavou A, Zhang MJ, Arcese W, et al. Effect of graft source on unrelated donor haemopoietic stem-cell transplantation in adults with acute leukaemia: a retrospective analysis. Lancet Oncol. 2010;11(7):653–60.

90. Milano F, Gooley T, Wood B, Woolfrey A, Flowers ME, Doney K, et al. Cord-blood transplantation in patients with minimal residual disease. N Engl J Med. 2016;375(10):944–53.
91. Keahi D, Cassaday R, Ermoian R, Dahlberg A, Delaney C, Milano F. Myeloablative cord blood transplantation yields excellent disease free survival in patients with acute lymphoblastic leukemia. Blood. 2016;128(22):4693.
92. Luznik L, Jalla S, Engstrom LW, Iannone R, Fuchs EJ. Durable engraftment of major histocompatibility complex-incompatible cells after nonmyeloablative conditioning with fludarabine, low-dose total body irradiation, and posttransplantation cyclophosphamide. Blood. 2001;98(12):3456–64.
93. Luznik L, O'Donnell PV, Symons HJ, Chen AR, Leffell MS, Zahurak M, et al. HLA-haploidentical bone marrow transplantation for hematologic malignancies using nonmyeloablative conditioning and high-dose, posttransplantation cyclophosphamide. Biol Blood Marrow Transplant. 2008;14(6):641–50.
94. Passweg JR, Baldomero H, Bader P, Basak GW, Bonini C, Duarte R, et al. Is the use of unrelated donor transplantation leveling off in Europe? The 2016 European Society for Blood and Marrow Transplant activity survey report. Bone Marrow Transplant. 2018;53(9):1139–48.
95. Aversa F, Tabilio A, Terenzi A, Velardi A, Falzetti F, Giannoni C, et al. Successful engraftment of T-cell-depleted haploidentical "three-loci" incompatible transplants in leukemia patients by addition of recombinant human granulocyte colony-stimulating factor mobilized peripheral blood progenitor cells to bone marrow inoculum. Blood. 1994;84(11):3948–55.
96. Srour SA, Milton DR, Bashey A, Karduss-Urueta A, Al Malki MM, Romee R, et al. Haploidentical transplantation with post-transplantation cyclophosphamide for high-risk acute lymphoblastic leukemia. Biol Blood Marrow Transplant. 2017;23(2):318–24.
97. Santoro N, Ruggeri A, Labopin M, Bacigalupo A, Ciceri F, Gulbas Z, et al. Unmanipulated haploidentical stem cell transplantation in adults with acute lymphoblastic leukemia: a study on behalf of the acute leukemia working party of the EBMT. J Hematol Oncol. 2017;10(1):113.
98. Shem-Tov N, Peczynski C, Labopin M, Itala-Remes M, Blaise D, Labussiere-Wallet H, et al. Haploidentical vs. unrelated allogeneic stem cell transplantation for acute lymphoblastic leukemia in first complete remission: on behalf of the ALWP of the EBMT. Leukemia. 2020;34(1):283–92.
99. Ruggeri A, Labopin M, Sanz G, Piemontese S, Arcese W, Bacigalupo A, et al. Comparison of outcomes after unrelated cord blood and unmanipulated haploidentical stem cell transplantation in adults with acute leukemia. Leukemia. 2015;29(9):1891–900.
100. Ruggeri L, Capanni M, Casucci M, Volpi I, Tosti A, Perruccio K, et al. Role of natural killer cell alloreactivity in HLA-mismatched hematopoietic stem cell transplantation. Blood. 1999;94(1):333–9.
101. Ruggeri L, Capanni M, Urbani E, Perruccio K, Shlomchik WD, Tosti A, et al. Effectiveness of donor natural killer cell alloreactivity in mismatched hematopoietic transplants. Science. 2002;295(5562):2097–100.
102. Leung W, Iyengar R, Turner V, Lang P, Bader P, Conn P, et al. Determinants of antileukemia effects of allogeneic NK cells. J Immunol. 2004;172(1):644–50.
103. Savani BN, Mielke S, Adams S, Uribe M, Rezvani K, Yong AS, et al. Rapid natural killer cell recovery determines outcome after T-cell-depleted HLA-identical stem cell transplantation in patients with myeloid leukemias but not with acute lymphoblastic leukemia. Leukemia. 2007;21(10):2145–52.
104. Bar M, Wood BL, Radich JP, Doney KC, Woolfrey AE, Delaney C, et al. Impact of minimal residual disease, detected by flow cytometry, on outcome of myeloablative hematopoietic cell transplantation for acute lymphoblastic leukemia. Leuk Res Treatment. 2014;2014:421723.
105. Zhou Y, Slack R, Jorgensen JL, Wang SA, Rondon G, de Lima M, et al. The effect of peritransplant minimal residual disease in adults with acute lymphoblastic leukemia undergoing allogeneic hematopoietic stem cell transplantation. Clin Lymphoma Myeloma Leuk. 2014;14(4):319–26.

106. Logan AC, Vashi N, Faham M, Carlton V, Kong K, Buno I, et al. Immunoglobulin and T cell receptor gene high-throughput sequencing quantifies minimal residual disease in acute lymphoblastic leukemia and predicts post-transplantation relapse and survival. Biol Blood Marrow Transplant. 2014;20(9):1307–13.
107. Advani AS, Jin T, Ramsingh G, Tiu R, Saber W, Theil K, et al. Time to post-remission therapy is an independent prognostic factor in adults with acute lymphoblastic leukemia. Leuk Lymphoma. 2008;49(8):1560–6.
108. Stock W, Johnson JL, Stone RM, Kolitz JE, Powell BL, Wetzler M, et al. Dose intensification of daunorubicin and cytarabine during treatment of adult acute lymphoblastic leukemia: results of cancer and leukemia group B study 19802. Cancer. 2013;119(1):90–8.
109. Ravandi F, O'Brien S, Thomas D, Faderl S, Jones D, Garris R, et al. First report of phase 2 study of dasatinib with hyper-CVAD for the frontline treatment of patients with Philadelphia chromosome-positive (Ph+) acute lymphoblastic leukemia. Blood. 2010;116(12):2070–7.
110. Bejanyan N, Zhang MJ, Wang HL, Lazaryan A, de Lima M, Marks DI, et al. Pretransplant consolidation is not beneficial for adults with ALL undergoing myeloablative allogeneic transplantation. Biol Blood Marrow Transplant. 2018;24(5):945–55.
111. Radich J, Gehly G, Lee A, Avery R, Bryant E, Edmands S, et al. Detection of bcr-abl transcripts in Philadelphia chromosome-positive acute lymphoblastic leukemia after marrow transplantation. Blood. 1997;89(7):2602–9.
112. Stirewalt DL, Guthrie KA, Beppu L, Bryant EM, Doney K, Gooley T, et al. Predictors of relapse and overall survival in Philadelphia chromosome-positive acute lymphoblastic leukemia after transplantation. Biol Blood Marrow Transplant. 2003;9(3):206–12.
113. Wassmann B, Pfeifer H, Stadler M, Bornhauser M, Bug G, Scheuring UJ, et al. Early molecular response to posttransplantation imatinib determines outcome in MRD+ Philadelphia-positive acute lymphoblastic leukemia (Ph+ ALL). Blood. 2005;106(2):458–63.
114. Carpenter PA, Snyder DS, Flowers ME, Sanders JE, Gooley TA, Martin PJ, et al. Prophylactic administration of imatinib after hematopoietic cell transplantation for high-risk Philadelphia chromosome-positive leukemia. Blood. 2007;109(7):2791–3.
115. Chen H, Liu KY, Xu LP, Liu DH, Chen YH, Zhao XY, et al. Administration of imatinib after allogeneic hematopoietic stem cell transplantation may improve disease-free survival for patients with Philadelphia chromosome-positive acute lymphoblastic leukemia. J Hematol Oncol. 2012;5:29.
116. Caocci G, Vacca A, Ledda A, Murgia F, Piras E, Greco M, et al. Prophylactic and preemptive therapy with dasatinib after hematopoietic stem cell transplantation for Philadelphia chromosome-positive acute lymphoblastic leukemia. Biol Blood Marrow Transplant. 2012;18(4):652–4.
117. Carpenter PA, Johnston L, Fernandez HF, Radich JP, Mauro MJ, Flowers MED, et al. Posttransplant feasibility study of nilotinib prophylaxis for high-risk Philadelphia chromosome positive leukemia. Blood. 2017;130(9):1170–2.
118. Brissot E, Labopin M, Beckers MM, Socie G, Rambaldi A, Volin L, et al. Tyrosine kinase inhibitors improve long-term outcome of allogeneic hematopoietic stem cell transplantation for adult patients with Philadelphia chromosome positive acute lymphoblastic leukemia. Haematologica. 2015;100(3):392–9.
119. Pfeifer H, Wassmann B, Bethge W, Dengler J, Bornhauser M, Stadler M, et al. Randomized comparison of prophylactic and minimal residual disease-triggered imatinib after allogeneic stem cell transplantation for BCR-ABL1-positive acute lymphoblastic leukemia. Leukemia. 2013;27(6):1254–62.
120. Giebel S, Czyz A, Ottmann O, Baron F, Brissot E, Ciceri F, et al. Use of tyrosine kinase inhibitors to prevent relapse after allogeneic hematopoietic stem cell transplantation for patients with Philadelphia chromosome-positive acute lymphoblastic leukemia: a position statement of the Acute Leukemia Working Party of the European Society for Blood and Marrow Transplantation. Cancer. 2016;122(19):2941–51.
121. Kebriaei P, Banerjee PP, Ganesh C, Kaplan M, Nandivada VD, Cortes AKN, et al. Blinatumomab is well tolerated maintenance therapy following allogeneic hematopoi-

etic cell transplantation for acute lymphoblastic leukemia. Biol Blood Marrow Transplant. 2020;26(3):S102–S3.
122. Poon LM, Hamdi A, Saliba R, Rondon G, Ledesma C, Kendrick M, et al. Outcomes of adults with acute lymphoblastic leukemia relapsing after allogeneic hematopoietic stem cell transplantation. Biol Blood Marrow Transplant. 2013;19(7):1059–64.
123. Hamdi A, Mawad R, Bassett R, di Stasi A, Ferro R, Afrough A, et al. Central nervous system relapse in adults with acute lymphoblastic leukemia after allogeneic hematopoietic stem cell transplantation. Biol Blood Marrow Transplant. 2014;20(11):1767–71.
124. Aldoss I, Al Malki MM, Stiller T, Cao T, Sanchez JF, Palmer J, et al. Implications and management of central nervous system involvement before allogeneic hematopoietic cell transplantation in acute lymphoblastic leukemia. Biol Blood Marrow Transplant. 2016;22(3):575–8.
125. Sauter CS, DeFilipp Z, Inamoto Y, Johnston L, Nagler A, Savani BN, et al. ASBMT statement on routine prophylaxis for central nervous system recurrence of acute lymphoblastic Leukemia following allogeneic hematopoietic cell transplantation. Biol Blood Marrow Transplant. 2019;25(3):e86–e8.
126. Gao RW, Dusenbery KE, Cao Q, Smith AR, Yuan J. Augmenting total body irradiation with a cranial boost before stem cell transplantation protects against post-transplant central nervous system relapse in acute lymphoblastic leukemia. Biol Blood Marrow Transplant. 2018;24(3):501–6.
127. Famoso JM, Grow JL, Laughlin B, Katsanis E, Stea B. The impact of low-dose cranial boost on the long-term outcomes of adult patients with high-risk acute lymphoblastic leukemia undergoing total body irradiation and allogeneic hematopoietic stem cell transplantation. Pract Radiat Oncol. 2019;9(3):e283–e9.
128. Su W, Thompson M, Sheu RD, Steinberg A, Isola L, Stock R, et al. Low-dose cranial boost in high-risk adult acute lymphoblastic leukemia patients undergoing bone marrow transplant. Pract Radiat Oncol. 2017;7(2):103–8.
129. Alexander BM, Wechsler D, Braun TM, Levine J, Herman J, Yanik G, et al. Utility of cranial boost in addition to total body irradiation in the treatment of high risk acute lymphoblastic leukemia. Int J Radiat Oncol Biol Phys. 2005;63(4):1191–6.
130. Curran E, Stock W. Taking a "BiTE out of ALL": blinatumomab approval for MRD-positive ALL. Blood. 2019;133(16):1715–9.
131. Kantarjian H, Stein A, Gokbuget N, Fielding AK, Schuh AC, Ribera JM, et al. Blinatumomab versus chemotherapy for advanced acute lymphoblastic leukemia. N Engl J Med. 2017;376(9):836–47.
132. Martinelli G, Boissel N, Chevallier P, Ottmann O, Gokbuget N, Topp MS, et al. Complete hematologic and molecular response in adult patients with relapsed/refractory Philadelphia chromosome-positive B-precursor acute lymphoblastic leukemia following treatment with blinatumomab: results from a phase II, single-arm. Multicenter Study J Clin Oncol. 2017;35(16).1795–802.
133. Gokbuget N, Dombret H, Bonifacio M, Reichle A, Graux C, Faul C, et al. Blinatumomab for minimal residual disease in adults with B-cell precursor acute lymphoblastic leukemia. Blood. 2018;131(14):1522–31.
134. Jabbour EJ, Gokbuget N, Kantarjian HM, Thomas X, Larson RA, Yoon SS, et al. Transplantation in adults with relapsed/refractory acute lymphoblastic leukemia who are treated with blinatumomab from a phase 3 study. Cancer. 2019;125(23):4181–92.
135. Brown PA, Ji L, Xu X, Devidas M, Hogan L, Borowitz MJ, et al. A randomized phase 3 trial of blinatumomab vs. chemotherapy as post-reinduction therapy in high and intermediate risk (HR/IR) first relapse of B-Acute Lymphoblastic Leukemia (B-ALL) in children and Adolescents/Young Adults (AYAs) demonstrates superior efficacy and tolerability of blinatumomab: a report from Childrens Oncology Group Study AALL1331. Blood. 2019;134(Sup plement_2):LBA-1-LBA.
136. Turtle CJ, Hanafi LA, Berger C, Gooley TA, Cherian S, Hudecek M, et al. CD19 CAR-T cells of defined CD4+:CD8+ composition in adult B cell ALL patients. J Clin Invest. 2016;126(6):2123–38.

137. Park JH, Riviere I, Gonen M, Wang X, Senechal B, Curran KJ, et al. Long-term follow-up of CD19 CAR therapy in acute lymphoblastic leukemia. N Engl J Med. 2018;378(5):449–59.
138. Shah NN, Fry TJ. Mechanisms of resistance to CAR T cell therapy. Nat Rev Clin Oncol. 2019;16(6):372–85.
139. Jacoby E. The role of allogeneic HSCT after CAR T cells for acute lymphoblastic leukemia. Bone Marrow Transplant. 2019;54(Suppl 2):810–4.
140. Shadman M, Gauthier J, Hay KA, Voutsinas JM, Milano F, Li A, et al. Safety of allogeneic hematopoietic cell transplant in adults after CD19-targeted CAR T-cell therapy. Blood Adv. 2019;3(20):3062–9.
141. Hay KA, Gauthier J, Hirayama AV, Voutsinas JM, Wu Q, Li D, et al. Factors associated with durable EFS in adult B-cell ALL patients achieving MRD-negative CR after CD19 CAR T-cell therapy. Blood. 2019;133(15):1652–63.
142. Kantarjian HM, DeAngelo DJ, Stelljes M, Martinelli G, Liedtke M, Stock W, et al. Inotuzumab ozogamicin versus standard therapy for acute lymphoblastic Leukemia. N Engl J Med. 2016;375(8):740–53.
143. Marks DI, Kebriaei P, Stelljes M, Gokbuget N, Kantarjian H, Advani AS, et al. Outcomes of allogeneic stem cell transplantation after inotuzumab ozogamicin treatment for relapsed or refractory acute lymphoblastic leukemia. Biol Blood Marrow Transplant. 2019;25(9):1720–9.
144. Kantarjian HM, DeAngelo DJ, Advani AS, Stelljes M, Kebriaei P, Cassaday RD, et al. Hepatic adverse event profile of inotuzumab ozogamicin in adult patients with relapsed or refractory acute lymphoblastic leukaemia: results from the open-label, randomised, phase 3 INO-VATE study. Lancet Haematol. 2017;4(8):e387–e98.
145. Kebriaei P, Cutler C, de Lima M, Giralt S, Lee SJ, Marks D, et al. Management of important adverse events associated with inotuzumab ozogamicin: expert panel review. Bone Marrow Transplant. 2018;53(4):449–56.
146. Hoelzer D, Bassan R, Dombret H, Fielding A, Ribera JM, Buske C, et al. Acute lymphoblastic leukaemia in adult patients: ESMO clinical practice guidelines for diagnosis, treatment and follow-up. Ann Oncol. 2016;27(suppl 5):v69–82.
147. Labar B, Suciu S, Muus P, Willemze R, Marie JP, Fillet G, et al. E07 stem cell transplantation in ALL: a donor versus no donor comparison in the EORTC ALL-4 study. Leuk Res. 2007;31:S15–S6.

Chapter 17
Hematopoietic Stem Cell Transplantation in Pediatric Acute Lymphoblastic Leukemia

Divya Subburaj and Kirk R. Schultz

History of HSCT in Pediatric ALL

In the 1970s, chemotherapy for leukemia in the pediatric population was relatively limited in its efficacy and allogeneic HSCT was considered an important part of high-risk leukemia treatment. The first report of allogeneic HSCT for children with ALL was published in 1975 in a young girl with relapsed ALL [1]. The first large report consisting of 100 patients was published in 1977, of which 46 had ALL and 34 were under the age of 20 years [2]. ALL was the first malignancy reported to have graft-versus-leukemia (GVL) effect post HSCT, where two boys developed remission after the onset of graft-versus-host disease (GvHD) [3]. The GVL effect induced by GvHD was described in 1979 where the relative relapse rate was 2.5 times less in allogeneic marrow recipients with GvHD [4]. Moreover, the authors were quoted stating "This apparent antileukemic effect was more marked in patients with lymphoblastic than non-lymphoblastic leukemia." Between 1976 and 1979, the modified Berlin-Frankfurt-Munster (BFM) regimen was used to treat 158 children and adolescents and achieved a 70% disease-free survival (DFS) [5]. The Children's Cancer Group (CCG) study treated 209 children with BFM-based chemotherapy and had a similar 4-year event free survival (EFS) of 62% [6].

By 1990, chemotherapy was established as the primary therapy for ALL in children. Its efficacy was similar to HSCT and the lower toxicity profile made it the preferred approach. Over the next few decades, there was a strong emphasis in the field of pediatric ALL to develop risk-based stratification, optimal chemotherapy

D. Subburaj
Pediatric Hematology/Oncology/BMT, BC Children's Hospital, Vancouver, BC, Canada

K. R. Schultz (✉)
Michael Cuccione Childhood Cancer Research Program, BC Children's Hospital and Research Institute, Vancouver, BC, Canada
e-mail: kschultz@mail.ubc.ca

M. R. Litzow, E. A. Raetz (eds.), *Clinical Management of Acute Lymphoblastic Leukemia*, https://doi.org/10.1007/978-3-030-85147-7_17

regimens and improved supportive care, which resulted in an improved 5-year EFS of greater than 85%. Recently, there has been an increased recognition for immune-mediated therapies including monoclonal antibodies, engineered T killer cell populations, and targeted therapies like tyrosine kinase inhibitors (TKIs) for the treatment of ALL. Although allogeneic HSCT continues to be one of the best forms of sustained immune therapy for ALL, its role is being redefined with the availability of novel modalities with potentially improved toxicity profile.

Current Indication for HSCT in Pediatric ALL

HSCT is still considered by many to be the final salvage therapy for ALL when conventional chemotherapy agents have failed. As part of immune therapy, the effects of allogeneic HSCT can involve multiple immune pathways including the T cell, B cell, NK cell, and innate immune response pathways. While newer immune therapies including CAR-T cells can induce dramatic initial responses, HSCT is still being utilized to consolidate remission. However, the two primary problems associated with HSCT in pediatrics include (a) long-term morbidity affecting growth and development including fertility and (b) chronic GvHD (cGvHD). These life-altering morbidities tend to move the position of allogeneic HSCT in ALL therapy to the last salvage option. Hence, we need to improve morbidity outcomes which can result in reconsideration of the role of HSCT in pediatric ALL therapy.

Criteria for HSCT in Pediatric ALL in CR1

Due to the success achieved with chemotherapy protocols, currently only 2–5% of pediatric ALL patients in CR1 receive allogeneic HSCT. The ability to assign risk categories in pediatric ALL has become increasingly sophisticated. They are generally based on the following criteria: (a) National Cancer Institute (NCI) risk assignment, age and white blood cell (WBC) count at presentation; (b) molecular and cytogenetic risk factors; and (c) response to therapy, MRD evaluation. The introduction of MRD evaluation at end of induction/consolidation therapy has changed our risk stratification process and subsequent therapeutic approaches.

Indications for considering allogeneic HSCT in CR1 include (a) end of induction (EOI) therapy failure (EOI marrow MRD >5% blasts or residual extramedullary disease) and (b) MRD+ disease at end of consolidation (EOC). The BFM 2000 trial measured MRD by PCR-based techniques, and positive MRD was defined as a level of $>10^{-3}$ on day 78 [7]. On the other hand, the COG AALL1131 (NCT02883049) and AALL1732 (NCT03959085) studies consider MRD >0.01% by flow cytometry as MRD+ at EOC. The involvement of extramedullary sites at diagnosis either in the central nervous system (CNS) or testes is not an indication for HSCT in CR1 as long as patients achieve complete disease remission with negative marrow MRD disease at EOC.

The indications for HSCT with MRD+ disease at EOI in combination with other high-risk cytogenetic features have been changing over the years. The criteria to assign allogeneic HSCT continue to be based on the expected EFS of chemotherapy versus HSCT in a particular risk group. Consideration for HSCT is usually based on an expected 10–20% improvement in 5-year EFS over chemotherapy. The current COG categories of standard-risk (SR) and high-risk (HR) ALL are expected to have a 5-year EFS of 90–95% and 88–90%, respectively. However, the 5-year EFS with chemotherapy for very high-risk (VHR) ALL has been much lower [8]. Historically, very high-risk features have included hypodiploidy, BCR-ABL1 or Philadelphia chromosome (Ph)-like ALL, Ph + ALL, *KMT2A*-rearranged infant ALL, and mixed-phenotype acute leukemia (MPAL) [9; Table 17.1]. Other cooperative groups have similarly categorized ALL; however, the BFM group has always used the initial response to prednisone as an important risk criterion.

The outcomes of HSCT continued to improve, and based on recent Center for International Blood and marrow Transplant Research (CIBMTR) data, children receiving a matched related donor for ALL in CR1 should expect a 5-year EFS of as high as 74% and those receiving an unrelated donor HSCT a 5-year EFS of 69% [10]. Based on the anticipated 15% improvement in the 5-year EFS rates with HSCT, offering it to children >2 years of age in CR1 for any risk category that has a 5-year EFS of <55% with chemotherapy should be beneficial. EOC MRD+ T-ALL

Table 17.1 Indications for HSCT

HSCT in CR1		
Category	**BFM-AIEOP**	**COG**
Induction failure	M3 marrow at day 33	EOI M3 marrow Or EOI MRD ≥5% blasts Or residual EM disease (for CNS, which includes CNS2 and CNS3)
Consolidation failure	**Matched sibling donor HSCT** MLL/KMT2A rearranged or Hypodiploid <44 chromosomes ***and*** MRD MR (EOC >10 $^{-4}$) or HR (>10^{-3}) **HSCT (any donor)** Poor prednisone response T-ALL *Or* B or T-ALL ***and*** MRD HR (EOC >10^{3})	For high-risk patients* EOC MRD ≥ 0.01% Or residual EM disease (for CNS, which includes CNS2 and CNS3) *high risk includes: iAMP21 Philadelphia chromosome+ ALL BCR-ABL-like ALL Hypodiploid <44 chromosomes MLL/KMT2A rearrangement Infant ALL MPAL

(continued)

Table 17.1 (continued)

HSCT in CR2		
	UK-ALL MRC and EBMT	**COG**
Late relapse	> 6 months from stopping therapy **B-ALL**, Combined/isolated marrow **and** MRD at EORI positive **T-ALL** Combined/isolated marrow	**B-ALL** ≥ 36 months from diagnosis – Marrow, end block 1 MRD ≥ 0.1% ≥ 18 months from diagnosis – isolated EM, end block 1 MRD ≥ 0.1% **any T-ALL/T-LL relapses**
Early relapse	**T- or B-ALL** (>18 months from diagnosis, < 6 months from stopping therapy) Combined/isolated marrow	**B-ALL** <36 months from diagnosis marrow **any T-ALL/T-LL relapses**
Very early relapse	**T- or B-ALL** (< 18 months from diagnosis) Combined/isolated medullary/isolated	**B-ALL** <18 months from diagnosis, marrow/isolated EM **any T-ALL/T-LL relapses**
Treatment failure	Induction failure	Failure to achieve the following at end block 1: M2 or better CNS remission (clearance of CSF blasts, i.e., CNS1)

EOI end of induction, *EORI* end of reinduction, *MRD* minimal residual disease, *EOCI* end of consolidation induction, *EM* extra medullary disease, *HR* high risk, *MR* medium risk, *MPAL* mixed-phenotype acute leukemia

or B-ALL, hypodiploidy, and BCR-ABL-like ALL with positive MRD generally fall in this category (Table 17.1). *KMT*2A-rearranged ALL as a sole adverse risk factor probably does not warrant HSCT; however, presence of *KMT2A* rearrangement with other adverse risk factors like older age, high WBC at presentation, and poor prednisone response does define a very high-risk subgroup for which HSCT may be recommended.

Recently, the CIBMTR developed a risk assignment algorithm for HSCT in ALL based on three factors – (a) ALL in CR1 or CR ≥ 2, (b) age, and (c) MRD status pre-HSCT (Table 17.2). Based on this algorithm, pediatric ALL-CR1 transplant outcomes (0–18 years) are considered "good" risk category for children over the age of 2 years with an expected leukemia-free survival (LFS) of about 70% and "moderate" risk for those under 2 years of age with an expected LFS of 50% [11].

The American Society for Transplantation and Cellular Therapy (ASTCT) developed an excellent evidence-based analysis of when HSCT should be considered for pediatric ALL [12]. Overall these analyses support the cooperative group recommendations, although they point out a lack of statistically significant supporting data for some of the categories.

Table 17.2 Adapted CIBMTR pediatric ALL risk index for allogeneic hematopoietic cell transplantation [40]

Variable	Number	Hazard ratio	Score
Age			
≥ 2 years < 2 years	579 35	1.00 1.77 (1.06–2.93)	0 3
Disease status			
First complete remission MRD (−)	148	1.00	0
First complete remission MRD (+)	72	1.04 (0.65–1.69)	0
First complete remission	13	2.66 (1.30–5.45)	
Second complete remission MRD (−)	254	1.51 (1.08–2.12)	2
Second complete remission MRD (+)	85	2.28 (1.49–3.34)	4
Second complete remission	21	1.87 (0.97–3.61)	
Relapse	21	1.58 (0.79–3.14)	2

Pediatric disease risk index (p-DRI)	**Age**	**Disease status pre-HSCT**	**Cytogenetic risk**	**Training cohort**	**Validation cohort**	**5-year LFS**
Good Score 0	≥ 2 years	1 CR MRD (−) 1 CR MRD (+)	Any cytogenetic risk	HR 1.00 *P* < 0.0001	HR 1.00 *P* < 0.0001	68% (63–72)
Intermediate Score 2–4	≥ 2 years	2 CR MRD (−) 2 CR MRD (+) Relapse	Any cytogenetic risk	HR 1.51 *P* = 0.004	HR 2.03 *P* < 0.0001	50% (45–54)
	< 2 years	1 CR MRD (−) 1 CR MRD (+)				
High Score ≥ 5	< 2 years	2 CR MRD (−) 2 CR MRD (+) Relapse	Any cytogenetic risk	HR 5.22 P < 0.0001	HR 6.65 P < 0.0001	15% (3–34)

*Based on N = 1228 CIBMTR database of ALL aged <18 years and transplanted between 2008 and 2017

MRD-Positive ALL-CR1

End of induction MRD positivity has emerged as the single major factor influencing survival in pediatric ALL. The *Associazione Italiana di Ematologia e Oncologia Pediatrica* and the *Berlin-Frankfurt-Munster* (AIEOP-BFM) 2000 (NCT00430118) study, a large prospective clinical trial, showed that MRD standard-risk (SR) children (MRD-negative disease at EOI and EOC) had a 5-year EFS of 95% compared to 55% in MRD high risk (HR) (MRD positive at EOI and EOC) [7]. The results showed that patients undergoing relatively intensive treatment, like the BFM-based chemotherapy, HSCT may not be indicated even in the presence of any other combination of risk factors if the MRD response proved to be favorable.

The COG AALL0331 (NCT00103285) trial showed that children with NCI standard-risk features at presentation, with an MRD >0.1% at EOI, could still be salvaged with intense chemotherapy-only approach, provided the EOC MRD was negative (6-year EFS of 90%) removing the need for HSCT in this group [13]. On the other hand, children with MRD+ disease at EOC did very poorly irrespective of cytogenetic factors. The presence of good prognostic markers like *ETV6-RUNX1* or trisomies of chromosomes 4 and 10 in NCI HR produced a dismal 5-year EFS of 43 ± 7% in children with EOC MRD+ disease [9]. The current COG AALL1731 (NCT03914625) study aims to improve outcomes of NCI SR patients who are MRD+ (0.1 to <1%) at EOC with addition of blinatumomab. Similarly, the NCI HR patients on AALL1732 who have EOC MRD >0.01% can move on to CAR-T trial AALL1721 (NCT03448393).

In the T-ALL cohort, MRD positivity at EOC constitutes the most important predictive factor for relapse. The BFM 2000 trial (NCT00430118) had an excellent outcome with a 7-year EFS of 80% if MRD was negative at EOC, compared to 50% for those who were still MRD positive, indicating that EOI MRD levels were irrelevant if MRD at EOC turned negative [14, 15]. Similar to B-ALL, children with T-ALL and MRD-positive disease at EOC should be considered for HSCT due to a higher relapse risk.

Philadelphia Chromosome-Positive (Ph+) ALL

Tyrosine kinase inhibitors (TKIs) have revolutionized the management of Ph + ALL. Pediatric studies showed that chemotherapy plus continuous TKI-based protocols achieved survival rates that were non-inferior to HSCT outcomes. The COG AALL0031 trial (NCT00022737) had an improved outcome with a 5-year DFS of 70% with a combination of intense chemotherapy, continuous TKI therapy (imatinib), and prophylactic cranial radiotherapy compared to a sibling donor HSCT with a DFS of 65% [16, 17]. The subsequent AALL0622 trial (NCT00720109) used dasatinib and risk stratified the Ph-positive ALL group as SR and HR based on EOI MRD levels [18]. The patients in HR groups were moved to the HSCT arm of the study after induction, and SR group patients continued on chemotherapy and TKI. Though the 5-year EFS for SR group was 60%, the OS was 87% as many could be salvaged with HSCT in CR2. The EsPhALL study (NCT00287105) and BFM 2000 (NCT00430118) trial recommended HSCT in Ph + ALL in a setting of matched related or unrelated donor. However, they found that MRD-negative patients treated with a TKI had a good DFS of 80%, similar to MSD (matched sibling donor) HSCT recipients [19]. Indications for HSCT in the current BFM and COG trails for children with Ph + ALL are persistent MRD positivity at end of consolidation therapy.

BCR-ABL-Like ALL

In 2009, the COG-St. Jude consortium and the Dutch group identified BCR-ABL-like ALL as a separate type of B-ALL with a gene expression profile similar to Ph + ALL, however lacking the classic BCR-ABL1 fusion protein. Though more commonly seen in young adults, Ph-like ALL can be seen in up to 12% of childhood ALL. Approximately half of the cases harbor rearrangement in the cytokine receptor CRLF2 (cytokine receptor-like factor 2), *IKZF1* deletions and intrachromosomal amplification of chromosome 21 (*iAMP21)* alterations are also frequently seen [20–22]. Among childhood and adolescent patients with *CRLF2* rearrangement, approximately half have concomitant activating mutations of the Janus kinase genes, *JAK1* or *JAK2*, which can be modified by *JAK2* inhibitors such as ruxolitinib. Around 10% have *ABL*-class gene fusions, and *ABL1* inhibitors like imatinib can be combined with conventional chemotherapy [21]. Most pediatric and adult studies showed higher MRD levels at EOI in BCR-ABL-like ALL when treated with conventional chemotherapy [23, 24]. Interestingly, the St. Jude Total Therapy Study XV which featured MRD-directed treatment had 40 patients with an overall 5-year EFS of 90% with only 15% of poor responders proceeding to HSCT [25]. The COG/Incyte AALL1521 trial (NCT02723994) aims to determine the role of ruxolitinib with conventional chemotherapy in children with BCR-ABL-like ALL with *JAK-STAT* pathway alterations. The role of HSCT if MRD+ at EOI needs to be determined as ruxolitinib is added only toward the end of induction. The outcomes of the study should shed light on the response rates of chemotherapy combined with targeted therapy, and HSCT should probably be reserved for patients who are MRD+ at EOC.

Hypodiploid ALL

Hypodiploid leukemia blast cells have less than 44 chromosomes which include distinct subtypes based on the chromosomal number – near haploidy (25–29 chromosomes), low hypodiploidy (33–39 chromosomes), high hypodiploidy (42–43 chromosomes) with complex karyotypes, and high hypodiploidy with 44 chromosomes [26, 27]. Among the various subtypes, low hypodiploid and near haploid fare worse due to a differential mutational profile [28]. Near-haploid ALL cases are characterized by genetic alterations in *IKZF3*, and low hypodiploid cases frequently carry germline *TP53* mutations [29]. Recent reports have shown a 10–15% improvement in overall survival with HSCT in hypodiploid ALL, though these differences were not statistically significant due to small numbers [28–31]. Patients treated on

AALL0331 (NCT00103285) and AALL0232 (NCT00075725) had a EFS and OS at 5 years of 29.4% ± 14.3% and 29.4% ± 14.3%, respectively with HSCT (n = 18), whereas EFS and OS were 16.7% ± 10.8% and 22.2% ± 13.9%, respectively with chemotherapy (n = 12, $P = 0.67$ for EFS and $P = 0.86$ for OS) among patients with EOI MRD >0.01% [32]. The retrospective analysis published in 2019 by Pui et al. showed that expected DFS was similar between chemotherapy and HSCT arm at approximately 70% in the EOI MRD-negative cohort. However, DFS with HSCT was higher at 55% compared to 40% with chemotherapy in the MRD+ group ($p = 0.29$) [28]. Outcomes with both chemotherapy and HSCT remain suboptimal, regardless of MRD response. The current open trials do not clearly specify the indication for HSCT in hypodiploid ALL due to a lack of significant benefit in past studies. There remains an urgent need for achieving better remission prior to HSCT with novel therapies.

Infant ALL

KMT2A (formerly *MLL – mixed-lineage leukemia*) rearrangements are most commonly observed in infant leukemias. The previous CCG and Pediatric Oncology Group (POG) trials did not find a survival advantage with HSCT over intensive chemotherapy in this cohort. Given that most children were young at the time of transplant, nearly half of them received a non-TBI (total body irradiation)-based conditioning in these trials. They also used single-agent prophylaxis for GVHD which might have contributed to the higher rates of grade 3 and 4 acute GVHD and transplant-related mortality (TRM), affecting the overall survival outcomes [33, 34]. On the other hand, HSCT showed a 64% reduction in risk of failure for high-risk infants (< 6 months of age, poor prednisone response) in the Interfant-99 trial (NCT00015873) [35]. However, the outcome in the subsequent Interfant-06 trial (NCT00550992) was poor as nearly half of the cohort experienced early relapse, prior to proceeding to transplant [36]. The role of HSCT in infant ALL in CR1 remains unclear. The results of the current St. Jude consortium TINI study (NCT02553460) that is investigating the role of *KMT2A* targeted agents bortezomib and vorinostat may help in defining the indications.

Mixed-Phenotype Acute Leukemia (MPAL)

Mixed-phenotypic leukemia is rare in children constituting 2–5% of acute leukemias, harboring immunophenotypic features of both lymphoid and myeloid leukemias. There has been no uniform protocol for treating MPAL in children so far; however, the current COG AALL1732 protocol has a separate MPAL stratum. The AMBI2012 registry study saw no significant benefit with HSCT in CR1; however, a trend toward improved EFS with HSCT was seen in those with EOI MRD ≥5%. The majority of the children on this study had a predominant B-lineage lymphoid component [37]. The COG consensus statement recommends upfront ALL-based chemotherapy irrespective of the blast phenotypes at presentation and recommends HSCT for those with poor response to induction and consolidation therapy [38].

Induction Failure

Induction failure with >5% blasts by MRD at the end of induction is rare, seen in less than 3% of pediatric and adolescent ALL. However, it is considered a very poor risk factor, and HSCT is generally indicated. Its prognostic significance becomes difficult, if patients achieve an MRD-negative remission post consolidation therapy, although outcomes following HSCT are encouraging for this cohort. A large European retrospective analysis on 44,017 pediatric ALL patients from 14 cooperative study groups between 1985 and 2000 documented an induction failure rate of 2.4%, with an overall 10-year survival rate of 32 ± 1%. The independent adverse prognostic factors were age > 10 years, M3 marrow (>25% blasts) at EOI, T-ALL, and the presence of a *KMT2A* rearrangement. HSCT was associated with a favorable trend for all categories except *KMT2A*-rearranged leukemia [39]. The AALL0031 study had a 4-year DFS of 44% for induction failure patients treated with intensive chemotherapy compared to 75 ± 19% ($P = 0.14$) in the transplant arm; however, this difference was not statistically significant due to small numbers [30].

Criteria for HSCT in Pediatric ALL in CR ≥2

HSCT plays a crucial role in a relapsed ALL setting, though the outcomes for ALL in CR2 are generally poor compared to CR1. At the time of relapse, patients are risk stratified based on duration of remission (CR1/CR2), immunophenotype, sites of relapse, and MRD at end of reinduction therapy (EORI). The COG protocols primarily use a flow-based MRD and a cutoff of 0.1%, and the EBMT and UK protocols use PCR-based MRD monitoring and aim for MRD $<10^{-4}$ at EORI. The current indications for allogeneic HSCT in CR2 are summarized in Table 17.1. Most cooperative groups recommend HSCT for relapsed high-risk ALL patients and chemotherapy-only approach for SR patients. More restricted criteria for HSCT are applied to standard-risk patients, especially those who present with late-onset relapse, B cell immunophenotype, isolated extramedullary involvement, and MRD-negative disease at EORI [40].

The results of ALL-REZ-BFM 2002 trial (NCT00114348) showed that patients with late marrow relapse had an EFS of 72% (95% CI 64% to 78%) and OS of 82%

(95% CI 75% to 87%). The majority of patients with MRD+ (> 10^{-3}) disease received HSCT and achieved an EFS of 81% vs. 68% for MRD >10^{-3} but < 10^{-2} and MRD >10^{-2} respectively at EORI [41].

The UKALLR3 (NCT00967057) trial evaluated 228 patients with late B-ALL marrow relapse, and nearly 97% achieved CR2 at EORI. One hundred and ten patients were MRD+ (>10^{-4}) at EORI, and 92 of them proceeded to HSCT with either a MSD or alternate donor. The 5-year progression-free survival (PFS) after transplant was 54% (95% CI 34–71) in the MRD+ cohort compared to 88% (95% CI 39–98) in MRD-negative cohort. Seventy patients with MRD level < 10^{-4} at EORI continued on chemotherapy with a 5-year PFS of 70% (95% CI 57–79). The 5-year survival was poor with PFS of 31% (95% CI 11–56) for children with MRD+ disease who went on to continue chemotherapy. The study suggested that HSCT be the preferred option for patients with late bone marrow relapse and MRD+ disease at EORI [42].

The COG AALL0433 trial (*NCT*00381680) accrued 275 children with either a late marrow relapse or an early isolated extramedullary relapse. Seventy-four patients underwent HSCT in CR2 (51 late marrow, 16 combined, and 7 isolated CNS relapses); 47 patients received matched sibling donor HSCT, and 27 underwent alternative donor transplant. The 3-year DFS was 77.5 ± 6.2% for HSCT vs. 66.9 ± 4.5% for chemotherapy ($p = 0.03$). However, this did not correspond to improved OS (81.5 ± 5.8% with HSCT vs. 85.8 ± 3.4% without, $p = 0.46$). In patients with MRD <0.1% at EORI, HSCT showed an improved 3-year DFS of 90.7 ± 6.5% vs. 74.1 ± 5.8% for chemotherapy ($p = 0.07$); however, the difference in 3-year OS again was not significant (95.5 ± 4.7% with HSCT vs. 93.1 ± 3.4% without, $p = 0.16$). In contrast to other studies, in patients with positive MRD >0.1%, HSCT did not show a benefit over chemotherapy (3-year DFS of 56.3 ± 13.2% with HSCT vs. 55.0 ± 11.1 with chemotherapy, $p = 0.23$) [43].

The outcomes for early bone marrow relapse have been uniformly poor. The older CCG1941 study highlighted that majority of treatment failures occurred before any HSCT procedure could be initiated and half of the patients with matched related donor either did not achieve a remission or relapsed and died before a HSCT was performed [44]. The ability to attain a MRD-negative remission using agents with a lower toxicity profile like blinatumomab has shown encouraging results in the recent COG AALL1331 relapsed ALL trial (NCT02101853). The study randomized 208 children with intermediate- and high-risk relapsed B- ALL to either receive intensive chemotherapy after Block 1 reinduction or two 4-week cycles of blinatumomab prior to HSCT. After a median follow-up of 1.4 years, those in blinatumomab group had higher 2-year DFS (59.3% vs. 41%), higher rates of undetectable MRD (70% vs. 21%), and a higher success rate of proceeding to stem cell transplant (73% vs. 45%). The blinatumomab arm also showed lower rates of infections, sepsis, and toxicity prior to HSCT [45].

The current CIBMTR risk assignment algorithm estimates that all HSCT in CR2 are either in the intermediate-risk or high-risk category. A score of 2 is given for

ALL-CR2 with MRD negativity and 4 for ALL-CR2 with MRD positivity. Age < 2 gets an additional score of 3. An intermediate score (2–4) yields an expected 5-year LFS of 50%, and a high risk score (≥5) has an expected 5-year LFS of 15% [46]. The poor LFS in the MRD+ disease emphasizes the need for alternative therapies such as CAR-T cells or blinatumomab prior to HSCT.

The Role of HSCT in Treatment of Relapsed T-ALL

Recently, the CIBMTR evaluated HSCT in 229 children with T-ALL in CR2 between 2000 and 2011. The donor sources included umbilical cord blood, matched sibling marrow, and unrelated donors with marrow or peripheral blood graft source. The 3-year DFS was 46% with a TRM of 13% and a relapse rate of 30%. The Multivariate analysis revealed that marrow relapse, with or without concurrent extramedullary relapse, were more likely to relapse post HSCT (hazard ratio, 3.94) compared to isolated extramedullary disease [47]. Although the ability of HSCT to treat refractory T-ALL does not appear to be as good as B-ALL, it still represents the only available salvage option for relapsed T-ALL.

The Role of HSCT in Treatment of Extramedullary Relapse

The incidence of CNS relapse is less than 5% in pediatric ALL; nonetheless, when relapse occurs, the CNS is involved in 22% to 40% of relapsed ALL cases [48, 49]. The probability of leukemia-free survival (LFS) at 5 years post HSCT for relapsed ALL was highest for patients with isolated CNS relapse at 91% (95% CI 51–99; $P < 0.01$) [50]. The Italian cooperative group evaluated the outcome of 281 children with extramedullary relapse between 1990 and 2015, and 167 had a relapse confined to the CNS, 73 to the testis, 14 to the mediastinum, and 27 to other organs. After reinduction therapy, 97 patients underwent autologous HSCT, and 184 received allogeneic HSCT. The 10-year overall survival was 54% with improved outcomes seen with TBI-based allogeneic transplants [51].

The 3-year EFS/OS for patients with very early isolated CNS relapse on the AALL0433 trial (*NCT*00381680) was 41.4% ± 9.2% and 51.7% ± 9.3%, respectively. The 3-year DFS/OS for transplanted patients (n = 7) was 71.4 ± 17.0% and 71.4 ± 17.1%, compared to 28.6 ± 9.9% and 42.9 ± 10.8% without HSCT (n = 21) ($p = 0.12$ for DFS, $p = 0.18$ for OS), respectively [43]. The isolated late CNS relapse cohort had the best outcome, and the relapse rate was higher for patients with early CNS relapse who continued on chemotherapy/radiation [52]. The current COG trials recommend HSCT for early extramedullary relapse (less than 18 months from initial diagnosis).

The Role of Second HSCT for Relapsed ALL

A second allogeneic HSCT can be potentially curative in children with relapsed ALL; however, it is limited significantly by higher level of morbidity and organ toxicity compared to the first transplant. If a second HSCT is considered, the interval between the first and second HSCT seems to significantly impact the TRM and possibly OS. The EBMT pediatric working committee in 2018 reviewed 214 patients who underwent second HSCT. The cumulative relapse rate for the cohort was 47%, non-relapse mortality was 22%, and 5-year LFS was 31%. Reduced intensity conditioning (RIC) was preferred second time around to reduce toxicity; however, it was associated with a poorer outcome. The use of the same or a different donor from first transplant did not seem to affect the outcome [53]. A retrospective study from Japan also had similar TRM and relapse rates at 18% and 44%, respectively. Younger age < 9 years, late relapse (180 days or more after first HSCT), CR prior to second HSCT, and myeloablative conditioning were found to be associated with longer survival [54].

The recent CIBMTR analysis reviewed 251 children and young adults with acute myelogenous or lymphoblastic leukemia who underwent a second HSCT, and ALL constituted 44% with a median interval of 17 months between the 2 transplants. Most of the patients were in CR pre-HSCT and received myeloablative conditioning regimen with >90% receiving an unrelated donor graft. The 8-year LFS for those in CR at the time of second transplant was 24% vs. 10% for those not in CR. Interestingly, the analysis found a lower relapse and a higher leukemia-free survival with (a) interval of >5 months between transplant and diagnosis of relapse, (b) using the same donor for both transplants, (c) a history of cGvHD, and (d) using either a non-myeloablative TBI-based regimens or a reduced intensity transplant with low-dose TBI [55–58].

The effect of immunophenotype, cytogenetic rearrangement, or the presence of medullary vs. extramedullary disease on the outcome of second transplant is also poorly understood. RIC was seen to be associated with higher relapse risk, and the question of different donor for second transplant is not well addressed in literature. The availability of CAR-T cell therapy for relapsed B-ALL post HSCT can help achieve good remission with lower toxicity [59]. The role of allogeneic HSCT particularly in the setting of post CAR-T cell therapy is still being established. It is possible that CAR-T cell therapy followed by a second HSCT can improve outcomes for multiple relapsed B-ALL. We need large multi-institutional studies to determine the impact of cytogenetic risk factors, conditioning regimens and the role of second HSCT post CAR-T cell therapy.

Factors Impacting Outcomes of HSCT in ALL

Preparative Regimen

TBI-based myeloablation continues to be the backbone of conditioning regimens in pediatric ALL transplant. The standard myeloablative regimen includes cyclophosphamide (Cy) at a dose of 120 mg/kg and TBI of 12 Gy [60]. A CIBMTR retrospective analysis showed that TBI/Cy-based regimens had the best outcomes and the sequence between TBI and Cy did not affect the outcome [61]. The long-term side effects of TBI, especially in very young children, have prompted studies to develop non-TBI-based regimens. Recently a large pediatric study performed by the International Allogeneic Stem Cell Transplantation in Children and Adolescents with Acute Lymphoblastic Leukaemia: ALL SCTped FORUM (NCT01949129 –.

For Omitting Radiation Under Majority Age) studied over 800 children and adolescents and demonstrated a clear survival advantage of TBI- regimens over non-TBI-based chemotherapy regimens [62]. Thus, the standard approach worldwide is to incorporate TBI in the conditioning to attain the best possible survival outcomes. The current PTCTC study for MRD Negative Children, Adolescents, and Young Adults with B-ALL [the EndRAD trial – NCT03509961] is evaluating whether very low MRD levels defined by deep sequencing prior to HSCT may allow for elimination of TBI in this low-risk patient group.

Donor Type and Graft Source

Matched sibling donors continue to be the preferred donor choice for transplant due to lower TRM and GvHD rates. Alternate donor sources include umbilical cord blood (UCB), unrelated donors, and haploidentical related donors. The retrospective EBMT-Eurocord registry study concluded that UCB had higher rates of engraftment failure (23% vs. 11%), higher grade 2–4 GvHD, and lower incidence of relapse compared to MUD, although there was no difference in DFS [63]. The outcome rates for mismatched unrelated marrow donors (MMUD) compared to MUD are lower due to the higher rates of GvHD and are being replaced by haploidentical related donors [64]. The use of bone marrow grafts compared to granulocyte colony-stimulating factor (G-CSF)-mobilized peripheral blood results in a significantly lower rate of cGvHD and better OS [65]. The novel mobilizing agents such as plerixafor, even when used in place of G-CSF, may also result in a similar rates of cGvHD [66]. Bone marrow grafts should continue to be the preferred donor source for both related and unrelated transplants.

There has been a recent shift in donor choices toward the use of haploidentical related donor, especially in the setting of absent MSD/MUD. The two approaches in haploidentical transplants include in vivo post-transplant cyclophosphamide (PT-Cy) and ex vivo T cell depleted haploidentical HSCT. The retrospective review by

AIEOP-GITMO looked at the feasibility of PT-Cy in children with hematological malignancies and found a non-inferior outcome with haplo-HSCT compared to other donor sources with an EFS of 61%, 1-year cumulative incidence of relapse (CIR) of 24%, and TRM of 9%. The authors contributed the slightly higher relapse rate to the high-risk nature of leukemia with 20% of the haplo cohort undergoing a second transplant [67]. The phase 2 study (NCT02120157) on PT-Cy haploidentical HSCT for acute leukemias/MDS in pediatrics reported a 1-year EFS of 65% in 32 patients. The study used TBI/Cy for ALLs followed by cyclophosphamide of 50 mg/kg on D + 3 and D + 4 and mycophenolate and tacrolimus GvHD prophylaxis starting on D + 5. Unmanipulated marrow product was the only type of graft source used in the study. The infused cell dose was found to be a major limiting factor affecting outcomes and recommended a minimum TNC of 2×10^8 cells/kg to avoid graft failure. The cohort had no grade 3/4 aGvHD, and cGvHD rate was documented at 11%. The 1-year relapse was slightly higher at 32% [68].

The alternate approach to PT-Cy in the haploidentical donor HSCT is to utilize ex vivo αβ T cell/CD19+ B cell depleted graft. A multicenter retrospective study on children with acute leukemia between 2010 and 2015 in 13 Italian centers compared 98 TCR αβ/CD19+ depleted haplo-HSCT to 127 MUD and 118 MMUD transplants. TBI was used in children >3 years of age, and anti-thymocyte globulin (ATG) was used in all three donor groups. Nearly two-thirds of the recipients in each group had ALL. The ex vivo depleted haplo-HSCT group received no post-transplant GvHD prophylaxis medications. Calcineurin inhibitors and short-term methotrexate were used in the MUD and MMUD cohort. Graft failure rate was 2% in all three groups; however, the neutrophil and platelet engraftment was faster in the ex vivo depleted haploidentical HSCT group. Reconstitution of CD3/CD4+ T-cells was better at 3 months in the MUD group; however, by 12 months, it was better in the haplo-HSCT group. The TRM rate was 8% in MUD, 9% in ex vivo depleted haplo-HSCT, and 28% in MMUD. The cumulative incidence of grade 3–4 aGvHD in the MUD vs. MMUD was 6% vs. 18%, respectively, compared to no grade 3–4 aGvHD in the ex vivo depleted haplo-HSCT recipients. The rate of CIR was 26%, 17%, and 29% in MUD, MMUD, and αβhaplo-HSCT recipients, respectively. The probability of 5-year LFS and cGvHD-free/relapse-free (GRFS) survival was equivalent among the MUD and αβhaplo-HSCT groups (67% and 61% in MUD vs. 62% and 58% in haplo, respectively); however, it was lower at 55% and 34% in the MMUD cohort [69].

The group also compared the results of the TCRαβ/CD19+ B cell depleted haploidentical transplants to 41 MSD transplants performed during the same time period. The probability of 5-year LFS for ex vivo depleted haploidentical donor vs. MSD was 70.7% vs. 68.1%, and GRFS was 70.7% vs. 63.2%, respectively. TBI-based conditioning was the only factor affecting the relapse risk in the haploidentical transplants [70].

The study showed that the outcome of ex vivo depleted haplo-HSCT was non-inferior to other alternate donor transplants and superior to MMUD with respect to engraftment, TRM, and GvHD. The marginally higher relapse rates were attributed to the high-risk nature of leukemia in the haploidentical cohort. The in vitro studies describe an early engraftment of donor-derived mature NK cells in the αβ depleted haplo-HSCT to exert a GVL effect and reduce early relapses [71]. One recent study suggested that a high $CD56^{dim}/CD56^{bright}$ NK cell ratio early after ex vivo TCR αβ/CD19 depleted transplant could lower relapse incidence [72].

The Impact of Pre-HSCT MRD on HSCT in ALL

MRD pre-HSCT has been established as a principal factor affecting the outcomes of transplant. The results of ALL-REZ BFM 2002 (NCT00114348) trial showed that EFS was worse in patients with MRD > 10^{-3} compared to patients with MRD < 10^{-3} before HSCT (50% vs. 81%, $P = 0.016$) [41, 73]. The high-risk relapsed ALL group had a similar outcome with EFS of 53% vs. 30% in the MRD-negative vs. MRD-positive groups, respectively. MRD prior to HSCT turned out as an independent prognostic factor in the multivariate analysis predicting adverse events after HSCT (risk ratio 2.4) [74]. The ASCT0431 trial also showed the presence of MRD of ≥0.1% pre-HSCT was associated with higher relapse risk (HR, 3.3) [75]. The FORUM study also showed that children with negative MRD by PCR (<10^{-6}) had the best outcome with a 2-year OS of 85% compared to 65% in patients with pre-transplant MRD >10^{-4}. Interestingly, the 2-year EFS was not different between the two cohorts [62].

Recently, studies have shown that both pre- and post-HSCT MRD seem to affect the EFS after HSCT. The ALL-BFM-SCT 2003 trial found that the discriminatory power of MRD detection 1 month post HSCT to predict the probability of relapse was more than 96% [76]. The Westhafen Intercontinental group for pediatric HSCT recently published a multicenter observational study on the role of MRD post HSCT and factors affecting CIR. Six hundred and sixteen pediatric subjects who underwent HSCT for ALL across North America and Europe were included. The post-HSCT MRD emerged as the most crucial factor influencing the relapse risk. The study found that patients with high pre-HSCT MRD levels had a reasonable chance of survival if they achieved MRD negativity early after HSCT. The other factor that could modify post-HSCT outcomes even in MRD+ patients was aGvHD. The study proposed and validated an integrated risk score (IRS) to risk-stratify patients into three risk groups based on (1) remission status, CR2 or more; (2) conditioning regimen TBI- vs. non-TBI-based regimen; and (3) pre-HSCT MRD (10^{-3} to 10^{-4} by qPCR or 0.1–0.01% by flow). The good outcome subgroup (IRS < 5) had CIR at 1 and 2 years of 16% (95% CI 11–21) and 21% (95% CI 15–27). The intermediate outcome subgroup (IRS 6–9) had CIR at 1 and 2 years of 32% (95% CI 20–44) and 38% (95% CI 30–56). The poor outcome group (IRS > 9) had CIR at 1 and 2 years of 41% (95% CI 30–53) and 47% (95% CI 35–59) [77].

GvHD and GVL Effect

The GVL effect by either acute or chronic GvHD was established in the early days of HSCT for pediatric ALL [3, 4]. A recent CIBMTR study explored the role of GVL in ALL by evaluating 5215 adult and pediatric patients from 287 centers. Grade 1 and 2 aGvHD without cGvHD provided the best survival advantage in pediatric ALL HSCT with a 17–24% lower risk of mortality compared to those with no GvHD. The DFS and OS were significantly worse for patients with grade 3 and 4 aGvHD with or without cGvHD, indicating that severe GvHD did not provide effective protection against relapse [78]. An earlier study also found patients with aGvHD to have lower relapse risk in ALL, and cGvHD had a protective effect against relapse in myeloid leukemias [79]. Interestingly, patients with Ph + ALL seemed to be particularly sensitive to GVL effect, with significantly fewer relapses in Ph + ALL compared to other subtypes of ALL [80]. The ASCT0431 study showed that pre-HSCT MRD and presence of aGvHD impacted the relapse risk. The lowest relapse rate was seen in patients with negative MRD pre-HSCT and aGvHD [81]. A few papers have reported the possible development of resistance to GVL in the ALL by biasing toward a Th2 response post HSCT resulting in relapse [82].

Post-Transplant Prophylaxis

The role of post-HSCT prophylaxis is unknown in pediatric ALL. MRD positivity and a drop in chimerism post HSCT are associated with an increased risk of relapse, although MRD appears to be the better predictor. The general consensus is to introduce pre-emptive or prophylactic approaches between 60 and 100 days after HSCT, prior to the majority of documented relapses [76]. Pre-emptive interventions like rapid withdrawal of immune suppression and use of targeted therapies such as blinatumomab early post HSCT may improve outcomes in MRD-positive disease. There are two pediatric pre-emptive trials in Canada and Europe evaluating the role of blinatumomab post HSCT. Routine evaluation of MRD post HSCT starting day +30 can identify patients at a higher risk of relapse, and a reasonable monitoring schedule of MRD status post HSCT would be day +30, +56–60, +90–100, 6 months, 9 months, and 12 months.

The role of TKI prophylaxis after HSCT for Ph + ALL is uncertain. The COG AALL0031 trial and a study from Fred Hutchinson Center evaluated the feasibility of addition of TKIs post HSCT; however, both studies were non-randomized and could not establish if TKI prophylaxis improved OS [30]. The current large pediatric EsPhALL/COG Ph + ALL trial, AALL1631 (NCT03007147), is again non-randomly assigning patients with HR Ph + ALL to receive a transplant and recommends imatinib post HSCT. However, even this large study may not have sufficient numbers to address the efficacy of TKI prophylaxis post HSCT. Imatinib is an immune suppressive agent and has been used to treat cGvHD [83]. Ideally, it should decrease rates of both cGvHD and relapse; however, data on its role post HSCT is lacking. A large CIBMTR registry study evaluating the impact of TKI post HSCT in chronic myeloid leukemia did not demonstrate survival advantage with the addition of TKI [84]. The efficacy of TKI prophylaxis post HSCT in pediatric Ph + ALL still remains questionable.

CNS Prophylaxis

The incidence of CNS relapse of leukemia after HSCT ranges from 2% to 5.5% in patients without previous CNS disease and 11% to 27% among patients with prior CNS involvement [85, 86]. Though intrathecal (IT) therapy pre-HSCT has reduced the rate of CNS relapse to less than 10%, evidence for the efficacy of prophylactic IT therapy post HSCT is limited in pediatrics [87]. The retrospective multicenter study by Gustafsson et al. in 2010 reviewed 397 post-allogeneic HSCT patients for ALL or AML between 1992 and 2006. The study did not find a statistically significant difference in the incidence of isolated or mixed CNS relapses between those who did and who did not receive IT prophylaxis post HSCT [88]. A survey was conducted by EBMT in 2005 to describe the current practice of IT prophylaxis in HSCT. Ninety centers participated, of which 42 (47%) had never used pre- or post-transplant IT prophylaxis, and pre-transplant IT therapy (close to HSCT) was given in 48 centers (53%), whereas only 29 centers (32%) were found to use post-transplant IT therapy. The EBMT study group (adult and pediatric) concluded that routine IT prophylaxis should not be given to patients without prior CNS involvement, but the study did not evaluate the efficacy of the therapy post HSCT [89]. The recent ASBMT statement also recognizes the lack of data on the role of routine post-HSCT CNS prophylaxis and urges for a well-designed study to answer the question [90]. Cranial radiation has been routinely used to treat CNS3 disease. A recent study looking at the role of cranial boost pre-HSCT found that none of the 30 children with prior CNS disease relapsed post TBI with cranial boost [91]. TBI combined with cranial boost is being routinely used as part of conditioning regimen in patients with prior CNS disease.

Long-Term Outcomes of HSCT

The 1-year post-transplant survival rates have improved dramatically over the last decade. Though the CIBMTR study concluded that the prospect for long-term survival is excellent at 85% for survivors beyond 2 years of allogeneic HSCT, life expectancy still remains lower than expected in them. The incidence of relapse and cumulative incidence of non-relapse mortality (NRM) at 10 years post HSCT for ALL are low; however, morbidity is significant. Development of chronic GvHD before 2 years was an important risk factor for late mortality post HSCT. Second cancers accounted for 2% to 10% of deaths in survivors [92]. Second malignancies including thyroid nodules, meningiomas, and carcinomas were seen in up to 20% of HSCT survivors [93]. The St. Jude cohort of survivors of childhood HSCT for leukemia showed that by the age of 25 years, the cumulative burden of chronic disease was 1.5 times higher for a HSCT survivor compared to 0.6 for a survivor treated with chemotherapy. There were higher rates of hypertension, dyslipidemia, abnormal glucose metabolism, and obesity among HSCT survivors indicating that the incidence of metabolic syndrome was higher in long-term childhood HSCT survivors [94].

While HSCT is a life-saving procedure, it comes with a risk of serious long-term complications, including cGvHD. Chronic GvHD is seen in 25% of pediatric HSCT survivors causing prolonged and often irreversible organ damage. The effects of residual cGvHD on children include stunted growth, poor lung functions, and joint deformities. In addition, metabolic syndrome, cardiovascular events, infection, and restricted mobility are amplified with cGvHD (Table 17.3). A recent retrospective study on 1246 adult HSCT patients from Sweden found that cGvHD was associated with considerable losses in workplace productivity and added to the financial burden of the society [95]. An analysis of children in British Columbia who received HSCT showed that drug and physician costs were at least two times higher for children who developed cGvHD compared to those who did not [96]. It also has devastating effects on the psychosocial functioning of survivors, significantly impairing their overall quality of life [97]. Data from the HSCT Survivor and Childhood Cancer Survivor Study revealed that allogeneic HSCT

Table 17.3 QOL issues and relative severity in pediatric and AYA HSCT and cancer survivors

Survivorship issue	Unique to HSCT survivors		Unique to cancer survivors
	Without cGvHD	With cGvHD	
Endocrine			
Infertility Hypothyroid.	+++ +	+++ +	+ +/−
Depression	++	+++	+
Vocational	++	+++	+
Dyslipidemia/metabolic syndrome	++	+++	+
Lack of worth	++	+++	+
Fatigue	+	+++	+/−
Pulmonary failure			
Bronchiolitis obliterans. Pulmonary fibrosis.	−++	+++ ++	+/− +/−
Restricted mobility	−	+++	+/−
Infections	++	+++	−
Secondary malignancy	++	+++	+
Cardiomyopathy	+	+	+
Sexual dysfunction	+	+, if mild cGvHD +++, if moderate cGvHD	+/−

recipients with active cGvHD had poorer general health, more pain, and greater functional and activity impairment compared to survivors treated with chemotherapy [98]. Few studies have specifically examined social attainment outcomes including employment, educational attainment, and relationship status in survivors of HSCT with cGvHD. Studies suggest that healthcare professionals' perceptions of pediatric and adolescent needs are significantly different from the actual needs expressed by survivors [99]. These discrepancies ultimately affect the delivery of follow-up care to survivors resulting in many survivors being lost to follow-up in adulthood. The pediatric transplant centers need to establish proactive long-term follow-up programs to help with transition of pediatric transplant survivors into adulthood.

HSCT in Era of CAR-T Cell Therapy

In August of 2017, FDA approved tisagenlecleucel, the anti CD19 CAR, for patients with relapsed and refractory B lymphoblastic disease. Seventy-five patients enrolled in the ELIANA trial (NCT02435849) received CAR-T cell therapy. The overall remission rate at 3 months was 81%, and the EFS rates were 73% at 6 months and 50% at 12 months [100]. The phase 1 NCI trial using anti-CD19 (NCT01593696) or anti-CD22 (NCT02315612) CAR-T cell protocol had 25 patients receive allogeneic HSCT after achieving MRD-negative status post CAR-T cell therapy. The 24-month CIR was reported at 13.5% after anti-CD19 and 11.3% after anti-CD22 CAR therapy. Up to 40% of patients developed aGvHD, with 12% having severe aGvHD. The paper concluded that CAR-T cells may have a synergistic effect on HSCT prior to the emergence of CD19/22 negative clones and reduce the subsequent relapse risk [101]. The role of HSCT post CAR-T cell is evolving as the current studies are non-randomized with a bias towards transplanting patients with higher risk of relapse.

Future of HSCT in ALL

HSCT continues to be the primary established immune therapy against hematopoietic malignancies for long-term remission While new targeted, potentially less-morbid immune therapies like CAR-T cells, bi-specific antibodies, and conjugated antibody therapies can give impressive initial responses, they often need to be consolidated with HSCT for durable remissions. These agents can be helpful in achieving MRD-negative remission in higher-risk ALL patients, and their lower toxicity profile reduces the comorbidities prior to HSCT, giving patients the best possible outcome post HSCT with a sustained remission and minimal morbidity. The best role for HSCT in treatment of ALL amidst the newer immune therapies needs to be determined through large multicenter cooperative trials.

References

1. Kolb H, Wündisch G, Bender-Götze C, Spitzer I, Brehm G, Rodt H, et al. Bone marrow transplantation in children with aplastic anemia and acute lymphatic leukemia. Blut Zeitschrift Für Die Gesamte Blutforschung. 1975;31(6):343–6.
2. Thomas E, Buckner C, Banaji M, Clift R, Fefer A, Flournoy N, et al. One hundred patients with acute leukemia treated by chemotherapy, total body irradiation, and allogeneic marrow transplantation. Blood. 1977;49(4):511–33.
3. Odem LF, August CS, Githens JH, Humbert JR, Morse H, Peakman D, et al. Remission of relapsed leukaemia during a graft-versus-host reaction. A "graft-versus-leukaemia reaction" in man? Lancet. 1978;2(8089):537–40.
4. Weiden P, Flournoy N, Thomas E, Prentice R, Fefer A, Buckner C, et al. Antileukemic effect of graft-versus-host disease in human recipients of allogeneic-marrow grafts. N Engl J Med. 1979;300(19):1068–73. https://doi.org/10.1056/nejm197905103001902.
5. Möricke A, Zimmermann M, Reiter A, Henze G, Schrauder A, Gadner H, et al. Long-term results of five consecutive trials in childhood acute lymphoblastic leukemia performed by the ALL-BFM study group from 1981 to 2000. Leukemia. 20091;24(2):265–84. https://doi.org/10.1038/leu.2009.257.
6. Gaynon P, Bleyer W, Steinherz P, Finklestein J, Littman P, Miller D, et al. Modified BFM therapy for children with previously untreated acute lymphoblastic Leukemia and Unfavorable prognostic features. J Pediatr Hematol Oncol. 1989;10(1):42–50. https://doi.org/10.1097/00043426-198821000-00009.
7. Conter V, Bartram C, Valsecchi M, Schrauder A, Panzer-Grümayer R, Möricke A, et al. Molecular response to treatment redefines all prognostic factors in children and adolescents with B-cell precursor acute lymphoblastic leukemia: results in 3184 patients of the AIEOP-BFM ALL 2000 study. Blood. 2010;115(16):3206–14.
8. Schultz KR, Pullen DJ, Sather HN, Shuster JJ, Devidas M, Borowitz MJ, et al. Risk- and response-based classification of childhood B-precursor acute lymphoblastic leukemia: a combined analysis of prognostic markers from the Pediatric Oncology Group (POG) and Children's Cancer Group (CCG). Blood. 2007;109(3):926–35.
9. Borowitz MJ, Devidas M, Hunger SP, Bowman WP, Carroll AJ, Carroll WL, et al. Clinical significance of minimal residual disease in childhood acute lymphoblastic leukemia and its relationship to other prognostic factors: a Children;s Oncology Group study. Blood. 2008;111(12):5477–85.
10. Satwani P, Sather H, Ozkaynak F, Heerema NA, Schultz KR, Sanders J, et al. Allogeneic bone marrow transplantation in first remission for children with ultra-high-risk features of acute lymphoblastic leukemia: a children's oncology group study report. Biol Blood Marrow Transplant. 2007;13(2):218–27.
11. D'Souza A, Fretham C. Current uses and outcomes of hematopoietic cell transplantation (HCT): CIBMTR summary slides, 2019. https://www.cibmtr.org/ReferenceCenter/SlidesReports/SummarySlides/Pages/index.aspx
12. Oliansky DM, Camitta B, Gaynon P, Nieder ML, Parsons SK, Pulsipher MA, et al. Role of cytotoxic therapy with hematopoietic stem cell transplantation in the treatment of pediatric acute lymphoblastic leukemia: update of the 2005 evidence-based review. Biol Blood Marrow Transplant. 2012;18(4):505–22.
13. Maloney K, Devidas M, Wang C, Mattano L, Friedmann A, Buckley P, et al. Outcome in children with standard-risk B-cell acute lymphoblastic leukemia: results of Children's Oncology Group Trial AALL0331. J Clin Oncol. 2020;38(6):602–12. https://doi.org/10.1200/jco.19.01086.
14. Schrappe M, Valsecchi M, Bartram C, Schrauder A, Panzer-Grümayer R, Möricke A, et al. Late MRD response determines relapse risk overall and in subsets of childhood T-cell ALL: results of the AIEOP-BFM-ALL 2000 study. Blood. 2011;118(8):2077–84.

15. Burke M, Verneris M, Le Rademacher J, He W, Abdel-Azim H, Abraham A, et al. Transplant outcomes for children with T cell acute lymphoblastic Leukemia in second remission: a report from the Center for International Blood and Marrow Transplant Research. Biol Blood Marrow. 2015;21(12):2154–9. https://doi.org/10.1016/j.bbmt.2015.08.023.
16. Schultz KR, Carroll A, Heerema NA, Bowman WP, Aledo A, Slayton WB, et al. Long-term follow-up of imatinib in pediatric Philadelphia chromosome-positive acute lymphoblastic leukemia: Children's Oncology Group study AALL0031. Leukemia. 2014;28(7):1467–71.
17. Schultz KR, Bowman WP, Aledo A, Slayton WB, Sather H, Devidas M, et al. Improved early event-free survival with imatinib in Philadelphia chromosome-positive acute lymphoblastic leukemia: a children's oncology group study. J Clin Oncol. 2009;27(31):5175–81.
18. Slayton WB, Schultz KR, Kairalla JA, Devidas M, Mi X, Pulsipher MA, et al. Dasatinib plus intensive chemotherapy in children, adolescents, and young adults with Philadelphia chromosome-positive acute lymphoblastic leukemia: results of Children's Oncology Group Trial AALL0622. J Clin Oncol. 2018;36(22):2306–14.
19. Biondi A, Schrappe M, De Lorenzo P, Castor A, Lucchini G, Gandemer V, et al. Imatinib after induction for treatment of children and adolescents with Philadelphia-chromosome-positive acute lymphoblastic leukaemia (EsPhALL): a randomised, open-label, intergroup study. Lancet Oncol. 2012;13(9):936–45. https://doi.org/10.1016/s1470-2045(12)70377-7.
20. Harvey RC, Mullighan CG, Chen IM, Wharton W, Mikhail FM, Caroll AJ, et al. Rearrangement of CRLF2 is associated with mutation of JAK kinases, alteration of IKZF1, Hispanic/Latino ethnicity, and a poor outcome in pediatric B- progenitor acute lymphoblastic leukemia. Blood. 2010;115:5312–21. [PubMed: 20139093].
21. Boer JM, Marchante JR, Evans WE, et al. BCR-ABL1-like cases in pediatric acute lymphoblastic leukemia: a comparison between DCOG/Erasmus MC and COG/St. Jude signatures. Haematologica. 2015;100(9):e354–7. https://doi.org/10.3324/haematol.2015.124941.
22. Mullighan CG, Su X, Zhang J, Radtke I, Philips LA, Miller CB, et al. Deletion of IKZF1 and prognosis in acute lymphoblastic leukemia. N Engl J Med. 2009;360:470–80. [PubMed: 19129520]
23. Den Boer ML, van Slegtenhorst M, De Menezes RX, Choek MS, Buijs-Gladinnes JG, Peters ST, et al. A subtype of childhood acute lymphoblastic leukaemia with poor treatment outcome: a genome-wide classification study. Lancet Oncol. 2009;10:125–34. [PubMed: 19138562]
24. Roberts KG, Pei D, Campana D, Payne-Turner D, Li Y, Cheng C, et al. Outcomes of children with BCR-ABL1–like acute lymphoblastic leukemia treated with risk-directed therapy based on the levels of minimal residual disease. J Clin Oncol. 2014;32:3012–20. [PubMed: 25049327]
25. Pui CH, Roberts KG, Yang JJ, Mullighan CG. Philadelphia chromosome-like acute lymphoblastic leukemia. Clin Lymphoma Myeloma Leuk. 2017;17(8):464–70. https://doi.org/10.1016/j.clml.2017.03.299.
26. Harrison CJ, Moorman AV, Broadfield ZJ, et al. Three distinct subgroups of hypodiploidy in acute lymphoblastic leukaemia. Br J Haematol. 2004;125:552–9.
27. Nachman JB, Heerema NA, Sather H, et al. Outcome of treatment in children with hypodiploid acute lymphoblastic leukemia. Blood. 2000;110:1112–5.
28. Pui CH, Rebora P, Schrappe M, Attarbaschi A, Baruchel A, Basso G, et al. Ponte di Legno Childhood ALL working group. Outcome of children with hypodiploid acute lymphoblastic leukemia: a retrospective multinational study. J Clin Oncol. 2019;37(10):770–9.
29. Safavi S, Paulsson K. Near-haploid and low-hypodiploid acute lymphoblastic leukemia: two distinct subtypes with consistently poor prognosis. Blood. 2017;129(4):420–3.
30. Schultz KR, Devidas M, Bowman WP, Aledo A, Slayton WB, Sather H, et al. Philadelphia chromosome-negative very high-risk acute lymphoblastic leukemia in children and adolescents: results from Children's Oncology Group Study AALL0031. Leukemia. 2014;28(4):964–7.

31. Mehta P, Eapen M, Zhang M, He W, Seber A, Kitko C, et al. Transplant outcomes for children with hypodiploid acute lymphoblastic leukemia: the CIBMTR experience. Biol Blood Marrow Transplant. 2014;20(2):S87. https://doi.org/10.1016/j.bbmt.2013.12.110.
32. McNeer JL, Devidas M, Dai Y, Carroll AJ, Heerema NA, Gastier-Foster JM. Hematopoietic stem-cell transplantation does not improve the poor outcome of children with hypodiploid acute lymphoblastic leukemia: a report from Children's Oncology Group. J Clin Oncol. 2019;37(10):780–9.
33. Pui CH, Gaynon PS, Boyett JM, Chessells JM, Baruchel A, Kamps W, et al. Outcome of treatment in childhood acute lymphoblastic leukaemia with rearrangements of the 11q23 chromosomal region. Lancet. 2002;359(9321):1909–15.
34. Dreyer Z, Dinndorf P, Camitta B, Sather H, La M, Devidas M, et al. Analysis of the role of hematopoietic stem-cell transplantation in infants with acute lymphoblastic Leukemia in first remission and MLL gene rearrangements: a report from the Children's Oncology Group. J Clin Oncol. 2011;29(2):214–22. https://doi.org/10.1200/jco.2009.26.8938.
35. Mann G, Attarbaschi A, Schrappe M, Lorenzo PD, Peters C, Hann I, et al. On behalf of the Interfant-99 study group; improved outcome with hematopoietic stem cell transplantation in a poor prognostic subgroup of infants with *mixed-lineage-leukemia(MLL)*–rearranged acute lymphoblastic leukemia: results from the Interfant-99 study. Blood. 2010;116(15):2644–50.
36. Peters R, De Lorenzo P, Ancliffe P, Aversa L, Brethon B, Biondi A, et al. Outcome of infants younger than 1 year with acute lymphoblastic leukemia treated with the interfant-06 protocol: results from an international phase III randomized study. J Clin Oncol. 2019;37(25):2246–56. https://doi.org/10.1200/jco.19.00261.
37. Hrusak O, de Haas V, Stancikova J, Vakrmanova B, Janotova I, Mejstrikova E, et al. International cooperative study identifies treatment strategy in childhood ambiguous lineage leukemia. Blood. 2018;132(3):264–76. https://doi.org/10.1182/blood-2017-12-821363.
38. Orgel E, Alexander TB, Wood BL, Kahwash SB, Devidas M, Dai Y, et al. Mixed-phenotype acute leukemia: a cohort and consensus research strategy from the Children's Oncology Group acute leukemia of ambiguous lineage task force. Cancer. 2020;126:593–601. https://doi.org/10.1002/cncr.32552.
39. Schrappe M, Hunger SP, Pui CH, Saha V, Gaynon PS, Baruchel A, et al. Outcomes after induction failure in childhood acute lymphoblastic leukemia. N Engl J Med. 2012;366(15):1371–81.
40. Locatelli F, Schrappe M, Bernardo ME, Rutella S. How I treat relapsed childhood acute lymphoblastic leukemia. Blood. 2012;120:2807–16.
41. Eckert C, Groeneveld-Krentz S, Kirschner-Schwabe R, Hagedorn N, Chen-Santel C, Bader P, et al. Improving stratification for children with late bone marrow B-cell acute lymphoblastic leukemia relapses with refined response classification and integration of genetics. J Clin Oncol. 2019;37:3493–07.
42. Parker C, Krishnan S, Hamadeh L, Irving J, Kuiper R, Révész T, et al. Outcomes of patients with childhood B-cell precursor acute lymphoblastic leukaemia with late bone marrow relapses: long-term follow-up of the ALLR3 open-label randomised trial. Lancet Haematol. 2019;6(4):e204–16. https://doi.org/10.1016/s2352-3026(19)30003-1.
43. Lew G, Chen Y, Lu X, Rheingold SR, Whitlock JA, Devidas M, et al. Outcomes after late bone marrow and very early central nervous system relapse of childhood B-acute lymphoblastic leukemia: a report from the Children's Oncology Group Phase III study AALL0433. Haematologica. 2020;105(5) https://doi.org/10.3324/haematol.2019.237230.
44. Gaynon P, Harris R, Altman A, Bostrom B, Breneman J, Hawks R, et al. Bone marrow transplantation versus prolonged intensive chemotherapy for children with acute lymphoblastic leukemia and an initial bone marrow relapse within 12 months of the completion of primary therapy: Children's Oncology Group Study CCG-1941. J Clin Oncol. 2006;24(19):3150–6. https://doi.org/10.1200/jco.2005.04.5856.
45. Brown P, Ji L, Xu X, Devidas M, Hogan LE, Borowitz MJ, et al. A randomized phase 3 trial of blinatumomab vs. chemotherapy as post-reinduction therapy in high and intermediate risk (HR/IR) first relapse of B-Acute Lymphoblastic Leukemia (B-ALL) in children and

Adolescents/Young Adults (AYAs) demonstrates superior efficacy and tolerability of blinatumomab: a report from Children's Oncology Group Study AALL1331. ASH Annual Meeting. December 2019. https://ash.confex.com/ash/2019/webprogram/Paper132435.html
46. Qayed M, Kitko CL, Ahn KW, Johnson MH, Schultz KR, Smith AR, et al. Development and validation of a pediatric disease risk index for allogeneic hematopoietic cell transplantation. ASCO 2020 meeting Qayed, M., et al. J Clin Oncol. 2020;38(15_suppl):7503.
47. Burke MJ, Verneris MR, Le Rademacher J, He W, Abdel-Azim H, Abraham AA, et al. Transplant outcomes for children with T cell acute lymphoblastic leukemia in second remission: a report from the Center for International Blood and Marrow Transplant Research. Biol Blood Marrow Transplant. 2015;21(12):2154–9.
48. Pui CH. Central nervous system disease in acute lymphoblastic leukemia: prophylaxis and treatment. Hematology Am Soc Hematol Educ Program. 2006:142–6.
49. Nguyen K, Cheng S-C, Raetz E, et al. Factors influencing survival after relapse from childhood ALL: a Children's Oncology Group Study. ASH Ann Meet Abstr. 2006;108:1855.
50. Harker-Murray PD, Thomas AJ, Wagner JE, Weisdorf D, Luo X, DeFor TE, Verneris MR, et al. Allogeneic hematopoietic cell transplantation in children with relapsed acute lymphoblastic leukemia isolated to the central nervous system. Biol Blood Marrow Transplant. 2008;14(6):685–92.
51. Gabelli M, Zecca M, Messina C, Carraro E, Buldini B, Rovelli AM, et al. Hematopoietic stem cell transplantation for isolated extramedullary relapse of acute lymphoblastic leukemia in children. Biol Blood Marrow Transplant. 2019;54(2):275–83.
52. Masurekar AN, Parker CA, Shanyinde M, Moorman AV, Hancock JP, Sutton R, et al. Outcome of central nervous system relapses in childhood acute lymphoblastic leukaemia – prospective open cohort analyses of the ALLR3 trial. PLoS One. 2014;9(10):e108107.
53. Yaniv I, Krauss A, Beohou E, Dalissier A, Corbacioglu S, Zecca M, et al. Second hematopoietic stem cell transplantation for post-transplantation relapsed acute leukemia in children: a retrospective EBMT-PDWP study. Biol Blood Marrow Transplant. 2018;24((8)L):1629–42. https://doi.org/10.1016/j.bbmt.2018.03.002.
54. Kato M, Horikoshi Y, Okamoto Y, Takahashi Y, Hasegawa D, Koh K, et al. Second allogeneic hematopoietic SCT for relapsed ALL in children. Bone Marrow Transplant. 2012;47(10):1307–11. https://doi.org/10.1038/bmt.2012.29.
55. Hamidieh AA, Monzavi SM, Kaboutari M, Behfar M, Esfandbod M. Outcome analysis of pediatric patients with acute lymphoblastic leukemia treated with total body irradiation-free allogeneic hematopoietic stem cell transplantation: comparison of patients with and without central nervous system involvement. Biol Blood Marrow Transplant. 2017;23(12):2110–7.
56. Ruutu T, De Wreede L, Van Biezen A, Brand R, Mohty M, Dreger P, et al. Second allogeneic transplantation for relapse of malignant disease: retrospective analysis of outcome and predictive factors by the EBMT. Bone Marrow Transplant. 2015;50(12):1542. [PubMed: 26367221]
57. Christopeit M, Kuss O, Finke J, Bacher U, Beelen DW, Bornhäuser M, et al. Second allograft for hematologic relapse of acute leukemia after first allogeneic stem-cell transplantation from related and unrelated donors: the role of donor change. J Clin Oncol. 2013;31(26):3259–71. [PubMed: 23918951]
58. Eapen M, Giralt S, Horowitz M, Klein J, Wagner J, Zhang M, et al. Second transplant for acute and chronic leukemia relapsing after first HLA-identical sibling transplant. Bone Marrow Transplant. 2004;34(8):721. [PubMed: 15322568]
59. Maude SL, Laetsch TW, Buechner J, Rives S, Boyer M, Bittencourt H, et al. Tisagenlecleucel in children and young adults with B-cell lymphoblastic leukemia. N Engl J Med. 2018;378(5):439–48.
60. Kalaycio M, Bolwell B, Rybicki L, Absi A, Andresen S, Pohlman B, et al. BU- vs TBI-based conditioning for adult patients with ALL. Bone Marrow Transplant. 2010;46(11):1413–7.
61. Holter-Chakrabarty JL, Pierson N, Zhang MJ, Zhu X, Akpek G, Aljurf MD, et al. The sequence of cyclophosphamide and myeloablative total body irradiation in hematopoietic

cell transplantation for patients with acute leukemia. Biol Blood Marrow Transplant. 2015;21(7):1251–7.

62. Peters C. TBI or chemotherapy based conditioning for children and adolescents with all: a prospective randomized multicenter-study 'FORUM' on behalf of the AIEOP-BFM-ALL-SG, IBFM-SG, INTREALL-SG and EBMT-PD-WP EHA Library. Peters C. 06/12/20; 294922; S102.
63. Rocha V, Kabbara N, Ionescu I, Ruggeri A, Purtill D, Gluckman E. Pediatric related and unrelated cord blood transplantation for malignant diseases. Bone Marrow Transplant. 2009;44:653–9.
64. Brunstein C, Fuchs E, Carter S, Karanes C, Costa L, Wu J, et al. Alternative donor transplantation after reduced intensity conditioning: results of parallel phase 2 trials using partially HLA-mismatched related bone marrow or unrelated double umbilical cord blood grafts. Blood. 2011;118(2):282–8.
65. Keesler DA, St Martin A, Bonfim C, Seber A, Zhang MJ, Eapen M. Bone marrow versus peripheral blood from unrelated donors for children and adolescents with acute Leukemia. Biol Blood Marrow Transplant. 2018;24(12):2487–92.
66. Couban S, Wong PC, Schultz KR. The case for plerixafor to replace filgrastim as the optimal agent to mobilize peripheral blood donors for allogeneic hematopoietic cell transplantation. Exp Hematol. 2019 Feb;70:1–9.
67. Berger M, Lanino E, Cesaro S, Zecca M, Vassallo E, Faraci M, et al. Feasibility and outcome of haploidentical hematopoietic stem cell transplantation with post-transplant high-dose cyclophosphamide for children and adolescents with hematologic malignancies: an AIEOP-GITMO retrospective multicenter study. Biol Blood Marrow Transplant. 2016;22(5):902–9.
68. Symons HJ, Cluster A, Caywood E, Dalal DEJ, Egeler RM, Huo JS et al. Haploidentical BMT using fully myeloablative conditioning, T cell replete bone marrow grafts, and post-transplant cyclophosphamide (PT/cy) has limited toxicity and promising efficacy in the first prospective multicenter trial for pediatric, adolescent, and young adult patients with high risk acute leukemias and myelodysplastic syndrome. ASTCT meeting February 2020.
69. Bertaina A, Zecca M, Buldini B, Sacchi N, Algeri M, Saglio F, et al. Unrelated donor vs HLA-haploidentical α/β T-cell– and B-cell–depleted HSCT in children with acute leukemia. Blood. 2018;132(24):2594–607. https://doi.org/10.1182/blood-2018-07-861575.
70. Locatelli F, Merli P, Pagliara D, Li Pira G, Falco M, Pende D, et al. Outcome of children with acute leukemia given HLA-haploidentical HSCT after αβ T-cell and B-cell depletion. Blood. 2017;130(5):677–85. https://doi.org/10.1182/blood-2017-04-779769.
71. Moretta L, Locatelli F, Pende D, Marcenaro E, Mingari MC, Moretta A. Killer Ig-like receptor- mediated control of natural killer cell alloreactivity in haploidentical hematopoietic stem cell transplantation. Blood. 2011;117(3):764–71.
72. Diaz MA, Zubicaray J, Molina B, Abad L, Castillo A, Sebastian E, et al. Haploidentical stem cell transplantation in children with hematological malignancies using $\alpha\beta^+$ T-cell receptor and $CD19^+$ cell depleted grafts: high $CD56^{dim}/CD56^{bright}$ NK cell ratio early following transplantation is associated with lower relapse incidence and better outcome. Front Immunol. 2019;10:2504.
73. Bader P, Kreyenberg H, Henze G, Eckert C, Reising M, Willasch A, et al. Prognostic value of minimal residual disease quantification before allogeneic stem-cell transplantation in relapsed childhood acute lymphoblastic leukemia: the ALL-REZ BFM study group. J Clin Oncol. 2008;27:377–84.
74. Eckert C, Henze G, Seeger K, Hagedorn N, Mann G, Panzer-Grumayer R, et al. Use of allogeneic hematopoietic stem-cell transplantation based on minimal residual disease response improves outcomes for children with relapsed acute lymphoblastic leukemia in the intermediate-risk group. J Clin Oncol. 2013;31:2736–42.
75. Pulsipher MA, Carlson CS, Mark K, Wall DA, Schultz KR, Bunin N, et al. Striking predictive power for relapse and decreased survival associated with detectable minimal residual disease by IGH VDJ deep sequencing of bone marrow pre- and post-allogeneic transplant in children

with B-lineage ALL: a subanalysis of the COG ASCT0431/PBMTC ONC051 study. Blood. 2013;122(21):919.

76. Bader P, Kreyenberg H, von Stackelberg A, Eckert C, Salzmann-Manrique E, Meisel R, et al. Monitoring of minimal residual disease after allogeneic stem-cell transplantation in relapsed childhood acute lymphoblastic leukemia allows for the identification of impending relapse: results of the ALL-BFM-SCT 2003 trial. J Clin Oncol. 2015;33(11):1275–84.
77. Bader P, Salzmann-Manrique E, Balduzzi A, Dalle JH, Woolfrey AE, Bar M, et al. More precisely defining risk peri-HCT in pediatric ALL: pre- vs post-MRD measures, serial positivity, and risk modeling. Blood Adv. 2019;3(21):3393–405.
78. Yeshurun M, Weisdorf D, Rowe J, Tallman M, Zhang M, Wang H, et al. The impact of the graft-versus-leukemia effect on survival in acute lymphoblastic leukemia. Blood Adv. 2019;3(4):670–80. https://doi.org/10.1182/bloodadvances.2018027003.
79. Horowitz M, Gale R, Sondel P, Goldman J, Kersey J, Kolb H, et al. Graft-versus-leukemia reactions after bone marrow transplantation. Blood. 1990;75(3):555–62.
80. Cornelissen J, Carston M, Kollman C, King R, Dekker A, Löwenberg B, et al. Unrelated marrow transplantation for adult patients with poor-risk acute lymphoblastic leukemia: strong graft-versus-leukemia effect and risk factors determining outcome. Blood. 2001;97(6):1572–7. https://doi.org/10.1182/Blood.v97.6.1572.
81. Pulsipher MA, Langholz B, Wall DA, Schultz KR, Bunin N, Carroll WL, et al. The addition of sirolimus to tacrolimus/methotrexate GVHD prophylaxis in children with ALL: a phase 3 Children's Oncology Group/pediatric Blood and Marrow Transplant Consortium trial. Blood. 2014;123(13):2017–25.
82. Reid GS, Terrett L, Alessandri AJ, Grubb S, Stork L, Seibel N, et al. Altered patterns of T cell cytokine production induced by relapsed pre-B ALL cells. Leuk Res. 2003;27(12):1135–42.
83. Olivieri A, Cimminiello M, Corradini P, Mordini N, Fedele R, Selleri C, et al. Long-term outcome and prospective validation of NIH response criteria in 39 patients receiving imatinib for steroid refractory chronic GVHD. Blood. 2013;122(25):4111–8.
84. DeFilipp Z, Ancheta R, Liu Y, Hu Z, Gale R, Snyder D, et al. Maintenance tyrosine kinase inhibitors following allogeneic hematopoietic stem cell transplantation for chronic myelogenous leukemia: a Center for International Blood and Marrow Transplant Research Study. Biol Blood Marrow Transplant. 2020;26(3):472–9. https://doi.org/10.1016/j.bbmt.2019.10.017.
85. Ganem G, Kuentz M, Bernaudin F, Gharbi A, Cordonnier C, Lemerle S, et al. Central nervous system relapses after bone marrow transplantation for acute lymphoblastic leukemia in remission. Cancer. 1989;64:1796–801.
86. Pui CH. Central nervous system disease in acute lymphoblastic leukemia: prophylaxis and treatment. Hematology Am Soc Hematol Educ Program. 2006:142–6.
87. Rubin J, Vettenranta K, Vettenranta J, Bierings M, Abrahamsson J, Békássy A, et al. Use of intrathecal chemoprophylaxis in children after SCT and the risk of central nervous system relapse. Bone Marrow Transplant. 2010;46(3):372–8. https://doi.org/10.1038/bmt.2010.121.
88. Rubin J, Vettenranta K, Vettenranta J, Bierings M, Abrahamsson J, Bekassy AN, et al. Use of intrathecal chemoprophylaxis in children after SCT and the risk of central nervous system relapse. Bone Marrow Transplant. 2011;46:372–8. https://doi.org/10.1038/bmt.2010.121.
89. Ruutu T, Corradini P, Gratwohl A, Holler E, Apperley J, Dini G, et al. Use of intrathecal prophylaxis in allogeneic haematopoietic stem cell transplantation for malignant blood diseases: a survey of the European Group for Blood and Marrow Transplantation (EBMT). Bone Marrow Transplant. 2005;35:121–4.
90. Sauter CS, DeFilipp Z, Inamoto Y, Johnston L, Nagler A, Savani BN, et al. ASBMT statement on routine prophylaxis for central nervous system recurrence of acute lymphoblastic leukemia following allogeneic hematopoietic cell transplantation. Biol Blood Marrow Transplant. 2009;25(3):e86–8.
91. Gao RW, Dusenbery KE, Cao Q, Smith AR, Yuan J. Augmenting total body irradiation with a cranial boost before stem cell transplantation protects against post-transplant central

nervous system relapse in acute lymphoblastic leukemia. Biol Blood Marrow Transplant. 2018;24(3):501–6.

92. Wingard J, Majhail N, Brazauskas R, Wang Z, Sobocinski K, Jacobsohn D, et al. Long-term survival and late deaths after allogeneic hematopoietic cell transplantation. J Clin Oncol. 2011;29(16):2230–9. https://doi.org/10.1200/jco.2010.33.7212.
93. Bhatia S, Davies SM, Baker SK, Pulsipher MA, Hansen JA, NCI, NHLBI first international consensus conference on late effects after pediatric hematopoietic cell transplantation: etiology and pathogenesis of late effects after HCT performed in childhood--methodologic challenges. Biol Blood Marrow Transplant. 2011;17(10):1428–35.
94. Eissa HM, Lu L, Baassiri M, Bhakta N, Ehrhardt MJ, Triplett BM, et al. Chronic disease burden and frailty in survivors of childhood HSCT: a report from the St. Jude Lifetime Cohort Study. Blood Adv. 2017;1(24):2243–6.
95. Schain F, Batyrbekova N, Liwing J, Prütz C, Simona B, Webb T, Remberger M, Mattsson J. Real-world study of healthcare utilization and long-term productivity loss in chronic graft versus host disease in Sweden. ISPO meeting 2019.
96. Schultz KR, Zhang Y, Mary L, McBride ML. High rate of health care utilization associated with chronic graft-versus-host disease among Canadian childhood cancer survivors treated with blood and marrow transplantation. EBMT meeting, Lisbon, March 18, 2018.
97. Thompson K, Dyson G, Holland L, Joubert L. An exploratory study of oncology specialists' understanding of the preferences of young people living with cancer. Soc Work Health Care. 2013;52(2–3):166–90.
98. Sun CL, Francisco L, Baker KS, Weisdorf DJ, Forman SJ, Bhatia S. Adverse psychological outcomes in long-term survivors of hematopoietic cell transplantation: a report from the Bone Marrow Transplant Survivor Study (BMTSS). Blood. 2011;118(17):4723–31.
99. Bhatt NS, Brazauskas R, Tecca HR, Carreras J, Burns LJ, Phelan R, et al. Post-transplantation employment status of adult survivors of childhood allogeneic hematopoietic cell transplant: a report from the Center for International Blood and Marrow Transplant Research (CIBMTR). Cancer. 2019;125(1):144–52.
100. Maude SL, Laetsch TW, Buechner J, Rives S, Boyer H, Bittencourt PB, et al. Tisagenlecleucel in children and young adults with B-cell lymphoblastic leukemia. N Engl J Med. 2018;378(5):439–48.
101. Shalabi H, Delbrook C, Stetler-Stevenson M, Yuan C, Steinberg S, Yates B, et al. Chimeric antigen receptor T-cell (CAR-T) therapy can render patients with ALL into PCR-negative remission and can be an effective bridge to transplant (HCT). Biol Blood Marrow Transplant. 2018;24(3):S25–6. https://doi.org/10.1016/j.bbmt.2017.12.018.

Index

M. R. Litzow, E. A. Raetz (eds.), *Clinical Management of Acute Lymphoblastic Leukemia*, https://doi.org/10.1007/978-3-030-85147-7